AF677515

LIBRARY OF CONGRESS
SURPLUS
LIBRARY OF CONGRESS
DUPLICATE

NEURO-PSYCHOPHARMACOLOGY

NEURO-PSYCHOPHARMACOLOGY

Proceedings of the 11th Congress of the Collegium Internationale Neuro-Psychopharmacologicum
Vienna, July 9-14, 1978

Editors:

B. SALETU
Vienna, Austria

P. BERNER
Vienna, Austria

L. HOLLISTER
Palo Alto, USA

PERGAMON PRESS

OXFORD · NEW YORK · TORONTO · SYDNEY · PARIS · FRANKFURT

RM315
C58
1979
c.1

U.K.	Pergamon Press Ltd., Headington Hill Hall, Oxford OX3 0BW, England
U.S.A.	Pergamon Press Inc., Maxwell House, Fairview Park, Elmsford, New York 10523, U.S.A.
CANADA	Pergamon of Canada, Suite 104, 150 Consumers Road, Willowdale, Ontario M2J 1P9, Canada
AUSTRALIA	Pergamon Press (Aust.) Pty. Ltd., P.O. Box 544, Potts Point, N.S.W. 2011, Australia
FRANCE	Pergamon Press SARL, 24 rue des Ecoles, 75240 Paris, Cedex 05, France
FEDERAL REPUBLIC OF GERMANY	Pergamon Press GmbH, 6242 Kronberg-Taunus, Pferdstrasse 1, Federal Republic of Germany

Copyright © 1979 Collegium Internationale
Neuro-Psychopharmacologicum

All Rights Reserved. No part of this publication may be reproduced, stored in a retrieval system or transmitted in any form or by any means: electronic, electrostatic, magnetic tape, mechanical, photocopying, recording or otherwise, without permission in writing from the copyright holders.

First edition 1979

British Library Cataloguing in Publication Data

Collegium Internationale Neuro-
Psychopharmacologicum. *Congress, 11th, Vienna, 1978*
Neuro-psychopharmacology.
1. Neuropsychopharmacology
I. Title II. Saletu, B III. Berner, P
IV. Hollister, Leo E
615'.78 RM315 79-40552
ISBN 0-08-023089-X

In order to make this volume available as economically and as rapidly as possible the authors' typescripts have been reproduced in their original forms. This method unfortunately has its typographical limitations but it is hoped that they in no way distract the reader.

*Printed and bound in Great Britain by
William Clowes (Beccles) Limited, Beccles and London*

Contents

NEUROPEPTIDES AND PSYCHIATRY

BIOLOGICAL MONITORING OF PSYCHOTROPIC DRUGS TREATMENT

CIRCADIAN RHYTHMS AND PSYCHOTROPIC DRUGS

C. I. N. P. COMMITTEES

EXECUTIVE COMMITTEE

President	L. HOLLISTER, Palo Alto, U.S.A.
Past President	P. DENIKER, Paris, France
President-Elect	A. CARLSSON, Göteborg, Sweden
Vice-Presidents	M. LADER, London, England
	H. VAN PRAGG, Utrecht, The Netherlands
Secretary	J. ANGST, Zurich, Switzerland
Treasurer	P. JANSSEN, Beerse, Belgium

COUNCILLORS	E. COSTA, Washington, U.S.A.
	S. GARATTINI, Milan, Italy
	A. HERZ, Munich, Germany
	O. RAFAELSEN, Copenhagen, Denmark
	P. SIMON, Paris, France
	F. SULSER, Nashville, U.S.A.
	Z. VOTAVA, Strbske Plese, Chechoslovakia

NOMINATING COMMITTEE

Chairman	H. HIPPIUS, Munich, Germany

MEMBERSHIP COMMITTEE

Chairman	M. HAMILTON, Leeds, England
Members	D. GINESTET, Paris, France
	N. MATUSSEK, Munich, Germany

PUBLICATION COMMITTEE

Chairman	C. STEFANIS, Athens, Greece
Members	J. BOISSIER, Paris, France
	E. CUENCA, Cadiz, Spain
	A. LEEDS, Rockville, U.S.A.
	M. SANDLER, London, England

FINANCE COMMITTEE

Chairman	M. LADER, London, England
Members	J. ANGST, Zurich, Switzerland
	A. CARLSSON, Göteborg, Sweden
	P. DENIKER, Paris, France
	S. GARATTINI, Milan, Italy
	H. HIPPIUS, Munich, Germany
	L. HOLLISTER, Palo Alto, U.S.A.
	H. LEHMANN, Montreal, Canada

11th C. I. N. P. CONGRESS COMMITTEES

SCIENTIFIC PROGRAM COMMITTEE

Chairman	P. BERNER
Members	R. BATTEGAY, Basle, Switzerland
	B. DAVIES, Victoria, Australia
	J. ELKES, Baltimore, U.S.A.
	S. GERSHON, New York, U.S.A.
	J. GLOWINSKI, Paris, France
	L. GRAM, Copenhagen, Denmark
	M. KAROBATH, Vienna, Austria
	G. LANGER, Vienna, Austria
	C. RADOUCO-THOMAS, Quebec, Canada
	B. SALETU, Vienna, Austria
	T. SILVERSTONE, London, England

ORGANIZING COMMITTEE

Chairman	B. SALETU
Members	P. BERNER, Vienna, Austria
	W. BIRKMAYER, Vienna, Austria
	G. HARRER, Salzburg, Austria
	G. HOFFMANN, Linz, Austria
	O. HORNYKIEWICZ, Vienna, Austria
	H. KONZETT, Innsbruck, Austria
	O. KRAUPP, Vienna, Austria
	K. KRYSPIN-EXNER, Innsbruck, Austria
	H. LECHNER, Graz, Austria
	F. LEMBECK, Graz, Austria
	Ch. STUMPF, Vienna, Austria
	H. VESELY, Vienna, Austria
	A. VILLENEUVE, Quebec, Canada

LADIES COMMITTEE

M. SALETU
C. BERNER
M. CHRISTIAN
R. CSERVENKA
A. LAHNSTEINER
M. KAROBATH

ACKNOWLEDGEMENTS

The C. I. N. P. wishes to thank the following pharmaceutical companies for their valuable contributions:

Abbott Laboratories, Chicago, Ill., U.S.A.
A. H. Robins, Richmond Va., U.S.A.
Burrough Wellcome Co., Research Triangle Park, N.C., U.S.A.
Chemie Linz AG, Linz, Austria
Chemiewerke Homburg, Frankfurt, Germany
Chemische Fabrik von Heyden, Munich, Germany
CIBA-GEIGY Corp., Summit, N.J., U.S.A.
CILAG-Chemie G. m. b. H., Vienna, Austria
CILAG-Chemie AG, Schaffhausen, Switzerland
COMESA KG, Vienna, Austria
Cyanamid of Canada Ltd., Montreal, Canada
E. Merck, Darmstadt, Germany
F. Angelini A. C. R. A. F., Rome, Italy
Gist-Brocades NV, Delft, The Netherlands
Hoechst Austria AG, Vienna, Austria
Hoechst-Roussel Pharmaceuticals Inc., Somerville, N.J., U.S.A.
Hoffmann-La Roche Ltd., Quebec, Canada
Hoffmann-La Roche Inc., Nutley, N.J., U.S.A.
Hoffmann-La Roche AG, Grenzach-Wyhlen, Germany
Hoffmann-La Roche & Co. AG, Basle, Switzerland
ICI-Pharma, Heidelberg, Germany
Lederle Laboratories, Pearl River, N.Y., U.S.A.
LEO Aktiebolaget, Helsingborg, Finland
McNeil Laboratories, Fort Washington, Pa., U.S.A.
Merck Sharp & Dohme Research Laboratories, West Point, Pa., U.S.A.
Merrell-National Laboratories, Cincinnati, Ohio, U.S.A.
Organon International BV, Oss, The Netherlands
Paul Martini Stiftung, Frankfurt, Germany
Philips-Duphar B.V., Amsterdam, The Netherlands
Sandoz Inc., East Hanover, N.J., U.S.A.
Sandoz Ltd., Basle, Switzerland
Solco Basel AG, Birsfelden, Switzerland
Smith Kline & French Laboratories, Philadelphia, Pa., U.S.A.
The Upjohn Company, Kalamazoo, Mich., U.S.A.
Troponwerke G. m. b. H. & Co. KG, Cologne, Germany
Warner-Lambert/Parke-Davis, Ann Arbor, Mich., U.S.A.
Wellcome Research Laboratories, England
Vienna Tourist Board, Vienna, Austria

Presidential Address

LEO E. HOLLISTER

Professor of Medicine, Psychiatry and Pharmacology, Stanford University
School of Medicine and Veterans Administration Hospital,
Palo Alto, CA. 94304, U.S.A.

Dr. Saletu, Dean Kraupp, Professor Berner, Esteemed Colleagues:

Welcome to the Eleventh Congress of the Collegium Internationale Neuropsychopharmacologicum. We anticipate a week in which our brains will be filled with new information, in which our stomachs will be filled with good food, and in which our spirits will be lightened by the gemütlichkeit that no visitor to Vienna can escape.

The enormous job of putting together a meeting such as this has undoubtedly involved more persons than I could possibly name. We owe especial thanks to Professor Peter Berner for arranging the excellent scientific program that awaits us and to Dr. Berndt Saletu for making the innumerable arrangements that were necessary to accommodate us physically. Such a vast undertaking is not expected to run perfectly so that if any of you have encountered difficulties along the way, please understand the complexity of the organization of such a Congress. We also wish to thank our numerous supporting members (all of whom have been recognized on the program, I hope) without whose support this Congress would have truly been impossible.

Approximately twenty-five years ago, the modern era of neuropsychopharmacology began with the successful treatment of schizophrenia with chlorpromazine. The immediate past-President of the C.I.N.P., Professor Pierre Deniker, was a participant in this epoch-making event, which led, among many other things, to the formation of the C.I.N.P. twenty years ago. Few of us would have guessed then how well this new, multidisciplinary field would fare over the succeeding years. Our field has attracted the interest of clinicians and basic scientists from many specialties and many disciplines. Meetings such as this foster the communication between such diverse groups necessary for the integration of knowledge that will allow us better to understand and better to treat disorders of the central nervous system, whether manifested by psychiatric, neurologic, endocrine or other disorders.

We may well be proud of the many new drugs that have been developed during the past quarter century that have ameliorated the course of these disorders for many patients. Present antipsychotic drugs embrace perhaps 200 or more compounds marketed throughout the world, involving a multiplicity of chemical structures. The tricyclic antidepressants are less numerous, but in recent years the number of chemical structures has been expanded to include new bicyclic and tetracyclic structures. A new division of monoamine oxidase inhibitors may allow more specific utilization of these drugs for treating depression and Parkinson's disease. The benzodiazepines have advantages that have made most of the barbiturates obsolete; indeed, their rapid proliferation may make this class of compounds even more plentiful than was the case with barbiturates. Lithium has replaced bromide as an ion therapy in psychiatry; its unique ability to modulate the course of manic-depressive disorder being a far greater contribution to treatment than anything offered by the bromide ion.

The drug-induced model of Parkinson's disease ultimately led to a completely new approach to treating this disorder. Treatment directed at increasing dopaminergic transmission, either with levodopa or with amantadine, has been added to the more conventional approach of treating with drugs that reduce cholinergic activity. Levodopa-induced dyskinesia and tardive dyskinesia from antipsychotic drugs both may be partial models for Huntington's disease. These models have stimulated new approaches to the treatment of this disorder, either by decreasing dopamine receptor sensitivity or by increasing cholinergic activity. We were well advised to use the compound term, neuropsychopharmacology, for describing our field and for naming this college some two decades ago.

Progress in the basic sciences of neuropharmacology has been even more impressive than it has been in the clinical applications. Twenty-five years ago, the only established central nervous system neurotransmitter was acetylcholine. Soon after the introduction of antipsychotic drugs, the so-called biogenic amines, serotonin, norepinephrine and dopamine, became considered as putative neurotransmitters. The mechanisms by which these biogenic amines are synthesized, transported, stored, released, recaptured and metabolized have been rather well worked out. Their selective distribution in the brain was delineated by simple yet elegant histochemical techniques. The effects of drugs on these systems led to the formulation both of the amine hypothesis of depression and the dopamine hypothesis of schizophrenia. These hypotheses, among others, can be tested in various ways, the first time that this essential aspect of the scientific method has been applicable to study of the pathogenesis of psychiatric disorders. More recently, attention has been focused on receptors for these neurotransmitters and the changes that may occur in these receptors during treatment with psychotherapeutic drugs.

One might say that the many advances in the basic sciences are overwhelming. Scarcely do we begin to understand the possible function of one or two neurotransmitters before additional ones are discovered. We are still uncertain about the role in the brain of some old neurotransmitters, such as histamine and epinephrine, not to mention the many new biogenic amines found in the brain that may have a role as neurotransmitters. Amino acids and peptides are present in abundance in the brain, and like the biogenic amines, are selectively distributed. The various endorphins are currently of greatest interest, as their action may relate to that of a classic drug, morphine, that acts on the central nervous system. Far less clear is why gastrointestinal hormones, such as gastrin and somatostatin, should be in the brain, or for that matter, whether the various releasing hormones may have functions other than mediating control of the pituitary by the brain.

Proliferation of receptors continues. It is likely that more than one type of receptor exists in the brain for most of the known neurotransmitters. Is it likely that specific receptors may be found for the very many centrally-acting drugs, such as seems to be the case for morphine, and that for each of these receptors for different types of drugs we may also expect to find an endogenous ligand? Does the finding of specific binding sites for benzodiazepines in the brain mean that God works for Hofmann-La Roche? Or does it simply mean that Art imitates Nature and that chlordiazepoxide is a weak imitator of Nature's own antianxiety drug, which too often seems to be present in too low a quantity for many of our patients?

Thus, it is the basic sciences, as usual, that raise more questions than they answer. And here is where one of the major current problems lies. We must continue to try to make sense of old discoveries while adding confusion through new discoveries. The structure and function of the brain gets ever more complex, the more we know about it. Yet somewhere, there must be a synthesis that reduces the complexity. A biology that can code all the genetic information with four nucleotides, or make all the necessary proteins with a mere 20 amino acids, certainly does not require the anticipation of making receptors for every centrally acting drug that has been invented to date as well as those still to be invented. This problem is a never-ending one and is the reason that, for the true scientist, work never ceases to be a fascinating challenge.

From the viewpoint of the clinician, a major current problem is the development of better drugs than those that we have. The treatment of schizophrenia has improved immeasurably during the 20-year life span of the C.I.N.P., yet most improvements in antipsychotic drugs have been largely technical. Many current drugs are better than chlorpromazine, either due to more specific pharmacologic actions or by having fewer unwanted pharmacological actions. Yet, so far as we know, they still work in relatively similar ways. Our batteries of pharmacologic screening tests are designed to find new chemicals that mimic the drugs we already have rather than to discover distinctly new approaches to treatment. We must find some way to get out from this circular trap.

Tardive dyskinesia associated with antipsychotic drug treatment is a problem that continues to be troubling. We haven't made a great deal of practical progress either in preventing its occurrence or in treating it effectively. Thus, this complication has become a major consideration in the use of these drugs. As it may occur in non-schizophrenic patients treated with relatively small doses of antipsychotics, it now seems prudent to restrict their clinical use to patients with definite psychotic disorders about which there would be no argument concerning the propriety of their use. One might tend to be somewhat more conservative about doses and duration of treatment. So many treatments have been reported to improve tardive dyskinesia that it may take some time before we know which ones are practical. The implications of tardive dyskinesia go beyond the neurological disorder. If the mechanism of tardive dyskinesia is a compensatory dopaminergic receptor supersensitivity, why should it not also occur in the mesolimbic system as it does in the nigrostriatal system? Some evidence has accumulated that such receptor supersensitivity does indeed occur in the mesolimbic system. What, then, are the implications for the schizophrenic patient? Could it mean that the patients develop tolerance/dependence to antipsychotic drugs in a way similar to the patient in chronic pain treated with opiates? Are schizophrenic patients destined to require ever higher doses of these drugs to maintain their improvement and will discontinuation of antipsychotic drugs result in a worse situation than was present when they started treatment? These questions are highly pertinent to our use of antipsychotic drugs and we must find the answers soon.

Treatment of major depressions with drugs has always been more controversial than treatment of schizophrenia. While there now seems to be little doubt that tricyclics, and to a lesser extent the monoamine oxidase inhibitors, are effective in some patients, we still have problems in choosing the right drug for the right patient. Much clinical evidence suggests that in the case of the tricyclics, specific antidepressant effects are limited to those types of depression termed "endogenous," a category not always consistently defined and diagnosed. Within the endogenous group, preliminary work suggests that one can make biochemical distinctions based on the involved neurotransmitter and select in advance the type of tricyclic most suited for an individual patient. Should such biochemical typology of endogenous depression be confirmed, the clinical implications would be exciting. The failure of many patients to respond to antidepressant drugs, either rapidly or completely enough to indicate that improvement is clearly drug-related, indicates the serious limitations of presently available drugs in the overall treatment of this syndrome. The application of pharmacokinetic principles to the exploitation of these drugs is another technical aspect which may enhance somewhat their yield of therapeutic successes. Nonetheless, we still do not have alternative approaches to the treatment of depression from those available twenty years ago. Once again, we are in some kind of circular trap.

Our treatment of manic-depressive disorder has been vastly improved by lithium, especially in the prevention of recurrences of mania or depression. Yet, it has not appreciably changed in the past decade. We do not have hypotheses about the mode of action of this simple material on both the manic and depressive phases of this illness that are nearly as tenable as those for the mode of action of antipsychotic or antidepressant drugs. The great success of lithium may have stultified research into other methods of treatment for manic-depressive disorder. Recent indications that longterm, or even sometimes short-term, treatment with lithium may be associated with irreversible renal damage mandate that alternative approaches to treatment of manic-depressive disorder be explored. We can never be content with the status quo.

Some of our problems are ones of omission. We lack effective drugs for many common psychiatric disorders. Senile brain disease, also known as Alzheimer's disease, remains a puzzle. Despite the fact that an increasing proportion of people in developed countries live long enough to become vulnerable to this disorder, we know very little about its pathogenesis and have few, if any, drugs of even limited value. Research into this disorder and into pharmacologic approaches to its treatment needs much more effort than the present level. A similar situation applies to mental subnormality. Although a few specific causes have been unraveled during the past twenty-five years, the cause of the deficient mental state remains unknown in the vast majority of afflicted persons. No presently available pharmacological treatment has done more than curb associated behavioral disturbances. Substance abuse is a major problem in many countries and, if past history is any guide, it will remain so for a long while. We are not sure why people smoke or why once started, the habit is so difficult to control. Possibly no other substance abuse is so life-threatening as smoking, yet relatively little effort has gone into developing drug treatments. Alcohol abuse has long been treated with aversive drugs, such as disulfiram, but little other progress has been made. With this drug, also, the ravages on health are considerable. One can hardly overemphasize the scourge of opiate addiction. Our major pharmacologic approach to treatment has been to supplant one opiate drug for another. Recently, effective, long-acting narcotic antagonists have become available as therapeutic agents. These are seemingly perfect drugs, in that their effects are highly predictable. The paradox is that patients won't take them. One would like to think that problems created by drugs might be amenable to treatment with drugs, but perhaps such reasoning is too naive. In any case, these problems require our continued efforts.

Some of our current problems are in the social sphere. For a variety of reasons, it is becoming increasingly difficult in many countries, most of all my own, to do clinical research. No one would argue against proper ethical constraints to protect human subjects, although what is proper is often difficult to define. Superficially, it would seem reasonable to expect that before a drug were put into man, testing in animals should be rather extensive. Yet, animal trials may not be predictive, either in terms of therapeutic efficacy or of toxicity, of the results to be obtained in man. We need to get drugs into man earlier than is presently possible, for often a very limited human experience with a drug may settle issues of whether or not the drug should be developed further. This issue is even more critical when drugs or chemicals are used as probes for studying the pathogenesis of disease states. Often none of these drugs or chemicals has any potential commercial value, so the funds for extensive studies of animal toxicity are not available. Without such preliminary studies, it may be impossible to use the drug in man to test a particular hypothesis. The future of neuropsychopharmacology's sister discipline, biological psychiatry, is heavily dependent upon the resolution of this problem.

Finally, our right to treat patients with drugs is being challenged. Our success with drug therapy in psychiatry has offended many who, for various reasons and with various motivations, abhor the use of drugs. The possibility of adverse effects from these drugs, especially tardive dyskinesia, has given impetus to make mandatory the consent of patients or their protectors prior to any use of drugs in psychiatric patients. In at least one state in the United States, such a law has been passed. It remains to be seen whether it can be implemented without serious disadvantage for those patients it presumably is meant to protect. The implications of such laws are even more ominous: A different set of standards is applied to the use of psychotherapeutic drugs than to any other class of drugs. Consent does not have to be obtained for the use of digoxin to treat patients with congestive heart failure, even though the adverse consequences of digoxin are at least as severe as those of antipsychotic drugs. For inexplicable reasons, the civil liberties of psychiatric patients are deemed to be more important than those of cardiac patients.

One may speculate that in today's climate it is easier to pervert the uses of psychiatry than that of any other medical specialty. Egregious examples of the misuse of psychiatry for political purposes are well documented. Drugs, which in the lay person's mind can easily be construed as means of controlling thoughts, are a logical target of such fears. Our problem is that we are neglecting to assure the public that psychotherapeutic drugs are not used for nefarious purposes. Drugs that remove the nagging hallucinations of schizophrenia, that disperse the dark cloud of melancholy, that calm the frenzied activity of mania, or that relieve the unknown apprehension of anxiety, are more properly liberating agents than they are means of restraint. Our problem is to defend our right to use these valuable agents that so many here have done so much to develop. If we do not act soon, our hands may be tied before we know it, and our patients will suffer.

Contrary to what you might suppose from my recital of this litany of problems for our field, I am quite optimistic about its future. We have been fortunate in attracting outstanding persons from many medical and scientific fields to this common ground of neuropsychopharmacology. Our progress over this past quarter century has been great. The fruits of our efforts are plainly visible. The challenges of understanding the brain and how drugs work on it continue to attract some of the best and brightest of our young colleagues. Present problems are the challenges that will advance our science, but their solutions will engender still more problems. The process is never-ending, but so is the search for knowledge.

Now we shall adjourn to the scientific portion of our meeting. If this Eleventh C.I.N.P. Congress is a success, you will become aware of even more problems than those few that I have selected to call to your attention. At the same time, you will be stimulated by contacts with your peers to attempt solutions for present problems. In the long run, our patients will benefit, just as they have from the efforts of neuropsychopharmacologists during the two decades that the C.I.N.P. has

been meeting. May you all have an interesting, informative and enjoyable time at this 1978 Congress in Vienna.

ECT in Depression: Biochemical Effects and Mode of Action

Summary

J.-O. OTTOSSON

Department of Psychiatry I., Göteborg University, Göteborg, Sweden

The reason for the restriction to the antidepressive action of ECT is that to an increasing extent ECT has become a treatment of depression where it is superior to drugs, whereas it is less and less used in mania and schizophrenia where there are equivalent or better alternatives. The main topics were blood-brain barrier (BBB), neuroendocrinology and monoamines.

1. In ECT given according to anesthesiological principles there is a marginally and reversibly increased diffusion of small and large molecules but no break down of the BBB. Electronmicroscopy showed no damage neither of vascular structures nor of brain cells. Similar changes occurred after the administration of carbon dioxide and therefore increased cerebral blood flow seems to be the common denominator.

The absence of damage or irreversible changes after ECT is in line with other studies showing that the antidepressive action is not dependent on or belonging to an organic syndrome. Organic signs may be evoked with intensive treatment given without consideration to anesthesiological principles but in modern use of ECT the goal is to obtain the antidepressive action in as pure a culture as possible.

2. Endocrine studies have shown a hypothalamic dysfunction in endogenous depression manifesting itself e.g. in hypersecretion of corticotropin releasing hormone, ACTH and cortisol which is due to loss of inhibiting hypothalamic control, and decreased reactivity of the growth hormone and luteinizing hormone systems. These changes partly normalize after recovery. In acute experiments ECT increases the reactivity of the neuroendocrine systems. The findings give a pathophysiological basis of the hypothalamic symptoms such as anorexia, decreased libido, sleep disturbance and changed diurnal rhythm which occupy a key position in endogenous depression as positive indicators of a rapid and convincing response to ECT. It is important for the understanding of the pathophysiology of depression and the mode of action of ECT that the hypothalamic dysfunction can be seen as a consequence of reduced monoaminerg activity.

3. Monoamine research in animals has concentrated on cumulative and sustained effects after series of ECT which are the obvious criteria if they shall be parallels to the antidepressive effect. There are two groups of findings: (i) increased synthesis of norepinephrine (but not of serotonin and dopamine), (ii) increased sensitivity of serotonin and dopamine and possibly also norepinephrine receptors. The clinical report of lowered 5-HIAA in CSF after a series of treatments may be

explained as a feed-back effect of increased sensitivity of serotonin receptors.

The findings imply that the action of ECT fits with the amine hypothesis, the emphasis being both on increased output of amines and increased amine receptor sensitivity. A distinction has been made between low output and low sensitivity depression. Whereas there is direct evidence of low output depression both regarding serotonin and dopamine, possibly also norepinephrine, the evidence of low sensitivity depression is mainly indirect. However, whatever the basic disturbance, ECT has possibilities of counteracting it. E.g. both a depression due to low output of serotonin and low sensitivity of serotonin receptors, if such exists, may be alleviated by increasing the sensitivity of serotonin receptors. This feature of ECT as a broad spectrum therapy may explain its higher recovery rate in comparison to the more specifically acting antidepressant drugs.

To conclude, recent research in ECT has given strong argument against those who claim that ECT is merely an empiric and even damaging treatment. The knowledge of its mode of action is approaching that of the antidepressant drugs. ECT is on its way of becoming a rational antidepressive treatment as concerns the knowledge both of the pathophysiology of endogenous depression and the mode of action of the treatment.

Long Lasting Effects of ECT on Monoaminergic Mechanisms

KJELL MODIGH

Department of Pharmacology, University of Göteborg, Göteborg, Sweden

ABSTRACT

Effects of electroconvulsive therapy (ECT), generally administered as one electroconvulsion daily for seven days (ECS x VII), on monoaminergic mechanisms were studied in vivo in rats and mice between one and ten days after the last ECS (day 1 - day 10). The results indicate increased synthesis of noradrenaline (NA) persisting at least until day 6 and a slightly reduced uptake of NA at the level of the cell membranes. The synthesis and uptake of dopamine (DA) and 5-hydroxytryptamine were not significantly affected by ECSxVII at any of the time intervals studied. ECS x VII potentiated behavioural and growth hormone (GH) releasing effects of DA-receptor agonists. The potentiation, which persisted at least until day 11, is indicative of increased sensitivity in postsynaptic DA receptors. Preliminary results from clinical investigations of these postsynaptic effects reveal no significant effect of ECT on apomorphine-induced release of hGH, but a palliative effect of ECT, given in combination with L-DOPA, on extrapyramidal symptoms in therapy resistant cases of Parkinson´s disease.

KEY WORDS

ECT, monoamine synthesis, monoamine uptake, monoamine receptors, animal behaviour, growth hormone, mental depression, Parkinson´s disease.

INTRODUCTION

The unknown mechanisms for the antidepressant effect of electroconvulsive therapy (ECT) is a challenging riddle. When it is solved, we have probably increased our understanding of affective disorders considerably and also gained information which will help to improve antidepressant therapy.

Many investigations have focused on the question whether ECT facilitates the neurotransmission in central monoaminergic neurons. The rational for this is of course the well known monoamine hypotheses of affective disorders and the presumed mode of action of antidepressant drugs. It was early established in animal experiments that the turnover of brain monoamines is increased immediately after electroconvulsions (ECS) (Ebert and coworkers, 1973; Engel and coworkers, 1968 and 1971; Schildkraut and Draskoczy, 1974; Shields, 1972).

The mechanisms mediating the antidepressant effect of ECT would however be expected to be longlasting and require multiple ECS to develop, since the clinical experience is that the treatment generally gives longlasting or permanent relief from antidepressant symptoms and that repeated ECS are required (cf. Kety, 1974). We have therefore in a series of animal experiments imitated the clinical use of ECT by administering multiple ECS over a period of several days and searched for longlasting effects on pre- and postsynaptic monoaminergic mechanisms. The evidence for such longlasting effects was, when we initiated these studies, limited to the findings of increased turnover of noradrenaline (NA) (Ebert and coworkers, 1973; Kety and coworkers, 1967; Ladisich and coworkers, 1969; Schildkraut and Draskoczy, 1974) and increased tyrosine hydroxylase activity in NA-rich areas of the brain (Musacchio and coworkers, 1969) around 24 h after the last of series of ECS and increased activity of brain monoamine oxidase (MAO) persisting for several weeks after the last of multiple ECS (Pryor and Otis, 1970; Pryor and coworkers, 1972).

METHODS

Male Sprague-Dawley rats and albino mice (N.M.R.I. strain) were used. ECS was delivered through alligator clip electrodes attached to the animals' ears. Brain concentrations of monoamines and their precursors were measured spectrophotofluorimetrically after purification on a strong cation exchange column. Blood samples for determination of growth hormone (GH) concentrations were taken from cannulae inserted into the aorta 4-7 days before the acute experiments. Plasma GH was determined by radio immuno assay using a double antibody technique. Motor activity was measured in activity meters based on photoconductive sensors. Apomorphine induced stereotyped behaviour was estimated semiquantitatively according to Costall and Naylor (1973). For detailed methodological descriptions see Modigh (1974, 1976) and Edén and Modigh (1977).

RESULTS AND DISCUSSION

Synthesis and Turnover

The tyrosine- and tryptophan hydroxylase activities, rate limiting in the synthesis of catecholamines (CA) and 5-hydroxytryptamine (5-HT), respectively, were estimated in vivo according to Carlsson and coworkers (1972) by measuring the accumulation of 3,4-dihydroxyphenylalanine (DOPA) and 5-hydroxytryptophan (5-HTP) respectively 30 min after administration of the decarboxylase inhibitor NSD 1015. ECT administered as one ECS daily for 7 days (ECS x VII) accelerated the DOPA accumulation significantly in NA-rich areas of the brain (hemispheres and brain stem) at all time intervals studied, i.e. from one (day 1) to seven days (day 7) after the last ECS. The DOPA accumulation in dopamine (DA) rich areas of the brain (striatum and limbic part) and the 5-HTP accumulation in all parts of the brain were not significantly changed by ECT at any of the time intervals studied (Fig. 1).

The utilization of brain monoamines was estimated by measuring their rates of depletion after synthesis inhibition. DL-α-methyl-p-tyrosine methylester HCl (H 44/68) and DL-α-propyldopacetamide (H 22/54) were used as inhibitors of CA and 5-HT synthesis, respectively. Animals pretreated with ECS x VII and tested at day 3 showed only a tendency ($p < 0.1$) to accelerated depletion of NA and normal depletion rates for DA and 5-HT (Fig. 2).

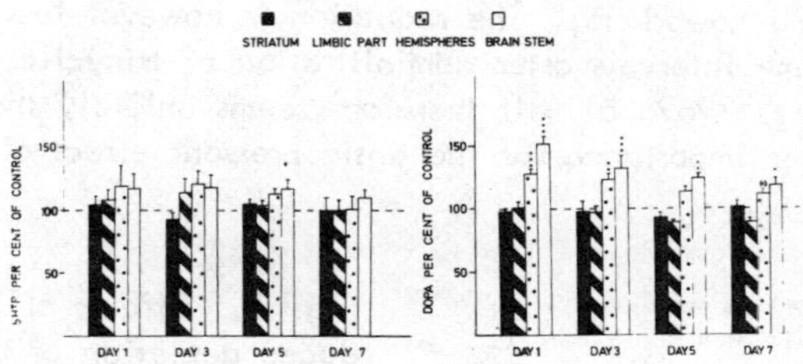

Fig. 1. Effect of ECS x VII on NSD 1015 induced accumulation of 5-HTP and DOPA in different parts of the rat brain. Each bar represents the mean of 5-6 determinations, expressed as per cent of control ± s.e.m. Statistically significant differences from control are indicated. *** $p<0.001$, ** $p<0.005$, * $p<0.05$ (from Modigh, 1976)

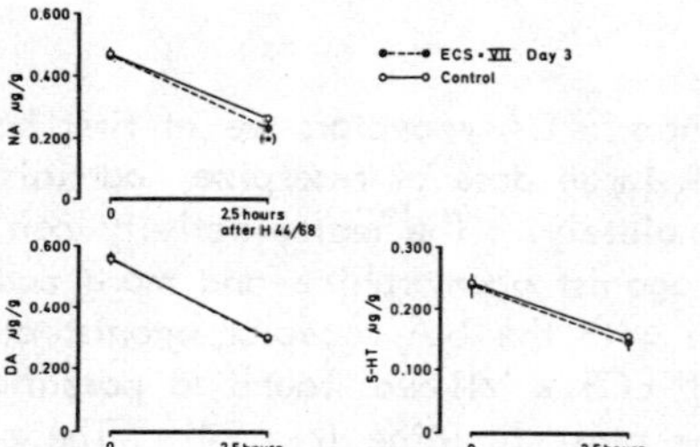

Fig. 2. Effects of ECS x VII on depletion of brain DA, NA and 5-HT after synthesis inhibition. Each point represents mean of 6-8 determinations ± s.e.m. Differences in amine concentrations between controls and ECS-treated rats were calculated by means of t-test. (*) $p<0.1$ (from Modigh, 1976).

The results indicate that ECT induces a fairly longlasting increase in NA synthesis and possibly also a slight increase of the impulse activity in NA neurons, since variations in rate of depletion of monoaminergic transmitters after synthesis inhibition generally reflect changes in nerve impulse flow (Andén and coworkers, 1969). The findings of unchanged synthesis and turnover of DA and 5-HT argue against longlasting generalized activation of DA and 5-HT neurons after ECT.

Uptake of Monoamines

A single ECS administered to mice was reported by Welch, Hendley and Turek (1974) to decrease the affinity for NA uptake, determined in synaptosome-rich homogenates of cerebral cortex. A decreased affinity for NA uptake was also found in a consecutive experiment on rats 18-24 h after the last of repeated ECS (Hendley, 1976). We have studied the effect of ECT on the monoamine uptake mechanisms at the level of the nerve cell membranes in vivo, according to Carlsson and coworkers (1969a,b). The model utilizes the displacing effects of monoamine analogues (H 77/77 and H 75/12) with affinity both for the uptake mechanisms at the cell membranes and for the uptake and binding mechanisms in the storage granules. The depletion of NA following administration of H 77/77 was slightly but significantly counteracted by ECS x VII on day 3, whereas the H 77/77 induced depletion of DA and the H 75/12 induced depletion of 5-HT were unaffected (Fig. 3). The results indicate a reduced uptake of NA after ECT in agreement with the reports by Hendley and coworkers. The reduction is however less pronounced than that obtainable at short time intervals after administration of tricyclic antidepressant drugs (cf. Carlsson and coworkers, 1969a,b). It therefore seems unlikely that inhibition of NA uptake per se is of major importance for the antidepressant effect of ECT.

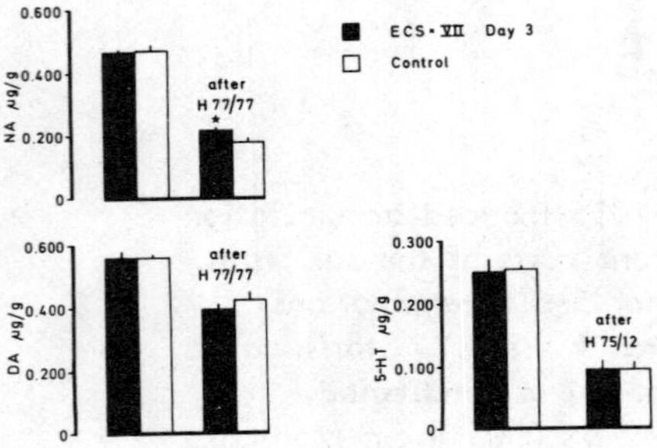

Fig. 3. Effects of ECSxVII on H 77/77 induced depletion of brain DA and NA and on H 75/12 induced depletion of brain 5-HT. Each bar represents the mean of 5-6 determinations + s.e.m. Statistical difference between ECS treated and control rats is indicated. * $p < 0.05$ (from Modigh, 1976).

Postsynaptic Mechanisms - Animal Experiments

In an attempt to investigate whether ECT affects postsynaptic CA receptors we at first hand utilized the behavioural model illustrated in Fig. 4. A large dose of reserpine, administered to mice, blocks their spontaneous motor activity completely. The motor activity can be restored partially by administration of the DA receptor agonist apomorphine and more completely by administration of apomorphine in combination with the NA receptor agonist clonidine (Andén and coworkers, 1973). Pretreatment with ECS x VII was found to potentiate the effects of apomorphine alone as well as apomorphine plus clonidine (Fig. 4). The potentiation required more than a single ECS to develop and persisted, in animals treated with

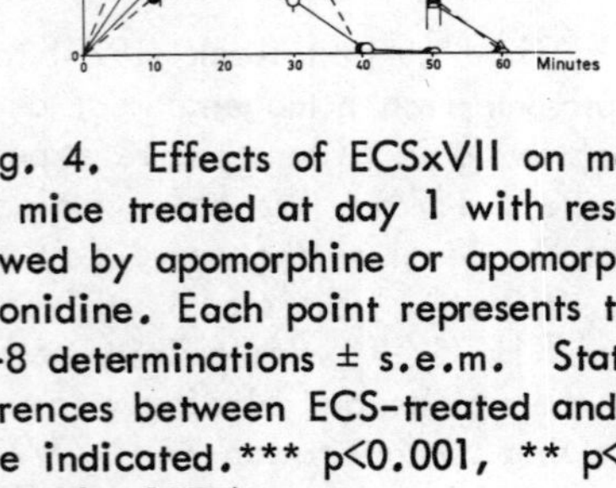

Fig. 4. Effects of ECSxVII on motor activity in mice treated at day 1 with reserpine followed by apomorphine or apomorphine plus clonidine. Each point represents the mean of 7-8 determinations ± s.e.m. Statistical differences between ECS-treated and control rats are indicated. *** $p<0.001$, ** $p<0.01$ (from Modigh, 1975).

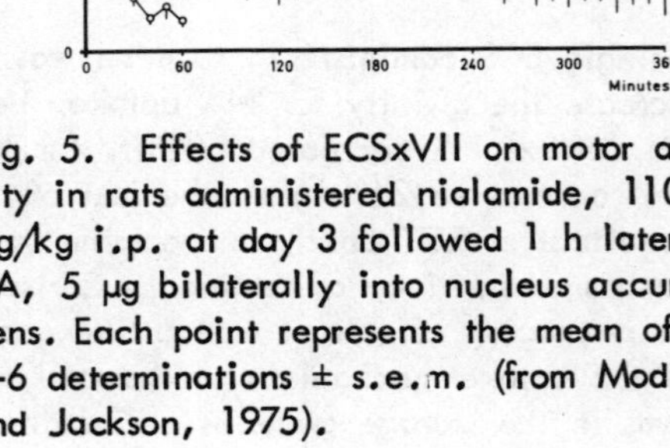

Fig. 5. Effects of ECSxVII on motor activity in rats administered nialamide, 110 mg/kg i.p. at day 3 followed 1 h later by DA, 5 μg bilaterally into nucleus accumbens. Each point represents the mean of 5-6 determinations ± s.e.m. (from Modigh and Jackson, 1975).

ECS x VII, till at least day 7. The effect of ECT to potentiate DA agonists could be demonstrated also in other, similar models. In Fig. 6 is shown the potentiating effect of ECS x VII on apomorphine induced stereotypies in rats at day 3. The potentiation remained statistically significant at day 10 (Fig. 7). In Fig. 5 is shown the potentiating effect of ECS x VII on the psychomotor stimulant effect of DA applied locally bilaterally into nucleus accumbens, indicating that the potentiation is not mediated by changes in permeability of the blood brain barrier (cf. Bolwig, this volume).

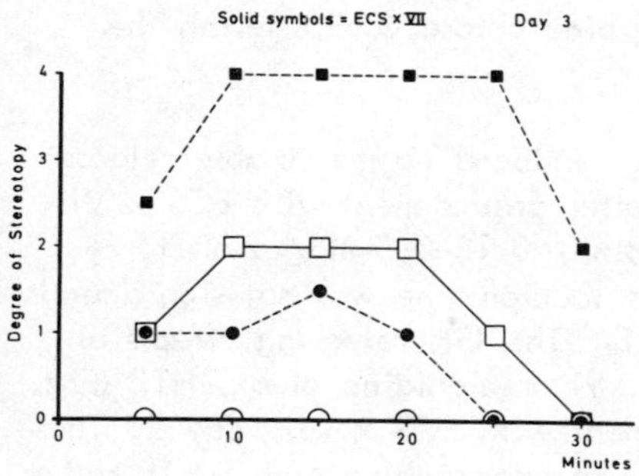

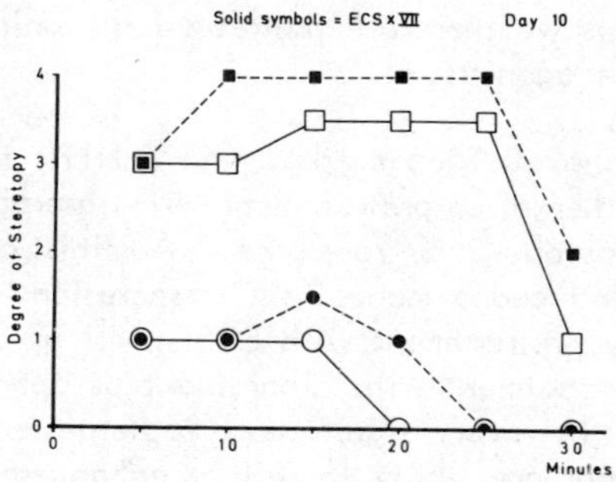

Figs 6 and 7. Effects of ECS x VII on apomorphine induced stereotypies in rats. Apomorphine 0.5 mg/kg (squares) or 1 mg/kg (circles) was administered 3 (Fig. 6) or 10 days (Fig. 7) after the last ECS. Shown are median scores in groups of 6 animals. Differences in stereotypies between experimental (E) and control (C) groups were estimated by nonparametric multivariate analysis. $p > 0.05$ was considered not significant (NS) (Montel and Valand, 1970).

			E - C
Day 3	apomorphine	0.5 mg/kg	$p < 0.01$
	"	1 mg/kg	$p < 0.01$
Day 10	"	0.5 mg/kg	NS
	"	1 mg/kg	$p < 0.05$

(Grabowska, M. and Modigh, K, unpublished results)

The potentiation of behavioural responses to DA agonists indicates that ECT increases the sensitivity of postsynaptic DA receptors or changes the structures connected to these receptors. No conclusions can be drawn regarding effects of ECT on NA receptors, since NA agonists have no measurable effect in these models when given alone. Grahame-Smith, Green and coworkers have in contemporary investigations, based on similar assumptions and experimental models as ours, confirmed the DA-agonist potentiating effect of ECT and also found that the treatment potentiates behavioural effects elicited by 5-HT agonists (Evans and coworkers, 1976, Green and coworkers, 1977) indicating that ECT may induce changes also in relation to postsynaptic 5-HT receptors. The exact nature of these postsynaptic changes remains to be clarified. They seem to differ from the receptor hypersensitivity observed after treatments which primarily led to decreased activation of postsynaptic DA receptors, since no longlasting changes appear to develop either in the dopaminergic adenylate cyclase system (Green and coworkers, 1977) or in dopaminergic receptor binding sites (Bergstrom and coworkers, 1978). Interesting in this respect is a recent report by Green and coworkers (1978) that the turnover of GABA is reduced after ECT. The reduction in turnover was interpreted to reflect a decreased inhibitory gabergic tone (see also Green, this volume).

Evaluation of whether the postsynaptic effects of ECT have relevance for the therapeutic effects of the treatment requires methods to study them clinically. We are at present investigating whether monoamine agonist induced release of GH is a useful model in this respect and as a first step we have evaluated this model in experiments on rats. The secretion of GH in rats is normally pulsatile, with peaks in plasma concentration at regular 3-4 h intervals during day and night (for review see Martin and coworkers, 1978). The frequent normal pulses of GH secretion make it difficult to evaluate drug induced secretory pulses. However, we found that the normal GH secretion could be blocked completely for 24 h by administration of reserpine in a high dose (10 mg/kg) and in the following experiments we therefore pretreated the animals with reserpine before administering the monoamine agonists.

Apomorphine, 0.25-5 mg/kg, and 5-HTP, 100-400 mg/kg, induced no measurable release of GH either after pretreatment with reserpine alone or after pretreatment with ECS x VII followed at day 2 by reserpine. Administration of clonidine, 0.15-0.5 mg/kg after reserpine, induced a moderate GH secretion. The response to clonidine was not significantly altered by pretreatment with ECS x VII at day 2 (Fig. 8). The GH releasing effects of combined treatment with clonidine plus apomorphine (Fig. 9) or clonidine plus 5-HTP (Fig. 10) were, however, significantly potentiated by pretreatment with ECS x VII, day 2. These potentiations are likely to reflect enhanced responsiveness to apomorphine and 5-HTP rather than to clonidine, since ECT did not potentiate the effect of clonidine alone. The results are thus in agreement with those from the behavioural experiments and provide suggestive evidence for increased sensitivity after ECT in DA- and 5-HT receptors involved in the regulation of GH secretion.

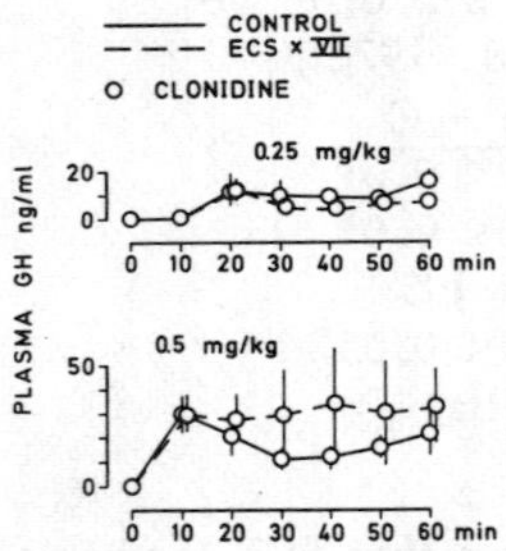

Fig. 8. Effects of various doses of clonidine on GH secretion in rats pretreated with reserpine alone (controls) or ECSxVII followed at day 2 by reserpine. Each point represents the mean of 6-7 determinations ± s.e.m. (from Balldin and coworkers, in manuscript 1978).

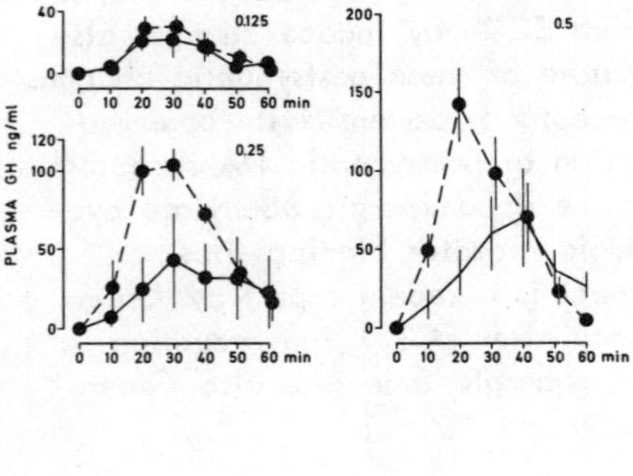

Fig. 9. Effects of combined treatment with various doses of clonidine and apomorphine on GH secretion in rats pretreated with reserpine alone (controls) or ECSxVII followed at day 2 by reserpine. Each point represents the mean of 3-6 determinations ± s.e.m. (from Edén and Modigh, 1977).

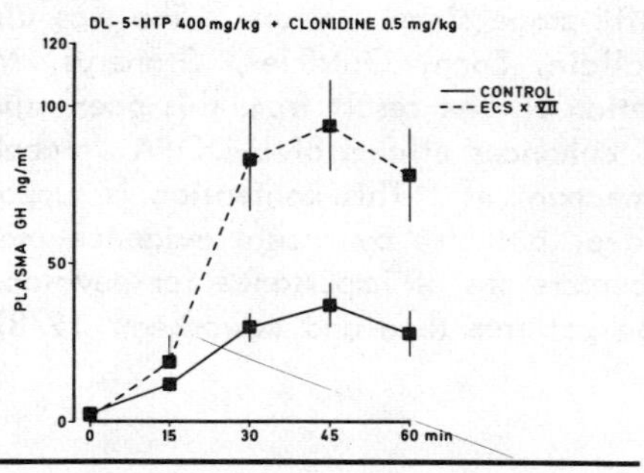

Fig. 10. Effect of combined treatment with clonidine and 5-HTP on GH secretion in rats pretreated with reserpine alone (controls) or ECSxVII followed at day 2 by reserpine. Each point represents the mean of 3-5 determinations ± s.e.m. (from Balldin and coworkers, in manuscript, 1978).

Postsynaptic Mechanisms - Clinical Investigations

The prerequisites for investigations of drug induced GH release in humans differ from those in rats, e.g. in that the physiological secretion of the hormone is very minute during day time. Moreover administration of DA agonists alone stimulates the hormone secretion in humans (for rev. see Martin and coworkers, 1978). We have therefore in clinical studies on depressed patients at first hand started to investigate whether ECT changes the hGH response to apomorphine, 0.18-0.24 mg administered intravenously. The apomorphine induced elevation of hGH in plasma is measured 1-4 days before and after a series of ECS. We have till now investigated nine patients in this way. The symptoms of depression were effectively relieved by ECT in all cases. Six of the patients showed higher maximal hGH responses after ECT than before, whereas the remaining three showed lower responses after ECT than before (Fig. 11). There is thus a tendency although not statistically significant towards enhanced apomorphine induced hGH responses after ECT.

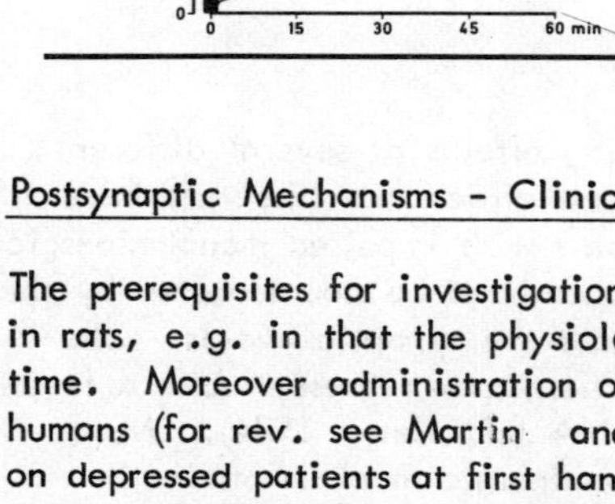

Fig. 11. Maximal hGH response to apomorphine in mentally depressed patients before (open symbols) and after ECT (solid symbols) (Balldin, Lindstedt, Modigh, Wallin, Wålinder, unpublished observation).

The question whether clinically administered ECT changes the responsiveness to DA agonists, can be approached also by studying the interaction between ECT and L-DOPA in treatment of patients with Parkinson's disease. ECT alone has been reported to alleviate extrapyramidal symptoms in patients suffering concomitantly from Parkinson's disease and depression (Lebensohn and Jenkins, 1975, Asnis, 1977). We have recently started to offer ECT to parkinsonian patients who have become partially refractory to L-DOPA, showing the "on-off" phenomenon. ECT is given according to the routines for treatment of depression, i.e. totally 6-8 ECS are given with a maximal frequency of 2 treatments weekly. The patients are maintained on earlier adjusted doses of L-DOPA during and after the ECT. Four patients have till now been treated in this way and we have noticed improvement in three of them.

The most remarkable improvement was seen in a 67 year old lady who had been treated with L-DOPA for 9 years and been in the "on-off" stage since 5 years. She was almost free from symptoms during 4 months after ECT (Balldin, Edén, Gottfries, Granerus, Modigh, Svanborg, Wallin, Wålinder, unpublished observation). The result from this open study strongly suggests that clinically administered ECT enhances effects of L-DOPA, probably by effects of ECT on postsynaptic dopaminergic mechanisms. This contention is supported not only by the animal experiments described above, but also by recent evidence indicating that adaptive changes in postsynaptic DA receptors are of importance for development of therapy residence in L-DOPA treated Parkinson patients (Lee and coworkers, 1978).

CONCLUDING REMARKS

The animal experiments reveal that ECT has fairly longlasting effects at several different levels of the monoaminergic neurotransmission. Most of these effects are likely to have stimulatory consequences when ECT is administered to patients with impaired monoaminergic nerve activity. In normal individuals, they may on the other hand be counteracted by the well developed system of feedback mechanisms which regulate the synaptic events. The sustained increase in MAO activity after ECT (see Introduction) may represent such a feedback phenomenon, compensating the increased turnover of NA (cf. Kety, 1974). Moreover, the general pattern of ECT induced changes of monoaminergic mechanisms in the animal experiments may reflect a balance between primary effects and antagonistic phenomena. Thus ECT was found to stimulate noradrenergic neurotransmission by effects on presynaptic mechanisms, whereas in the GH experiments, no evidence for increased sensitivity of NA receptors was found. On the contrary the NA receptor sensitivity, estimated as NA stimulated adenylate cyclase activity (Vetalani and coworkers, 1976), is decreased by ECT. On the other hand, the animal experiments provide evidence for longlasting facilitatory effects in relation to postsynaptic dopaminergic and serotonergic receptors after ECT but not for any longlasting facilitatory effects related to presynaptic mechanisms in DA and 5-HT neurons.

Whether the effects of ECT on monoaminergic mechanisms, observed in animal experiments, have relevance for the antidepressant effect of the treatment can be definitely evaluated only in clinical research. The stimulant effect on the synthesis and turnover of NA fits well into the NA hypothesis of depression and the facilitatory effect on the serotonergic neurotransmission via interference with postsynaptic mechanisms, fits well into the indolamine hypothesis of depression. None of these effects have, however, yet been refound clinically (cf. Goodwin, this volume). The effect of ECT, related to postsynaptic DA receptors, is likely to be of importance for alleviating psychomotor inhibition in depression. This view is supported inter alia by the finding of a positive correlation between deficiency on DA turnover and psychomotor inhibition in depressed patients (van Praag and Korf, 1975). The possibility that effects of ECT on DA receptors may have more general significance in the treatment of depression should also be considered. In this context it is note-worthy that after discontinuation of treatment with reserpine or haloperidol, which in animals has been shown to increase the sensitivity of DA receptors, depressive symptoms seem to be alleviated (Dalén and coworkers, 1973, Corsini and coworkers, 1975). The possibilities to further investigate the effect of ECT on DA receptors in clinical research seem propitious in view of the apparent effect of the treatment in therapy resistant cases of Parkinson's disease.

REFERENCES

Andén, N.-E., H. Corrodi, and K. Fuxe (1969) Turnover studies using synthesis inhibition. In G. Hooper (Ed.), Metabolism of Amines in the Brain, MacMillan, London, pp. 38-47.

Andén, N.-E., U. Strömbom, and T.H. Svensson (1973) Dopamine and noradrenaline receptor stimulation: reversal of reserpine-induced suppression of motor activity. Psychopharmacologia (Berl.), 29, 289-298.

Asnis, G. (1977) Parkinson's disease, depression and ECT: a review and case study. Am. J. Psychiat., 134, 191-195.

Balldin, J., P. Bolle, S. Edén, and K. Modigh (1978) Effects of electroconvulsive therapy on growth hormone secretion induced by catecholamine receptor agonists in reserpine-pretreated rats. In manuscript.

Bergstrom, D.A., S. Treiser, and K.J. Kellar (1978) Electroconvulsive shock: Effects on monaminergic receptor binding in rat brain. In: Catecholamines: Basic and Clinical Frontiers, Abstract 180. 4th International Catecholamine Symposium, Sept. 17-22, 1978, Pacific Grove, California.

Carlsson, A., H. Corrodi, K. Fuxe, and T. Hökfelt (1969a) Effects of some antidepressant drugs on the depletion of catecholamine stores caused by 4,α-dimethyl-metatyramine. Europ. J. Pharmacol., 5, 367-373.

Carlsson, A., H. Corrodi, K. Fuxe, and T. Hökfelt, (1969b) Effect of antidepressant drugs on the depletion of intraneuronal brain 5-hydroxytryptamine stores caused by 3-methyl-α-ethyl-metatyramine. Europ. J. Pharmacol., 5, 357-366.

Carlsson, A., J.N. Davis, W. Kehr, M. Lindqvist, and C.V. Atack (1972) Simultaneous measurement of tyrosine and tryptophan hydroxylase activities in brain in vivo using an inhibitor of the aromatic amino acid decarboxylase. Naunyn-Schmideberg's Arch. Pharmacol., 275, 153-168.

Corsini, G.U., C. Masala, M. Del Zompo, M.P. Piccardi, and A. Margoni (1975) Potentiation of the antidepressant effect of chlorimipramine following haloperidol withdrawal. Sixth Int. Congr. Pharmacol., Finnish Pharmacological Soc. Abstract 1080.

Costall, B., and R.J. Naylor (1973) The role of telencephalic dopaminergic systems in the mediation of apomorphine-stereotyped behaviour. European J. Pharmacol., 24, 8-24.

Dalén, P., T. Ljungberg, and U. Ungerstedt (1973) The modified amine hypothesis. Lancet, 1, 1196-1197.

Ebert, M.H., R.J. Baldessarini, J. Lipinski, and K. Berv (1973) Effects of electroconvulsive seizures on amine metabolism in the rat brain. Arch.gen.Psychiat., 29, 397-401.

Edén, S., and K. Modigh (1977) Effects of apomorphine and clonidine on rat plasma growth hormone after pretreatment with reserpine and electroconvulsive shocks. Brain Res., 129, 379-384.

Engel, J., L.C.F. Hanson, and B.-E. Roos (1971) Effect of electroshock on 5-HT metabolism in rat brain. Psychopharmacologia (Berl.), 20, 197-200.

Engel, J., L.C.F. Hanson, B.-E. Roos, and L.E. Strömbergsson (1968) Effect of electroshock on dopamine metabolism in rat brain. Psychopharmacologia (Berl.), 13, 140-144.

Evans, J.P.M., D.G. Grahame-Smith, A.R. Green, and A.F.C. Tordoff (1976) Electroconvulsive shock increases the behavioural responses of rats to brain 5-hydroxytryptamine accumulation and central nervous system stimulant drugs. Br. J. Pharmac., 56, 193-199.

Green, A.R., D.J. Heal, and D.G. Grahame-Smith (1977) Further observations on the effect of repeated electroconvulsive shock on the behavioural responses of rats produced by increases in the functional activity of brain 5-hydroxytryptamine and dopamine. Psychopharmacology, 52, 195-200.

Green, A.R., E. Peralta, J.S. Hong, C.C. Mao, C.K. Atterwill, and E. Costa (1978) Alterations in GABA metabolism and met-enkephalin content in rat brain following repeated electroconvulsive shocks. J. Neurochem. In press.

Hendley, E.D. (1976) Electroconvulsive shock and norepinephrine uptake kinetics in the rat brain. Psychopharmacol. Comm., 2, 17-25.

Kety, S.S. (1974) Biochemical and neurochemical effects of electroconvulsive shock. In M. Fink, S. Kety, J. McGaugh, and T.A. Williams (Eds.), Psychobiology of Convulsive Therapy. V.H. Winston & Sons, Washington, D.C.

Kety, S.S., F. Javoy, A.M. Therry, L. Julou, and J. Glowinski (1967) A sustained effect of electroconvulsive shock on the turnover of norepinephrine in the central nervous system of the rat. Proc. nat. Acad. Sci. (Wash.), 58, 1249-1254.

Ladisich, W., N. Steinhauff, and N. Matussek (1969) Chronic administration of electroconvulsive shock and norepinephrine metabolism in the rat brain. Psychopharmacologia (Berl.), 15, 296-304.

Lebensohn, Z.M., and R.B. Jenkins (1975) Improvement of Parkinsonism in depressed patients treated with ECT. Am. J. Psychiat., 132, 283-285.

Lee, T., P. Seeman, A. Rajput, I.J. Farley, and O. Hornykiewicz (1978) Receptor basis for dopaminergic supersensitivity in Parkinson's disease. Nature, 273, 59-60.

Martin, J.B., P. Brazeau, G.S. Tannenbaum, J.O. Willoughby, J. Epelbaum, L.C. Terry, and D. Durand (1978) Neuroendocrine organization of growth hormone regulation. In S. Reichlin, R.J. Baldessarini, and J.B. Martin (Eds.), The Hypothalamus. Raven Press, New York, pp. 329-357.

Modigh, K. (1975) Electroconvulsive shock and postsynaptic catecholamine effects: increased psychomotor stimulant action of apomorphine and clonidine in reserpine pretreated mice by repeated ECS. J. Neural Transmission, 36, 19-32.

Modigh, K., and D.M. Jackson (1975) Evidence for a sustained effect of ECS on neuronal structures connected to brain catecholamine neurons. In Sixth Int. Congr. Pharmacology, Finnish Pharmacol. Soc., Abstract 394.

Musacchio, J.M., L. Julou, S.S. Kety, and J. Glowinski (1969) Increase in rat brain tyrosine hydroxylase activity produced by electroconvulsive shock. Proc. nat. Acad. Sci. (Wash.), 63, 1117-1119.

Praag, H.M. van, and J. Korf (1975) Zur Diskussion: Central monoamine deficiency in depressions: Causative or secondary phenomenon? Pharmacopsych., 8, 322 326.

Pryor, G.T., and L.S. Otis (1970) Persisting effects of chronic electroshock seizures on brain and behavour in two strains of rats. Physiol. Behav., 5, 1053-1055.

Pryor, G.T., S. Peache, and M.K. Scott (1972) The effect of repeated electroconvulsive shock on avoidance conditioning and brain monoamine oxidase activity. Physiol. Behav., 9, 623-628.

Schildkraut, J.J., and P.R. Draskoczy (1974) Effects of electroconvulsive shock on noradrenaline turnover and metabolism: Basic and clinical studies. In M. Fink, S. Kety, J. McGaugh, and T.A. Williams (Eds.), Psychobiology of Convulsive Therapy. V.H. Winston & Sons, Washington, D.C.

Shields, P.J. (1972) Effects of electroconvulsive shock on the metabolism of 5-hydroxytryptamine in the rat brain. J. Pharm. Pharmacol., 24, 919-920.

Vetulani, J., R.J. Stawarz, J.V. Dingell, and F. Sulser (1976) A possible common mechanism of action of antidepressant treatments. Naunyn-Schmiedeberg's Arch. Pharmacol., 293, 109-114.

Welch, B.L., E.D. Hendley, and I. Turek (1974) Norepinephrine uptake into cerebral cortical synaptosomes after one fight or electroconvulsive shock. Science, 183, 220-221.

Enhanced Monoamine Behavioural Responses Following Repeated Electroconvulsive Shock to Rats and their Relevance to ECT

A. R. GREEN, D. W. COSTAIN, D. J. HEAL, C. K. ATTERWILL and D. G. GRAHAME-SMITH

MRC Clinical Pharmacology Unit, Radcliffe Infirmary, Oxford OX2 6HE, England

ABSTRACT

Following administration of a single electroconvulsive shock (ECS) daily for 8-10 days rats show enhanced behavioural responses to treatments thought to increase 5-hydroxytryptamine and dopamine function in the brain. Similar enhancement occurs following a single daily convulsion for 8-10 days produced by exposure to the inhalant convulsant drug flurothyl. Enhancement can be produced when the ECS is given in ways closely mimicking the clinical conditions thought necessary for the successful anti-depressant action of ECT. Thus unilateral and bilateral electrode placement and varying current conditions produce enhancement and the effect is seen when 5 ECS are administered spread out over 10 days or when the ECS is given after neuromuscular blockade. The possibility that ECT produces its anti-depressant effect by increasing post-synaptic monoaminergic-mediated responses is discussed. The mechanism of the enhancement has also been investigated. Changes in GABA concentration and synthesis following repeated ECS were found which suggested a decreased GABA inhibitory tone in the n.caudatus and n.accumbens. Behavioural data on neuroleptic-induced catalepsy support this suggestion.

Keywords: Electroconvulsive shock, electroconvulsive therapy, 5-hydroxytryptamine, dopamine, GABA, behaviour, catalepsy.

INTRODUCTION

Despite the continued success of electroconvulsive therapy (ECT) in treating severe endogenous depression (Royal College of Psychiatrists, 1977; Turek and Hanlon, 1977; Drugs and Therapeutics Bulletin, 1977) there is a paucity of data on its possible therapeutic mechanism. The difficulties in studying brain function in man means that we must to a great extent rely on animal data in order to clarify the possible mode of action of ECT.

In this paper we report work performed in our laboratory on the biochemical and behavioural changes produced in rats following repeated electroconvulsive shock (ECS) and discuss its possible relevance to the antidepressant mechanism of ECT.

METHODS

Two main approaches have been used: measurement of the effects of ECS on behav-

ioural changes produced by increases in the functional activity of 5-hydroxytryptamine (5-HT) and dopamine (DA) in the brain and various biochemical analyses of putative neurotransmitters.

Changes in 5-HT function were assessed by examination of the hyperactivity response which follows administration of a monoamine oxidase inhibitor (tranylcypromine in our experiments) and L-tryptophan (Grahame-Smith, 1971). Changes in dopamine function were assessed by measuring the hyperactivity response to tranylcypromine and L-dopa (Green and Kelly, 1976) or the circling response in unilateral nigro-striatal lesioned rats to methamphetamine or apomorphine (Ungerstedt, 1971). Post-synaptic changes in monoamine function were examined by use of appropriate monoamine agonists which by-pass pre-synaptic events and directly stimulate the post-synaptic monoamine receptor. Further details on these approaches are given elsewhere (Green and Grahame-Smith, 1976; Grahame-Smith, Green and Costain, 1978).

Electroconvulsive shocks were delivered through ear-clip electrodes from either an Edison portable ECT unit or a Theratronics small animal electroplexy unit. The shock was normally 50 Hz sinusoidal 150 v for 1 s given to rats lightly anaesthetised with halothane, control rats receiving halothane only.

Activity was measured with LKB Animex activity meters.

RESULTS

Following administration of a single ECS daily for 10 days the rats showed an enhanced hyperactivity response to tranylcypromine/L-tryptophan and tranylcypromine/L-dopa when tested 24 h following the final shock (Fig. 1). The rates of brain 5-HT and DA synthesis were the same in both the ECS and control groups, suggesting that the enhancement was due to a post-synaptic change in the 5-HT and DA systems mediating the behavioural responses. This was confirmed by the observations that responses to the 5-HT agonist 5-methoxy N,N-dimethyltryptamine, the DA releasing drug methamphetamine and the DA agonist apomorphine were also enhanced (Evans and colleagues, 1976; Green, Heal and Grahame-Smith, 1977). It was also found that circling in unilateral nigro-striatal lesioned rats to both methamphetamine and apomorphine was similarly enhanced by ECS pretreatment (Green and colleagues, 1977).

Taken together with the data of Modigh (1975, 1976) showing enhanced noradrenergic responses after ECS, this data suggested to us a possible explanation for the anti-depressant action of ECT. Evidence suggests that most current antidepressant treatments have in common the action of increasing the availability of monoamine transmitters to the receptor; thereby presumably increasing the monoaminergic response. Our hypothesis is that ECT also produces an increase in the post-synaptic amine response but that it does so by increasing, in some way, the size of the post-synaptic response to the same amount of released transmitter.

If one is to promote such a hypothesis, the enhanced behavioural responses seen after ECS in rats should be produced under conditions similar to the clinical conditions that have developed empirically over the years and which are thought necessary for successful treatment with ECT. This we have tried to do and the results are now discussed.

(a) A single ECT has little clinical effect; repeated shocks given over a period are usually necessary for successful anti-depressant therapy. Normally 2-3 ECT per week are given for a total of 6-8 treatments. Single ECS administration to rats has no enhancing effect on the 5-HT behavioural syndrome but enhancement is produced by 5 ECS spaced out over 10 days or 8 ECS spaced out over 17 days (Costain and colleagues, 1979; Fig. 2, Table 1).

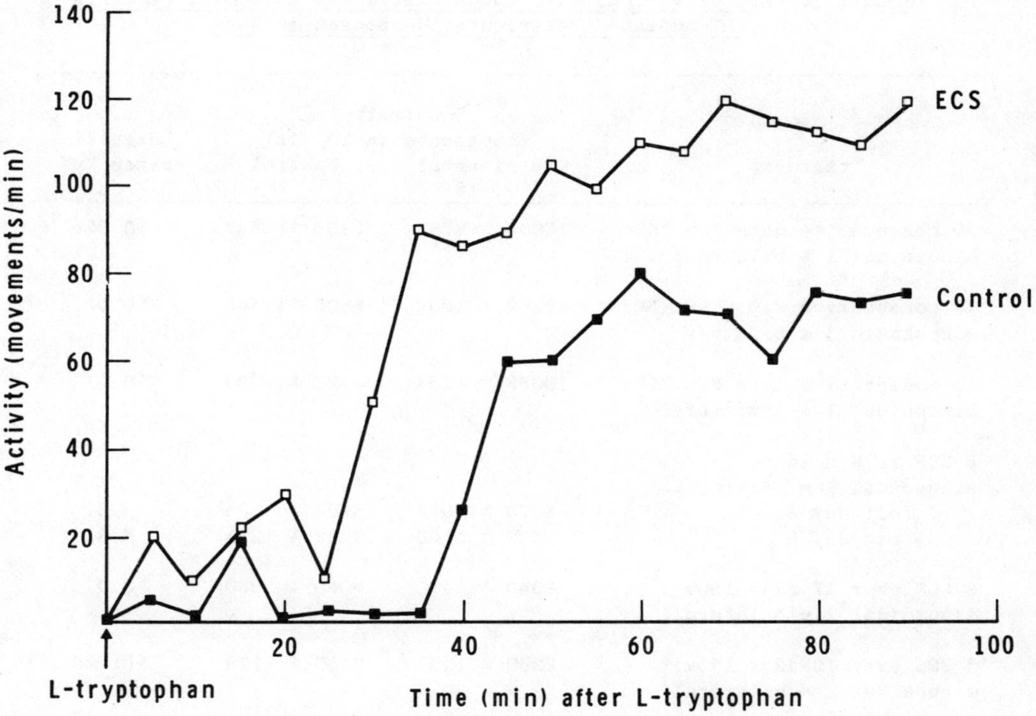

Fig. 1. Effect of repeated ECS on the hyperactivity following tranylcypromine and L-tryptophan. Rats were given a single ECS each day for 10 days. Twenty-four hours after the final shock they were injected with tranylcypromine (20 mg/kg) and L-tryptophan (50 mg/kg) 30 min later. Figure shows the hyperactivity following the tryptophan in the control (halolane anaesthesia only) group (■) and the ECS group (□).

Furthermore multiple ECT (ECT given several times in 1 day) has little effect clinically and has no effect on our animal behavioural model (Table 1).

(b) It appears that ECT is probably effective whether given through bilaterally or unilaterally placed electrodes and whether the current is alternating sinusoidal alternating pulsatile or unidirectional pulsatile. These varying electrode placements and current conditions all enhance the 5-HT hyperactivity when treatment is given over 10 days (Table 1).

(c) Sub-convulsive shocks are believed to be clinically ineffective, while introduction of neuromuscular blocking drugs to protect the patients in no way altered the therapeutic response. Similarly sub-convulsive shocks do not produce enhanced responses (Green and colleagues, 1977) while enhancement is produced in animals given a neuromuscular blocking drug before the ECS (Table 1).

(d) Clinically the method of inducing the seizure is not important, the number and frequency of the seizures being the important variables. In agreement it was found that the inhalant convulsant flurothyl ("Indoklon") used successfully in the clinic in place of ECT, produces enhanced rat behavioural responses (Green, 1978a; Fig. 3).

TABLE 1 Effect of Various Electroconvulsive Shock (ECS) Treatments on 5-HT-mediated Behavioural Responses in Rats

Treatment	Activity (movements in 90 min) Experimental	Control	Significance "p" =
10 consecutive days ECS 150v sinusoidal 1 s bilateral	10006 ± 761	6108 ± 847	<0.025
10 consecutive days ECS 150v monophasic 1 s bilateral	9587 ± 1804	6605 ± 1546	<0.05
10 consecutive days ECS 150v sinusoidal 1 s unilateral	10069 ± 1154	6422 ± 229	<0.01
8 ECS in 8 h 150v sinusoidal 1 s bilateral			
Test day 3	8970 ± 675	8664 ± 834	N.S.
Test day 9	9569 ± 1160	9293 ± 1249	N.S.
8 ECS over 17 days 150v sinusoidal 1 s bilateral	9340 ± 470	6080 ± 930	<0.01
5 ECS over 10 days 150v sinusoidal 1 s bilateral	9260 ± 1197	6400 ± 779	<0.025
5 ECS over 10 days 150v sinusoidal 1 s bilateral + Fazadinium pretreatment	8408 ± 1358	5610 ± 390	<0.025
10 consecutive days foot shock 150v biphasic	8042 ± 2936	8052 ± 806	N.S.
10 consecutive days hypoxia	6513 ± 1407	5605 ± 742	N.S.

Results show mean ± S.D. of at least 3 experiments. Significance assessed by students 't' test (unpaired). Fazadinium = neuromuscular blocker.

(e) Finally one should try to exclude non-specific effects of the shock. We find that production of hypoxia in rats daily for 10 days has no effect on the behavioural responses (Table 1). Furthermore while it has been reported that there are reversible changes in the blood-brain barrier following ECS, this is unlikely to explain any of our data, as ECS enhances the responses following injection of dopamine directly into the brain (thereby by-passing the blood-brain barrier) (Heal and Green, 1978). We also feel that "stress" is not likely to be the cause of the changes we observe. Sub-convulsive shocks presumably are very stressful but have no effect on the behavioural responses nor does the administration of a potentially convulsive shock when applied to the feet (Table 1).

One problem with our data is that the enhanced responses are only seen for about 6 days following the final shock (Green and colleagues, 1977). ECT, in contrast, generally has a long-term effect. We can perhaps suggest that in the rats we are disturbing the function of a normal brain, which then returns to normal, whereas ECT is presumably reverting to normal an abnormally functioning brain.

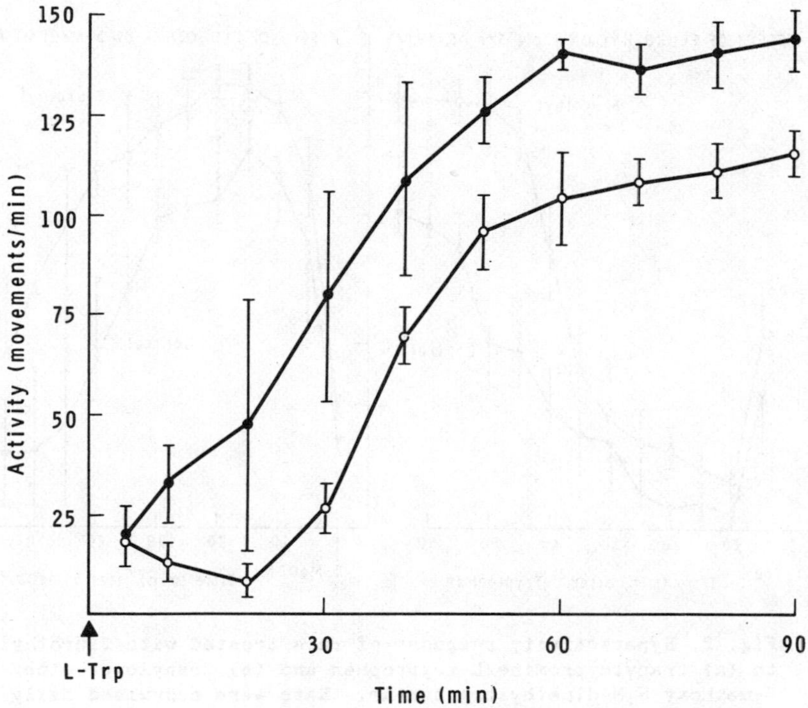

Fig. 2. The effect of 5 ECS spread out over 10 days on the hyperactivity response to tranylcypromine/L-tryptophan. Rats were given ECS 5 x (●-●) or anaesthesia (control) (O-O) spread out over 10 days (see Methods). Twenty-four hours following the final shock both groups were given tranylcypromine (10 mg kg^{-1}) followed 30 min later by L-tryptophan (50 mg kg^{-1}). The figure shows activity following L-tryptophan and results are expressed as mean ± S.D. (bars). Total movements during the 90 min period are shown in Table 1.

TABLE 2 Tissue GABA Concentration and GABA Fractional Rate Constant

	N.accumbens		N.caudatus	
	GABA	k_{GABA}	GABA	k_{GABA}
Control	48 ± 4	24 ± 3	25 ± 1	17 ± 1
ECS x 10	79 ± 10*	12 ± 2**	37 ± 4**	11 ± 1†
Sub-con x 10	48 ± 3	26 ± 1	24 ± 2	17 ± 1
ECS x 1	51 ± 4	27 ± 2	23 ± 2	19 ± 5
Sub-con x 1	44 ± 4	27 ± 2	24 ± 2	21 ± 7

ECS: electroconvulsive shock, sub-con: sub-convulsive shock. Results expressed as mean ± S.E.M. of 4-7 determinations. GABA concentration given in nmol/mg protein. *p<0.05 **p<0.01 † p<0.001 compared to control.

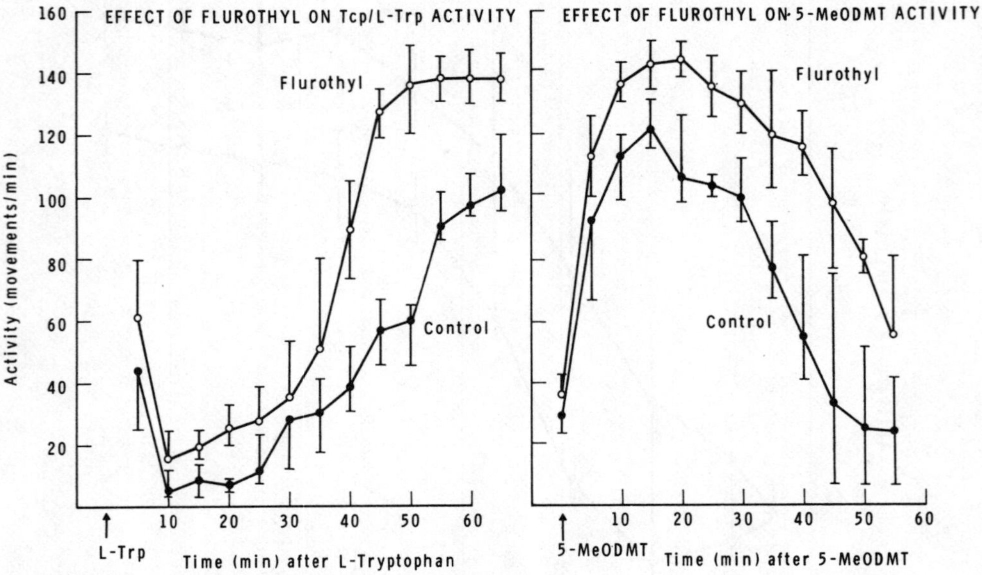

Fig. 3. Hyperactivity response of rats treated with flurothyl to (a) tranylcypromine/L-tryptophan and (b) tranylcypromine/ 5-methoxy N,N-dimethyltryptamine. Rats were convulsed daily for 10 days by exposure to flurothyl. Twenty-four hours after the final convulsion the rats were injected with tranylcypromine (20 mg/kg) followed 30 min later by either L-tryptophan (L-Tryp) 50 mg/kg or 5-methoxy N,N-dimethyltryptamine (5-MeODMT) (2 mg/kg). Results show activity response following L-tryptophan or 5-MeODMT. The mean and range of 3 separate observations (control) and 2 observations (flurothyl) is shown. (●) Control (untreated). (O) flurothyl-treated. Total movements ± s.e.mean during 60 min after L-tryptophan: control 2443 ± 267 (3), flurothyl 4077 ± 352 (2), $P < 0.025$. Total movements ± s.e.mean during 60 min following 5-MeODMT: control 4316 ± 325 (3), flurothyl 6327 ± 487 (2), $P < 0.025$.

The question arises as to the mechanism producing the enhanced post-synaptic monoaminergic responses. We do have some indications.

The behavioural responses used can be altered by alteration of brain GABA function, decreasing GABA function increasing the responses while increasing GABA function decreases the behavioural changes (Green, Tordoff and Bloomfield, 1976; Cott and Engel, 1977).

When rats were given 10 days ECS and GABA functions examined 24 hr after the final shock it was found that brain GABA concentrations had risen in the n.accumbens and n.caudatus, while the rate of GABA synthesis was markedly inhibited in these areas (Green and colleagues, 1978; Table 2). No consistent changes were seen in the substantia nigra. This data was interpreted as indicating that GABA release was inhibited in these regions and GABA function had been partly "switched-off". A decreased GABA inhibitory tone in interneurones in these areas would certainly be expected to increase behavioural responses (Heal and colleagues, 1978) and enhanced

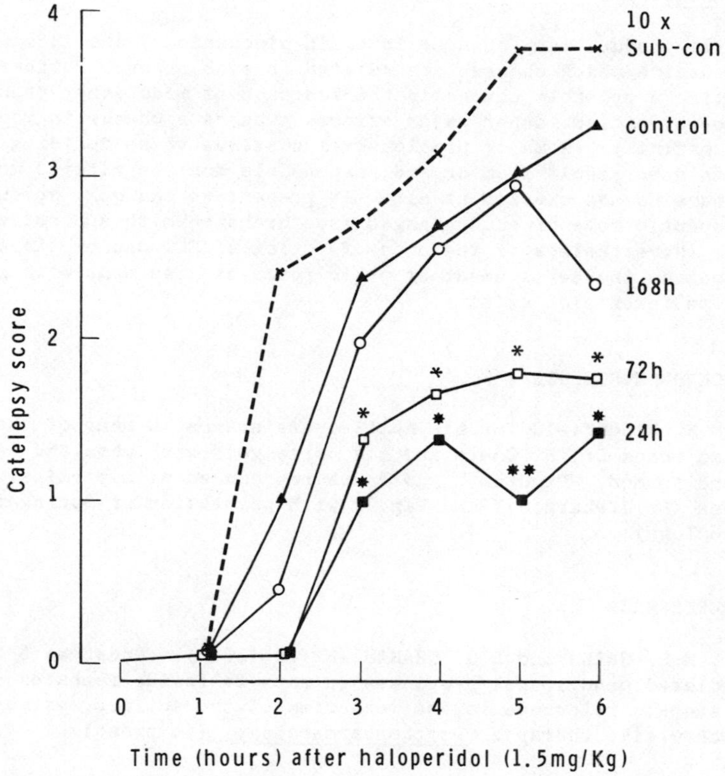

Fig. 4. Cataleptic response to haloperidol at various times following a single electroconvulsive shock given daily for 10 days (ECS x 10). Rats were given a single ECS daily for 10 days and the cataleptic response during 6 h following haloperidol (1.5 mg kg^{-1}) measured 24 h (■) 72 h (□) and 168 h (O) after the final shock. Anaesthetic only (control) response (▲) and the cataleptic response 24 h after the final shock of 10 sub-convulsive shocks (one daily for 10 days) (X) also shown. Significantly different from the control response. $^*p < 0.01$ $^{**}p < 0.001$.

behavioural responses following repeated ECS are, of course, seen (Green and colleagues, 1977; Heal and Green, 1978). It is important to note that conditions not producing behavioural enhancement (sub-convulsive shocks, 1 ECS) do not change GABA function (Table 2).

We have also recently observed that neuroleptic-induced catalepsy (which is also increased by increasing GABA function and decreased by decreased GABA function) is altered by catalepsy in a way consistent with our interpretation of the GABA biochemical data. A single ECS attenuates catalepsy 24 h after the shock, but not 48 h later. Five daily ECS attenuates the cataleptic response for up to 48 h while 10 daily ECS diminishes the responses for over 3 days but not more than 7 days (Green and colleagues, 1979) (Fig. 4). Again sub-convulsive shocks have no effect on the cataleptogenic response.

CONCLUSIONS

Clearly ECS will produce many changes in brain biochemistry and function and the problem is to decide which changes are related to each other. Furthermore our data, whilst indicating a probable change in the function of modulatory transmitters such as GABA, in no way exclude other major effects such as a change in monoamine receptor number or affinity. A major problem will continue to be deciding whether the various changes seen result from or are responsible for the altered monoaminergic response, or have no association at all. At present we can only speculate on the possible therapeutic role of such changes (see Grahame-Smith and colleagues, 1978; Green, 1978b). Nevertheless if the mode of action of ECT can be clarified it may go some way towards the development of other forms of treatment with similar efficacy and perhaps fewer side effects.

ACKNOWLEDGEMENTS

We thank Mr. M.R. Bloomfield for his skilled assistance in many of these experiments. We also thank Dr. E. Costa and his colleagues with whom the GABA turnover studies were performed. Figures 1 and 3 are reproduced with permission of Macmillan Press (Br.J.Pharmac.) and Fig. 2 with permission of Springer-Verlag (Psychopharmacology).

REFERENCES

COSTAIN, D.W., A.R. GREEN and D.G. GRAHAME-SMITH (1979). Enhanced 5-hydroxytryptamine-mediated behavioural responses in rats following repeated electroconvulsive shock: relevance to the mechanism of the antidepressive effect of electroconvulsive therapy. Psychopharmacology, (in press).

COTT, J. and J. ENGEL (1977). Suppression by GABAergic drugs of the locomotor stimulation induced by morphine, amphetamine and apomorphine: evidence for both pre- and post-synaptic inhibition of catecholamine systems. J.Neural Trans., 40, 253-268.

DRUG THER. BULL. (1977). When should ECT be used? Drug Ther.Bull., 15, 2-4.

EVANS, J.P.M., D.G. GRAHAME-SMITH, A.R. GREEN and A.F.C. TORDOFF (1976). Electroconvulsive shock increases the behavioural responses of rats to brain 5-hydroxytryptamine accumulation and central nervous system stimulant drugs. Br.J.Pharmac., 56, 193-199.

GRAHAME-SMITH, D.G. (1971). Studies in vivo on the relationship between brain tryptophan, brain 5-HT synthesis and hyperactivity in rats treated with a monoamine oxidase inhibitor and L-tryptophan. J.Neurochem., 18, 1053-1066.

GRAHAME-SMITH, D.G., A.R. GREEN and D.W. COSTAIN (1978). Mechanism of the antidepressant action of electroconvulsive therapy. Lancet, i, 254-257.

GREEN, A.R. (1978a). Repeated exposure of rats to the convulsant agent flurothyl enhances 5-hydroxytryptamine and dopamine mediated behavioural responses. Br.J.Pharmac., 62, 325-331.

GREEN, A.R. (1978b). ECT - How does it work? Trends in Neurosci., 1, 53-54.

GREEN, A.R., M.R. BLOOMFIELD, C.K. ATTERWILL and D.W. COSTAIN (1979). Electroconvulsive shock reduces the cataleptogenic effect of both haloperidol and arecoline in rats. (Submitted for publication).

GREEN, A.R. and D.G. GRAHAME-SMITH (1976). Effects of drugs on the processes regulating the functional activity of brain 5-hydroxytryptamine. Nature, 260, 487-491.

GREEN, A.R., D.J. HEAL and D.G. GRAHAME-SMITH (1977). Further observations on the effect of repeated electroconvulsive shock on the behavioural responses of rats produced by increases in the functional activity of brain 5-hydroxytryptamine and dopamine. Psychopharmacology, 52, 195-200.

GREEN, A.R. and P.H. KELLY (1976). Evidence concerning the involvement of 5-hydroxytryptamine in the locomotor activity produced by amphetamine or tranylcypromine plus L-dopa. Br.J.Pharmac., 57, 141-147.

GREEN, A.R., E. PERALTA, J.S. HONG, C.C. MAO, C.K. ATTERWILL and E. COSTA (1978). Alterations in GABA metabolism and met-enkephalin content in rat brain following repeated electroconvulsive shocks. J.Neurochem., 31, 607-611.

GREEN, A.R., A.F.C. TORDOFF and M.R. BLOOMFIELD (1976). Elevation of brain GABA concentrations with amino-oxyacetic acid; effect on the hyperactivity syndrome produced by increased 5-hydroxytryptamine synthesis in rats. J.Neural Trans., 39, 103-112.

HEAL, D.J. and A.R. GREEN (1978). Repeated electroconvulsive shock increases the behavioural responses of rats to injection of both dopamine and dibutyryl cyclic AMP into the nucleus accumbens. (Submitted for publication).

HEAL, D.J., A.G. PHILLIPS and A.R. GREEN (1978). Studies on the locomotor activity produced by injection of dibutyryl cyclic 3'5'AMP into the nucleus accumbens of rats. Neuropharmacology, 17, 265-270.

MODIGH, K. (1975). Electroconvulsive shock and post-synaptic catecholamine effects: Increased psychomotor stimulant action of apomorphine and clonidine in reserpine pretreated mice by repeated ECS. J.Neural Transm., 36, 19-32.

MODIGH, K. (1976). Long-term effects of electroconvulsive shock therapy on synthesis turnover and uptake of brain monoamines. Psychopharmacology, 49, 179-185.

ROYAL COLLEGE OF PSYCHIATRISTS. (1977). The Royal College of Psychiatrists memorandum on the use of electroconvulsive therapy. Br.J.Psychiat., 131, 261-272.

TUREK, I.S. and T.E. HANLON (1977). The effectiveness and safety of electroconvulsive therapy (ECT). J.Nerv.Ment.Dis., 164, 419-431.

UNGERSTEDT, U. (1971). Postsynaptic supersensitivity after 6-hydroxydopamine induced degeneration of the nigrostriatal dopamine system in the rat brain. Acta Physiol.Scand., 83 Suppl.367, 49-68.

ECT Effects on Mineral Metabolism and Neuroendocrine Function

PETER E. STOKES

Chief, Division of Psychobiology, Department of Psychiatry, Payne Whitney Clinic, New York Hospital, Cornell Medical Center, New York, New York 10021

ABSTRACT

This chapter reviews the current status of studies in calcium metabolism in depression treated by ECT. Metabolic balance studies, urinary calcium excretion, blood and cerebrospinal fluid calcium concentrations are discussed in relation to pre, immediately post and late post-ECT measurements. Inadequate and somewhat conflicting data make a definitive conclusion impossible at this time. There is a general consensus that calcium metabolism tends to be negative during depression and moves toward a positive balance, with decreased urinary calcium, after successful treatment. Reported serum calcium changes are contradictory, with earlier results from several studies showing an immediate and transient increase in serum levels (in some reports followed by an immediate rebound decrease) with return to pretreatment values within hours. A single more recent (and apparently better controlled) study of seven cases reports an immediate post-ECT decrease in serum and cerebrospinal fluid calcium but apparently only after a few ECT and coinciding with lessening of depression. Late post-ECT values appear to return to or toward normal. All data are consistent in finding pretreatment serum and cerebrospinal fluid calcium levels within normal limits. Potential neuroendocrine and non-hormonal mechanisms which could contribute to these changes are discussed.
Keywords: electroshock, depression, calcium metabolism

INTRODUCTION

The purpose of this chapter is to review the current status of inquiries into the relationship of calcium metabolism to depressive illness.

First there will be a brief discussion of the rationale for interest in calcium metabolism in psychiatric disorders and the difficulties inherent in clinical investigation of calcium metabolism in regard to the CNS. In the subsequent review of data from studies in the literature, attention will be given to studies of calcium balance, urinary calcium excretion, and changes in serum and cerebrospinal fluid (CSF) calcium levels in depressed patients before, during and after recovery from depression. A synopsis of potential mechanisms that may be involved in the changes in calcium metabolism in relation to ECT in depressed patients follows, including some discussion of what mechanisms may be most important. Last are a few suggestions about what is needed in future investigations.

PROBLEMS INHERENT TO CLINICAL INVESTIGATION OF CALCIUM METABOLISM IN PSYCHIATRIC PATIENTS

Clinical investigation of mineral changes in the CNS of humans is obviously fraught with the difficulties existent with all human studies of CNS substances in that one is forced to use indirect techniques to measure phenomena within an inaccessible biological compartment. Three compartments which may indirectly reflect CNS chemical events and are available for biochemical analysis are the urine, blood and CSF. However the latter two have large amounts of endogenous minerals within them. The CSF is derived from the blood plasma and is essentially returned to the intravascular compartment by reabsorption. Urinary minerals are the net result of glomerular filtration and tubular reabsorption or excretion, but the load of mineral presented is largely from tissues other than the CNS. The concentration of calcium for example is twice as great in plasma as in CSF. Calcium is ubiquitous in its distribution though mainly extracellular. One tissue, bone, contains greater than 99% of total body calcium. Furthermore, this bone calcium is in constant equilibrium with that in the intravascular volume. Consequently only a very small fraction (certainly less than 1%) of the filtered load of calcium presented to the kidney via the blood stream is even potentially derived from CNS tissues. As such, changes in urinary calcium, even on a fixed calcium diet,are by themselves not very useful for assessing calcium changes within the CNS.

Measurements of blood mineral content are fraught with difficulties of interpretation parallel to those evident for urine mineral analysis as a parameter of CNS mineral metabolism. To some degree however these problems are potentially partially soluble by using a technique similar to the Fick principle of measurement of simultaneous venous and arterial blood concentrations of the substance under study. This has in fact been done in studies of cerebral metabolism performed in this unit on patients receiving ECT (Posner, Plum and Van Poznak, 1969). When combined with blood flow measurements and clearance rates or secretory rates, the amount of substance in question being removed from or taken up into the blood by the tissue or organ in question can be calculated. This technique allows one to calculate the net uptake or excretion of a particular substance by the tissue (brain) supplied by the arterial capillary bed and venous outflow of that partiular tissue. If no net change occurs in the concentration or amount of substance measured, one cannot by this technique alone rule out the existence of simultameous and equal transport of the substance into and out of the tissue being studied. The addition of tracer techniques could help solve this problem.

Even measurement of CSF constituents, which at first view would appear to be a most direct means for assessing CNS metabolism, is in fact complicated. CSF is itself a derivative of plasma, in part an ultrafiltrate and in part formed by secretory functions of the choroid plexus as well as by passive diffusion (and active secretion) of substances from CNS cells adjacent to the ventricular system. The CSF that reaches the lumbar sac of the spinal cord has of course also been exposed to the cells of the cord and the capillary bed of the spinal cord and meninges. Thus exchanges could occur from CSF to cord cells and vice versa as well as across the capillary bed in either direction.

It is apparent from prior studies (Graziani, Escriva and Katzman, 1965) that CSF calcium is derived in the main from plasma calcium and that the CSF calcium is not solely a product of unbound serum calcium but is in equilibrium with total serum calcium. In fact, experimentally induced acute elevations in serum calcium were associated with increased exchangeable total calcium concentration in most tissues including peripheral nerves but, at least acutely, not in brain (Wallach and coworkers, 1964). The acute increases in serum calcium did not produce significantly detectable changes in total or exchangeable brain calcium, sodium or potassium. The increases in peripheral nerve calcium are similar to that described in the giant axon of the squid, and confirm the finding that in most tissues calcium uptake is proportional to extracellular calcium but this has not been shown to be true for brain. In fact it has been shown in rats and cats that very little calcium moves from the CSF to brain during 3 hours of perfusion of the ventricular system of these live animals with artificial CSF whose electrolyte, osmotic, and pH characteristics closely mimic endogenous CSF (Graziani, Escriva and Katzman, 1965). Less than 10% or radiolabelled CSF calcium was found in the brains of these animals, and what had entered was localized to the one millimeter or less of brain tissue adjacent to the ventricular system and surface of the midbrain, pons, medulla and upper cervical spinal cord. These are the sub-arachnoid areas most extensively perfused by the CSF. There appears to be specific inhibition of calcium movement into brain tissue. Little of CSF calcium is derived from brain, probably less than 15%, but this net transfer of calcium into CSF is a result of simultaneous two way exchange of calcium between CSF and brain.

Changes in calcium metabolism have been examined in human CSF for more than half a century (Sholberg and Goodall, 1926). However, there is still a relative paucity of data available on this subject as compared to that on other ions, in part related to the relative difficulty in obtaining repetitive samples of CSF and the technical laboriousness required to perform precise calcium analyses. This latter problem has been somewhat alleviated by the introduction of precise and reproducible techniques including atomic absorption spectroscopy and more precise titrimetric methods. All techniques, including the old standard Clark and Collip method, appear to give essentially comparable results however when performed with exacting care (Bradbury and colleagues, 1968).

RATIONALE FOR STUDIES OF CALCIUM METABOLISM IN PSYCHIATRIC PATIENTS

Despite these difficulties, it is understandable and pertinent that electrolyte and mineral concentrations of body fluids closest to the CNS be investigated for potential abnormalities in patients with psychiatric disturbances. Calcium, potassium and sodium all have known functions in normal nerve cell transmission. These functions include maintenance of normal transmembranal charge and electrical potential differences as well as a role in activation of certain active metabolic processes of the cell such as activation of Na-K sensitive ATP-ase and cyclic AMP. Furthermore it is reasonable to assume that the CSF approximates brain extracellular fluid (ECF) and as such is a source for estimating changes in this organ's ECF and by implication its neurons. Of course it must be noted that changes in CSF mineral concentration may not accurately or totally reflect transient larger potential changes in ion concentration within specific brain centers immediately after ECT.

From a clinical viewpoint it is also understandable that interest has existed for some time in mineral and electrolyte metabolism in patients with psychiatric disturbances. It is clear that certain types of primary endocrine disturbances can present clinically with pronounced psychiatric syndromes including a picture of affective disease, cognitive disorders and organic mental syndromes. Patients with hyper- and hypoparathyroidism or hypercalcemia based on other causes (sarcoidosis, vitamin D intoxication, cancer, etc.) have been repetitively reported as demonstrating a variety of psychiatric disorders (Whybrow and Hurwitz, 1976). Similarly patients with Addisons disease, Cushings disease and Cushings Syndrome (spontaneous or iatrogenic) have been noted to fequently present with severe affective disease (Horwith and Stokes, 1960; Whybrow and Hurwitz, 1976). While recent data implicate hypothalamic peptides and the pituitary and peripheral hormones as potentially important, newly recognized substances in the geneses of these psychiatric disorders associated with endocrine diseases, it appears appropriate at this writing to consider that their overt development is biochemically multifactorial and superimposed on a susceptible background of genetic predisposition or genetic propensity modulated by early experience and current environment.

DATA REVIEW

The remainder of this report will concentrate on calcium changes observed in psychiatric patients undergoing ECT.

Before discusssing CSF calcium changes, some attention to blood, urinary and total body alterations in calcium content is appropriate as background for approaching the CSF changes with better comprehension.

Studies from this laboratory have demonstrated small changes in total body calcium balance in small numbers of depressed hospitalized psychiatric patients (Faragalla and Flach, 1970; Flach, Liang and Stokes, 1960). In most of these patients serum and urinary calcium levels decreased after ECT (or antidepressant drug therapy), producing a net increase in calcium retention associated with improvement in depression. With the use of radiocalcium tracer techniques these studies demonstrated increased net gut absorption of calcium and decreased urinary calcium, correlating with clinical improvement after ECT. The increased retention of calcium associated with ECT was due to a markedly (20-40%) decreased bone resorption. In contrast, treatment with imipramine was associated with increased calcium retention associated with increased bone formation in three of four patients. No significant changes in calcium pool size were apparent. It is of interest that some years earlier Malm (1958), studying calcium metabolism in normal man, noted decreased calcium retention in two subjects during periods of "depression."

Changes in the blood and CSF concentration of calcium in animals and humans in association with ECT have been reported. The data however are often conflicting. Early studies (Eiduson, Brill and Crumpton, 1960; Henry and Ebeling, 1925; Katzenelbogen, 1935, 1938; Weston and Howard, 1922) found the concentrations of calcium, sodium and potassium in the CSF and blood of schizophrenic and manic depressive patients, as well as patients with personality disorders, to be within the range of that reported for hospitalized normals (Shaw and Wolley, 1951). A number of studies have reported a fall in blood calcium levels in heterogeneous populations of psychiatric patients after clinical improvement from "depression." Gour and Chaudhry (1957) found increased serum calcium (by as much as 2 mg/100ml) "immediately" after the first ECT in 15 hospitalized patients variously diagnosed as manic depressive, schizophrenic or melancholic. This post-ECT hypercalcemia slowly returned to normal within two to four hours after the shock. Serum calcium then fell below the pre-ECT levels to reach a nadir ten hours post-ECT and returned to pre-ECT levels 24 hours after shock. No statement was made as to whether the ECT was modified or given without either muscle relaxants or anesthesia. Furthermore, no mention was made of the time of day when ECT was given and no data in non-shocked patients were presented in order to control for diurnal or post-prandial variations in the reported post-ECT serum calcium levels. After a course of ten ECT, the resting serum calcium levels 48 hours after the last ECT were similar to those observed before therapy. The depressed group (melancholia) had the greatest serum calcium rise immediately after ECT and the lowest serum calcium levels ten hours post-ECT. These patients also showed the greatest clinical improvement after ECT, as might be expected, and the authors suggested that the degree of immediate hypercalcemia and subsequent fall in serum calcium could be used as a biological index of prognostic value regarding future response to a full course of ECT. This suggestion has not been tested in subsequent studies. The duration and degree of hypercalcemia observed are too great to be explained totally on the basis of ECT-induced altered permeability of the vascular capillary bed with resultant hemoconcentration. However this must be considered since no data on serum protein or osmoles were provided. Methodological problems with all of the above studies include lack of uniform clinical criteria for defining diagnostic groups and degree of improvement. Many of these studies were carried out prior to the now widely accepted operational criteria for categorization of patients and the use of validated rating scales.

In contrast to the sharp and rather marked serum calcium increases observed immediately after ECT in an earlier report (Gour and Chaudhry, 1957), discussed above, a recent study of serum calcium changes after each ECT in a single patient found no change in serum calcium as measured shortly after the initial ECTs (Carman and others, 1977). As the course of ECT continued, significant, apparently shortlived (90 minute) decreases in serum calcium occurred. These began to occur at the time of onset of clinical antidepressant effect of the course of ECT. The decreases were most marked at five minutes and persisted with gradual diminution for up to 90 minutes after each ECT. There were no changes in concentration of other serum ions measured simultaneously. A group of seven patients was studied on a different protocol by these same authors. All patients met Research Diagnostic Criteria for primary affective disorder (Spitzer, Endicott and Robins, 1975). Significant progressive post-ECT serum calcium decreases occurred in these seven patients during the course of ECT as measured in samples taken at 7 a.m., 2 1/2 hours prior to ECT (more than 24 hours post-ECT) but again these post-ECT changes did not occur until the ECT antidepressant effect had started. This longer term hypocalcemic response was also transient and one week after completing the course of ECT the serum had returned to or toward pre-ECT levels in all but one of the seven cases studied. While all seven cases revealed a decrease in a.m. resting serum calcium after the onset of an antidepressant effect of the ECT, some of these patients showed minimal changes and a few had rather marked decrements, thus weighting the mean serum calcium change.

Cisternal CSF calcium concentration has been reported to be elevated by 23% ($p < .01$) one hour after an initial ECT and to again be elevated when sampled one hour after two or three subsequent ECT (Essman, 1973). An extensive study of the effects of ECT on human CSF concentrations of calcium, sodium, potassium and protein in 66 male chronic schizophrenics and 30 male patients with schizoaffective or depressive disorders confirmed the normal ranges of concentration of these substances (Eiduson, Brill and Crumpton, 1960), as reported in earlier studies of inpatients with functional psychiatric disorders prior to ECT. This study also found no change in concentration or shift in the CSF distribution of concentrations of these cations two weeks or one month after a course of 20 ECT. It was observed that those patients who improved with ECT had lower CSF calcium values before the course of ECT than those patients who did not improve. However, as noted by these authors, it is possible that the difference in initial CSF calcium values could have occurred by chance alone, in view of the twenty biochemical variables analyzed statistically. An important conclusion of these data was that clinical improvement following ECT was not associated with a significant change in group mean values or the range of distribution of levels of these CSF cations when measurements were made two and four weeks after completing a course of ECT. No mention was made of the direction of change, if any, in calcium levels in individual cases pre to post-ECT

Recently CSF calcium levels were reported to be within the range of normal in 21 endogenous depressed patients and not significantly changed by a course of drug therapy or modified ECT (Bjorum, Plenge and Rafaelsen, 1972). Blood calcium was reported by this same group to show "minute changes with a trend" toward decreased serum calcium after recovery from depression. No data on blood or CSF calcium levels immediately before and after individual ECTs were provided. No significant differences in a.m. resting serum calcium levels in "retarded" versus "nonretarded" depressives were noted. However methological difficulties, including the technique of storage of calcium samples and a lack of description of exactly when the CSF samples were obtained in relation to time of ECT, limit the interpretations that can be made from this report. Earlier studies had reported no change from pre-ECT levels in CSF calcium two and four weeks after a course of ECT in schizophrenic patients (Eiduson, Brill and Crumpton, 1969), or after metrazol induced convulsions (Katzenelbogen and colleagues, 1939) or in patients with epileptic seizures (Ueno and others, 1961). In light of the above reports is interesting that a well designed study (Carman and co-workers, 1977) did find CSF calcium changes in association with the antidepressant effect of ECT in a small number of carefully diagnosed, depressed patients. These patients were studied under controlled conditions while off other drugs. These authors report that CSF calcium in the six cases of depression studied all showed a decrease one hour after the last ECT (average number of ECT: 4.2) as compared to pre-ECT calcium ($p<.05$). Inspection of the individual data reveals that one patient contributed very remarkably to the observed mean decrease in CSF calcium post-ECT and two others had very minimal changes. It is of further note that in four patients who remained improved and drug free these acute post-ECT CSF calcium levels remained below pre-ECT values even two weeks after completion of the course of ECT. No significant changes in CSF protein or magnesium were observed, suggesting a relative specificity of the effect of ECT on CSF calcium level.

There is at present no evident explanation for the conflicting serum and CSF changes noted in the different studies reviewed above, other than the unsatisfactory caveat that noncomparable experimental protocols and patient populations may be responsible for these different results.

MECHANISMS ACCOUNTING FOR OBSERVED CHANGES IN CALCIUM METABOLISM

The mechanisms of these changes in calcium metabolism are not clear at this time but probably are multiple. Possible factors are alterations in parathyroid hormone and calcitonin and the effects of hyperactivity of the hypothalamic pituitary adrenocortical (HPAC) system often observed in depression (Stokes, 1972). Other hormonal factors may also be important, including vitamin D metabolism, growth hormone and thyroid hormone. Conceivably changes in calcium levels in some depressed patients could be related to markedly decreased physical activity.

Previous work from this medical center demonstrated hypercalcemia and negative calcium balance in normal men encased in total body casts (Deitrick, Whedon and Shorr, 1949). These abnormalities were reversed by passive mobilization on an oscillating bed (Whedon, Deitrick and Shorr, 1948). However later work by this same group was not able to reverse the hypercalciuria of poliomyelitis patients by passive ambulation (oscillating bed) or by various degrees of active ambulation (Whedon and Shorr, 1957). In another series of studies from this center it was shown that ambulatory patients with bulbar poliomyelitis developed hypercalciuria while patients with spinal poliomyelitis did not (Dunning and Plum, 1962; Plum and Dunning, 1958). These data taken together all argue against decreased activity (Deitrick, Whedon and Shorr, 1948) as a complete explanation for the negative calcium balance and relative hypercalciuria described in depressed patients. It has also been pointed out that in tuberculosis without bone involvement renal calculi develope commonly only in those patients with meningeal and CNS tuberculosis (Dunning and Plum, 1962). Thus it would appear that it is reasonable to look for some disturbance in CNS function and to a resultant brain mediated humeral or neurohumeral role in the disturbed calcium metabolism of depression, as originally suggested for the hypercalciuria and demineralization associated with poliomyelitis (Dunning and Plum, 1962).

Brain (hypothalamic) control of HPAC activity is well documented (Joseph and Knigge, 1976), and it is well established that hypercortisolemia occurs in a majority of patients with severe depressive illness (Stokes, 1972), especially those with the endogenomorphic type of depression (Carroll, 1976). It is notable that the calcium balance and serum calcium changes noted above, as well as the CSF changes, all occurred in association with clinical improvement, a time when the hypercortisolemia of depression also subsides. Furthermore ECT itself has been demonstrated to induce pronounced transient changes in plasma cortisol (Stokes, 1972) and ACTH (Allen and colleagues, 1974; Stokes, unpublished). Hypercalcemia from causes other than hyperparathyrodism, e.g. sarcoidosis, vitamin D intoxication and cancer, is diminished or abolished by administration of cortisone in animals and in humans (Harrison and Harrison, 1960). It has been demonstrated in cortisone treated rats that their decreased intestinal active calcium transport will not be returned to normal levels even by the administration of 1,25-dihydroxycholecaliferol, the final active metabolite of vitamin D (Favus, Walling and Kimbere, 1973). This evidence and the fact that intestinal mucosal calcium binding protein and 1,25-dihydroxycholecalciferol levels were normal in cortisone treated rats support the proposal that glucocorticoids apparently decrease intestinal calcium absorption by inducing alterations in the intestinal mucosal cell, making the calcium transport system relatively unresponsive to vitamin D. Many studies with balance and radiocalcium techniques demonstrate decreased calcium absorption in man after treatment with glucocortoid (Bunim and co-workers, 1958; Gallagher and colleagues, 1973; Slater and others, 1959). It is now generally accepted that hypercortisolemia contributes to negative calcium balance via the inhibitory effect of cortisol on vitamin D induced gut absorption of calcium (Harrison and Harrison, 1960). Massive doses of vitamin D can increase calcium absorption in glucocorticoid treated humans (Gallagher and co-workers, 1973). Increased calcium excretion via the kidney is also associated with glucocorticoid administration and occurs in Cushings syndrome (Edwards and Hodgkinson, 1965; Molinatti, Camanni and Olivetti, 1960; Pechet, Bowers and Bartter, 1959). The hypercalciuria may result from a glucocorticoid effect on the renal tubule similar to that on the intestinal mucosal cell.

Obviously calcium metabolism and extracellular fluid calcium levels are importantly influenced by parathyroid hormone (PTH) and calcitonin (CT). PTH has been shown to increase intestinal calcium absorption in man and requires vitamin D for this action (Dowdle, Schachter and Schenker, 1960; Wills and co-workers, 1972).

One must also consider the role of diurnal variation in serum (and CSF) calcium values in assessing calcium changes post-ECT or during recovery from depression. In general most recent investigators have found a diurnal variation in urinary calcium excretion with a trough in the late evening hours and peak excretion in the late morning in fasting subjects or in those on a normal calcium intake of evenly spaced meals (Min, Jones and Flink, 1966). The mechanism for this cyclical variation in urinary excretion of calcium is not clear but may be related to diurnal alterations in glomerular filtration rate associated with the diurnal rhythm of plasma cortisol (Doe, Vennes and Flink, 1960). Data regarding diurnal plasma calcium variation is scant, but fluctuations in dietary intake can influence serum calcium levels and urinary excretion. The position of the fasting human subject (supine or standing) may also alter serum calcium concentrations by as much as five to ten percent (Husdan, Rapoport and Locke, 1973).

In view of the extreme complexity of control of calcium metabolism it is not possible at this time to contruct a unifying suggestion for the causes of calcium change reported following ECT or in association with recovery from depression.

Some interesting suggestions have been made as to the possible role of PTH and CT on the observed decrease in serum and CSF calcium (Carman and colleagues, 1977; Gerner and others, 1977). CT causes lowered serum calcium (Roycroft and Talmadge, 1973) similar in degree and time course to that reported after the onset of improvement in ECT for depression (Carman and co-workers, 1977) and induces changes in bone metabolism similar to that observed in depressed patients after successful antidepressant treatment (Faragalla and Flach, 1970). Measurement of serum PTH in one case immediately following ECT showed a modest increase in PTH during a concomitant sudden small decrease in total plasma calcium. CT was not measured but it was suggested that repetitive bursts of CT after each ECT (if they occur) may gradually inhibit renal synthesis of 1,25-dihydroxycholecalciferol and thus diminish serum and CSF calcium after the cumulative effects of a series of ECT. It is of further interest that lithium, a known inhibitor of brain adenyl cyclase, can inhibit the expected hypercalcemia of infused PTH, although in drug free subjects no change in affect occurred during these infusions (Gerner and colleagues, 1977). The therapeutic effect of lithium may be related, at least in part, to its ability to stabilize and slightly elevate (at least acutely) calcium levels in patients and animals (Andreoli, Villani and Brambilla, 1972; Mellerup and others, 1970; Tupin and co-workers, 1968).

CONCLUSION

It is apparent that in subsequent studies careful attention must be given to patient selection with proper emphasis on an operational approach to diagnostic categorization. Only by this technique can sufficient clinical homogeneity of subjects be obtained. The design of the study must allow for control of calcium changes in blood and CSF that might result from variables other than ECT, such as diet, diurnal variation of calcium level, and the influence of other drugs, hormones or endocrine disease. More data are needed under these controlled conditions regarding serum and CSF calcium changes in relation to the pretreatment diagnosis and behavioral state, the immediate and late effects of ECT and the relationship, if any, of state changes (i.e., recovery from depression) to calcium levels. Treatment modalities must be carefully controlled and described as to method, dosage, duration, etc. Until careful replications of reports of ECT induced changes in calcium metabolism occur, it will be premature to try to specify underlying mechanisms of action.

REFERENCES

Allen, J.P., D. Denny, J.W. Kendall and P.H. Blachly (1974). Corticotrophin release during ECT in man. Am. J. Psychiat., 131, 1225-1228.

Andreoli, V.M., F. Villani and G. Brambilla (1972). Increased calcium and magnesium excretion induced by lithium carbonate. Psychopharmacologia, 25, 77-85.

Bjorum, N., P. Plenge and O.J. Rafaelsen (1972). Electrolytes in cerebrospinal fluid in endogenous depression. Acta psychiat. neurol. scand., 48, 533-539.

Bradbury, M.W.B., C.R. Kleeman, H. Bagdoyan and A. Berberian (1968). The calcium and magnesium content of skeletal muscle, brain, and cerebrospinal fluid as determined by atomic absorption flame photometry. J. Lab. clin. Med., 7, 884-892.

Bunim, J.J., R.L. Black, L. Lutwak, R.C. Peterson and G.D. Whedon (1958). Studies on dexamethasone: a new synthetic steroid in rheumatoid arthritis. A preliminary report. Arthritis Rheum., 1, 313-331.

Carman, J.S., R.M. Post, F.K. Goodwin and W.E. Bunney (1977). Calcium and electroconvulsive therapy of severe depressive illness. Biol. Psychiat., 12, 5-17.

Carroll, B.J. (1976). Limbic system-adrenal cortex regulation in depression and schizophrenia. Psychosom. Med., 38, 106-121.

Cochran, M., M. Peacock, G. Sachs and B.E.C. Nordin (1970). Renal effects of calcitonin. Br. med. J., 1, 135-137.

Deftos, L.J., D. Burton, B.D. Catherwood, H.G. Bone, J.G. Parthemore, R. Guillemin, W. Watkins and R.Y. Moore (1978). Demonstration by immunoperoxidase histochemistry of calcitonin in the anterior lobe of the rat pituitary. J. clin. Endocr. Metab., 47, 457-460.

Deitrick, J.E., G.D. Whedon and E. Shorr (1948). Effects of immobilization upon

various metabolic and physiologic functions of normal men. Am. J. Med., 4, 3-36.
Doe, R.P., J.A. Vennes and M.D. Flink (1960). Diurnal variation of 17-hydroxycorticosteroids, sodium, potassium, magnesium and creatinine in normal subjects and in cases of treated adrenal insufficiency and Cushing's syndrome. J. clin. Endocr. Metab., 20, 253-265.
Dowdle, E.B., D. Schachter and H. Schenker (1960). Requirement for vitamin D for the active transport of calcium by the intestine. Am. J. Physiol., 198, 269-274.
Dunning, M.F. and F. Plum (1962). Hypercalciuria following poliomyelitis. Archs int. Med., 99, 716-731.
Edwards, A.N. and A. Hodgkinson (1965). Metabolic studies in patients with idiopathic hypercalciuria. Clin. Sci., 29, 143-154.
Eiduson, S., N.Q. Brill and E. Crumpton (1960). The effect of electro-convulsive therapy on spinal fluid constituents. J. ment. Sci., 106, 692-698.
Essman, W.B. (1973). Neurochemistry of Cerebral Electroshock. Halsted Press, New York. Chap. 4, pp. 23-31.
Faragalla, F.F. and F.F. Flach (1970). Studies of mineral metabolism in mental depression. J. nerv. ment. Dis., 151, 120-129.
Favus, M.J., M.W. Walling and D.V. Kimbere (1973). Effects of 1,25 dihydroxycholecalciferol on intestinal calcium transport in cortisone-treated rats. J. clin. Invest., 52, 1680-1685.
Flach, F.F., E. Liang and P.E. Stokes (1960). The effect of electric convulsive treatments on nitrogen, calcium, and phosphorus metabolism in psychiatric patients. J. ment. Sci., 106, 638-647.
Gallagher, J.C., J. Aaron, A. Horsman, R. Wilkinson and B.E.C. Nordin (1973). Corticosteroid osteoporosis. In B.E.C. Nordin (Ed.), Clinics in Endocrinology and Metabolism. Osteoporosis, Vol. 2(2). Saunders, London. pp. 355-368.
Gerner, R.H., R.M. Post, A.M. Spiegel and D.L. Murphy (1977). Effects of parathormone and lithium treatment on calcium and mood in depressed patients. Biol. Psychiat., 12, 145-151.
Gour, K.N. and Chaudhry (1957). Study of calcium metabolism in electric convulsive therapy (E.C.T.) in certain mental diseases. J. ment. Sci., 103, 275-285.
Graziani, L., A. Escriva and R. Katzman (1965). Exchange of calcium between blood, brain, and cerebrospinal fluid. Am. J. Physiol., 208, 1058-1064.
Gudmundsson, T.V., I. MacIntyre and H.A. Soliman (1966). The isolation of thyrocalcitonin and a study of its effects in the rat. Proc. R. Soc., Series B, 164, 460-477.
Harrison, H.E. and H.C. Harrison (1960). Transfer of ^{45}Ca across intestinal wall in vitro in relation to action of vitamin D and cortisol. Am. J. Physiol., 199, 265-271.
Henry, G.W. and W.E. Ebeling (1925). Blood calcium and phosphorus in the personality disorders. Archs Neurol. Psychiat., Chicago, 16, 48-54.
Horwith, M. and P.E. Stokes (1960). Cushing's syndrome: experience with total adrenalectomy. Advances in Internal Medicine, Vol. 10. Yearbook Medical Publishers, New York. pp. 259-295.
Husdan, H., A. Rapoport and S. Locke (1973). Influence of posture on the serum concentration of calcium. Metabolism, 22, 787-797.
Isaac, R., R.E. Merceron, G. Caillens, J.P. Raymond and R. Andraillou (1978). Effect of parathyroid hormone on plasma prolactin in man. J. clin. Endocr. Metab., 47, 18-23.
Joseph, S.A. and K.M. Knigge (1976). The endocrine hypothalamus: recent anatomical studies. In S. Reichlin, R.J. Baldessarini and J.B. Martin (Eds.), The Hypothalamus. Raven Press, New York. pp. 15-47.
Katzenelbogen, S. (1935). The Cerebrospinal Fluid and its Relation to Blood. Johns Hopkins Press, Baltimore.
Katzenelbogen, S., M.W. Brody, M. Hayman and E. Margolin (1939). Metrazol convulsions in man. Am. J. Psychiat., 95, 1343-1348.
Komendantova, M.V., A.I. Briskin, A.G. Bakunyaeva and G.P. Milogradova (1973). Influence of thyrocalcitonin on conditional reflexes and the cerebral electrical

Krepke, D.F., P. Lauie, D. Parker, L. Huey and L.J. Deftos (1978). Plasma parathyroid hormone and calcium are related to sleep stage cycles. J. clin. Endocr. Metab., 47, 1021-1027.

Malm, O.J. (1958). Calcium requirements and absorption adaptation in adult men. Scand. J. clin. Lab. Invest. (Suppl. 36), 10, 1-290.

Mellerup, E.T., P. Plenge, R. Ziegler and O.J. Rafaelsen (1970). Lithium effects on calcium metabolism in rats. Int. Pharmacopsychiat., 5, 258-264.

Min, H.K., J.E. Jones and E.B. Flink (1966). Circadian variations in renal excretion of magnesium, calcium, phosphorus, sodium and potassium-during frequent feeding and fasting. Fedn Proc. Fedn Am. Socs exp. Biol., 25, 917-921.

Molinatti, G.M., F. Camanni and M. Olivetti (1960). A study on the metabolism of calcium in the hyperadrenocortical syndrome. Acta endocr., Copnh., 34, 323-334.

Pechet, M.M., B. Bowers and F.C. Bartter (1959). Metabolic studies with a new series of 1,4-diene steroids. Effects on normal subjects of prednisone, prednisolone and 9-fluoroprednisolone. J. clin. Invest., 38, 681-690.

Plum, F. and F. Dunning (1958). The effects of therapeutic mobilization on hypercalciuria following acute poliomyelitis. Archs int. Med., 101, 528-536.

Posner, J.B., F. Plum and A.V. Van Posnak (1969). Cerebral metabolism during electrically induced seizures in man. Archs Neurol., Chicago, 20, 388-395.

Roycroft, J. and R.V. Talmadge (1973). Changes due to age in the hypocalcemic and hypophosphatemic effects of salmon calcitonin in growing rats. Proc. Soc. exp. Biol. Med., 144, 17-21.

Shaw, C.W. and H.L. Wolley (1951). Sodium and potassium concentration in human cerebrospinal fluid. J. Lab. clin. Med., 38, 574-576.

Sholberg, H.L. and E. Goodall (1926). The phosphorus and calcium content of the blood-plasma and cerebro-spinal fluid in the psychoses. J. ment. Sci., 72, 51-58.

Slater, J.D.H., P.E. Heffron, A. Vernet and J.D.N. Nabarro (1959). Clinical and metabolic effects of dexamethasone. Lancet, i, 173-177.

Spanos, E.K., K.W. Colston, I.M.S. Evans, L.S. Galante, S.J. Macauley and I. MacIntyre (1976). Effect of prolactin on vitamin D metabolism. Molec. cell. Endocr., 5, 163-167.

Spitzer, R.L., J. Endicott and E. Robins (1975). Clinical criteria for psychiatric diagnosis and DSM-III. Am. J. Psychiat., 132, 1187-1192.

Stokes, P.E. (1972). Studies on the control of adrenocortical function in depression. In T.A. Williams, M.M. Katz and J.A. Shields (Eds.), Recent Advances in the Psychobiology of the Depressive Illnesses. U.S. Government Printing Office, DHEW Publication No. (HSM) 70-9053, Washington, D.C. pp. 199-220.

Tupin, J.P., G.K. Schlagenhauf and D.L. Creson (1968). Lithium effects on electrolyte excretion. Am. J. Psychiat., 125, 536-543.

Ueno, Y., N. Aoki, T. Yabuki and F. Kuraishi (1961). Electrolyte metabolism in blood and cerebrospinal fluid in psychoses. Folia psychiat. neurol. Jap., 15, 536-543.

Wallach, S., J.V. Bellavia, J. Schorr and D.L. Reizenstein (1964). Tissue distribution of electrolytes, Ca^{47}, and Mg^{28} in acute hypercalcemia. Am. J. Physiol., 207, 553-560.

Weston, P.G. and M.Q. Howard (1922). The determination of sodium, potassium, calcium and magnesium in the blood of patients suffering from manic-depressive insanity. Archs Neurol. Psychiat., Chicago, 8, 179-183.

Whedon, G.D., J.E. Deitrick and E. Shorr (1949). Modification of the effects of immobilization upon metabolic and physiologic functions of normal men by the use of an oscillating bed. Am. J. Med., 6, 684-711.

Whedon, G.D. and E. Shorr (1957). Metabolic studies in paralytic acute anterior poliomyelitis. J. clin. Invest., 36, 941-965.

Whybrow, P.C. and T. Hurwitz (1976). Psychological disturbances associated with endocrine disease and hormone therapy. In E.J. Sachar (Ed.), Hormones, Behavior and Psychopathology. Raven Press, New York. pp. 125-143.

Wills, M.R., J.B. Phillips, R.C. Day and E.C. Bateman (1972). Phytic acid and nutritional rickets in immigrants. Lancet, i, 771-773.

Convulsive Therapy in Depression: A Neurohumoral and Neuroendocrine Theory

MAX FINK

Department of Psychiatry and Behavioral Science, School of Medicine, SUNY at Stony Brook, Stony Brook, New York

Aided, in part, by the International Association for Psychiatric Research, Inc.

Much has been learned about the convulsive therapy process since its introduction forty years ago. While early theories focussed on the psychologic factors of stress, punishment, amnesia, and psychologic defenses, on the neurophysiologic aspects of seizures, or on peripheral events, recent theories emphasize the biochemical changes in the central nervous system.* With an increase in the usage of convulsive therapy and improvements in treatment methods, the aspects of the treatment process which are essential to a good therapeutic outcome have been defined, allowing its mode of action to be understood in the same framework as the effects of drugs on the CNS.

Essential features of ECT.

Since its introduction in 1935, many types of mentally ill and many modifications of the treatment process have been examined. Convulsive therapy has three behavioral effects: antidepressant, antipsychotic, and antimanic. Of these, the antidepressant is best defined. Convulsive therapy is specific for psychotic (primary) depression, relieving this syndrome after four to eight inductions. Seizures in the brain, best defined by characteristic EEG patterns of at least 20 seconds duration are essential; while convulsions of the body musculature, anoxemia, or peripheral biochemical events contribute little to therapeutic efficacy. Seizure inductions must be spaced, and only occasionally are a series of seizures in one sitting or one day sufficient for a clinical antidepressant effect. Clinical efficacy is not related to the mode of

---

* The citations for this summary are extensive and will not be cited in the text. Interested readers are referred to some recent reviews listed in the references.

seizure induction, with an equivalence for electrical and chemical inductions; nor is efficacy enhanced or hindered by anesthesia, muscle relaxation or paralysis, anticholinergic drugs, or hyperoxygenation, although these procedures may reduce some of the unpleasant consequences of the treatments.

The effects of repeated seizures are additive --- with the biochemical events persisting for minutes after the first seizure and for progressively longer periods with more seizures, so that some measures remain altered for days after a series of four to eight seizures.

The principal effects on behavior are seen in patients with severe depressive mood. But efficacy is enhanced if the symptoms of hypothalamic dysfunction --- insomnia, anorexia, weight loss, reduced secretions, loss of libido --- are prominent. While antipsychotic and antimanic effects are observed, these require more seizures, more frequently induced, with a specificity that is much less.

Biochemical effects.

When convulsive therapy was introduced, the effects of insulin on brain function were just being recognized, and the first theories emphasized the effects of the 'shock therapies' on hypothalamic functions. As the applications and the theories of ECT became focussed on other systems, ECT was seen to increase the permeability of the blood-brain barrier, and to alter the metabolism of some minerals, notable calcium.

Neurohumoral effects are profound. The early studies were indirect, inferring from the effects of intravenous epinephrine and subcutaneous methacholine on blood pressure that the responsivity to these neurohumoral stimulants was reduced in depression and reversed by ECT. Plasma levels of norepinephrine and epinephrine were elevated by ECT. Turnover and synthesis of serotonin, norepinephrine, epinephrine, and dopamine increased; and both spinal fluid and brain levels of these neurohumors increased with treatment. These changes were accompanied by increases in tyrosine hydroxylase and monamine oxidase. But the significance of these findings is unclear, considering that barbiturate anesthesia inhibited them.

Recent studies find that serotonin, 5-HIAA, and typtrophan increase with ECS, suggesting that the turnover of 5-HT is increased. They also find a sustained increase in the activity of noradrenergic neurons (but not those which are dopaminergic or serotonininergic); and increased post-synaptic sensitivity to dopamine and serotonin. Human studies, however, are less secure, with various authors finding some changes in serotonin and dopamine turnover. Increases are also reported in brain and CSF acetylcholine, and plasma and CSF cholinesterase. These changes are blocked by anticholinergic drugs.

Neuroendocrine effects are also extensive. While the adrenals liberate steroids and blood levels of 17-hydroxycorticosteroid are elevated with ECT, the successful treatment of a patient without adrenals suggested that these changes were secondary. After ECT, pituitary and hypothalamic functions are enhanced. ACTH is liberated, but its direct administration to depressed patients fails to elicit a behavioral improvement. Plasma prolactin, serum growth hormone and glucose, and CSF endorphin levels increase with ECT, and in males, so do serum levels of FSH and LH.

Other evidence of the effects on hypothalamic and pituitary functions can be inferred from studies of these systems in patients with depression. The normal response of the pituitary and hypothalamus to various stressors is reduced in depression and enhanced after recovery. Thus, GH response to hypoglycemia and to *l*-Dopa is reduced in depression and returns to normal with ECT; as do the TSH response to TRH and the suppression of cortisol excretion by dexamethasone.

A Theory of ECT

From these data we can derive a testable theory of the mode of action of convulsive therapy. Hypothalamic activity is altered by induced convulsions both by direct stimulation of hypothalamic cells and by increasing the functional neurotransmitter activity levels in the brain; thereby releasing substances, most probably peptide hormones, which affect the vegetative functions of the body and the endocrine glands. Specific substances are released which modify mood and the behaviors associated with mood disturbances. The biochemical events which precede and accompany the seizure are the trigger for increased neurohumoral activity.

But since the efficacy of ECT is not dependent on the mode of induction, we would add that in ECT, the direct stimulation of the electric currents augment, but are not necessary for, the changes in hypothalamic functions.

For depression, we can infer that hypothalamic dysfunction, most probably hypofunction, with a failure to release mood regulating peptides in adequate amounts is the near-final pathway in endogenous depression. From this inference, I anticipate that the replacement of ECT by the direct administration of mood modifying peptides is probable within the next few years. The observations that such peptides as TRH, FK 33-584, des-tyr-γ-endorphin, and β-endorphin affect mood and thought processes encourage this conclusion.

There is much evidence to support such a theory. Vegetative systems are disturbed in patients with depressive psychoses, and return to normal levels with treatment. The modulating centers for the vegetative functions of sleep, feeding, reproduction, temperature regulation are located in brain stem and hypothalamus and it is here that seizures seem to have their most direct and most lasting effects.

Seizure induction is necessary for a therapeutic result. Seizures must be bilateral and generalized in the brain. The principal site from which such diffuse effects in the brain can be derived is the brain stem. Following successful convulsive therapy, regardless of the mode of induction (chemical or electrical; unilateral or bilateral electrodes) we find persistent symmetric, bilateral EEG slow waves, derived most probably from brain stem loci.

The abnormal neuroendocrine functions of depressed patients revert to normal with convulsive therapy. Similarly, the measures of neurohumor modifiers (norepinephrine, acetylcholine, serotonin) show these to be reduced in depression and enhanced after ECT. While these data are fragmentary, the findings in the studies of the effects of ECT parallel those reported in studies with the tricyclic antidepressants. From this view, convulsive therapy is seen as a special case in pharmacotherapy.

Other changes induced by ECT are consistent with this hypothesis. The increased permeability of the blood brain barrier allows substances, including peptides, to diffuse more readily to remote nervous centers. The reduction in plasma and CSF calcium suggests that intracellular calcium is increased-- a necessary step in the liberation of hormonal substances from endocrine glands.

Conclusion

The present theory finds convulsive therapy to be a special case in pharmacotherapy, acting throught the increased liberation of hypothalamic peptides which are the regulators of mood and other vegetative systems of the body. Increases in the turnover of neruohumors, in the permeability of the blood brain barrier, and in the intracellular incorporation of calcium are supporting processes.

Recent theories of ECT suggest that hypothalamic dysfunction is the core process in endogenous depression, and that this syndrome is distinct in its pathophysiology from neurotic (anxious) depression. The studies also indicate that the pathophysiology of catatonia, particularly the varieties labelled 'pernicious', or secondary to toxic or infectious causes, may have features similar to that of endogenous depression.

References

Fink, M.: Efficacy and safety of induced seizures (EST) in man. Comprehens. Psychiat. 19: 1-18, 1978.

Fink, M.: Convulsive Therapy: Theory and Practice. New York, Raven Press, 1979.

Fink, M., Kety, S., McGaugh, J. and Williams, T. (Eds.): Psychobiology of Convulsive Therapy. Washington, D.C., V.H. Winston & Sons, 312 pp., 1974.

Frankel, F. (Ed.): Report of the Task Force on Convulsive Therapy. Washington, D.C., American Psychiatric Association, 1978.

Genetic Aspects of Psychopharmacology

The HLA System and the Celinical Response to Treatment with Haloperidol

C. L. CAZZULLO, E. SMERALDI, L. BELLODI, F. NEGRI and P. BONARA*

Institute of Clinical Psychiatry, University of Milano Medical School
*Institute of Internal Medicine IV, Laboratory of Cellular Immunology

ABSTRACT

In a previous work we found a highly significant positive correlation between clinical responsiveness to chlorpromazine and some HLA alleles, more precisely A 1. We also reported that the products of this HLA allele and related cross-reacting alleles (A 1 CRAG antigens) are able to bind the drug on the cell membrane. Since haloperidol also shows this in vitro property, in the present study we tested whether or not the clinical response to haloperidol is related in the schizophrenic patients to the presence or absence of the antigens able to interact with the drug in vitro.
In a group of 16 patients divided according to the CRAG A 1 positive or negative typing, clinical responses to haloperidol were quantitatively evaluated after 5 mg/day and 10 mg/day treatment. The scores of positive subjects were significantly lower after treatment, indicating that they responded to a greater degree, at least for psychotic hostility, hyperactivity and formal thought disorders. The implications of these data are briefly discussed.

INTRODUCTION

Many factors have already been shown to influence in different ways the clinical effects of psychotropic drugs, so that we can assume that there will be great person-to-person differences in response to treatment. To arrive at insights which will predict drug response we must study and better understand this heterogeneity, which at the moment decreases the sensitivity of our clinical observations and which obscures, without explaining the psychotropic effects of the drugs (ref. 1). Differences in individual pharmacokinetics, as one source of individual differences in responsiveness to drug treatment have been extensively studied so far. However, in this field, conflicting results have been reported as to the pharmacokinetics of neuroleptics.

In this paper we are going to discuss data about a possible role of the membrane structures controlled by the HLA genetic system in the generation of this variability. For a good review of the HLA system see ref. 2. Some of our studies have suggested that some A-locus membrane structures, more precisely the HLA-A 1 antigen and, to a lesser extent some other specificities (CRAG A 1 antigens) cross-reacting with it i.e., A 3, A 10 and A 11 are able to bind several psychotropic drugs and neurotransmitters (ref. 3,4). This was demonstrated by the fact that specific anti-HLA antisera could no longer be absorbed into cells carrying CRAG A 1 antigens after preincubation with some psychotropic drugs, as shown by a lesser or absent decreases in cytotoxic titres than when the antisera were absorbed with untreated cells. In other words, it seems that of the 18 possibilities on the cell membrane surface, depending on the allelic constitution of the A locus of the subject, only these four antigens are able to bind the psychotropic drugs so-far tested, - chlorpromazine haloperidol sulpiride - with different affinities for different molecules (ref. 4). Nevertheless, the specificity of the binding we observed is suggested by the drug concentrations at which the interference can be observed and, more important, by the fact that no interaction was demonstrated between the same drugs and antigens other than CRAG A 1, even with specificities present on the same cell membranes (ref. 5).

Thus previous investigation on the psychotropic effects of chlorpromazine (CPZ) seems to support the idea that HLA molecules may be involved in the individual differences in response to psychotropic drugs. Two facts must be stressed:

1) in mice, the major one of the two loci controlling the sensitivity to CPZ is in the H 2 chromosomal region, which is analogous to the human HLA one (ref. 6). This locus is considered to exist in two allelic forms: the one related to a high sensitivity to CPZ should correspond, at least from a pharmacological point of view, to the allele A 1 at the locus HLA-A in humans;
2) A 1 positive schizophrenic subjects seem to have a better clinical response to CPZ treatment than do A 1 negative ones (ref. 7).

However, before accepting that this kind of investigation will be valuable for predicting the clinical response to drug, we had first to exclude the possibility that the results obtained were due merely to chance. To rule out this possibility, we tested whether or not the clinical response to haloperidol which binds <u>in vitro</u> to cells with A 10 and A 11 antigens (ref. 4), would differ in its effects in psychiatric patients according to the presence or absence of these antigens.

MATERIALS AND METHODS

We studied 16 chronic schizophrenic patients (11 males and 5 females), all with more than 10 years of illness. These patients were selected from those hospitalized in the Psychiatric Hospital of our country. All patients consented to take part in the study and were free to withdraw at any time. The criteria adopted for the diagnosis of chronic Schizophrenia are reported elsewere (ref. 8) and are largely the same as those of Woodruff et al. (ref. 9).

At the beginning of our study, none of our patients had taken any drug for at least three weeks. They were then given haloperidol 5 mg/day for two weeks and then 10 mg/day for two weeks, and no other medications. The psychopathological patterns in our sample were evaluated by two independent psychiatrists, using the Comprehensive Psychopathological Rating Scale (ref. 10); three times for each subject, before treatment, two weeks after the beginning of the study and at the end of it.

The typing of the patients according to HLA system, performed independent of and without knowledge the clinical analysis, by the usual techniques in our laboratory, led us to classify the patients into CRAG A 1 positive subjects (8 subjects) and CRAG A 1 negatives ones (8 subjects). For each subject, the scores for each item were combined according to symptomatological clusters and a log transformation was submitted to analysis of variance according to a mixed factorial design, in order to statistically evaluate the differences in psychopathological patterns between the group with A 1 CRAG antigens and without, the effect of treatment and dose on the symptoms of the combined subjects, and the interactions between HLA typing and responses to treatment or to dose.

RESULTS

The results obtained in the statistical analysis are reported in the table. In this table, the values of the left hand column under "Fisher indices" refer to the effect of the presence or absence of the CRAG A 1 antigens on the psychopathological patterns of the patients. None of the symptoms we considered was significantly different in the two groups, so our patients can be considered to be fairly homogeneous from a symptomatological point of view.

Since we are considering the differences in the individual responses to haloperidol, first of all we must be certain that our patients improved after treatment. The effects of treatment in our sample were shown in the second column under indices of significance. There was a significant improvement ($p < 0.01$) in autism, psychotic hostility, hallucinations, formal thought disorders (mainly non-dissociative ones) and changes in ego reality. Nevertheless, against our expectations, in this study delusions did not seem to significantly decrease with treatment. Perhaps this odd result may be explained by the fact that our schizophrenic patients are severely chronic and characterized by very long histories of hospitalization. Their delusional systems, when present, are very firmly structured and unlikely to respond easily and appreciably to treatment lasting only one month.

The third source of variation analyzed was the effect of two different doses of haloperidol (5 mg vs. 10 mg). No significant

TABLE Comparison of clinical responses to haloperidol in A 1 CRAG positive and negative patients. Analysis of variance according to a mixed factorial design.

Symptoms	Sources of variation: Fisher's Indices				
	Effect of group A1+vs.A1-	Effect of treatment	Effect of dose	Interaction group x treatment	Interaction group x dose
Flatness of affect	.6	3.63	.05	0.	3.17
Autism	.34	11.98**	.01	1.62	.48
Changes of ego reality	.01	9.32**	1.41	.09	.12
Reduced psychomotor activity	.37	.13	.08	1.07	.15
Hyperactivity	2.93	1.71	.01	3.96	4.64*
Psychotic hostility	.01	49.17**	.35	16.35**	3.39
Hallucinations	.64	9.47**	.05	.95	.15
Delusions	2.5	2.01	.26	0.	1.52
Thought disord.	.78	15.52**	.01	.95	9.70**
dissociative	1.26	6.45*	0.	.70	.55
non dissocia.	.16	14.06**	1.13	.27	10.99**
Anxiety	1.77	.41	.36	.01	.90

* $p < 0.05$
** $p < 0.01$

differences in any cluster of symptoms considered were observed. The failure to demonstrate any dose effect might be due to the fact that we considered only the doses, of the drug, while the plasma drug levels would be a more precise index of concentrations at the receptor sites, or, more probably to the fact that even the minor dose adopted (5 mg/day) has a good clinical effect, at least in the italian psychiatric population and therefore is often the full dosage of haloperidol given in common psychiatric practice.

Finally, we considered the differences between responses to treatment and to dose, respectively, with our schizophrenic subjects divided according to the presence or absence of A 1 CRAG antigens. These differences were evaluated from the indices of the interactions reported in the last two columns of the table. For hostility which is a good index of individual psychotic condition, we observed that A 1 CRAG positive subjects showed greater improvement than A 1 CRAG negative patients did. This was observed during the first period of treatment as well as in the following two weeks of therapy (10 mg/day), but with a significant interaction only for group x treatment, not for group x dose.

The two groups of patients had, on the contrary, different clinical responses to each period of treatment when hyperactivity and formal thought disorders were taken into account. In fact, only A 1 CRAG positive patients displayed a decrease in the first item during the second period of treatment, whereas neither groups improved significantly during the first period of the treatment. As for the second item, that is, formal thought disorders, the A 1 CRAG positive patients displayed a progressive constant improvement in the symptomatology, whereas A 1 CRAG negative subjects settled to a steady state after an initial moderate improvement.

DISCUSSION

The results of this study require some comment. First of all it must be emphasized that in our study there was a greater decrease in the scores in the presence of the relevant antigens, of a only few psychopathological manifestations, but these can be considered to be meaningful clues from a phenomenological point of view, particularly psychotic hostility and thinking disorders. Two additional facts must be stressed. Differences in the psychopharmacological effects are difficult to evaluate during the course treatment with only one drug and without comparison between drug and placebo, at least from a mathematical point of view. Also, the experimental design we adopted did not take into account a possible effect of duration of treatment. It is possible, in fact, that a longer period of treatment would cause a further improvement in those symptoms which are more established so that the differences in the responses according to HLA type might become larger.

The present data cannot exclude that HLA typing is somehow correlated to the individual pharmacokinetic characteristics and influences in this way the clinical responsiveness to the psychotropic drugs. At present, studies directly comparing psychopharmacodynamics, clinical responses and HLA typing are not available. However, in the case of haloperidol, the range of individual variations in plasma levels after identical doses of the drug narrows when we consider only the free diffusible fraction, which is virtually constant over a broad range of total concentration (ref. 11). For this reason, and because there are not indications of psychoactive metabolites, we believe it to be unlikely that the bioavailability of the drug can explain the differences we evidence in our study.

The important role played by individual sensitivity to the drug is supported by the fact that, even when the serum levels of free haloperidol are similar in various individuals, a biological response to the drug, such as prolactin release, shows individual variability. Indeed, we think that the HLA induced modulation of the clinical effect applies at the central receptor level. In fact, as we have already said, A 1 CRAG antigens are able to bind the drug and they are present outside the Central Nervous System in great amounts, are present, in fact, on the membrane surfaces of all nucleated cells and even in plasma and body fluids. In spite of haloperidol's weaker affinity for the HLA antigens than for the specific receptors, the antigens could extract an important proportion of the drug from specific psychopharmacological action. This mechanism might explain some normal and abnormal states in animals and man (ref. 12), but it appears to contrast with the results obtained in vivo for both CPZ and haloperidol, which seem to suggest that those subjects who have on their cells the relevant antigens respond better to psychoactive drugs than individuals who lack it. Since a purely passive peripheral interference cannot satisfactorily explain the data, we have hypothesized that the drug bound to the HLA antigen on nerve cells also has some pharmacological activity, and thus that this additional effect is present only in those subjects who have A 1 CRAG antigens and who for this reason, seem to display better clinica clinical responses.

REFERENCES

1) Klett C.L. (1978). Models for the management of heterogeneity: an interdependency between problems of research design, sensitivity and opportunities for predictive insight. In M.A. Lipton, A. Di Mascio and K.F. Killam (Eds.), Psychopharmacology: a generation of progress, Raven Press, New York, pp. 821-825

2) Payne R. (1977). The HLA complex: genetics and implications in the immune response. In J. Dausset and A Svejgaard (Eds.), HLA and disease, Munksgaard, Copenhagen, pp. 20-29

3) Smeraldi E. and Scorza-Smeraldi R. (1976). Interference between anti-HLA antibodies and chlorpromazine. Nature, 260, 532-33

4) Scorza-Smeraldi R., Smeraldi E., Fabio G., Bellodi L., Sacchetti E. and Rugarli C. (1977). Interference between anti-HLA-antibodies and adrenergic receptor-binding drugs. Tissue Antigens, 9, 163-166

5) Smeraldi E., Scorza-Smeraldi R., Fabio G. and Negri F. Interference between anti-HLA antibodies and CPZ metabolites. Submitted for publication.

6) Castellano C., Eleftheriou B.E., Bailey D.W. and Oliverio A.

We would like to thank Dr. G. Malagoli for allowing us access to his hospitalized patients.

(1974). Chlorpromazine and avoidance: a genetic analysis. Psychopharmacologia (Berl.), 34, 309-316

7) Smeraldi E., Bellodi L., Sacchetti E. and Cazzullo C.L. (1976). The HLA system and the clinical response to treatment with chlorpromazine. Br. J. Psychiat., 129, 486-489

8) Smeraldi E., Bellodi L., Scorza-Smeraldi R., Fabio G. and Sacchetti E. (1976). HLA-SD antigens and schizophrenia: statistical and genetical considerations. Tissue Antigens, 8, 191-196

9) Woodruff R.A., Goodwin D.W. and GUZE S.B. (1974). Psychiatric Diagnosis. Oxford University Press.

10) Asberg M., Perris C., Schalling D. and Sedvall G. (1978). The CPRS - development and applications of a psychiatric rating scale. Acta Psychiat. Scand., suppl. 271

11) Forsman A. (1978). Pharmacokinetics and pharmacodynamics of haloperidol in man. Paper read at 11th C.I.N.P. Congress, Vienna, July 9-14

12) Svejgaard A. and Ryder L.P. (1976). Interaction of HLA molecules with non-immunological ligands as an explanation of HLA and disease associations. Lancet , ii, 547-549

Genetic Components in the Mechanism of Action of Lithium: HLA-Antigens and the Response to Prophylactic Lithium

C. PERRIS*, E. STRANDMAN* and L. WÄHLBY**

*Department of Psychiatry, Umeå University, Umeå, Sweden
**Blood Center, Umeå University, Umeå, Sweden

ABSTRACT

82 consecutive patients on continous lithium treatment checked at the out-patient clinic of the psychiatry department of the Umeå university were typed for HLA-antigens. By comparing the group of those who did not relapse on lithium therapy (n=48) with the group of those who did relapse (n=34) there was a significant higher frequency of the HLA-A3 antigen among those who did relapse, and none of those who did not relapse was found to have the HLA-B18 antigen. In 42 patients the RBC/plasma lithium ratio has also been calculated. When the patients in this latter series were divided into two groups above and below the median value of the RBC/plasma ratio, a heterogeneity among the groups as regards the antigens B35 and B40 emerged. The results suggest a possible interference between HLA-antigens and response to lithium treatment.

Key words: HLA-antigens and lithium, lithium treatment, lithium and genetics

The aim of this report is to present the findings of some initial investigations which might contribute in illustrating a possible genetic component in the mechanism of action of lithium.

During the last ten years, several investigations have been published suggesting that the therapeutic action of lithium might largely depend upon its distribution across cell membranes (Duhm and co-workers, 1976; Greil and co-workers, 1976; Mendels and Frazer, 1975; Naylor and co-workers, 1976), and that this distribution might be genetically controlled (Dorus and co-workers, 1974; Schless and co-workers, 1975).

In particular, Mendels and Frazer (1975) have proposed that manic-depressive patients have a disturbance in some aspect of the cell membrane function governing the passage of electrolytes into and out of the erythrocyte resulting in an increased concentration of lithium within the cell. The authors hypothesize that the dysfunction in this system is parallelled by a similar change in neuronal membrances at some critical site in the central nervous system (CNS). Also family studies carried out by Mendlewicz (1976) seem to suggest the importance of genetic factors for the intra- and extracellular distribution of lithium.

The HLA system is one of the most complex genetic systems in man. All HLA phenotypes are individually rare and it is difficult to find unrelated individuals, who have identical HLA phenotypes. All of the antigens are inherited as co-dominant characters which are present from early fetal life and do not change with age (Svejgaard and co-workers, 1975). HLA genes are located in the chormosomal region MHC (major histocompatibility complex) whose loci seem to behave as a functional unit controlling the structures of the outer as well as the inner cellular membranes (Ceppellini, 1972).

Since HLA antigens are assumed to control membrane functioning, and since lithium effect depends upon its distribution across the cell membrane it seems justified to assume that HLA antigens may be in some way associated with the effect of lithium. To test this hypothesis response to lithium treatment and HLA typing were taken into account in an unselected series of 82 patients who had been on lithium for several years, and who had been typed for HLA in the course of genetic studies (Beckman and co-workers, 1978a, 1978b, 1978c, 1978d; Perris, 1978). According to diagnosis, the series could be subdivided in the following subgroups: 33 were bipolar manic-depressive patients, 29 were unipolar depressive and 20 were patients who had suffered from cycloid psychosis. The composition of the series is presented in Table 1.

TABLE 1 The Series

Group	Without relapses	With relapses	Total
Bipolar	21	12	33
Unipolar	20	9	29
Cycloid	7	13	20
	48	34	82

These patients resided in the area served by our hospital during treatment with lithium, and were seen periodically at our out-patients department. The two psychiatrists (CP and ES) revised the records of all patients being unaware of the HLA results. The patients were thus divided into those who had never shown any relapse since lithium treatment was started, and those who had shown at least one relapse requiring treatment during the follow-up period which ranged from one to about ten years. The plasma levels were adequate in both groups (.06 - 1.0 mmol/l). Patients who had been treated with lithium for some years, and had shown satisfactory plasma levels at the periodical check-ups but in whom lithium had been stopped because of lack of morbidity suppressive effect were included in the second group, i.e. that of patients with relapses. The distribution of HLA antigens in these two groups is shown in Tables 2 and 3.

TABLE 2 Per cent Distribution

Antigen	Without relapses n=48	With relapses n=34
A1	6.3	4.3
A2	17.0	17.2
A3	4.0	11.2**
A9	5.1	5.2
A10	22.9	11.8
A11	1.1	3.4
Aw19	2.9	1.7
A28	3.4	1.7

** $p < .01$

TABLE 3 Per cent Distribution

Antigen	Without relapses n=48	With relapses n=34
B5	0.6	2.6
B7	9.1	8.6
B8	6.9	2.6
B12	13.1	10.3
B13	2.3	3.4
Bw15	5.1	4.3
Bw17	1.1	0.9
B18	0.0	2.6
B22	0.0	0.9
B27	5.7	8.6
Bw35	2.3	2.6
Bw40	6.9	4.3

On comparing the two groups we found a significantly higher frequency of the A3 antigen among the patients who had had relapses. It is also noteworthy that all the three patients with the B18 antigen belong to the same group. Table 4 shows the A3 distribution in the diagnostic subgroups.

TABLE 4 A3 Antigen: Per cent Distribution

Group	Without relapses	With relapses
Bipolar n=33	1.4	9.1**
Unipolar n=29	5.3	13.8
Cycloid n=20	6.5	11.6

** $p < .01$

Thus it seems that A3 when present, on the cell membrane, alone or in some particular combination might disturb the system which controls the lithium distribution across the mambrane, especially in bipolar patients. However, our results must be viewed with caution with regard to the relatively small number of patients involved. This applies in particular to B18 which is a relatively rare antigen, also in the general population.

Scorza-Smeraldi and Smeraldi (pers. communic., 1978) following another approach have recently found in an in vitro study that HLA antigens are one of the factors contributing to lithium uptake in the red blood cells. In particular they found that about 70 per cent of the individuals who showed a high RBC/plasma lithium had the antigen B35. Challenged by this finding we have re-analyzed the data of 42 patients who had participated in previous studies of lithium in plasma and in RBC (von Knorring and co-workers, 1976a, 1976b) and who had also been typed for HLA. According to their RBC/plasma lithium the patients were divided into two groups above and below the median (RBC/plasma lithium x 100 = 50). The figures for this second part of the study are summarized in Tables 5 and 6.

TABLE 5 RBC/Plasma Li and HLA

Antigen	Median	n=18	Median	n=24	Contr. n=449
A1	4	22.2	4	16.7	20.7
A2	10	55.6	17	70.8	61.5
A3	6	33.3	10	41.7	29.6
A9	4	22.2	4	16.7	17.4
A10	4	22.2	3	12.5	10.7
A11	1	5.6	2	8.3	11.6
A28	2	11.1	3	12.5	13.4
Aw19	2	11.1	2	8.3	9.6

TABLE 6 RBC/Plasma Li and HLA

Antigen	Median	n=18	Median	n=24	Contr. n=449
B5	3	16.7	4	16.7	11.8
B7	6	33.3	8	33.3	39.0
B8	4	22.2	6	25.0	22.1
B12	8	44.4	8	33.3	29.2
B13	–	–	–	–	1.1
Bw15	4	22.2	7	29.2	23.8
B17	–	–	–	–	2.2
B18	1	5.6	1	4.2	4.7
Bw22	–	–	–	–	2.4
B27	3	16.7	5	20.8	16.7
Bw35	5	27.8	1	4.2**	8.9*
Bw40	2	11.1	7	29.2**	17.4

* $p < .05$
** $p < .10 > .05$

It is evident that there is a heterogeneity among the groups especially as regards the antigens B35 and B40. In particular it must be noted that five of our six patients with the antigen B35 belong to the group with an RBC/plasma lithium above the median, and that seven of the nine patients with the antigen Bw40 belong to the group with an RBC/plasma lithium below the median.

Although the difference is not statistically significant in our series, the results concerning B35 point in the same direction as those of Scorza-Smeraldi and Smeraldi (cit.). However, we were still unable to find any significant correlation between RBC/plasma lithium and therapeutic response. In fact three of the five patients with an high RBC/plasma lithium and the antigen B35 had shown relapses. This lack of correlation is in line with our previous results (von Knorring and co-workers, 1978a).

Although preliminary in their nature, and limited by the small number of patients who have been investigated, the results of our investigation seem to support the hypothesis that genetic factors might play an important role in determining the effect of lithium. Further studies of the HLA antigens could prove to be a challenging approach to the identification of some of these factors.

REFERENCES

Beckman, G., L. Beckman, B. Cedergren, C. Perris, and E. Strandman (1978a). Serum protein and red cell enzyme polymorphisms in affective disorders. Hum. Hered., 28, 41-47.

Beckman, G., L. Beckman, C. Perris, and E. Strandman (1978b). No association of red cell adenylate kinase phenotypes with affective disorders. Hum. Genet., 41, 355-357.

Beckman, L., B. Cedergren, C. Perris, and E. Strandman (1978c). Blood groups and affective disorders. Hum. Hered., 28, 48-55.

Beckman, L., C. Perris, E. Strandman, and L. Wählby (1978d). HLA antigens and affective disorders. Hum. Hered., 28, 96-99.

Ceppellini, R. (1972). HLA types and disease entities. In McDevitt and Landy (Ed.s), Genetic Control of Immune Responsiveness. Academic Press, New York.

Dorus, E., G.N. Pandey, A. Frazer, and J. Mendels (1974). Genetic determinent of lithium ion distribution. I. An in vitro monozygotic-dizygotic twin study. Arch. gen. Psychiat., 31, 463-465.

Duhm, J., F. Eisenried, B.F. Becker, and W. Greil (1976). Studies on the lithium transport across the red cell membrane. Pflügers Arch. ges. Physiol., 364, 147-155.

Greil, W., F. Eisenried, B.F. Becker, and J. Duhm (1976). Interindividual differences of the Na+ dependent Li+ countertransport system and of the Li+ distribution ratio across the red cell membrane in Li+ treated patients. 10th Congress CINP, Quebec.

von Knorring, L., L. Oreland, C. Perris, and S. Runeberg (1976a). Lithium RBC/plasma ratio in subgroups of patients with affective disorders. Neuropsychobiology, 2, 74-80.

von Knorring, L., L. Oreland, C. Perris, and Å. Wiberg (1976b). Evaluation of the lithium RBC/plasma ratio as a predictor of the prophylactic effect of lithium treatment in affective disorders. Pharmakopsych., 9, 81-84.

Mendels, J., and A. Frazer (1975). Lithium distribution in depressed patients: Implications for an alteration in cell membrane function in depression. In J. Mendels (Ed.), Psychobiology of Depression. Spectrum Publ. Inc., New York. Chapter 7.

Mendlewicz, J. (1976). Lithium et équipement génétique. L'Evolution Psychiatrique, 3, 551-556.

Naylor, G.J., B.A.T. Dick, and E.G. Dick (1976). Erythrocyte membrane cation carrier, relapse rate of manic-depressive illness and response to lithium. Psychol. Med., 6, 257-264.

Perris, C. (1977). Recent perspectives in the genetics of affective disorders. Read at the VIth World Congress of Psychiatry, Honolulu, Hawaii, Aug. 28 - Sept. 3.

Schless, A.P., A. Frazer, J. Mendels, G.N. Pandey, and V.J. Theodorides (1975). Genetic determinent of lithium ion metabolism. II. An in vivo study of lithium ion distribution across erythrocyte membranes. Arch. gen. Psychiat.,32, 337-340.

Svejgaard, A., M. Hauge, C. Jersild, P. Platz, L.P. Ryder, L. Staub Nielsen, and M. Thomsen (1975). The HLA system. An introductory survey. Monogr. hum. Genet., 7, Karger, Basel.

Supported in part by a grant from the Torsten and Ragnar Söderberg's Fund.

Genetics and Lithium Ion Metabolism in Affective Disorders

J. MENDLEWICZ, P. VERBANCK and P. LINKOWSKI

University of Brussels, Belgium

ABSTRACT

In order to investigate genetic variables in lithium prophylaxis and lithium distribution across the erythrocyte in manic-depression, we have examined fourty two pairs of monozygotic (N=25) and dizygotic (N=17) twins with manic-depression. Concordant twins as a group show better lithium prophylaxis than do discordant twins.
Lithium distribution across the red blood cell (RBC) was assessed by estimating lithium RBC/plasma ratios. The lithium ratios' intra pair differences in both groups of twins were minimal with a high heritability index suggesting that genetic factors play a role in lithium ion distribution. A high linear correlation was found between lithium ratio and plasma lithium and there was no difference in lithium ratios according to sex, affective state and response to lithium. The distribution of lithium ratios was homogenous in the lithium responders' population, suggesting biological heterogeneity of lithium distribution in lithium failures. The implications of these results are discussed as they relate to the genetic determinants of lithium prophylaxis in manic-depressive illness.

INTRODUCTION

Heredity is of importance in drug metabolism and drug response (Mendlewicz and others, 1975). Heredity also contributes to a large extent to the etiology of major psychoses such as schizophrenia and manic-depression (Heston, 1970; Mendlewicz and Rainer, 1977). The prophylactic efficacy of lithium salts in manic-depressive illness is now well documented (Schou, 1968) but its mode of action remains to be clarified. Recent genetic studies have shown a positive correlation between long-term lithium response in manic-depression and the patient's genetic background (Mendlewicz and others, 1972; Mendlewicz and others, 1973; Mendlewicz and Verbanck, 1978; Prien and others, 1974; Taylor and Abrams, 1975; Cazullo and Smeraldi, in press; Kupfer and others, 1975). This observation emphasizes the importance of lithium action at the receptor level as a possible indicator of biological disturbances in membrane factors in manic-depressive illness (Mendels and Frazer, 1973).
This question has recently been investigated in manic-depressive patients by studying lithium distribution across the red blood cell (RBC). The ratio of RBC lithium concentration to plasma lithium

concentration, ie. the lithium ratio is now being the subject of much controversy concerning its use as a potential clinical or research indicator. Some authors have reported the lithium RBC/plasma ratios to be significantly higher in depressed manic-depressive patients who were lithium responders as compared to lithium failures (Mendels and Frazer, 1973; Cazullo and others, 1975). Other investigators have shown correlations between the erythrocyte/plasma lithium ratios and clinical affective state in bipolar (manic-depressive) and unipolar (depressive) patients (Elizur and others, 1972; Ramsey and others, 1976; Soucek and others, 1974; Lyttkens and others, 1973). These results however are disputed by other laboratories who were unable to confirm such findings (Lee and others, 1975; Rybakowski and others, 1974; Von Knorring and others, 1976).

Furthermore, there are conflicting results concerning the relationship between extra and intracellular lithium concentration in erythrocytes, thus making it difficult to interpret clinical studies based on lithium ratio estimations (Ratey and Mallinger, 1977).

In this paper, the mechanism of lithium distribution across the RBC membrane and the importance of genetic factors are further investigated with relation to lithium prophylaxis in a homogenous group of manic-depressive twins.

SAMPLE AND METHODS

A group of 71 pairs of twins with a diagnosis of affective illness has been ascertained in Brussels. Among this group, 42 twin probands were identified as having been treated with lithium carbonate during at least two years for manic-depression. All subjects were available and willing to participate in the present investigation, after being informed as to the nature of the study. These twins were selected through a Belgian Twin Register (N=11) containing the names of 597 twins, and through private and hospital referrals (N=31).

There were 25 pairs of monozygotic twins and 17 pairs of dizygotic twins. The age distribution varies between 23 and 66 years. Zygocity was determined by estimating similarity in physical traits, history of similar appearance to parents and teachers since early childhood and serological determinations. The zygocity determinations were performed blindly: ie. without knowledge of the lithium response and the co-twin diagnosis.

The diagnoses of primary affective illness, either of the bipolar (manic-depressive) type or unipolar (depressive) type were made according to Feighner's criteria (Feighner and others, 1972), using a modified form of the semi-structured interview, Current and Past Psychopathology Scales (CAPPS) (Endicott and Spitzer, 1972).

The proband twin and co-twin diagnoses were done by different investigators. At the time of the study, all twin probands were treated with lithium salts for at least two years. Serum lithium levels were monitored once every six weeks and dosage was regulated to maintain a serum lithium level between 0.8 mEq/liter and 1.3 mEq/liter. A patient was considered to be a lithium prophylaxis failure during this two year period, if he or she required additional medication (other than lithium) or hospitalization for a manic or depressive episode.

Details of the method and results of our twin study have been presented elsewhere (Mendlewicz and Verbanck, 1978). At the time of the study, all manic-depressive twins had been normothymic for at least three weeks. A lithium wash-out period was institute 8 days before the experiment which consisted of the administration of a single dose of 900 mg of lithium carbonate at 9 A.M. during one week. The same regimen was applied to the co-twins. The plasma and RBC lithium determinations were done in duplicate by atomic absorption spectrophotometry (Perkin-Elmer, 305-B) four hours after lithium administration and the results included in Tables 2 and 3 are the means of three weekly determinations. The lithium distribution between intra-cellular and extra-cellular compartment was assessed by estimating the lithium ratio: Li RBC/Li Plasma. Statistical analysis was performed by using the X 2 test with Yates correction, the t student test for means comparison, the F test for comparing variance and the Rankit test for the analysis of lithium ratios distributions, (Delaunois, 1973, Vol. 1; Delaunois, 1973, Vol. 2).

RESULTS

A. Lithium Prophylaxis and Genetic Background

TABLE I

Lithium Prophylaxis in Bipolar Twins

LITHIUM PROPHYLAXIS IN MZ BIPOLAR PROBANDS	CO-TWIN			
	BIPOLAR	UNIPOLAR	NORMAL	TOTAL
RESPONDER	12	2	2	16
NON RESPONDER	2	0	7	9
TOTAL	14	2	9	25

LITHIUM PROPHYLAXIS IN DZ BIPOLAR PROBANDS	CO-TWIN			
	BIPOLAR	UNIPOLAR	NORMAL	TOTAL
RESPONDER	4	1	3	8
NON RESPONDER	0	0	9	9
TOTAL	4	1	12	17

Table I, shows the results of lithium prophylaxis in 25 bipolar monozygotic twin probands and 17 bipolar dizygotic probands according to the co-twin diagnosis. Among the 16 bipolar monozygotic twins benefiting from lithium treatment, 12 have a co-twin who is manic-depressive (ie. they are concordant for the illness), while only 2 pairs of twins are concordant for manic-depression among the 9 lithium failures. Out of 8 lithium responders in the dizygotic group, 4 pairs were concordant for bipolar illness, while there was no concordant pair among the 9 lithium failures. Concordant twins as a group show significantly better lithium prophylaxis than do discordant twins (X2 = 10.79, with Yates' correction, d.f. = 1, $p < 0.02$). The presence of unipolar illness in co-twins does not differentiate between responders or failures to lithium treatment. These twin data confirm and extend previous family studies from our laboratory and by others, (Mendlewicz and others, 1972; Mendlewicz and others, 1973; Mendlewicz and Verbanck, 1978; Prien and others, 1974; Taylor and Abrams, 1975; Cazullo and Smeraldi, in press; Kupfer and others, 1975) demonstrating an association between the presence of bipolar heredity and succes to lithium prophylaxis. These results indicate that genetic factors play a role in the mechanisms of action of lithium salts.

B. Lithium Ratio, Affective Diagnosis and Lithium Prophylaxis

TABLE II

LITHIUM DISTRIBUTION IN BIPOLAR MONOZYGOTIC TWINS

TWIN (PROBAND)	SEX	PROPHYLAXIS	Li/PLASMA mEq/L	Li/RBC mEq/L	Li RATIO (PROBAND)	Li RATIO (CO-TWIN)
I. CONCORDANT PAIRS : BP-BP						
1	F	+	.61 ± .07	.47 ± .03	.77	.83
2	M	+	.58 ± .08	.41 ± .05	.71	.65
3	M	+	.68 ± .05	.42 ± .03	.62	.56
4	F	_	.46 ± .09	.51 ± .01	1.11	1.10
5	M	_	.71 ± .08	.41 ± .02	.59	.54
6	F	+	.64 ± .09	.41 ± .01	.64	.67
7	F	+	.71 ± .11	.34 ± .02	.47	.52
8	M	+	.58 ± .12	.32 ± .01	.55	.53
9	F	+	.59 ± .09	.41 ± .01	.69	.77
10	F	+	.67 ± .08	.52 ± .02	.77	.78
11	M	+	.80 ± .11	.42 ± .02	.52	.55
12	F	+	.62 ± .07	.67 ± .01	1.08	1.08
13	M	+	.76 ± .01	.59 ± .02	.79	.81
14	F	+	.59 ± .08	.49 ± .02	.83	.82
II. CONCORDANT PAIRS : BP-UP						
1	F	+	.47 ± .06	.21 ± .02	.45	.46
2	M	+	.61 ± .09	.33 ± .01	.54	.58
III. DISCORDANT PAIRS						
1	M	_	.82 ± .11	.14 ± .03	.17	.20
2	F	_	.73 ± .06	.23 ± .02	.31	.29
3	F	_	.69 ± .05	.20 ± .01	.28	.32
4	M	_	.77 ± .06	.24 ± .01	.24	.31
5	M	+	.65 ± .09	.29 ± .01	.44	.44
6	F	_	.88 ± .09	.18 ± .02	.20	.22
7	F	_	.83 ± .11	.19 ± .01	.22	.23
8	F	_	.72 ± .08	.22 ± .01	.30	.24
9	F	+	.69 ± .12	.33 ± .02	.47	.44

TABLE III

LITHIUM DISTRIBUTION IN BIPOLAR DIZYGOTIC TWINS

TWIN (PROBAND)	SEX	PROPHYLAXIS	LI/PLASMA MEQ/L	LI/RBC MEQ/L	LI RATIO (PROBAND)	LI RATIO (CO-TWIN)
I. CONCORDANT PAIRS : BP-BP						
1	M	+	.70 ± .09	.29 ± .04	.41	.32
2	F	+	.57 ± .10	.37 ± .01	.65	.51
3	F	+	.62 ± .14	.27 ± .04	.44	.43
4	M	+	.82 ± .08	.18 ± .03	.22	.30
I. CONCORDANT PAIRS : BP-UP						
1	M	+	.60 ± .07	.47 ± .02	.78	.81
III. DISCORDANT PAIRS						
1	M	_	.59 ± .08	.53 ± .03	.90	1.13
2	F	_	.21 ± .12	.42 ± .04	2.00	1.44
3	F	+	.51 ± .09	.42 ± .02	.82	.69
4	M	+	.39 ± .09	.54 ± .02	1.38	1.14
5	F	_	.27 ± .08	.52 ± .01	1.93	1.97
6	F	_	.70 ± .09	.33 ± .02	.47	.66
7	M	_	.69 ± .07	.31 ± .02	.45	.38
8	F	_	.89 ± .09	.24 ± .01	.27	.36
9	M	+	.51 ± .07	.31 ± .02	.61	.66
10	M	_	.41 ± .08	.61 ± .02	1.49	1.17
11	M	_	.51 ± .07	.42 ± .02	.82	.84
12	F	_	.67 ± .06	.39 ± .03	.58	.69

Table II and III illustrate the lithium values for plasma, RBC and the lithium RBC/plasma ratios in monozygotic and dizygotic bipolar twins in relation to twin concordance and lithium prophylaxis. The results included in these tables are the means of three weekly determinations and are expressed in mEq/liter. The analysis of lithium ratios does not show any significant difference between monozygotic and dizygotic twins (t=0.35, N.S.). There was no difference in lithium ratios between unipolar and bipolar patients (t=0.12, N.S.), nor was there any significant difference between responders and failures to lithium prophylaxis (t=0.25, N.S.). Furthermore, we were unable to confirm reports from Lyttkens and others (1973) and Rybakowski and others (1977) of a sexual difference in the distribution of lithium ratios. In our sample, there was no difference in ratios according to sex (t=0.04, N.S.). Our resutls indicate that lithium ratios are not related to affective subgroups and are of little value in the assessement of lithium maintenance therapy. However, as can be seen from figure 1 and 2, lithium responders as a group show a more homogenous pattern of lithium distribution across the red blood cell than do lithium non responders according to the F test ($F=4.73$, d.f. $_{2440}$, $p < 0.001$).

Figure 1

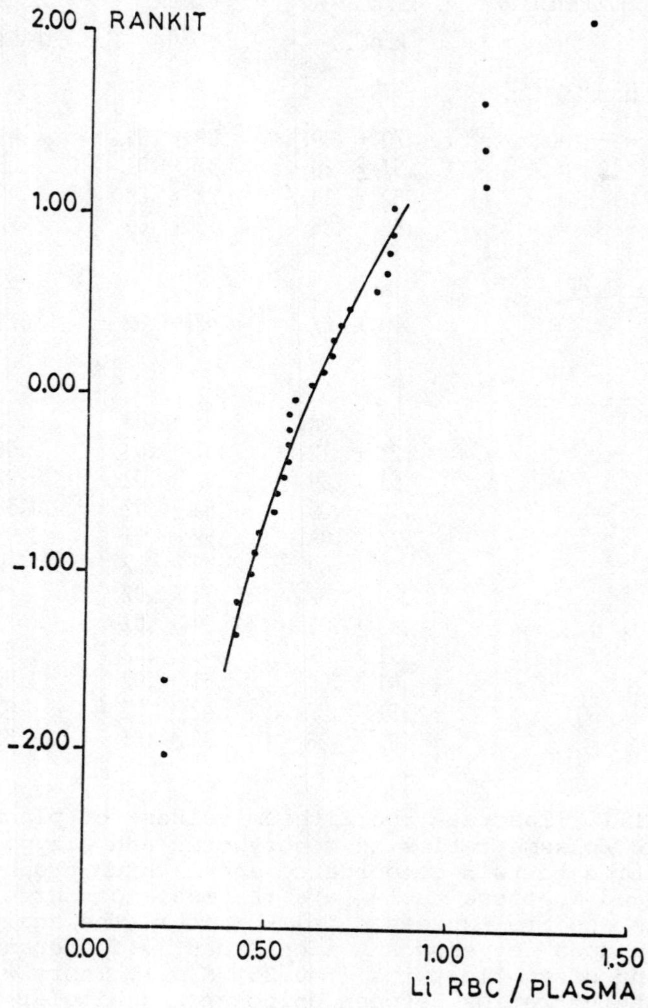

Figure 2

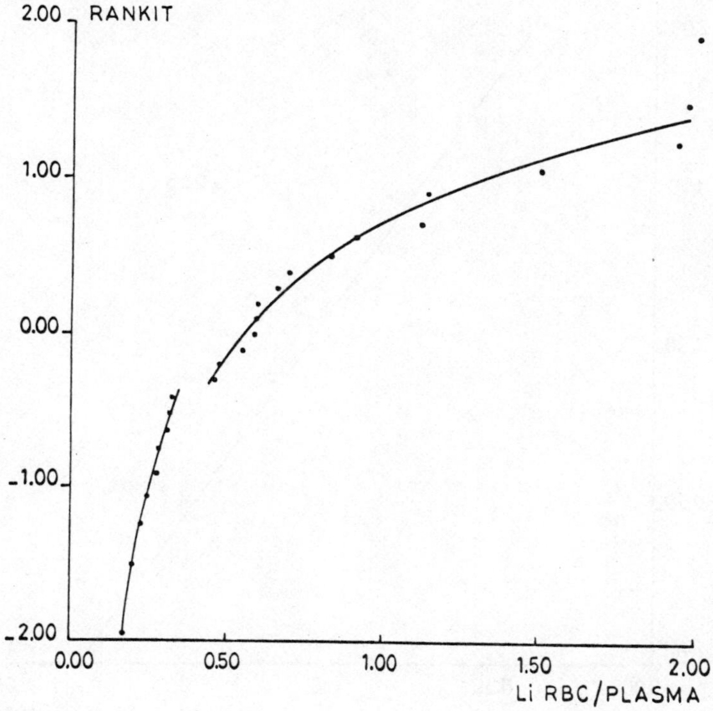

Furthermore, applying a rank test to the distribution of lithium ratios in lithium responders (Figure 1) and non responders (Figure 2), there is indication of the existence of two subgroups in the non responders' population. This observation is in line with some reports suggesting that manic-depression and its response to lithium are heterogenous (Mendlewicz and others, 1972; Jenner and Lee, 1976; Mendlewicz and Verbanck, 1977).

However, in contrast with Jenner and Lee's suggestion (1976) that the lithium responders' group appears to be heterogenous, our data indicate the opposite, ie. the group of lithium failures is more likely to be heterogenous.

C. Extra and Intracellular Lithium Concentrations

Figure 3

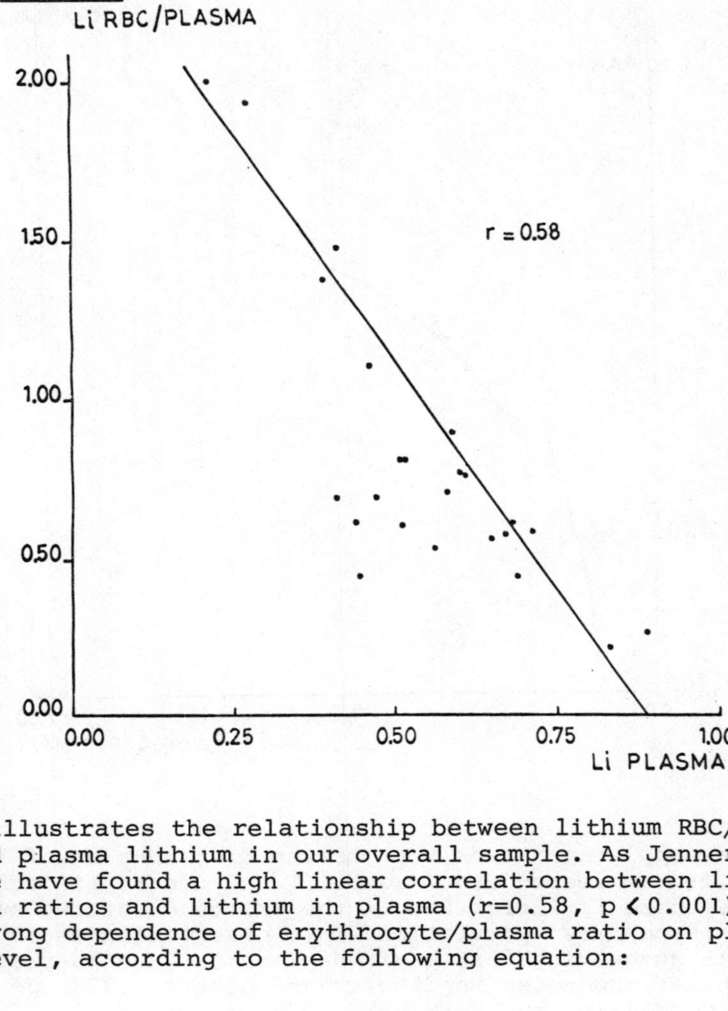

Figure 3 illustrates the relationship between lithium RBC/plasma ratios and plasma lithium in our overall sample. As Jenner and Lee (1976), we have found a high linear correlation between lithium RBC/plasma ratios and lithium in plasma ($r=0.58$, $p < 0.001$), suggesting a strong dependence of erythrocyte/plasma ratio on plasma lithium level, according to the following equation:

$$Li_{RBC} = a\ Li^2_{plasma} + b\ Li_{plasma}$$

These data indicate that the use of lithium ratios alone will not substantially contribute to our understanding of the mode of action of this ion in affective illness. Nevertheless, the factors governing accumulation of lithium ion by the erythrocyte and the genetic mechanism operating in lithium distribution across the RBC membrane deserve further investigation.

Figure 4

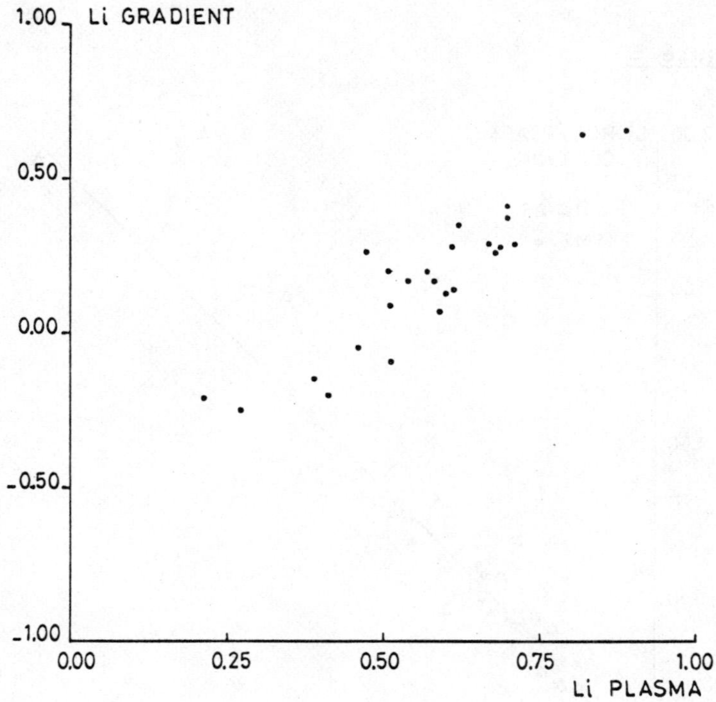

Figure 4 shows the concentration gradients between plasma and erythrocyte in relation to the plasma lithium concentration. The gradients are first negative for small lithium plasma concentrations (indicating lithium RBC intrusion) and become positive for higher lithium plasma concentrations (consistant with lithium extrusion from the RBC). These data suggest that the erythrocyte tends to maintain a constant concentration of lithium in its inner compartment, perhaps through a Na+- depend lithium countertransport system as described by some authors for human erythrocyte (Greil and others 1977; Haas and others, 1975). This active lithium efflux from RBC against an electrochemical gradient occurs by means of a countercurrent exchange with sodium. This mechanism has recently been implicated in the genetic determination and in the large interindividual variation of lithium distribution across the RBC in lithium treated patients (Greil and others, 1977). This interindividual variations of lithium ratios and the genetic factor are illustrated in Table II and III, by the small intrapair differences of lithium ratios in both monozygotic and dizygotic twins (which are of the same order of magnitude as those published by Dorus and others, 1975). Furthermore, the individual lithium ratios do not vary with time as has been shown before (Mendlewicz and Verbanck, 1978). In order to further study the importance of genetic factors in the establishment of lithium distribution across the RBC, we have compared lithium ratios in pairs of monozygotic and dizygotic brothers in our homogenous twin sample. When the values of the lithium ratios for each twin pair were plotted for both Monozygotic and Dizygotic twins, the points for each Monozygotic twins clustered about a 45° line from the origin, an observation indicating a strong genetic influence (Figure 5).

Figure 5

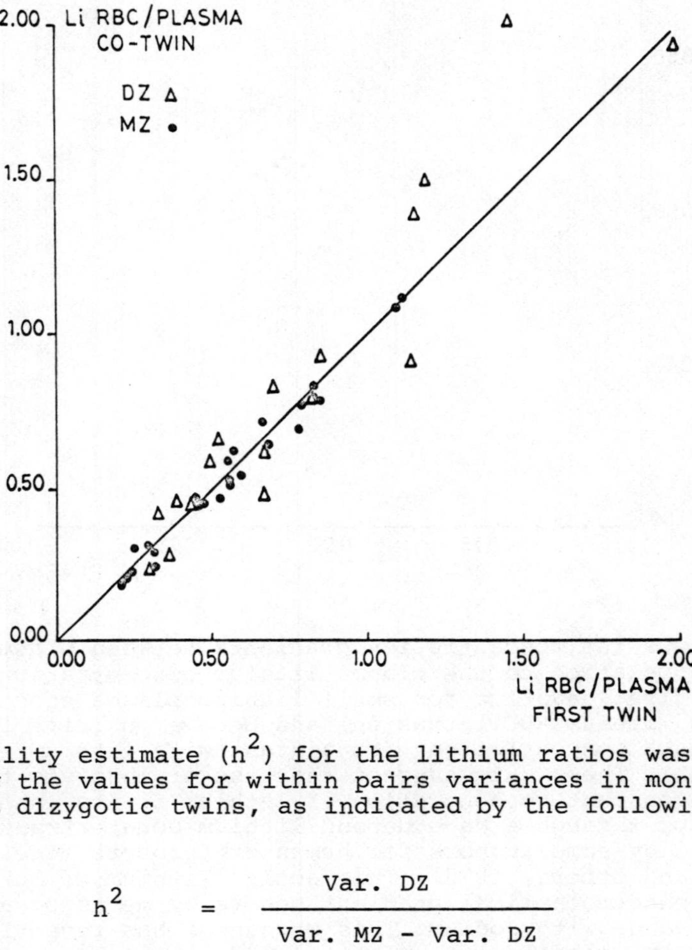

The heritability estimate (h^2) for the lithium ratios was obtained by comparing the values for within pairs variances in monozygotic twins versus dizygotic twins, as indicated by the following equation:

$$h^2 = \frac{\text{Var. DZ}}{\text{Var. MZ - Var. DZ}}$$

The heritability estimate (h^2) was found to be very high in our sample ($h\ 2= 0.97$, $F_{33/49}= 33.10$, $p < 0.001$) and of the same order of magnitude as the one reported by Dorus and others, 1975. This result emphasizes the genetic determination of lithium membrane-transport.

DISCUSSION

Our present study assessing the efficacy of lithium prophylaxis in monozygotic and dizygotic manic-depressive twins indicates that concordant twins are significantly better lithium responders than discordant twins. Although lithium prophylaxis was assessed in probands on a retrospective basis, the study was designed as to keep the investigators blind to zygocity and to clinical status of the co-twin. These twin data confirm previous family studies demonstrating that manic-depressive patients characterized by a positive heredity for manic-depression have statistically a better chance to respond favorably to long-term lithium treatment (Mendlewicz and others, 1972; Mendlewicz and others, 1973; Mendlewicz and Verbanck, 1978; Prien and others, 1974; Taylor and Abrams, 1975; Cazullo and Smeraldi, in press, Kupfer and others, 1975). These results suggest that the patient's genetic make-up could serve as a predicting factor for lithium prophylaxis. According to our study, the estimation of lithium/RBC plasma ratios cannot be used as a psychobiological measure to either differentiate between bipolar and unipolar forms of affective illness, or to predict lithium response in manic-depression. The lack of agreement between studies on the relationship between lithium ratio, clinical status and lithium response may due to methodological problems limiting the interpretation to some studies, as has been pointed out by Jenner and Lee (1976). The samples studied are not always homogenous, sometimes ill-defined and the use of small patients' populations may lead to erroneous associations. In our own preliminary work dealing with a limited group of monozygotic manic-depressive twins (N=8), there was an apparent positive relationship between the lithium ratio and long-term lithium response (Mendlewicz and Verbanck, 1978). However, when we extended our series to 42 pairs, including dizygotic twins, this relationship was no longer present. In our study, there is a high linear correlation between lithium ratio and plasma lithium, indicating that peripheral pharmacokinetic parameters such as intestinal absorption, renal excretion and lithium space distribution play a role in the determination of the lithium ratio. Our lithium kinetic data and the evidence in favor of genetic factors involved in lithium membrane distribution presented in this study can not be solely explained by a passive diffusion model as proposed by Marini (1977). Our results, however, are consistant with the concept of a lithium extrusion mechanism from red blood cells (Mendels and Frazer, 1973; Greil and others, 1977; Haas and others, 1975). Wether this lithium countertransport mechanism is involved in the genetic determinants of lithium ion distribution across the red blood cell membrane, remains to be proven.

ACKNOWLEDGMENTS

This work has been supported by grants from the University of Brussels and the Fondation Interuniversitaire pour la Recherche sur le Processus de Vieillissement.

REFERENCES

Cazullo, C.L., Smeraldi, E., Sachetti, E., and Bottinelli, S. (1975). Intracellular lithium concentration and clinical response. Brit. J. Psychiat., 126, 298-300.

Cazullo, C.L., Smeraldi, L. (in press). HLA system, Psychiatry and Psychopharmacology. Progress in Neuropsychopharmacology.

Delaunois, A.L. (1973). Biostatistics in Pharmacology. Pergamon Press, Oxford, Vol. 1.

Delaunois, A.L. (1973). Biostatistics in Pharmacology. Pergamon Press, Oxford, Vol. 2.

Dorus, E., Pandey, G.N., Davis, J.M. (1975). Genetic determinants of lithium ion distribution. An in vivo monozygotic-dizygotic twin study. Arch. Gen. Psychiat., 32, 1097-1100.

Elizur, A., Shopsin, B., Gershon, S. and Ehlenberger, A. (1972). Intra-extracellular lithium ratios and clinical course in affective states. Clinical Pharmacology and Therapeutics, 13, 947-952.

Endicott, J., Spitzer, R.L. (1972). Current and Past Psychopathology Scales: Rationale reliability and validity. Arch. Gen. Psychiat., 27, 678-687.

Feighner, J.P., Robins, E., Guze, S.B., Woodruff, R.A., Jr., Winokur, G. and Munoz, R. (1972). Diagnostic criteria for use in Psychiatric Research. Arch. Gen. Psychiat., 26, 57-63.

Greil, W., Eisenried, F., Becker, B.F. and Duhm, J. (1977). Interindividual differences in the Na+ dependent Li+ countertransport system and the Li+ distribution ratio across the red cell membrane among Li+ treated patients. Psychopharmacology, 53, 19-26.

Haas, M., Schooler, J. and Tosteson, D.C. (1975). Coupling of lithium to sodium transport in human red cells. Nature, 258, 425-427.

Heston, L.L. (1970). The genetics of schizophrenic and schizoid disease. Science. 167, 249-256.

Jenner, F.A. and Lee, C.R. (1976). Intracellular lithium and clinical response. Lancet, ii, 641-642.

Kupfer, D.J., Dickar, D., Himmelhoch, J.M. and Detre, T.P. (1975). Are there two types of unipolar depression ?. Arch. Gen. Psychiat. 32, 866-871.

Lee, C.R., Hill, S.E., Dimitrakoudi, M., Jenner, F.A. and Pollit, P. (1975). The relationship of plasma to erythrocyte lithium levels in patients taking lithium carbonate. Brit. J. Psychiat., 127, 596-598.

Lyttkens, L., Soderberg, U. and Wetterberg, L. (1973). Increased lithium erythrocyte/Plasma ratio in manic-depressive psychosis. Lancet, i, 40.

Marini, J.L. (1977). On the significance of the erythocyte lithium to plasma lithium ratio. Brit. J. Psychiat., 130, 139-143.

Mendels, J. and Frazer, A. (1973). Intracellular lithium concentration and clinical response: toward a membrane theory of depression. Journal of Psychiatric Research, 10, 9-18.

Mendlewicz, J., Fieve, R.R., Stallone, F., Shelley, E. and Fleiss, J.L. (1972). Genetic history as a predictor of lithium response in manic-depressive illness. Lancet, i, 599-600.

Mendlewicz, J., Fieve, R.R., Stallone, F. (1973). Relationship between the effectiveness of lithium therapy and family history. American J. Psychiat., 130, 9, 1011-1013.

Mendlewicz, J., (1975). Genetics and Psychopharmacology. In Modern Problems of Pharmacopsychiatry (Ed.), Vol. 10. (Series eds.) T.A. Ban, F.A. Freyhan, P. Pichot, W. Poldinger, S. Karger A.G. (Publ.).

Mendlewicz, J. and Verbanck, P. (1977). Lithium ratio and clinical response in manic-depressive illness. Lancet, i, 41.

Mendlewicz, J. and Rainer, J.D. (1977). Adoption study supporting genetic transmission in manic-depressive illness. Nature, 268, 327-329.

Mendlewicz, J. and Verbanck, P. (1978). A pharmacogenetic approach to study lithium treatment in manic-depressive illness In Neuropsychopharmacology, (Eds.) P. Deniker, C. Radouco-Thomas, A. Villeneuve, Pergamon Press Ltd., Oxford, 1, 817-823.

Prien, R.F., Caffey, E.H., Klett, C.J. (1974). Factors associated with treatment success in lithium carbonate prophylaxis. Arch. Gen. Psychiat., 31, 189-192.

Ramsey, T.A., Frazer, A., Dyson, W.L., Mendels, J. (1976). Intracellular lithium and clinical response. Brit. J. Psychiat., 128, 103-104.

Ratey, J.J., Mallinger, A.G. (1977). The relationship between extra and intracellular lithium concentration in human red blood cell: an in vitro study. Brit. J. Psychiat., 131, 59-62.

Rybakowski, J., Chlopocka, M., Kapelski, Z., Henacka, B., Szajnerman, Z., Kasprzak, K. (1974). Red blood cell lithium index in patients with affective disorders in the course of lithium prophylaxis. International Pharmacopsychiatry, 9, 166-171.

Rybakowski, J. (1977). Pharmacogenetic aspects of red blood cell lithium index in manic-depressive psychosis. Biol. Psychiat., 12, 3, 425.

Schou, M. (1968). Lithium in psychiatric therapy and prophylaxis. Journal of Psychiatric Research, 6, 67.

Soucek, K., Zvolsky, P., Kralik, R., Filip, V., Vinarova, E., Dostal, T. (1974). The levels of lithium in serum and red blood cells and its ratios in manic-depressive patients. Activitas Nervosa Superior, (Praha), 16, 193-195.

Táylor, M.A., Abrams, R. (1975). Acute Mania. Arch. Gen. Psychiat., 32, 863-865.

Von Knorring, L., Oreland, L., Perris, C., Runeberg, S. (1976). Lithium RBC/plasma ratio in subgroups of patients with affective disorders. Neuropsychobiology, 2, 74-80.

LEGEND FOR ILLUSTRATION

Figure 1. Lithium RBC/plasma distribution in lithium responders

Figure 2. Lithium RBC/plasma distribution in lithium non responders

Figure 3. Lithium RBC/plasma ratios in relation to plasma lithium

Figure 4. Lithium ratios in MZ and DZ twins

Figure 5. Lithium gradient in relation to plasma lithium

Pharmacogenetics and the Pharmacologic Challenge Strategy in Clinical Research: Studies of D-Amphetamine and Arecoline

E. S. GERSHON*, J. N. NURNBERGER*, N. SITARAM and J. C. GILLIN****

*Section on Psychogenetics, Biological Psychiatry Branch, National Institute of Mental Health, Bethesda, Maryland
**Unit on Sleep Studies, Biological Psychiatry Branch, National Institute of Mental Health, Bethesda, Maryland

ABSTRACT

Pharmacogenetics of drug response and use of brief pharmacologic challenges to identify an underlying biological abnormality are two investigative approaches to major psychiatric illness. We report here high intraclass correlation of behavior and mood response to d-amphetamine in 4 monozygotic twin pairs, suggesting genetic variation in CNS catecholamine systems on which the drug acts. In a separate study, a cholinergic muscaranic agonist Arecoline produced rapid induction of REM sleep in 5 Bipolar patients (drug free and in remission) but not in 7 normal controls. This suggests chronically greater sensitivity of a cholinergic system in Bipolar patients. Replication and extension of this finding to pedigrees of Bipolar patients are planned.

KEYWORDS

pharmacogenetics; d-amphetamine; Arecoline; Bipolar manic-depressive illness; rapid eye movement (REM) sleep; twin studies; sleep studies

INTRODUCTION

Two uses of pharmacogenetics in etiological and genetic research in psychiatry are (1) pharmacogenetics of drug response, including behavioral, biochemical, endocrine, and neurophysiologic responses to psychoactive agents, as suggested by Kalow (1975), and (2) use of brief pharmacologic challenges to identify an underlying defect associated with vulnerability to psychiatric illness (analagous to the glucose tolerance test in diabetes). The goal of these studies is to identify genetic variants that are part of the pathophysiologic process which produces vulnerability to major psychiatric illness. As we have reviewed elsewhere (Gershon, 1978), "a characteristic can be investigated as a possible genetic marker of vulnerability to an illness if it meets certain prior qualifications: 1. The characteristic must be associated with an increased likelihood of the psychiatric illness. (The converse, that persons with the illness should generally show the characteristic, need not be true since there may be biologic heterogeneity in the illness). 2. It must be heritable and must not be a secondary effect of the illness. 3. it must be observable (or evocable) in the well state, so that it is possible to determine its presence independently of the illness and to evaluate well relatives." Pharmacogenetic studies of drug response can satisfy the second requirement, and pharmacologic challenge studies comparing normals with patients in remission can satisfy the first and third requirements. To be a valid marker, after satisfying these prior qualifications, the pharmacologic challenge would then have to distinguish ill from well persons within pedigrees of appropriate patients.

We present here, preliminary results of work in progress to illustrate each strategy: (1) the pharmacogenetics of behavioral response to d-amphetamine in monozygotic twins and (2) studies of rapid eye movement (REM) sleep induction by a cholinergic agonist (Arecoline) in Bipolar manic-depressive patients in the well state as compared with normal controls. Our choice of drugs is determined by current hypotheses that alterations in monoamine and cholinergic neuron systems are associated with vulnerability to affective disorders.

D-amphetamine is an indirect post-synaptic agonist of dopamine and norepinephrine CNS neurons, and generally is a psychomotor stimulant. Tecce and Cole (1974) reported that there is great variability in the response to a single oral dose of 10 mg d-amphetamine, ranging from excitement to sleepiness, which suggests the possibility of genetically controlled variation in behavioral and biologic response to amphetamine. To study the degree of genetic control of this variation, we are administering d-amphetamine intravenously to a series of normal monozygotic (MZ) and dizygotic (DZ) twins, studying correlations between twins in behavior (mood and behavioral scale, motor activity), endocrine response (growth hormone, prolactin, cortisol), measures of catecholamine response, and pharmacokinetics of amphetamine.

Arecoline is a specific muscarinic cholinergic agonist (Baker and others, 1971) in low doses. It has been found to trigger the onset of REM sleep when infused during nonREM sleep in normal subjects, and this induction is blocked by scopolamine, a central muscarinic blocking agent (Sitaram, Moore and Gillin, in press). These findings are of particular interest in primary affective disorder, in view of the findings of Kupfer (1976) that the latency to onset of REM sleep is significantly shortened in depressed patients with primary affective disorder, and in view of the cholinergic/adrenergic balance hypothesis of affective disorders (Janowsky and others, 1972). The early REM onset in depression returns to normal with improvement, but we hypothesize that the sensitivity to REM induction persists into the well state, and will differentiate the response to Arecoline in primary affective disorder patients as compared with normal controls.

METHODS

Subjects. Patients with Bipolar manic-depressive illness (according to diagnostic criteria of Mazure and Gershon, in press) were studied in remission, after having had no psychotropic agents for 14 days. Normal controls (including twins) were carefully screened for preexisting medical or psychiatric disorder. Zygosity determination for twins was performed using multiple red cell phenotyping.

Mood and behavior response. A 20 item scale was constructed, incorporating items that appeared to us characteristic of amphetamine response during infusions in previous studies. Items were depression, crying, increased speech, decreased speech, elation, grandiosity, demanding contact, hyperactivity, decreased activity, distractibility, quality of language and speech, impulsivity, sexual preoccupations, delusions, hallucinations, sleepiness, anxiety. Each item was scored on a zero to eight point scale. Overall reliability for all items was 90%. All amphetamine infusions were video taped from 20 minutes before the infusion to 60 minutes after. Video tapes were blindly rated by two raters. The final score is the difference between amphetamine and placebo ratings for each time point. Results are presented here only for the overall (total) score on this scale. Activity was measured using an electronic patient activity monitor (Colburn, Smith and Guarini, 1976).

Drug Administration. D-amphetamine 0.3 mg/kg was administered intravenously at approximately 9:00 a.m. with one or two infusion days assigned to active drug and the remaining day for each subject assigned to placebo, in a double blind randomized crossover design. Subjects followed an acid-ash diet for three days prior to the infusion to reduce the effects of variation in urinary PH on pharmacokinetics of amphetamine (Davis and others, 1971).

Arecoline was administered 1 mg intravenously for all subjects after pretreatment with 0.3 mg methscopolamine intravenously. After an adaptation and one or two baseline nights, subjects were studied on two experimental nights when they slept with an intravenous catheter. An infusion of either placebo (normal saline) or Arecoline 1.0 mg was administered in random order about 25 minutes after the end of the first REM period. Subjects were pretreated with 0.3 mg methscopolamine IV given at sleep onset on both the placebo and arecoline night. Methscopolamine itself has been reported not to affect sleep EEG (Sagales, Erill and Domino, 1969). Daytime Arecoline was given in the morning between 8:00 and 11:00 a.m. All daytime infusions were performed double blind.

During the Arecoline study, all-night polygraphic recordings were made of EEG, electro-oculogram, and submental electromyogram. Sleep records were scored according to standard criteria (Rechtschaffen and Kales, 1968) without knowledge of whether the patient received placebo or Arecoline.

RESULTS

Pharmacogenetics of response to amphetamine. Total mood and behavior score responses were generally similar over time in MZ twin pairs (Fig. 1). The intraclass correlation between pair members (of amphetamine minus placebo session scores) is significantly positive during the four minutes following infusion (r=.79) and between 24 and 60 minutes after the infusion (r=.82 to .91) (Table 1).

TABLE 1 Intraclass Correlation of Mood and Behavior Response to Amphetamine in Monozygotic Twins

Time	-8	-4	0	+4	+8	+12	+24	+36	+48	+60
Intraclass r	.32	.31	.79*	.53	.69	.69	.82*	.85*	.91**	.89**

* $p < .05$
** $p < .01$

For each time point, the correlation is calculated between pair members for Amphetamine-Placebo session scores.

These results suggest heritable variation in the behavioral response to amphetamine. This is the first evidence suggestive of genetically controlled variation in behavioral response to sympathomimetic agents. The interviewer's clinical observations confirmed the suggestion of heritable variation. In pair 1 both members became excited and had greatly disorganized speech to the point of incoherence after the infusion of active drug, whereas in pair 4, both members showed no mood effect after the same amphetamine dose.

However, an increased number of MZ twin pairs and a series of DZ twins would be needed to firmly establish the heritability of the behavioral response to amphetamine. Should our current results be confirmed in a larger series, it would be of interest to compare Bipolar patients with controls to see if the response of the Bipolar patients was distinguishable from the controls, as an application of the pharmacologic challenge strategy.

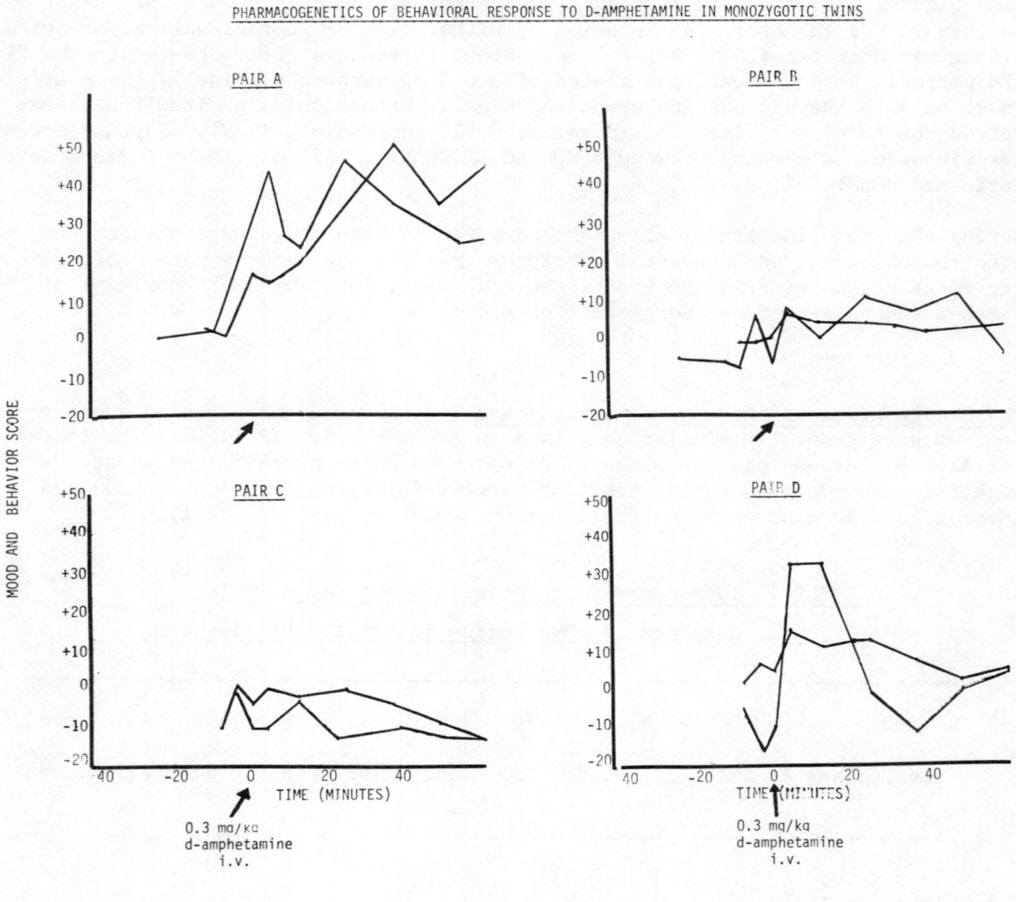

Fig. 1. Pharmacogenetics of behavioral response to d-amphetamine in monozygotic twins.

The activity response to amphetamine over 24 hours is also of interest, although at this time complete data is available only on two pairs of twins, so statistical comparisons are not possible. No apparent difference in daytime activity between the pairs was found before or after amphetamine, but a differential effect on night-time activity (1:00 to 6:00 a.m.) was noted, corresponding to a differential effect of amphetamine in producing insomnia (Fig. 2, Table 2). Pharmacokinetic data on amphetamine in this series is not yet available, so we do not know if the difference in activity represents differences in the rate of elimination of amphetamine.

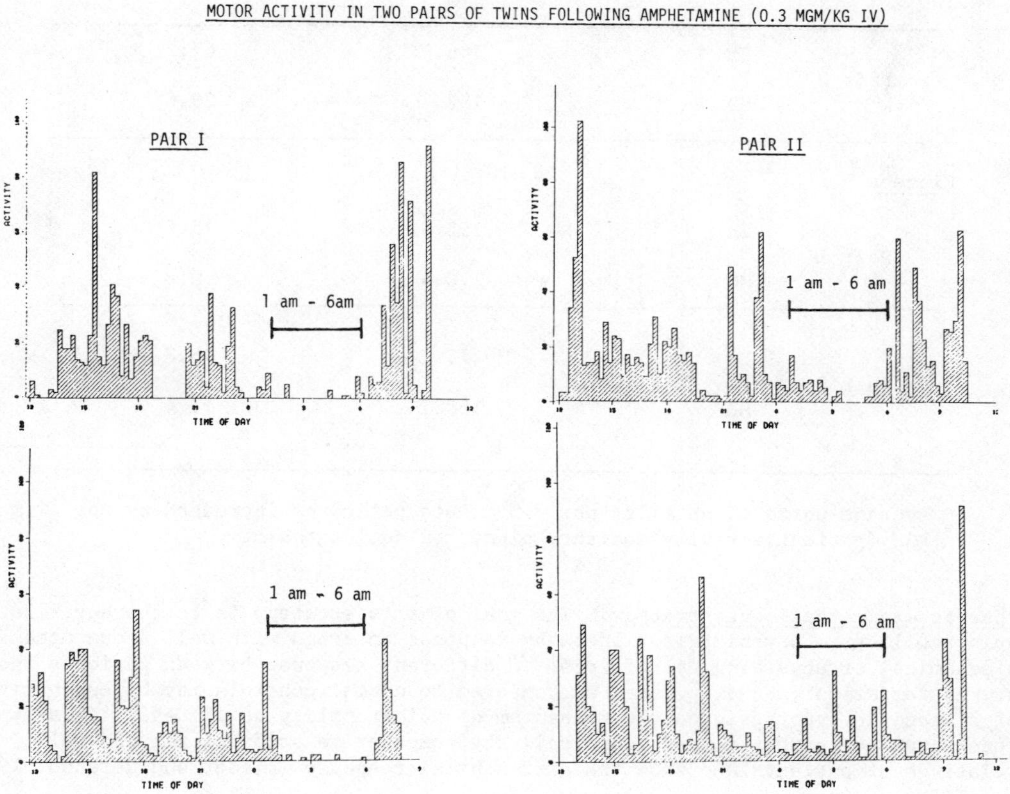

Fig. 2. Motor Activity in two pairs of twins following amphetamine (0.3 mgm/kg IV)

TABLE 2 Mean Waking and Sleeping Activity of Identical Twin Pairs With and Without Amphetamine

		1:00-8:00 p.m.	1:00-6:00 a.m.
Amphetamine (0.3 mg/kg IV)			
Pair 1	EN	139.4 *	11.2
	MN	141.1	9.6
Pair 2	EM	166.9	67.2
	MD	153.4	29.6
Placebo			
Pair 1	EN	195.0	15.6
	MN	170.4	6.8
Pair 2	EM	72.1	15.8
	MD	150.1	11.4

* Average units of activity per 7.5 minute period as increased by the PAM (patient activity monitor) placed on dominant arm.

Pharmacologic challenge strategy. The goal of this strategy is to characterize vulnerability to psychiatric illness by response to drugs with well documented biochemical or physiological effects. A different response between patients who are in remission (and drug free) as compared to normal controls may be supportive of a specific hypothesis on the mechanism of vulnerability to illness. This hypothesis can be further tested genetically by comparative study of ill and well relatives of patients who show the differential response (Rieder and Gershon, 1978).

For example, based on current hypotheses on the role of monoaminergic and cholinergic neurotransmitters in these disorders, we can consider several hypotheses on the nature of the pre-clinical vulnerable state. One class of hypotheses would be that there are chronic alterations in receptor sensitivity in patients predisposed to illness. As a specific example, we hypothesize in primary affective disorder that there is increased sensitivity or increase in numbers of acetyl choline receptors associated with REM induction, leading to decreased latency of REM sleep in the depressed state, and to increased sensitivity to cholinergic stimulation in the well state. Data on this latter hypothesis is offered here from an ongoing study at NIMH by Drs. Sitaram, Nurnberger, Gershon and Gillin comparing the effect of small doses of Arecoline in normal controls and in Bipolar patients who are in remission.

The effect of Arecoline 1 mg in inducing the onset of the second REM period was significantly greater in 5 euthymic Bipolar patients than in 7 normal controls (Table 3). There were no placebo differences in time to next REM period between patients and controls.

Four of the five patients had been treated only with lithium prior to drug withdrawal, and the fifth had lithium and amitryptiline. This suggests that the increased sensitivity to cholinergic agonists in the Bipolar patients was not produced as a result of long-term drug treatment with cholinergic antagonists, a mechanism reported elsewhere (Sitaram, Moore and Gillin, in press).

Daytime infusions of 3 mg Arecoline intravenously produced no striking changes in the mood and behavior scale in any subject. Some dizziness was experienced by all subjects during the first few minutes after infusion.

TABLE 3 Arecoline Effect on REM Induction in Bipolar Patients

(Euthymic, Off Drugs)

	Placebo	Arecoline (1 mgm I.V.)
Normals (N=7)	58.0 ± 4.88 min*	38.57 ± 10.26
Bipolars (N=5)	51.4 ± 7.21	9.4 ± 1.57**

* Time from infusion (at 25 minutes after first REM period) to onset of second REM period.

** $p < .05$ vs normals
$p < .01$ vs placebo (paired t-test)

DISCUSSION

Pharmacogenetics of drug response and pharmacologic challenge strategies have not been previously applied to genetic studies of affective illness. Advances in biochemical pharmacology of drugs affecting CNS monoamines and acetyl choline may offer significant opportunities for genetic study of affective illness. The goal of these studies is to identify genetically controlled pharmacologic responses which segregate with psychiatric illness within pedigrees, and thus would serve as genetic markers of vulnerability to illness. Prior to undertaking pedigree studies, the pharmacologic response must first be demonstrated to be under genetic control and to distinguish patients from normal controls.

The mood and behavior response to d-amphetamine is highly correlated between monozygotic twins, which suggests that variation in response is under genetic control. The behavioral responses to amphetamine are thought to be produced by release of stored catecholamines which act on post-synaptic receptors (Cooper, Bloom and Roth, 1978). Genetic variation in the amount of releasable catecholamines, in susceptibility of cellular and vesicular membranes to amphetamine, or in sensitivity of post-synaptic receptor sites may be responsible for the observed heritable response, although other explanations are possible. Since the half-life of d-amphetamine in persons with acid urine is approximately 9 hours (Davis and others, 1971), much longer than the period of mood and behavior observations (1 hour), it is unlikely that genetic variation in pharmacokinetics of drug disposition accounts for these observations.

The possibility that shared environmental factors account for the similarity between monozygotic twins can be tested by comparison with dizygotic twins. Study of dizygotic twins and expansion of the number of pairs of monozygotic twins tested is underway.

The significantly greater REM-inducing effect of Arecoline in Bipolar patients compared to controls suggests that the patients have chronically increased sensitivity to cholinergic stimulation of the REM generating system. We speculate that this is due to increased numbers or sensitivity of cholinergic muscarinic receptors, but we hasten to note that the current experiment is not a direct test of this hypothesis. Changes distal to the involved cholinergic neurons may be producing the changes in response to cholinergic stimulation. Other neurotransmitter systems affect REM latency; as reviewed elsewhere, norepinephrine appears to inhibit REM sleep and increase REM latency (Mendelson and others, 1977).

These data on Arecoline show significantly different responses between Bipolar patients and controls, but because the number of persons studied is small, these are to be considered a preliminary report of work in progress. If these results are confirmed in the final report of this study, we would become interested in the genetics of variation in REM induction in the population, and then in the segregation of increased sensitivity to Arecoline REM induction in pedigrees of Bipolar patients.

The pharmacologic methods described here are offered to illustrate some of the steps in demonstrating whether pharmacologic response characteristics are transmitted in pedigrees along with a psychiatric illness. This method also offers a test of the etiologic mechanism producing the illness. If a genetic characteristic is consistently transmitted in pedigrees along with Bipolar illness; that is, if all ill relatives show the same response characteristic as the patient introducing the pedigree, even though some well relatives also display the characteristic, then one may conclude that the characteristic is necessary for manifestation of the illness (Rieder and Gershon, 1978). If exceptions are found, so that most but not all cases of illness in relatives are associated with the characteristic, the characteristic would be considered a contributory but not a necessary part of the predisposition to illness. Where the distribution of the characteristic in the pedigree is entirely unrelated to the distribution of illness, the characteristic is demonstrated to have no etiologic significance in the production of illness.

REFERENCES

Baker, R.W., C.H. Chothia, P. Pauling, and T.J. Petcher (1971). Structure and activity of muscarinic stimulants. Nature, 230, 439-445.

Colburn, T.R., B. Smith, J.J. Guarini (1976). An ambulatory activity monitor with solid state memory. Biomed. Sci. Instrument. 12, 117-122.

Cooper, J.R., F.E. Bloom, and R.H. Roth (1978). The Biochemical Basis of Neuropharmacology. Third Edition. Oxford University Press, New York.

Davis, J.M., I.J. Kopin, L. Lemberger, and J. Axelrod (1971). Effects of urinary pH on amphetamine metabolism. Ann. N.Y. Acad. Sci. 179, 493-501.

Gershon, E.S., S.D. Targum, L.R. Kessler, C.M. Mazure, and W.E. Bunney, Jr. (1977). Genetic studies and biologic strategies in the affective disorders. Prog. Med. Genet., New Series, Vol. II, 101-164.

Janowsky, D.S., J.M. Davis, M.K. El-Youssef, and H.J. Sekerke (1972). A cholinergic-adrenergic hypothesis of mania and depression. Lancet 2, 632-635.

Kalow, W., and A.E. LeBlanc (1975). Implications of psychopharmacogenetics Research. In D.B. Elefheriou (Ed.), Psychopharmacogenetics. Plenum Press, New York.

Kupfer, D.J. (1976). REM Latency: a psychobiologic marker for primary depressive disease. Biol Psychiat. 11, 159-174.

Mazure, C., and E.S. Gershon (in press). Blindness and reliability in lifetime psychiatric diagnosis. Arch. Gen. Psychiatry.

Mendelson, W.B., J.C. Gillin, and R.J. Wyatt (1977). Human Sleep and its Disorders. Plenum Press, New York.

Rechtschaffen, A., and A. Kales. A Manual of Standardized Terminology Techniques and Scoring for Sleep Stages of Human Subjects, NIH Publication 204, Government Printing Office, Washington, D.C.

Rieder, R.O., and E.S. Gershon (1978). Genetic strategies in biological psychiatry. Arch. Gen. Psychiatry, 35, 866-876.

Sagales, T., S. Erill, and E.F. Domino (1969). Differential effects of scopolamine and chlorpromazine on REM and NREM sleep in normal male subjects. Clin. Pharmacol. Ther. 10, 522-529, 1969.

Sitaram, N., A.M. Moore, and J.C. Gillin (in press). Induction and resetting of REM sleep rhythm in normal man by arecholine: blockade by scopolamine. Nature.

Tecce, J.J., and J.O. Cole (1974). Amphetamine effects in man: paradoxical drowsiness and lowered electrical brain activity (CNV). Science, 185, 451-453.

Functional Activitiy of Brain Monoamine Oxidase

M. B. H. YOUDIM

Technion, Faculty of Medicine, Department of Pharmacology, Haifa, Israel

ABSTRACT

A characteristic behaviour, namely hyperactivity syndrome, is observed when rats are pretreated with an irreversible non-specific monoamine oxidase (MAO) inhibitor e.g. tranylcypromine followed by L-tryptophan or L-Dopa (L-3,4-dihydroxyphenylalanine). The occurrence of hyperactivity is dependent on the increased rates of brain 5-hydroxytryptamine (5-HT) or dopamine (DA) synthesis as a result of MAO inhibition. The extent of MAO inhibition required is 85% of total enzyme activity, because with selective MAO inhibitors clorgyline and deprenyl, which can fully inhibit either MAO 'type A' or 'type B' respectively, hyperactivity syndrome with L-tryptophan or L-Dopa are not observed. The pharmacological and behavioural changes are seen only when the remaining 15% of total 'functionally active MAO' is inhibited. The relevance of this finding to the use of MAO inhibitors as antidepressants, alone or in combination with 5-HT precursors and in the potentiation of antiakinetic property of L-Dopa in parkinson's disease is highly pertinent.

INTRODUCTION

Biogenic monoamine neurotransmitters, dopamine (DA), 5-hydroxytryptamine (5-HT) and nor-adrenaline (NA) have been suggested as playing a role in animal behaviour as well as in psychiatric and certain neurological disorders. Support for a link between monoamines and behaviour is provided by the behavioural effects often achieved with drugs which interfere with monoamine metabolism and function (see Usdin et al. 1977). Alteration in monoamine metabolism can be induced by drugs during their synthesis as well as during their degradation. Aberration in the function of any of the enzymes involved could finally result in a malfunction of those neuronal pathways in which the respective monoamine neurotransmitter plays a role. It is therefore important that the functional activity of these enzymes should be well understood.

Prominent among the monoamine enzymes is the flavin linked mitochondrial membrane MAO which catalyses the oxidative deamination of the monoamines DA, 5-HT and NA (Youdim, 1975a, 1976).

Intraneuronal MAO is considered to be important in regulating functionally active pool of monoamine neurotransmitters in the central nervous system, thus keeping their cytoplasmic concentration in the neuron low (Youdim, 1975b). Under conditions when MAO activity is changed, either increased or decreased, the concentration of cytoplasmic neuronal amines as well as amine storage capacity of granules could alter(Trendelenberg et al. 1972). It is for this reason that much attention has been paid to what regulates the activity of MAO *in vivo* and in disease states such as endogenous depression and schizophrenia (Youdim & Holzbauer, 1976; Ask et al. 1978).

In this paper I wish to discuss the 'functional activity of MAO' in relation to 5-HT and DA metabolism, in animal behavioural syndromes produced by the increase of latter amines in the brain and its relevance to clinical conditions, namely endogenous depression, schizophrenia and Parkinson's disease.

MULTIPLE FORMS OF MAO AND SELECTIVE INHIBITORS

The demonstration that soluble preparations of MAO from liver and brain could be resolved into a number of discrete bands of enzyme activity by gel electrophoresis led to the suggestion that there might be multiple forms of the enzyme (Youdim & Sandler, 1967 Youdim et al. 1969; Houslay et al. 1976) having different substrate and inhibitor specificities. The controversy that electrophoretically separated forms of MAO may be artefacts of the solubilization procedure, causing enzyme molecule with different amounts of membrane lipid material bound to them to be liberated remains unresolved (Salach & Youdim, 1978). The relevance of these results to the situation within the cell is not clear.

The use of selective inhibitors has provided useful information on the situation that is likely to exist within the cell and there is considerable body of evidence to indicate that there are two major species of enzyme activity in the mitochondria from a number of sources including the brain which can be identified *in vitro* and *in vivo* (Youdim & Sourkes, 1965; Johnston, 1968; Knoll & Magyar, 1972; Squires, 1972; Houslay et al., 1976; Bakhle & Youdim, 1976, 1978). In certain studies these two enzyme systems have been referred to as MAO 'type A' and 'type B'. 'Type A' enzyme is selectively inhibited by clorgyline and oxidatively deaminates 5-HT and NA, while 'type B' species are responsible for oxidative deamination of such amines as benzylamine, phenylethylamine and tryptamine and is selectively inactivated by deprenyl. Tyramine and DA are substrates for both enzyme forms and biphasic inhibition curves are obtained. In view of the interest in the therapeutic use of these drugs their *in vivo* action on 5-HT and DA functional activity in terms of MAO inhibition has been investigated.

THE ROLE OF 5-HT, DA AND MAO IN THE PRODUCTION OF HYPERACTIVITY SYNDROME

Everett et al. (1963) and Grahame-Smith (1971) respectively showed that DA and 5-HT could be increased significantly in rat brain without any overt behavioural changes by giving either L-Dopa or L-tryptophan. However, a characteristic behavioural syndrome, which could be measured as hyperactivity and stereotypity by an activity meter, resulted if the animals were pretreated with the irreversible non-selective MAO inhibitor pargyline or tranylcypromine. Their conclusion was that this demonstrated the ability of intraneuronal MAO to catabolize the increased DA or 5-HT being synthesized, thereby preventing the amine being released into synaptic cleft, stimulating the receptors and producing the behavioural changes. When an MAO inhibitor was administered, this intraneuronal catabolism was prevented and the increased amine 'spilt-over' onto the receptor, resulting in the marked alteration of behaviour. Using these behavioural models together with biochemical measurements the action of various drugs on the functional activity of MAO has been investigated (Green & Youdim, 1975).

A. 5-HYDROXYTRYPTAMINE (5-HT)

It was felt that if the hyperactivity syndrome was the result of increased 5-HT synthesis as suggested by Grahame-Smith (1971) then hyperactivity that would be seen after clorgyline, a selecttive inhibitor of 5-HT deamination, plus L-tryptophan but not deprenyl plus L-tryptophan. For comparison a study was also made of the action of non-selective MAO inhibitor tranylcypromine plus L-tryptophan. This inhibitor inactivates 'type A' and 'type B' MAO equally (Green & Youdim, 1975).

Table I summarizes the results obtained in rats following MAO inhibitors and L-tryptophan. At doses indicated neither clorgyline nor deprenyl administered before L-tryptophan resulted in hyperactivity, while with tranylcypromine at 2.5 mg/kg and higher followed L-tryptophan, the characteristic hyperactivity was observed. However, when clorgyline and deprenyl were injected together at a dose of 2.5 mg/kg and higher of each before L-tryptophan the animals displayed the hyperactivity syndrome (Green & Youdim, 1975). The explaination for the difference between selective inhibitors and tranylcypromine lies in their ability to inhibit MAO and thus raise the brain levels of 5-HT (Table I). No dose of either clorgyline or deprenyl produced as large a rise in brain 5-HT concentration as that seen after tranylcypromine (2.5 mg/kg) and L-tryptophan. However, comparable changes in these parameters were seen when clorgyline plus deprenyl (2.5 mg/kg of each) were given. It is most important to note that in contrast to tranylcypromine no dose of clorgyline or deprenyl fully inhibited both MAO 'type A' and 'type B'. The results indicate the selective action of these drugs on the various forms of MAO. When both clorgyline and deprenyl (2.5 mg/kg of each) were given, both forms of MAO were fully inhibited. Our studies indicate that in the rat brain the ratio of MAO A to B is 1:1 and inorder to observe 5-HT functional activity due to increased brain 5-HT as expressed by hyperactivity syndrome, total brain MAO has to be inhibited by at least 85%.

B. DOPAMINE (DA)

We have examined the hyperactivity syndrome to L-Dopa and MAO inhibitors (Green et al. 1977) similar to those reported for 5-HT and have obtained almost identical results. In another set of experiments when rats were given L-Dopa (50 mg/kg) ½, 6, 12, 18, 24, 36 and 48 hours after tranylcypromine (20 mg/kg), they displayed characteristic behavioural syndrome and locomotor activity only at ½, 6 and 12 hour. During this time there was a marked increase in DA and NA and the inhibition of MAO was above 85%, using 5-HT, DA and phenylethylamine as substrates. MAO inhibition was markedly less than 85% at 18 hour. Neither clorgyline nor deprenyl could potentiate the functional activity of L-Dopa leading to hyperactivity. This is best explained by the fact that DA is substrate

TABLE I. Effect of MAO inhibitors on brain MAO activity and brain 5-HT with or without subsequent L-tryptophan injection

Injection(mg/kg)	Brain 5-HT (ug 5-HT/g brain)		MAO Activity % Inhibition		H*
	Saline	Tryptophan	5-HT	PEA	
Saline	0.49±0.01	0.80±0.05	0	0	-
Tranylcypromine					
1.0	0.60±0.03	0.75±0.14	85±5	85±5	-
5.0	0.77±0.02	1.12±0.14	100	100	+
10.0	0.79±0.05	1.18±0.07	100	100	+
Clogyline					
1.0	0.60±0.05	0.90±0.10	61±7	19±7	-
5.0	0.65±0.04	0.91±0.10	98±2	29±10	-
10.0	0.69±0.03	0.90±0.09	99±1	67±8	-
Deprenyl					
1.0	0.51±0.01	0.73±0.09	23±7	58±5	-
5.0	0.56±0.03	0.77±0.07	31±4	91±4	-
10.0	0.57±0.02	0.78±0.12	44±8	98±2	-
Clorgyline + deprenyl					
1.0 + 1.0	0.68±0.03	0.68±0.08	84±7	76±20	-
2.5 + 2.5	0.76±0.05	1.14±0.14	97±14	87±13	+

*H, hyperactivity; 5-HT, 5-hydroxytryptamine; PEA, phenylethylamine. Wistar rats were injected with saline or one of the inhibitors at the concentrations indicated. 30 min later they were given saline or L-tryptophan (100 mg/kg) i.p. They were placed on Animex activity meters and their activity recorded for the next 90 min on groups of 3 animals. At the end of this period the animals were killed by decapitation, brain 5-HT and brain MAO 'type A' and 'type B' activities were determined using 5-HT and PEA as substrates. The results are expressed as mean ± S.E.M. and are from 6 to 12 animals.

for MAO 'type A' and 'type B' in the rat brain (Green et al., 1977). and when one form of the enzyme is inhibited the amine can still be deaminated by the other.

C. FUNCTIONAL ACTIVITY OF MONOAMINE OXIDASE (MAO)

The experiments with the selective inhibitors clorgyline and deprenyl (Table I) show that while *in vitro* clorgyline totally inhibits MAO 'type A', *in vivo* 5-HT can be still be metabolized by the remaining MAO 'type B'. The lack of hyperactivity indicates that in animals treated with L-tryptophan and clorgyline 5-HT functional activity has not been increased because the amine is continuously metabolized by MAO B, and the rate of 5-HT synthesis is significantly lower than that observed in rats treated with tranylcypromine and L-tryptophan. The results clearly demonstrate that the total enzyme must be inhibited by around 85% before changes in 5-HT and DA functional activity are observed and that inhibition of MAO B does not alter 5-HT or DA functional activity nor greatly increase the rate of amine synthesis. The enhancement of 5-HT or DA functional activity is observed only when both MAO A and B are inhibited in the presynaptic nerve endings by about 85% as seen when clorgyline and deprenyl (2.5 mg/kg of each) are given (Green & and Youdim, 1975).

MAO ACTIVITY IN PSYCHIATRIC DISEASES

The amine theory of affective disorders suggests that there might be an abnormality of catecholamine and or indoleamine metabolism (see Usdin et al., 1977). This has led many investigators to examine the activities of several enzymes involved in monoamine metabolism, including MAO, in schizophrenic patients and in patients suffering from bipolar and unipolar depression. For the studies on MAO, the human platelet enzyme has been the only source of material. It has been reported that platelet MAO activity is low in schizophrenics (Murphy & Wyatt, 1972) and suggested that this enzyme is a 'genetic marker' for vulnerability to the schizophrenic disorder (Wyatt et al., 1973). The situation at present is rather confusing and controversial because there is noagreement (see Table II). Any change in MAO activity that might have been observed with the platelet enzyme is rather meagre and the studies made so have not shown no differences in brain MAO in any of the chronic schizophrenic patient groups including the study in which MAO 'type A' an and 'type B' were measured. Therefore there is a situation in which some workers find highly significant differences in platelet MAO activity between their control group and patient populations and others do not. The factors which may account for these differences require careful examination.

In any attempt to seek a causal link between mental disorders and MAO activity in blood platelets or brain tissues many factors have to be taken into account which are often beyond the control of the investigation and in the case of post mortem material can usually not even be established. They include the time at which blood samples were taken or the time lapse between death and removal of the brain and the temperature at which these samples were kept, drugs administered during the agonal period, preceeding long term drug treatment (e.g. phenothiazines), a possible history of alcoholism (Gottfries et al. 1975) and the nutritional state of the patients e.g. iron-deficiency (Youdim et al., 1975, 1976).

We have found that nutritional iron to be important for MAO activity and that iron-deficiency in man significantly lowers MAO activity in the platelets. Where the serum concentration of iron could be restored to normal by iron therapy, the blood platelet MAO activity returned to normal. The discrepency between platelet MAO activity and brain enzyme becomes more evident when one examines MAO activity in rats made iron-deficient. Here it has been shown that although MAO activity is lowered significantly in peripheral tissues, brain enzyme activity is unchanged. Thus brain MAO activity is highly resistant to change.

TABLE II. Platelet MAO activity in schizophrenic patients

Authors		MAO Activity	
		Unchanged	Decreased
Murphy & Wyatt,	1972		+
Meltzer & Stahl,	1974		+
Shasken & Becker,	1974	+	
Nies et al.,	1974		+
Utena et al.,	1968	+	
Vogel et al.,	1969	+	
Domino et al.,	1974	+	
Schwartz et al.,	1974	+	
Friedman et al.,	1974	+	
Wyatt et al.,	1975		+
Gottfries et al.,	1975		+
Zeller et al.,	1975	+	+
Carpenter et al.,	1975	+	
Takahashi et al.,	1975	+	
Crow et al.,	1976	+	
Murphy et al.,	1976		+
Domino & Khanna,	1976		+
Owen et al.,	1976	+	
Belmaker et al.,	1976	+	
Youdim & Orr,	1976	+	
Berrettini et al.,	1976		+
Schildkraut et al.,	1976		+
Becker & Shaskan,	1977	+	
Joseph et al.,	1977	+	
Barchas et al.,	1978		+

The picture becomes even more complicated when one considers that in a number of pathological conditions MAO activity is lowered. For example some forms of migraine (e.g. cases in which the headache attacks were provoked by chocolate) were accompanied by a decrease in platelet MAO activity (Sandler et al., 1974). Anselmi et al. (1974) observed lower platelet MAO activity in patients suffering from essential hypertension. Pregnancy toxicosis also decreases tissue and platelet MAO activity (Sandler & Conway, 1962), as may hyperthyroidism (Levene et al.1962) and arthritis (Haddox et al., 1964).

Discrepancies between different teams in their observations on MAO activity in psychiatric disorders may thus be due to differences in the MAO assay methods (Tipton & Youdim, 1976; Ask et al., 1978), the substrates used, the procedure for preparation of the platelets, in the mode of disecting the brain regions and in addition, to other pathological afflictions of patients often unknown to the researcher.There is one other very important factor which must be also considered, and that is the differences in medications. The few studies so far done on platelet MAO activity from drug free schizophrenics must be extended taking into account the above suggestions.

THE CLINICAL USE OF MAO 'TYPE B' INHIBITORS IN THE TREATMENT OF DEPRESSION AND PARKINSON'S DISEASE

The clinical use of irreversible MAO inhibitors as anti-depressants or as agents to potentiate the action of L-Dopa in the treatment of Parkinson's disease had a drawback when it was discovered that they provoke hypertensive crises (cheese effect) in certain patients who had ingested food rich in vasoactive substances such as tyramine (see Youdim, 1977 for review). Thus an MAO inhibitor without the cheese effect has always been thought to be desirable. When multiple forms of MAO, with different substrate specificities and inhibitor sensitivities were described (Youdim et al., 1969), the possibility of tailoring specific inhibitors selectively to prevent the deamination of some monoamines, while allowing the degradation of others (e.g. tyramine) to proceed was suggested by Youdim et al. (1971). L-Deprenyl, an inhibitor of MAO 'type B' without cheese effect (Knoll & Magyar, 1972) has properties which make it a suitable drug.

The distribution of MAO 'type A' and 'type B' in various tissues of human is not uniform. In contrast to rat brain which contains A and B type MAO in the ratio of 1:1, human brain enzyme is predominently (80%)'type B' (Squires, 1972; Youdim, 1977). Substrate specificity of human brain MAO confirms this notion because benzylamine, phenylethylamine and dopamine are most actively deaminated substrates, while 5-HT, a substrate for 'type A' MAO, the least (Collins et al., 1970; Glover et al., 1977; Riederer et al., 1978). Further support for these findings comes from inhibitor studies where we have shown that deprenil is by far the most active inhibitor of human brain enzyme in comparison to clorgyline, tranylcypromine and harmaline. In these respects human brain MAO closely resembles that of the platelet enzyme (Glover et al., 1977; Youdim et al., 1976; Riederer et al., 1978).

In an attempt to increase the effectiveness of L-Dopa in Parkinson's disease, deprenyl, MAO 'type B' inhibitor has been used in addition to Madopar (L-Dopa combined with the peripheral Dopa decarboxilase inhibitor Benserazide) (Birkmayer et al., 1975, 1977). The addition of this specific MAO inhibitor provided definite improvement over the treatment with Madopar alone, especially during the so called 'off-periods'. Confirmation of these results has recently been reported by others (see Yahr & Birkmayer, 1978). The potentiation of L-Dopa effect is related to the inhibition of brain MAO by more than 80%(Riederer et al., 1978). It is noteworthy that the platelet MAO which has been used as a peripheral marker of brain MAO is also inhibited to the same extent (Birkmayer et al., 1977) and confirmed by Elsworth et al. (1978). These results encouraged us to investigate the possible potentiation of the anti-depressant property of L-5-hydroxytryptophan (5-HTP) by deprenyl. In an open trial study deprenyl given to unipolar and bipolar depressed patients receiving 5-HTP resulted in a significant reduction of patients Hamilton Score (Mendlewicz & Youdim, 1978). Those patients that showed good anti-depressant response to the combination of drugs had platelet MAO inhibition of more than 85%, while in non-respoders the inhibition of MAO actvity was significantly below this figure. The observation that hyperactivity syndrome in rat due to the accumulation of brain 5-HT following MAO inhibitor and L-tryptophan or 5-HTP is dependent on the inhibition of brain MAO activity by more than 85%, suggests that this enzyme is present in the brain grossly in excess of normal requirement (Green & Youdim, 1975; Green et al., 1977). This has been suggested as the reason why successful therapy of deprssive illness by MAO inhibitors was difficult to achieve (Green & Youdim, 1976). Confirmation of this hypothesis receives support from the studies of Mendlewicz and Youdim.(1978) in which patients who did not respond to the 5-HTP plus deprenyl combination had platelet MAO inhibition below the 80% mark.

REFERENCES

Anselmi, R., Buffoni, F., Curradi, C., Del Bianco, P.L., and Secuteri, F. (1974). Brit. J. Parmacol. 52, 460P.

Ask, A.L., Book, J.A., Heyden, T. Ross, S.B., Unge, C., Wetterberg, L., Eiduson, S., and Kobayashi, K. (1978). Clin. Gen. in press.

Bakhle, Y.S., and Youdim, M.B.H. (1976). Brit. J. Pharmacol. 56, 125-127.

Bakhle, Y.S., and Youdim, M.B.H. (1978). Brit. J. Pharmacol. in press.

Barchas, J.D., Berger, P.A., Elliot, G.R., Erdelyi, E. and Wyatt, R.J. (1977). In: E. Usdin, N. Weiner and M.B.H. Youdim (Eds.), Structure and Function of Monoamine Enzymes, Dekker, New York. pp. 863-9o4.

Becker, R.E., and Shaskan, E.G. (1977). Am. J. Psychiat. 134, 512-517.

Belmaker, R.H., Ebbesen, K., Epstein, R., and Rimon, R. (1976). Brit. J. Psychiat. 129, 227-232.

Berrettini, W.H., Vogel, W.H. and Clause, R. (1977). Am. J. Psychiat. 134, 805-806.

Birkmayer, W., Riederer, P., Youdim, M.B.H., and Linauer, W. (1975). J. Neural Transmn. 36, 303-326.

Birkmayer, W., Riederer, P., Ambrozi, L., and Youdim, M.B.H. (1977). Lancet I, 439-443.

Carpenter, W.T., Muphy, D.L., and Wyatt, R.J. (1975). Am. J. Psychiat. 132, 438-441.

Collins, G.G.S., Sandler, M., Williams, E.D., and Youdim, M.B.H. (1970). Nature, 225, 817-820.

Crow, T.J., Johnstone, E.C., and Owen, F.R. (1976). In: G.W.E. Wolstenholme and J. Knight (Eds.), Monoamine Oxidase and Its Inhibition. Elsevier, Amsterdam, pp. 353-363.

Domino, E.F., and Khana, S.S. (1976). Am. J. Psychiat. 133, 323-326.

Domino, E.F., Krause, R.R., and Bowers, J. (1974). Arch. Gen. Psychiat. 29, 195-201.

Elsworth, J.D., Glover, V., Reynolds, G.P., Sandler, M., Lees, A.J. Phuapradit, P., Shaw, K.M., Stern, G.M. and Kumar, P. (1978). Psychopharmacology, 57, 33-38.

Everett, G.M., Wiegand, R.G., and Rinaldi, F.U. (1963). Anna. N. Y. Acad. Sci. 107, 1068-1080.

Friedman, E., Shopsin, B., Sathananthan, G., and Gershon, S. (1974). Am. J. Psychiat. 131, 1392-1394
Glover, V., Sandler, M., Owen, F. and Riley, G.J. (1977). Nature, 265, 80-81.
Gottfries, C.G., Oreland, L., Wiberg, A. and Winblad, B. (1975). J. Neurochem. 25, 667-674.
Grahame-Smith, D.G. (1971). J. Neurochem. 18, 1053-1061.
Green, A.R. and Youdim, M.B.H. (1975). Brit. J. Pharmacol. 55, 415-422.
Green, A.R. and Youdim, M.B.H. (1976). In: G.W.E. Wlostenholme and J. Knight (Eds.). Monoamine Oxidase and Its Inhibition. Elsevier, Amsterdam. pp. 231-246.
Green, A.R., Mitchell, B.D., Tordoff, F.C. and Youdim, M.B.H. (1977). Brit. J. Pharmacol. 60, 343-349.
Haddox, G.H., Saslaw, M.S., Seligman, B. and Stauffer, S. (1964). Biochim. Biophys. Acta, 81, 184-187.
Houslay, M.D., Tipton, K.F. and Youdim, M.B.H. (1976). Life Sci. 19, 467-483.
Johoston, J.P. (1968). Biochem. Pharmacol. 17, 1285-1297.
Joseph, M.H., Owen, F., Baker, H.F. and Bourne, R.C. (1977). Psycholog. Med. 7, 159-162.
Knoll, J. and Magyar, K. (1972). Adv. Biochem. Psychopharmacol. 5, 393-408.
Levene, R.J., Oates, J.A., Vendsalu, A. and Sjoerdsma, A. (1962). J. Clin. Endocr. Metab. 22, 1242-1250.
Mendlewicz, J. and Youdim, M.B.H. (1978). J. Neural Transmn., in press.
Meltzer, H.Y. and Stahl, S.M. (1974). Res. Commun. Chem. Path. Pharmacol. 7, 419-431.
Murphy, D.L., Donnelly, C.H., Miller, L. and Wyatt, RLJ. (1976). Arch. Gen. Psychiat. 33, 1377-1381.
Nies, A., Robinson, D.S., Harris, L.S. and Lamborn, K.R. (1974). Adv. Biochem. Psychpharmacol. 12, 59-85.
Owen, F. Bourne, R.T., Crow, T.J., Johonstone, E.C., Bailey, A.R. and Hershon, H. (1976). Arch. Gen. Psychiat. 33, 1370-1373.
Riederer, P., Youdim, M.B.H., Birkmayer, W. and Jellinger, K. (1978). In: P.J. Roberts, G.N. Woodruff and L.L. Iversen (Eds.). Dopamine. Raven Press, New York. pp. 377-382.
Salach, J.I. and Youdim, M.B.H. (1978). Mol.Pharmacol. in press.
Sandler, M. and Conway, J. (1962). LancetI, 1096-1098.
Sandler, M., Youdim, M.B.H. and Hanington, E. (1974). Nature, 250, 335-337.
Shaskan, E.G. and Becker, R.E. (1974). Nature, 253, 659-660.
Schildkraut, J.J., Herzog, J.M., Oruslak, P.J., Edelman, S.E. and Fraizer, S.H. (1976). Am. J. Psychiat. 133, 438-440.
Schwartz, M.A., Aikens, A.M. and Wyatt, R.J. (1974). Psychopharmacologia, 38, 319-328.
Takahashi, S., Yamane, H. and Tani, N. (1975). Folia Psychiat. Neurol. Jap. 29, 207-214.
Tipton, K.F. and Youdim, M.B.H. (1976). In: G.W.E. Wolstenholme and J. Knight (Eds.). Monoamine Oxidase and Its Inhibition. Elsevier, Amsterdam. pp. 393-403.
Trendelenberg, U., Draskoizy, P.R. and Grafe, K. (1972). Adv. Biochem. Psychopharmacol. 5, 371-378.
Usdin, E., Hamburg, D. and Barchas, J. (1977). Neuroregulators and Psychiatric Disorders. Oxford, New York.
Utena, H., Kanamura, H., Suda, S., Nakamura, R., Machiyama, Y. and Takahashi, R. (1968). Proc. Jap. Acad. 44, 1078-1083.

Vogel, W.H., Orfei, V. and Centuary, B. (1969). J. Pharmacol. exp. Ther. 165, 195-203.

Wyatt, R.J. and Murphy, D.L. (1975). In: D.X. Freedman (Ed.). Biology of the Major Psychosis. Raven Press, New York. pp. 289-297.

Wyatt, R.J., Murphy, D.L., Belmaker, R., Cohen, s., Donnelly, C.H. and Pollin, W. (1973). Science, 179, 916-918.

Yahr, M. and Birkmayer, W. (1978). Inhibition of MAO-type B (deprenyl) in treatment of Parkinsonism. Spriger, Vienna. in press.

Youdim, M.B.H. (1975a). In: H.K.F. Blaschko (Ed.). International Review of Science, Vol. 12. Butterworth, London. pp. 169-210.

Youdim, M.B.H. (1975b). In: J. Mendlewicz (Ed.). Modern Problems of Pharmacopsychiatry. Genetics and Psychopharmacology. Karger, Basel. pp. 65-88.

Youdim, M.B.H. (1976). In: T.P. Singer (Ed.). Flavins and Flavoproteins. Elsevier, Amsterdam. pp. 593-604.

Youdim, M.B.H. (1977). In: E. Usdin, D. Hamburg and J. Barchas (Eds.). Neuroregulators and Psychiatric Disorders. Oxford, New York. pp. 57-67.

Youdim, M.B.H. and Holzbauer, M. (1976). J. Neural Transmn. 38, 193-230.

Youdim, M.B.H. and Orr, M. (1966). unpublished data.

Youdim, M.B.H. and Sandler, M. (1967). Biochem. J. 105, 43P.

Youdim, M.B.H. and Sourkes, T.L. (1965). Can. J. Biochem. 43, 1305-1318.

Youdim, M.B.H., Collins, G.G.S. and Sandler, M. (1969). Nature, 223, 626-628.

Youdim, M.B.H., Collins, G.G.S. and Sandler, M. (1971). Biochem. J. 121, 34P-36P.

Youdim, M.B.H., Grahame-Smith, D.G. and Woods, H.F. (1976). Clin. Sci. Mol. Med. 50, 479-485.

Youdim, M.B.H., Woods, H.F., Mitchell, B.D., Grahame-Smith, D.G. and Callender, S. (1975). Clin. Sci. Mol. Med. 48, 289-295.

Zeller, E.A., Boshes, J.M., Davis, J.M. and Thorner, M. (1975). Lancet I. 1385.

Biochemical Genetics and Platelet MAO

R. H. BELMAKER and R. P. EBSTEIN

Jerusalem Mental Health Center-Ezrath Nashim, POB 140, Jerusalem, Israel

ABSTRACT

Low platelet monoamine oxidase activity has been associated with schizophrenia in some studies but not in others. It is suggested that population differences in genetic enzyme mutant forms might explain the conflicting reports. Work on platelet MAO in schizophrenia with polyacrilamide gel electrophoresis, with amphetamine inhibition constant, and with Michaelis binding constant is described.

Keywords: Platelet monoamine oxidase, Electrophoresis, Amphetamine, Michaelis constant.

INTRODUCTION

The finding of low platelet monoamine oxidase (MAO) in schizophrenic patients by Murphy and Wyatt in 1972 has since generated a large number of attempts at replication. These are reviewed elsewhere (Buchsbaum, 1978). An attempt at a transcultural replication in Jerusalem (Belmaker and colleagues, 1976) was unable to find evidence for reduced platelet MAO in schizophrenic patients (Table 1). A repeat study in Jerusalem with an independent control group and an independent chronic schizophrenic patient group with first degree schizophrenic relatives, again failed to find low platelet MAO in schizophrenia (Belmaker and colleagues, 1977).

One possible explanation of these conflicting results would be the existence of population differences in an underlying, qualitative enzyme abnormality. Sickle disease hemoglobin is a major cause of anemia in East Africa but hemoglobin C disease is a common cause of anemia in West Africa (Harris, 1975). Research in East Africa associating red cell sickling and anemia might not be replicable in West Africa. Another example exists in the numerous mutant forms of glucose-6-phosphate-dehydrogenase (G6PD), some of which have reduced enzyme activity when measured in vitro whereas others have normal or even increased enzyme activity (Yoshida, 1973). Thus research on hemolytic anemia, even research on hemolytic anemia when G6PD deficiency is strongly suspected, might not always elucidate a simple reduction in red cell G6PD activity. More sophisticated biochemical study is needed to positively identify G6PD mutants.

TABLE 1 Platelet MAO Activity in the Jerusalem Study

	Platelet MAO* benzylamine substrate		Platelet MAO tryptamine substrate		Plasma MAO*** benzylamine substrate	
	N	nm/hr/10^8 plate	N**	nm/hr/10^9 plate	N	nm/hr/cc
Manic-depressive	27	12.7±5.5	21	5.2±1.5	27	23.0±7.1
Male	9	13.0±6.1	6	5.3±1.7	9	20.9±6.4
Female	18	12.6±5.2	15	5.1±1.4	18	24.0±7.1
Schizophrenic	18	9.9±2.7	15	4.7±1.3	18	22.2±6.1
Male	12	8.9±2.3	10	4.5±0.8	12	21.5±7.1
Female	6	11.7±2.3	5	5.1±1.8	6	23.7±2.4
Control	19	8.8±2.9	15	4.4±1.3	19	23.4±4.8
Male	10	7.8±1.8	8	4.0±1.0	10	22.6±4.8
Female	9	10.0±3.3	7	5.0±1.4	9	24.3±4.7

Values represent mean ± standard deviation.

* Total MAO activity minus pargyline-insensitive plasma MAO activity.

** Several subjects assayed with benzylamine were not repeated with tryptamine because of insufficiency of sample.

*** Pargyline-insensitive MAO activity.

The technique of polyacrylamide gel electrophoresis (PAGE) is capable of revealing qualitative differences between proteins arising from genetic variation at the molecular level. Such variant enzymes are often detectable by differences in their rate of migration during electrophoresis. Harris (1975) has estimated that over 25% of enzyme proteins will show genetic mutant forms or polymorphism in a manner detectable by electrophoresis. We therefore decided to examine, using PAGE, platelet MAO from manic-depressive and schizophrenic patients.

Figure 1 shows the mean PAGE pattern for each group for 10 manic-depressive, 12 schizophrenic, and 11 normal individuals. After PAGE two peaks of platelet MAO activity are detectable, one migrating 8-10 mm and the other broader peak migrating 24-32 mm into the gel in the time allotted. There are, however, no differences in the rate of migration of either band between the groups examined, and no individual was found with a peak in a reproducibly altered position on the gel at the pH used (pH 8.3). The increased platelet MAO activity found in manic-depressive patients in Jerusalem (Belmaker and colleagues, 1976) is clearly apparent even after PAGE in both electrophoretic peaks. However, this increased height of each peak of the manic-depressives does not give any information about mutant forms, since no variation in the rate of migration of the peaks was observed. No individual patient was observed to have an absence of either electrophoretic peak of platelet MAO.

This lack of success in finding rate variants of platelet MAO in PAGE should not be accepted as conclusive. The technical problems are formidable, as platelet MAO is a relatively large molecule (mol. wt. 235,000) and is also membrane-bound (Collins and Sandler, 1971). The quantity of MAO enzyme activity available by peripheral venipuncture in individual psychiatric patients is too small to allow purification before PAGE. In the above-described study the platelet MAO was solubilized for PAGE as gently as possible, with 5 seconds of sonication in 1% Triton X-100 as detergent, but no Triton was used in the gel or buffer solution itself. We were afraid that an excess of Triton would coat all proteins present and prevent the appearance of differences in migration rate due to small

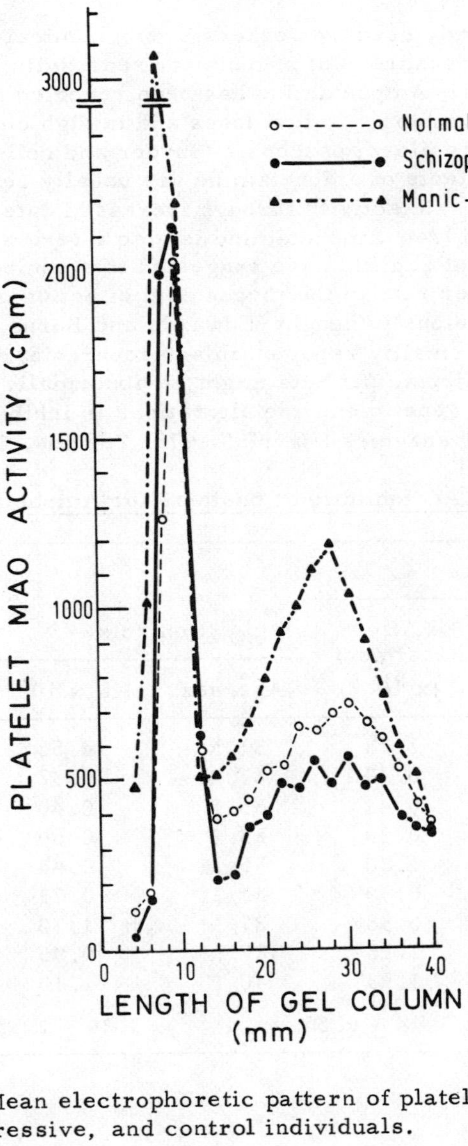

Fig. 1. Mean electrophoretic pattern of platelet MAO from schizophrenic, manic-depressive, and control individuals.

charge differences. However, it is possible that even the minimal amount of Triton used obscured charge differences and resulted in electrophoretic mobility dependent solely on size. New methods need to be developed to "clean" MAO of its lipid attachments without coating the enzyme with Triton-like detergents. Electrophoresis of such a clean enzyme might yield more information about the characteristics of the enzyme, including possible mutant forms. Another important consideration that moderates the negative impact of this study is the influence of pH on PAGE (Harris, 1975). Some mutant enzyme forms become apparent in PAGE at specific pH levels only, and further electrophoretic screening of human platelet MAO at pH levels other than pH 8.3 is therefore necessary (Belmaker and Ebstein, 1977).

Another recent approach, frequently used by workers in biochemical genetics outside of psychiatry, has been measurement of inhibitor sensitivity of platelet MAO from schizophrenic patients. Amphetamine has been reported to specifically exacerbate schizophrenic symptoms in low doses and in high chronic dosages to cause a de novo schizophreniform psychosis (Snyder and colleagues, 1974). While these behavioral effects of amphetamine are usually related to its ability to enhance brain dopaminergic activity through increased catecholamine release (Snyder and colleagues, 1974), amphetamine is also a reversible MAO inhibitor (Sharman, 1976). Recent reports have suggested that competitive inhibition of MAO may play a greater role in the mechanism of action of some psychoactive compounds than previously thought (Edwards and Burns, 1975). Because of the platelet MAO abnormality reported in schizophrenia, we hypothesized that platelet MAO of schizophrenic patients might be abnormally sensitive to inhibition by amphetamine. Such genetic enzyme alterations in inhibitor sensitivity have been reported for other enzymes (Harris, 1975; Yoshida, 1973).

TABLE 2 Platelet MAO Inhibition Constants for Amphetamine

Schizophrenic patients				Controls	
Patient	Age, sex	Ki Before treatment ($x\ 10^{-5}$)	Ki After treatment ($x\ 10^{-5}$)	Age, sex	Ki ($x\ 10^{-5}$)
BY	28, M	0.59	1.78	31, M	4.56
PA	29, M	0.43	0.42	27, M	0.32
ZS	40, F	0.54	0.41	35, F	0.40
IE	22, F	1.27	0.88	23, F	0.60
LY	39, M	1.12	1.80	35, M	0.44
CR	39, M	0.68	0.99	33, M	0.73
PI	21, M	1.80	0.88	21, M	1.70
AE	23, M	1.21	1.26	27, M	0.95
SS	38, F	2.15	1.83	40, F	1.10
$x \pm SD$		0.85 ± 0.54	1.14 ± 0.56		1.20 ± 1.33

Sensitivity to amphetamine inhibition has been shown in monkey brain to be a property of MAO that varies between individuals on a genetic basis (Omenn and Cheung, 1976).

Table 2 summarizes the inhibition of platelet MAO by d-amphetamine in 9 chronic schizophrenic patients and matched controls. No significant difference in sensitivity to amphetamine was found in the schizophrenic group before and after phenothiazine therapy. No significant difference was found between the schizophrenic patients and their age- and sex-matched controls. The range of Ki (the inhibition constant of the platelet MAO for amphetamine) in the schizophrenic and control groups was similar.

A POSSIBLE MICHAELIS CONSTANT ABNORMALITY

Berretini, Vogel and Clouse (1977) were the first to report an abnormal Km (Michaelis binding constant) of platelet MAO from schizophrenic patients. Km determinations are less subject to artifactual influences of platelet-count, non-platelet protein contamination, and enzymatic degradation than are determinations of simple platelet MAO enzyme activity. In response to the study of Berretini, Vogel and Clouse (1977) we reanalyzed our data (Reches, Ebstein and Belmaker, 1977) to extract the Km (Dixon and Webb, 1964) of platelet MAO using benzylamine as substrate (Belmaker and colleagues, 1976) at pH 9.2, for chronic schizophrenic patients and age- and sex-matched normal controls. The results are shown in Table 3.

The Km of platelet MAO from the drug-free schizophrenic patients is significantly higher than the Km for matched controls. Chlorpromazine treatment (300 mg daily for 10 days) lowered the Km values of the schizophrenic patients in the direction of normality.

TABLE 3 Km ($\times 10^{-7}$) of Platelet MAO in Schizophrenic Patients and Controls

No.	Schizophrenic patients: Drug-free	Schizophrenic patients: After chlorpromazine	Controls
1	32	49	17
2	28	26	17
3	32	23	12
4	99	55	36
5	88	199	22
6	39	54	18
7	220	57	167
8	64	69	65
9	229	202	81
Mean ± S.E.M.	92.3 ± 26.4*	81.6 ± 23.0	48.3 ± 16.9*

* $p < 0.025$ (paired t-test)

Berretini, Vogel and Clouse (1977) reported a lower, not higher, Km of platelet MAO from schizophrenic patients. These discrepant results may indicate that platelet MAO in schizophrenia has both low and high Km variants in different human populations. This could explain why some laboratories but not others have found that simple platelet MAO activity is low in schizophrenia as some laboratories (including our own) have used high substrate concentrations that are advisable in biochemical research but which would "cover-up" a high-Km mutant if it existed and perhaps prevent its detection.

Progress in biochemical genetics (Harris, 1975) suggests that resolution of the platelet MAO controversy does not depend on innumerable further attempts to replicate whether simple platelet MAO activity is low in schizophrenia. Such research would never have given an answer as to whether G6PD activity is low in anemia (Belmaker and Ebstein, 1977). The G6PD mutant forms in Iraqi Jews in Israel and in American blacks are different, and may not be revealed by the same techniques. Sophisticated biochemical examination of human platelet MAO, as to Michaelis constant, electrophoretic mobility at different pH levels, and sensitivity to many inhibitors, is called for, both in normal and in behaviorally disturbed subjects.

REFERENCES

Belmaker, R.H., R.P. Ebstein, K. Ebbesen, and R. Rimon (1976). Platelet monoamine oxidase in schizophrenia and manic-depressive illness. Brit. J. Psychiat., 129, 227-232.

Belmaker, R.H., R.P. Ebstein, R. Rimon, R.J. Wyatt, and D.L. Murphy (1976). Electrophoresis of platelet monoamine oxidase in schizophrenia and manic-depressive illness. Acta psychiat. scand., 54, 67-72.

Belmaker, R.H., and R.P. Ebstein (1977). The search for genetic polymorphisms of human biogenic amine-related enzymes. In E. Gershon, R.H. Belmaker, M. Rosenbaum, and S. Kety (Eds.), The Impact of Biology on Modern Psychiatry, Plenum Press, New York. pp. 241-260.

Belmaker, R.H., A. Galon, L. Perez, and R.P. Ebstein (1977). Platelet MAO in schizophrenics with and without family history of schizophrenia. Brit. J. Psychiat., 131, 551-552.

Belmaker, R.H., A. Reches, and R.P. Ebstein (1977). Platelet monoamine oxidase in schizophrenia. Lancet, 2, 821.

Berretini, W.H., W.H. Vogel, and R. Clouse (1977). Platelet monoamine oxidase in chronic schizophrenia. Am. J. Psychiat., 134, 805-806.

Buchsbaum, M. (1978). In preparation.

Collins, G.G.S., and M. Sandler (1971). Human blood platelet monoamine oxidase. Biochem. Pharmacol., 20, 289-296.

Dixon, M., and E.C. Webb (1964). Enzymes, Academic Press, New York. pp. 330.

Edwards, D.J., and M.O. Burns (1975). Effect of tricyclic antidepressants upon human platelet monoamine oxidase. Life Sci., 15, 2045-2058.

Harris, H. (1975). The Principles of Human Biochemical Genetics, 2nd ed. North-Holland Publishing Co., Amsterdam.

Murphy, D.L., and R.J. Wyatt (1972). Reduced MAO activity in blood platelets from schizophrenic patients. Nature, 238, 225-226.

Omenn, G. S., and S. Cheung (1976). Pharmacogenetic studies of monoamine oxidase in human and macaque brain. Proc. Am. Soc. Neurochem., Vancouver.

Reches, A., R. P. Ebstein, and R. H. Belmaker (1977). d-Amphetamine inhibition of platelet MAO in schizophrenia. Biol. Psychiat., 12, 655-660.

Sharman, D. F. (1976). Can the intra- and extrahomoneural metabolism of catecholamines be distinguished in the mammalian central nervous system. In Monoamine Oxidase and Its Inhibition, Ciba Foundation Symposium 39 (new series), Elsvier Excerpta Medica North-Holland, Amsterdam. pp. 203-229.

Snyder, S. H., S. P. Banerjee, H. I. Yamamura, and D. Greenberg (1974). Drugs, neurotransmitters and schizophrenia. Science, 184, 1243-1253.

Yoshida, A. (1973). Hemolytic anemia and G6PD deficiency. Science, 179, 532-537.

Biological Research in Depression and Mania

Serotonin in Depressive Illness - Studies of CSF 5-HIAA

MARIE ÅSBERG* and LEIF BERTILSSON**

*Department of Psychiatry, Karolinska Hospital, S-104 01 Stockholm 60
**Department of Clinical Pharmacology, Huddinge Hospital, S-141 86 Huddinge, Sweden

ABSTRACT

The concentration of 5-hydroxyindoleacetic acid (5-HIAA) in lumbar spinal fluid (CSF) is a commonly used estimate of serotonin turnover in man. Valid comparisons between controls and psychiatric patients using this estimate necessitates sensitive and precise analytical methods and attention to factors such as age, body height and drug treatment. When these factors are taken into account, there is a small but significant difference between depressed patients and controls. There is however no simple association between a low CSF 5-HIAA and depressive illness. The repeated demonstration of a bimodal distribution of CSF 5-HIAA in depressive illness suggests the existence of a subgroup of depressed patients with a disturbance of serotonin functions. A low CSF 5-HIAA is associated with an increased tendency to attempt suicide also in non-depressed individuals and with a different reaction to antidepressant drugs.

Key words: Serotonin, depressive illness, 5-hydroxyindoleacetic acid, cerebrospinal fluid, biochemical subgroups, tricyclic antidepressants, suicide.

INTRODUCTION

Are disturbances of serotonin turnover of any importance in depressive illness? The question has been researched for over a decade, but is still not definitely answered. This is perhaps not surprising, considering the difficulties in obtaining estimates of serotonin function in depressed patients, of obtaining adequate controls and also in defining comparable groups of depressed patients in different centers.

There have been several good reviews of the available evidence in this field (see for instance Murphy and co-workers, 1978 and Cowdry and Goodwin, 1978) and in this presentation we will limit ourselves to cerebrospinal fluid studies. Methodological problems will be discussed, and we will also present recent findings indicating a role for serotonin in some, but probably not all cases of depressive illness.

RESULTS AND DISCUSSION

CSF 5-HIAA as an Estimate of Serotonin Turnover

The most commonly used technique for assessing serotonin turnover in depressed patients is to measure concentrations of its main metabolite, 5-hydroxyindoleacetic acid (5-HIAA) in the lumbar cerebrospinal fluid (CSF). This is, of course, a very indirect measure, but as yet the most easily available one in a living patient.

The concentration of 5-HIAA in CSF depends not only on synthesis rate of the metabolite, but also on the active transport mechanism which removes the metabolite from CSF. Many investigators have tried to get rid of this additional source of variation between individuals, which is presumably of less interest in psychiatric disorders, by blocking the active transport with probenecid. This approach is theoretically attractive, but creates certain new problems, for instance how to deal with interindividual variability in probenecid metabolism (Sjöström, 1972, van Praag and co-workers, 1973a, Goodwin and co-workers, 1973). Probenecid may also alter the availability of tryptophan to brain, since it lowers tryptophan levels in plasma, possibly by displacing the amino acid from albumin (van Praag and co-workers, 1973b). Another obvious disadvantage with the probenecid technique is the increased discomfort to the patients, which makes large scale investigations difficult.

One advantage of the probenecid technique is that the concentrations of 5-HIAA will be higher, and differences between patients and controls are likely to be magnified. This places less heavy demands on the analytic techniques. We have, however, chosen not to use probenecid but rather to apply mass fragmentography for the 5-HIAA assessments, which ensures specificity and a very high analytical precision (Bertilsson and co-workers, 1972). It has recently been shown (Sjöquist and Johansson, 1978) that the correlation between mass fragmentographic and fluorometric assessments of 5-HIAA is quite poor ($r = 0.55$, $n = 17$).

The origin of 5-HIAA in CSF is another problem which has caused much debate. There is evidence that some of the 5-HIAA in lumbar CSF is derived from the spinal cord, rather than from the brain (Bulat and Zivkovic, 1971, cf also Jakupcevic and co-workers, 1977). This does not in itself invalidate any findings with CSF 5-HIAA, since possible disturbances may be shared by cord and brain neurons.

Conclusions drawn from the baseline levels of a transmitter metabolite in CSF to transmitter function in the CNS must naturally remain very tenuous. There is, however, indirect evidence that CSF monoamine metabolite levels do indeed mirror some neuronal events.

Drugs which are known to interfere with monoamine transmission also seem to change monoamine metabolite levels in the CSF in a predictable way. Neuroleptic drugs, which are dopamine receptor blockers, raise CSF levels of the dopamine metabolite homovanillic acid (HVA), probably because of a receptor feedback mediated increase of transmitter synthesis (Sedvall and co-workers, 1975). The noradrenaline agonist clonidine decreases CSF levels of the noradrenaline metabolite, 4-hydroxy--3-methoxyphenyl glycol (HMPG), but leaves HVA and 5-HIAA unaffected (Bertilsson and co-workers, 1977). Zimelidine, a relatively pure inhibitor of serotonin uptake, decreases 5-HIAA levels (Siwers and co-workers, 1978).

Chlorimipramine, which is a potent inhibitor of serotonin uptake, causes a pronounced decrease in CSF 5-HIAA, much more so than the preferential noradrenaline uptake inhibitor nortriptyline, which causes a more marked decrease in HMPG (Bertilsson and co-workers, 1974). Interestingly, the magnitude of the decrease in 5-HIAA caused by chlorimipramine is linearly related to the extent of the serotonin uptake inhibition, measured in vitro in patient plasma (essentially a bioassay of the non-proteinbound fraction of the drug) (Åsberg and co-workers, 1977). The total plasma level of the drug is also linearly correlated to the decrease in 5-HIAA, but only up to a certain critical drug level. Higher levels have little effect on the metabolite (Bertilsson and co-workers, 1978).

Chlorimipramine is demethylated in the body, and the demethyl metabolite is a potent inhibitor of noradrenaline uptake. There is a significant positive correlation between the plasma level of this metabolite, and the decrease in HMPG (but not in 5-HIAA). The decrease is also significantly correlated to the antidepressant effect (Träskman and co-workers, 1978). The CSF monoamine metabolite changes are thus precise enough to allow differentiation between a drug and its endogenously formed metabolite.

CSF 5-HIAA in Depressives and Controls

While the majority of studies of probenecid induced accumulation of CSF 5-HIAA have shown a lower accumulation in depressives than in controls, there is much more conflict about baseline levels. Since the differences, if any, are likely to be smaller when probenecid is not used, it is important that the controls are adequately selected, and that the procedure is performed in an identical way in both groups of subjects. This is particularly important, since there is a concentration gradient of 5-HIAA in the CSF (Gerbode and Bowers, 1968, Jakupcevic and co-workers, loc.cit.). This means that if a smaller amount of CSF were drawn from patients than from volunteers, a spurious difference in CSF 5-HIAA between the two groups could very easily be demonstrated.

In our studies, we have consistently worked with payed healthy volunteers, recruited among hospital staff and blood donors. It can perhaps be questioned how representative such volunteers may be for the "normal" population. Ongoing studies of their personalities will hopefully tell us more about this. But this selection of volunteers carries with it even more mundane problems: the volunteers tend to be younger, and more often of male sex, than the depressives who are typically middle-aged and elderly women.

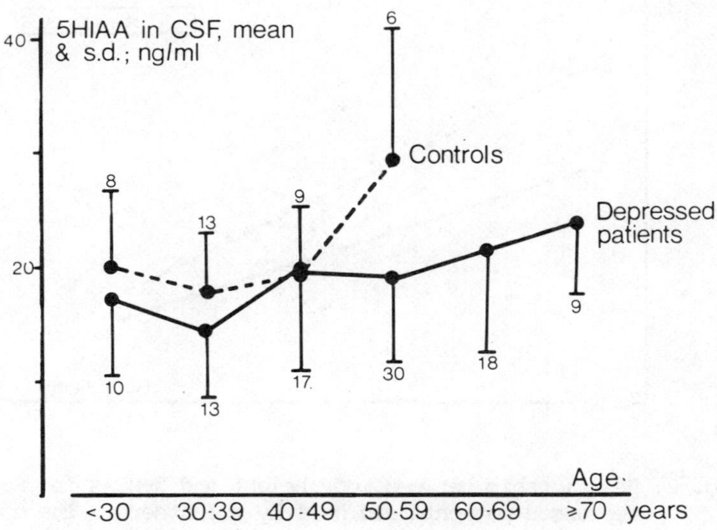

Fig. 1. CSF 5-HIAA in different age groups in controls (healthy volunteers) and depressed patients. The same amount of CSF was taken from each subject (13 ml) in the early morning after at least eight hours of fasting and bed rest. CSF was taken with a fine disposable needle with the subject in the sitting position. "Depression" was diagnosed according to the Newcastle inventory (Gurney and co-workers, 1972). 5-HIAA was analyzed according to the mass fragmentographic method described by Bertilsson and co-workers (1972).

Age and sex may both be important for CSF 5-HIAA. Most, but not all investigators report increasing levels in the higher age groups (Gottfries and co-workers, 1971, Åsberg and co-workers, 1973). In our volunteer material (Fig. 1), the association appears to be curvilinear with a rather steep rise above 50 years, in agreement with the findings of Bowers and Gerbode (1968) for neurological and psychiatric patients.

In our CSF studies, we have consistently found a tendency for women to have higher 5-HIAA than men (Åsberg and co-workers, 1978). A similar difference has been found for brain 5-HIAA by Gottfries and co-workers (1974). Once more, this sex difference is not found by all investigators. Coppen and co-workers (1972) for instance report slightly higher (although not significantly so) levels in men than in women.

In a recent study of psychotic patients Wode-Helgodt and Sedvall (1978) found that much of this sex difference could be accounted for by differences in body height. We find a similar association in depressed patients, obsessional patients and healthy volunteers. When this correlation is adjusted for by means of analysis of covariance, we find a significant difference between depressed patients and controls despite the difference in age (Fig. 2). The conflict among investigators who compare CSF 5-HIAA levels between depressed patients and controls

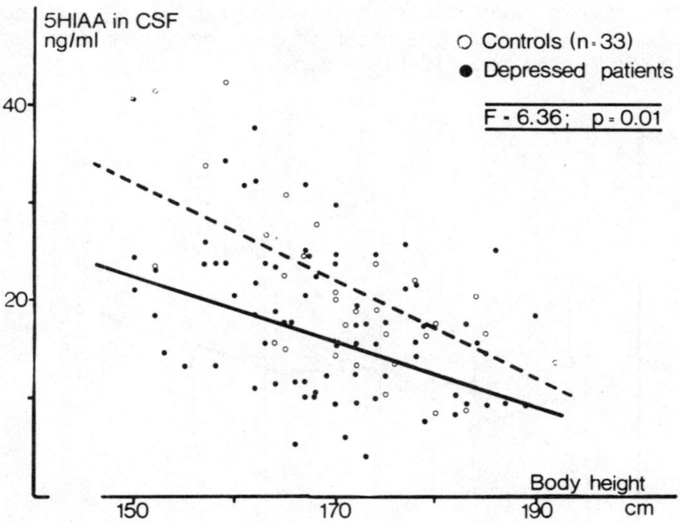

Fig. 2. Relationship between body height and 5-HIAA in CSF in depressed patients and healthy volunteers. The dotted line represents the regression line for controls, the unbroken line the regression in depressives. The difference is significant at the 1 per cent level according to analysis of covariance.

becomes more understandable in view of the fact that not even the importance of such variables as age and sex (which presumably can be measured with smaller experimental error than the presence of depressive illness!) are unanimously agreed on. In our opinion, this underlines the importance of attention to methodology in CSF studies.

We have tried to account for both body height and age differences by matching patients with volunteers. Such matching was possible for 27 pairs, and there was a significantly lower 5-HIAA in the depressive members of the pairs (Fig. 3).

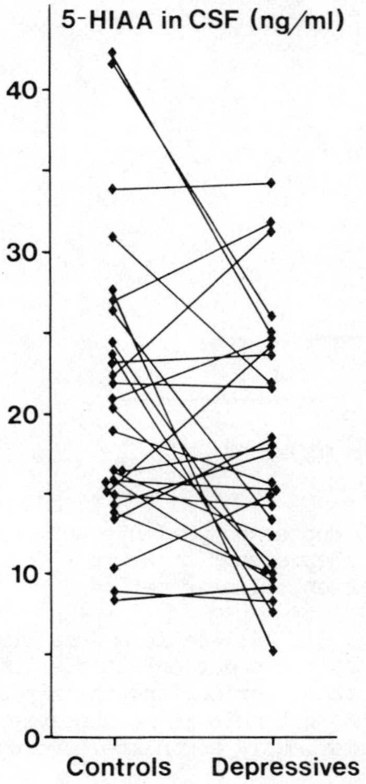

Fig. 3. CSF 5-HIAA in controls and depressives, matched for age (within 10 years) and height (within 10 cm). The difference is significant at the 5 per cent level (paired t-test; one-tailed).

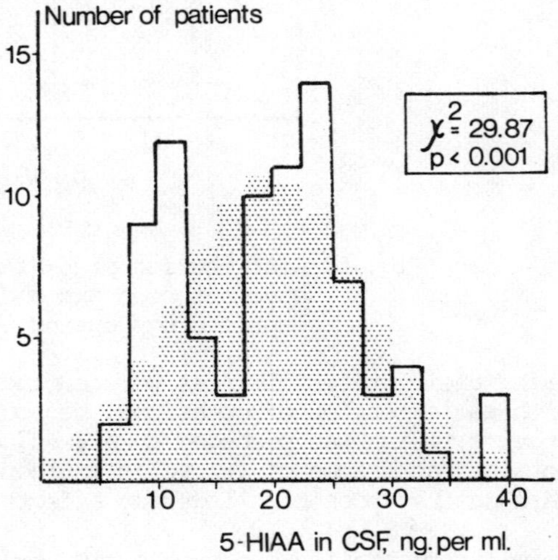

Fig. 4. Distribution of CSF 5-HIAA in 83 depressed patients. The shadowed area indicates the theoretical normal distribution, calculated from the mean and standard deviation of the observed distribution. The observed distribution deviates significantly from normality.

The mean differences between depressives and controls are, however, not very large and the majority of the patients have values within the "normal" range. The differences found in HVA levels between depressives and controls appear more impressive (depressives have significantly lower levels).

What is perhaps more interesting is that we have, in two consecutive patient groups, found a bimodal distribution of 5-HIAA concentrations (Åsberg and coworkers, 1973, Åsberg and co-workers, 1976a) (Fig. 4). This bimodality could not be explained by height or age, nor by previously given antidepressant drugs, since it was even more apparent when patients who had not received such drugs at all

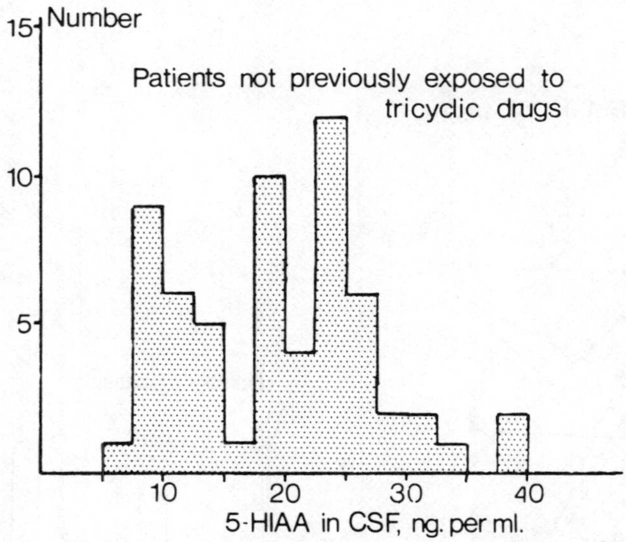

Fig. 5. Distribution of 5-HIAA in 60 depressed patients who have not been exposed to antidepressant or neuroleptic drugs during their present illness period.

during their present illness were excluded (Fig. 5). All patiens were drug free (with the exception of occasional bensodiazepines for sedation) at the lumbar puncture, which was preceded by a 4 - 7 days washout period, and their plasma contained no traces of tricyclic antidepressants, but this is no absolute safeguard against possible lingering effects from previously administered drugs.

A similar bimodality had previously been demonstrated by van Praag and Korf in 1971 for probenecid-induced accumulation of 5-HIAA. These authors (van Praag and co-workers, 1972) found an antidepressant effect of the serotonin precursor amino acid 5-hydroxy-tryptophan among patients with low pretreatment 5-HIAA, and suggest that they might have a disturbance of serotonin turnover. Our finding that patients with low pretreatment 5-HIAA do less well on treatment with the noradrenaline uptake inhibitor nortriptyline falls well in line with this contention (Åsberg and co-workers, 1973).

Low CSF 5-HIAA - State-Dependent or Constitutional?

It is not yet known whether the low 5-HIAA levels in CSF encountered in some depressed patients are a function of the illness, or whether they remain low when the patient has recovered.

In our volunteer studies, there is little change in CSF 5-HIAA over a period of three weeks ($r = 0.84$, $n = 16$). Studies in depressed patients are more difficult to perform, since they require that the patient is drug free. This is not often the case, since so many depressed patients receive long-term treatment. We have, however, been able to investigate a number of patients who have been readmitted for a second illness period and in these cases, the levels have remained fairly stable. Nine patients have also been investigated during remission, 3-6 years after their illness, and also here, the levels have remained quite stable (Fig. 6).

The number of patients is, however, as yet too small to allow any definite conclusions.

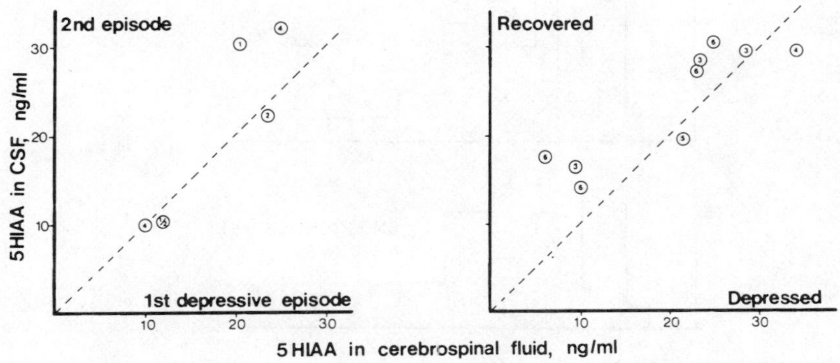

Fig. 6. Left: CSF 5-HIAA at first and second episode of depressive illness in 5 patients. Time interval between the two examinations is indicated in the circles (1/2 - 4 years). Right: CSF 5-HIAA in 9 depressed patients during depression and during remission. Time interval is indicated in the circles (3 - 6 years). All subjects were drug free at both lumbar punctures.

CSF 5-HIAA in Different Diagnostic Subtypes of Depression

Patient selection criteria apparently affect the shape of the distribution of CSF 5-HIAA. In our first studies (Fig. 4) the inclusion criteria were that the patient should be clinically judged to suffer from a primary depressive illness, which was thought severe enough to require antidepressant treatment. In a later patient group, we have the possibility of studying distributions when criteria of increasing severity are used. In Fig. 7, the upper panel shows the 5-HIAA distribution in patients diagnosed by the Newcastle inventory (Gurney and co-workers, 1972) as depressed (regardless of the treatment criterion). The mid panel shows the patients in this group who received a diagnosis of endogenous depression on the Newcastle Inventory, and the bottom panel shows the still smaller group who have received a WHO diagnosis of endogenous depression on release from hospital (in our present diagnostic tradition, this diagnosis is used only sparingly, and the Newcastle Inventory clearly overdiagnoses endogenous illness in comparison with the clinical diagnoses). As seen from the Figure, the shapes of the distributions change with the severity of criteria.

CSF 5-HIAA and Clinical Correlates

A 5-HIAA concentration below 15 ng/ml - the antimode in our depressed patients - is by no means exclusive to depressive illness. Such levels are not uncommon among healthy volunteers who lack any evidence of psychiatric disturbance as well as heredity for such illnesses. They also occur among patients with obsessive disorder, where a low CSF 5-HIAA predicts a poorer outcome on treatment with the serotonin uptake inhibitor chlorimipramine (Thorén and co-workers, unpublished data).

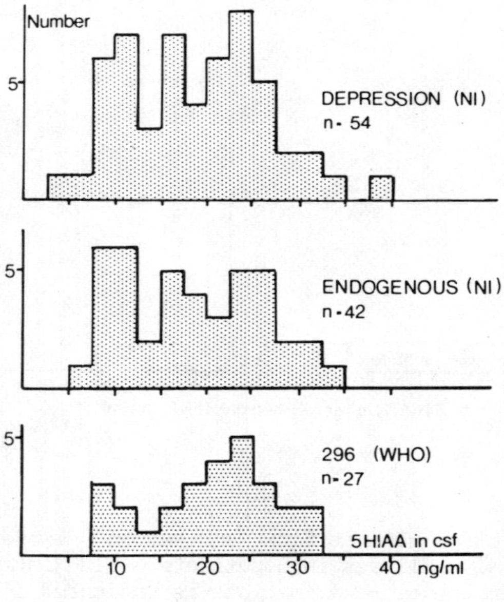

Fig. 7. Distribution of 5-HIAA in CSF in depressed patients diagnosed according to different criteria (see text).

One unexpected and interesting clinical correlate to a low CSF 5-HIAA in depressives was a significantly higher incidence of suicide attempts, particularly of an active, violent type in the low 5-HIAA group (Åsberg and co-workers, 1976b). We have recently replicated this finding and also showed that the association between a low CSF 5-HIAA and violent suicide attempts hold for non-depressed suicide attempters as well. It is, however, well known that men tend to make more violent suicide attempts and they also have lower 5-HIAA levels. We have therefore, in the comparison shown in Fig. 8, adjusted all 5-HIAA levels to a body height of 170 cm by means of the regression equation. Of the 44 suicide attempters (depressed or non-depressed) in this group, 6 were found at follow-up to have completed suicide. All of these, as well as all of those who made "violent" attempts (i.e. not drug over-doses or wrist cutting) had CSF 5-HIAA levels at the lower end of the distribution.

COMMENTS

"Depression" is a quite unspecific reaction pattern which may occur in several psychiatric as well as somatic conditions. Already for that reason, it seems less likely that the syndrome should always be associated with a reduced serotonin turnover. It is also clear from the studies reported by ourselves and others that there is no one-to-one relationship between a low CSF 5-HIAA and a depressive syndrome.

The existence of a group of depressed individuals with very low CSF 5-HIAA levels, the association with violent suicide attempts, also in non-depressed individuals, and the predictable changes in CSF 5-HIAA levels caused by antidepressant drugs, however, support the meaningfulness of the variable for psychiatric disturbances. Perhaps the association with clinical variables should be sought, not in a particular psychiatric syndrome but rather in some more subtle personality trait, which might predispose for manifest psychiatric disorder. Aggression or hostility is one such interesting candidate for study in view of the aggressive character of many suicide attempts, the classical psychoanalytical association between aggression and depression, and the many animal experiments that point to a role for a serotonin deficiency in certain forms of aggressive behaviour.

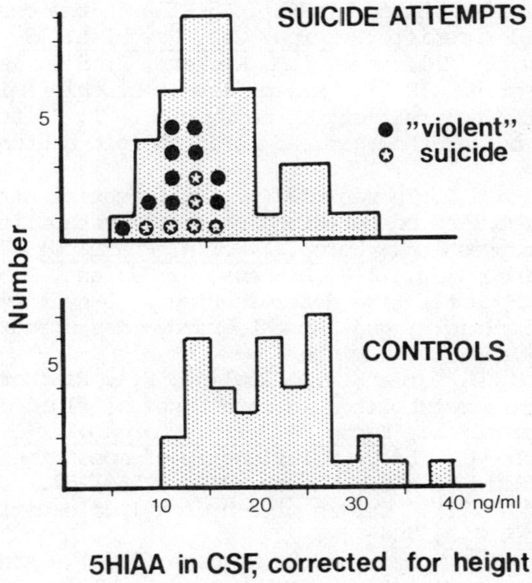

Fig. 8. CSF 5-HIAA adjusted to a body height of 170 cm (using the regression equation, see text) in 44 suicide attempters and 37 healthy controls. Black dots indicate suicide attempts by any other means than drug overdose or wrist cutting. Stars indicate patients who were found to have committed suicide at follow up. Follow up period varies from 3 months to 6 years.

ACKNOWLEDGEMENTS

The skilled assistance of the staff at the Psychiatric Clinic, Karolinska Hospital, and of Gunnel Tybring is gratefully acknowledged. The studies have been supported by The Tercentenary Fund of the Bank of Sweden (74/110), The Swedish Medical Research Council (29X-05015; 04X-03902; 21P-4676; 21X-05454) and by funds from the Karolinska Institute.

REFERENCES

Åsberg, M., L. Bertilsson, P. Thorén, and L. Träskman (1978). CSF monoamine metabolites in depressive illness. In S. Garattini (Ed.), Depressive Disorders, Schattauer Verlag, Stuttgart-New York, pp 293-305.

Åsberg, M., L. Bertilsson, D. Tuck, B. Cronholm, and F. Sjöqvist (1973). Indoleamine metabolites in the cerebrospinal fluid of depressed patients before and during treatment with nortriptyline. Clin. Pharmacol. Ther. 14, 277-286.

Åsberg, M., V.-A. Ringberger, F. Sjöqvist, P. Thorén, L. Träskman and J.R. Tuck (1977). Monoamine metabolites in cerebrospinal fluid and serotonin uptake inhibition during treatment with chlorimipramine. Clin. Pharmacol. Ther. 21, 201-207.

Åsberg, M., P. Thorén, L. Träskman, L. Bertilsson and V. Ringberger (1976a). "Serotonin depression" - a biochemical subgroup within the affective disorders? Science, 191, 478-480.

Åsberg, M., L. Träskman and P. Thorén (1976b). 5-HIAA in the cerebrospinal fluid - a biochemical suicide predictor? Arch. Gen. Psychiat. 33, 1193-1197.

Bertilsson, L., M. Åsberg, B. Mellström, L.M. Neckers, F. Sjöqvist, P. Thorén, L. Träskman and G. Tybring (1978). Plasma levels of chlorimipramine and its demethyl metabolite during treatment of depression. I. Differential effects of the two compounds on serotonergic and noradrenergic neurons. Submitted for publication.

Bertilsson, L., M. Åsberg and P. Thorén (1974). Differential effect of chlorimipramine and nortriptyline on cerebrospinal fluid metabolites of serotonin an noradrenaline in depression. Europ. J. clin. Pharmacol. 7, 365-368.

Bertilsson, L., A.J. Atkinson, Jr., J.R. Althaus, Å. Härfast, J.-E. Lindgren and B. Holmstedt (1972). Quantitative determination of 5-hydroxyindole-3-acetic acid in cerebrospinal fluid by gas chromatography-mass spectrometry. Anal. Chem. 44, 1434-1438.

Bertilsson, L., K. Haglund, J. Östman, M.D. Rawlins, V.A. Ringberger and F. Sjöqvist (1977). Monoamine metabolites in cerebrospinal fluid during treatment with clonidine or alprenolol. Europ. J. clin. Pharmacol. 11, 125-128.

Bowers, M.B. and F.A. Gerbode (1968). Relationship of monoamine metabolites in human cerebrospinal fluid to age. Nature, 219, 1256-1257.

Bulat, M. and B. Zivković (1971). Origin of 5-hydroxyindoleacetic acid in the spinal fluid. Science, 173, 738-740.

Coppen, A., A.J. Prange, P.C. Whybrow and R. Noguera (1972). Abnormalities of indoleamines in affective disorders. Arch. Gen. Psychiat. 26, 474-478.

Cowdry, R.W. and F.K. Goodwin (1978). Amine neurotransmitter studies and psychiatric illness: Toward more meaningful diagnostic concepts. In R.L. Spitzer and D.F. Klein (Eds.), Clinical Issues in Psychiatric Diagnosis, Raven Press, New York, pp. 281-304.

Gerbode, F.A. and M.B. Bowers (1968). Measurement of acid monoamine metabolites in human and animal cerebrospinal fluid. J. Neurochem. 15, 1053-1055.

Goodwin, F., R.M. Post, D.L. Dunner and E.K. Gordon (1973). Cerebrospinal fluid amine metabolites in affective illness: The probenecid technique. Am. J. Psychiatry, 130, 73-78.

Gottfries, C.G., I. Gottfries, B. Johansson, R. Olsson, T. Persson, B.-E. Roos and R. Sjöström (1971). Acid monoamine metabolites in human cerebrospinal fluid and their relations to age and sex. Neuropharmacology, 10, 665-672.

Gottfries, C.G., B.-E. Roos and B. Winblad (1974). Determination of 5-hydroxytryptamine, 5-hydroxyindoleacetic acid and homovanillic acid in brain tissue from an autopsy material. Acta psychiat. scand. 50, 496-507.

Gurney, C., M. Roth, R.F. Garside, T.A. Kerr and K. Schapira (1972). Studies in the classification of affective disorders. The relationship between anxiety states and depressive illnesses - II. Brit. J. Psychiat. 121, 162-166.

Jakupcević, M., Z. Lacković, D. Stefoski and M. Bulat (1977). Nonhomogenous distribution of 5-hydroxyindoleacetic acid and homovanillic acid in the lumbar cerebrospinal fluid of man. J. Neurol. Sci. 31, 165-171.

Murphy, D.L., I.C. Campbell and J.L. Costa (1978). The brain serotonergic system in the affective disorders. Prog. Neuro-Psychopharmac. 2, 1-31.

van Praag, H.M., F. Flentge, J. Korf, L.C.W. Dols and R. Schut (1973a). The influence of probenecid on the metabolism of serotonin, dopamine and their precursors in man. Psychopharmacologia, 33, 141-151.

van Praag, H.M. and J. Korf (1971). Endogenous depressions with and without disturbances in the 5-hydroxytryptamine metabolism: a biochemical classification? Psychopharmacologia, 19, 148-152.

van Praag, H.M., J. Korf, L.C.W. Dols and T. Schut (1972). A pilot study of the predictive value of the probenecid test in application of 5-hydroxytryptophan as an antidepressant. Psychopharmacologia, 25, 14-21.

van Praag, H.M., J. Korf and D. Schut (1973b). Cerebral monoamines and depression. Arch. Gen. Psychiatry, 28, 827-831.

Sedvall, G., G. Alfredsson, L. Bjerkenstedt, P. Eneroth, B. Fyrö, C. Härnryd, C.-G. Swahn, F.-A. Wiesel and B. Wode-Helgodt (1975). Selective effects of psychoactive drugs on levels of monoamine metabolites and prolactin in cerebrospinal fluid of psychiatric patients. Proc. Sixth International Congress Pharmacology, 3, 255-267.

Siwers, B., V.-A. Ringberger, J.R. Tuck and F. Sjöqvist (1977). Initial clinical trial based on biochemical methodology of zimelidine (a serotonin uptake inhibitor) in depressed patients. Clin. Pharmacol. Ther. 21, 194-200.

Sjöquist, B. and B. Johansson (1978). A comparison between fluorometric and mass fragmentographic determinations of homovanillic acid and 5-hydroxyindoleacetic acid in human cerebrospinal fluid. J. Neurochem. 31, 621-625.

Sjöström, R. (1972). Steady-state levels of probenecid and their relation to acid monoamine metabolites in human cerebrospinal fluid. Psychopharmacologia, 25, 96-100.

Träskman, L., M. Åsberg, L. Bertilsson, B. Cronholm, B. Mellström and P. Thorén (1978). Plasma levels of chlorimipramine and its demethyl metabolite during treatment of depression. II. Antidepressant effect in biochemical subgroups. Submitted for publication.

Wode-Helgodt, B. and G. Sedvall (1978). Correlations between height of subject and concentrations of monoamine metabolites in cerebrospinal fluid from psychotic men and women. Commun. in Psychopharmacology, 2, 177-183.

Obsessive-Compulsive Disorders: A Serotonergic Hypothesis

J. A. YARYURA-TOBIAS*, F. NEZIROGLU* and H. N. BHAGAVAN

*Division of Research, North Nassau Mental Health Center, Manhasset, New York 11030, U.S.A.

ABSTRACT

Obsessive-compulsive disorders are characterized by two main groups of symptoms, viz. (a) obsessions manifested by unpleasant and intrusive thoughts, images or melodies that dwell in the mind and cannot be repelled, and (b) compulsions, described by an urge to perform an act. Anxiety, depression, aggressive behavior, sexual pathology and family disturbances are secondary manifestations of obsessive-compulsive disorders. A high incidence of obsessive-compulsive symptoms observed in Gilles De La Tourette Syndrome, Lesch-Nyhan Syndrome, Parkinsonian Syndromes, Epilepsy, Primary Anorexia Nervosa, and certain forms of severe Self-Mutilation, suggested an organic pathology for obsessive-compulsive disorders. Based on the therapeutic efficacy of chlorimipramine, a potent serotonin re-uptake blocker, and L-tryptophan, a precursor of serotonin, a serotonergic theory for the physiopathology of obsessive-compulsive disorders was put forward. Biochemical data obtained from patients showed low blood levels of serotonin when compared to a control population ($p < .05$). Currently, clinical grouping of patients and biochemical studies of the indolamine pathway are being conducted.

KEYWORDS

Obsessions, Compulsions, Chlorimipramine, L-Tryptophan, Serotonin, Hypothalamus

INTRODUCTION

Obsessive-compulsive disorders (OCD) are a group of neuropsychiatric entities characterized by the presence of ideational and motor symptomatology. From this group of disorders, we have studied in depth obsessive-compulsive neurosis. What has traditionally been called obsessive-compulsive neurosis, we term true OCD in order to differentiate it from other types of illnesses which encompass obsessive-compulsive symptoms. In all the studies, The Research Diagnostic Criteria (Spitzer, Endicott, and Robins, 1977) was used for diagnostic purposes.

<u>Obsessions</u> are defined as intrusive thoughts, images or melodies that cannot be repelled from the mind, whereas <u>compulsions</u> are an urge or need to perform an ideational or motor act that cannot be postponed (see Table 1).

TABLE 1 Obsessive-Compulsive Symptoms

Ideational	Doubtful Intrusive Obstinate Magic
Motor	Iterative Ritualistic

The characteristics of obsessive-compulsive thoughts are best described by their magical quality, doubtfulness, unpleasantness, and unproductiveness. The motor symptomatology is basically iterative and can be seen in the performance of routine tasks, physiological activities, nonsensical acts, and movements (see Table 2). In addition, many of these patients manifest sexual disorders, aggressive behavior, and family constellation disturbances. As a result, symptoms of anxiety and depression become manifest; and at times, due to their intensity, they mask the primary symptoms.

TABLE 2 Motor Aspects of Compulsions

Routine	Double checking Cleaning Hand washing
Bizarre	Self-Mutilation
Physiological	Eating Drinking
Nonsensical	Touching Tapping Tics Grimacing Jumping

In spite of its bizarre behavior, reality testing is intact; yet a true OCD is commonly misdiagnosed as schizophrenia. Furthermore, the abnormal behavior embarrasses the patient who usually waits for an aggravation of symptoms to seek help. Due to the diversity of symptoms, it is also mistakingly diagnosed as panneurosis, anxiety neurosis, depressive neurosis, and rarely as manic depressive illness. The premorbid personality usually comprises rigidity of thought, aggressive behavior, meticulosity, and high verbal intellectual quotient.

From our true OCD sample, we have separated one subgroup with manic depressive illness, as previously mentioned by Kleist (1921); a second one comprising anorexia and self-mutilation (Yaryura-Tobias and Neziroglu, 1978), and a third one with perceptual changes (Neziroglu, 1976). A list of neuropsychiatric entities that present obsessive-compulsive symptoms can be seen in Table 3.

It is important to note in what entities common symptoms occur since it may lead to further conclusions regarding its biochemical basis and/or anatomical location.

TABLE 3 Clinical Symptoms with Obsessive-Compulsive Symptoms

True Obsessive-Compulsive Disorder
Gilles De La Tourette Syndrome
Primary Anorexia Nervosa
Anorectic-Mutilating Syndrome
Lesch-Nyhan Syndrome
Psychosis
Epilepsy
Mental Retardation
Parkinsonism
Schizophrenia
Manic Depressive Illness

The etiopathology of true OCD has been accepted as psychodynamic since the early work of Freud. Its treatment has embraced a wide variety of approaches including psychoanalysis, chemotherapy, behavioral therapy, and in the intractable patient, psychosurgery. Of all these therapeutic modalities, best results appeared to have been obtained by the use of behavioral therapy (Wolpe, 1958; Solyom, 1969; Marks, Rachman, and Hodgson, 1975; Rabavilas, Boulougouris, and Stefanis, 1976; Neziroglu and Yaryura-Tobias, 1977; Solyom and Sookman, 1977; Foa and Goldstein, in press) or by the use of chlorimipramine* (CLI) (Fernández and López-Ibor, 1967; Rack, 1970; Capstick, 1975; Yaryura-Tobias and Neziroglu, 1975; Yaryura-Tobias, Neziroglu, and Bergman, 1976).

We selected CLI as the treatment of choice for obsessive-compulsive symptoms (see Table 4), since its therapeutic efficacy surpassed other modes of therapy as compared to other reports in the literature primarily in terms of rate of recovery and total reduction of symptoms. Besides, its potent re-uptake blocking action on serotonin (5-HT) tacitly supported the foundation for the proposal of an organic theory of OCD.

TABLE 4 Sample Population with Obsessive-Compulsive Symptoms Period 1974-78

True Obsessive-Compulsive Disorders	150
Gilles De La Tourette Syndrome	60
Anorectic-Mutilating Syndrome	24
Lesch-Nyhan Syndrome	4
Schizophrenia	11
Mental Retardation	4
Epilepsy	4
Manic Depressive Subgroup	8
Perceptual Disorders Subgroup	29
Total	294

It was postulated that true OCD are the result of a serotonin disturbance (Yaryura-Tobias, 1976). To test this hypothesis, whole blood 5-HT levels and 24-hour urinary 5-hydroxyindoleacetic acid (5-HIAA) were measured in a control sample (N=11) and in true OCD patients (N=21) before and after treatment. Results indicated that patients had lower blood 5-HT values when compared to controls ($p < 0.01$) (Yaryura-Tobias and others, 1977). Since Tryptophan (Trp) is the precursor

*ANAFRANIL, T.M., Courtesy of CIBA-GEIGY, U.S.A.

of 5-HT and its availability regulates 5-HT synthesis in brain (Moir and Eccleston, 1968; Fernstrom and Wurtman, 1971), we administered L-Trp, niacinamide, and pyridoxine to seven true OCD patients. Niacinamide was given to inhibit the kynurenic pathway and thus make more Trp available for 5-HT synthesis (Scherer and Kramer, 1972). Results were moderately good (Yaryura-Tobias and Bhagavan, 1977).

Based on the report that the action of CLI is potentiated by Trp administration in the treatment of depression (Walinder and others, 1976), we treated approximately 100 patients by giving CLI, L-Trp, niacinamide, and pyridoxine (see Table 5). On this regimen, we were able to reduce the amount of CLI administered by 50 percent. We have also used in a group of five true OCD patients a combination of L-Trp and the MAOI tranylcypromine with negative results.

TABLE 5 Combined Treatment for Obsessive-Compulsive Disorders

Chlorimipramine	1 mg/kg body weight/day
L-Tryptophan*	50-100 mg/kg body weight/day
Niacinamide	15-30 mg/kg body weight/day
Pyridoxine	1.5-3.0 mg/kg body weight/day

*To be given on an empty stomach.

On the other hand, amytryptiline and desipramine, two tricyclical antidepressants, reported to be more selective for blocking norepinephrine (NE) uptake, have been considered efficacious for the treatment of true OCD symptoms (Ananth and Van Den Stenn, 1977). Contrariwise, some of our patients that have used these medications did not benefit from them. Nevertheless, we entertained the possibility of a NE-5-HT imbalance in the physiopathology of OCD, since both NE and 5-HT appear to be equally distributed in the hypothalamic area; for us an anatomical region theoretically involved in the pathology of OCD. Therefore, we decided to use Nisoxetine Hydrochloride*, a non-tricyclical antidepressant with specific NE blocking activity. Our results were negative after a double-blind placebo ten-week study with 24 true OCD patients. These findings pointed out, once again, a predominant serotonergic involvement in OCD.

Further clinical evidence of CLI activity on serotonin levels are given by some of its side effects (see Table 6) which are similar to the pharmacological actions of 5-HT (see Table 7).

TABLE 6 Main Side Effects of Chlorimipramine Therapy

Dry mouth	Antidiuretic effect
Perspiration	Sedation
Nausea	Sleepiness
Hypotension	Delayed Ejaculation

It is of interest to mention that the hypothalamus appears to regulate some of the functions already mentioned as side effects: sexual drive, glucose metabolism, sleep mechanism, aggressive behavior, thirst, and appetite. As previously indicated, in this region, high concentrations of norepinephrine and serotonin are found. Furthermore, the psychosurgical treatment of true OCD, Gilles De La Tourette Syndrome, Primary Anorexia Nervosa, and Self-Mutilation has been directed

*Courtesy of ELI LILLY, U.S.A.

TABLE 7 Pharmacological Actions of 5-HT

Vasodilation (Due to Histamine Liberation)
Orthostatic Hypotension (Bezold-Jarisch Reflex)
Antidiuretic (Renal Vascular Response)
Decrease in Pain Threshold
Antiaggressive
Psychotomimetic Precursor

towards ablations in or around the hypothalamic region (Sano, 1960; Hassler and Dieckmann, 1970; Nadvornik and others, 1972; Laitinen and Livingston, 1973; Bridges and Goktepe, 1973; Post and Schurr, 1977). Therefore, these surgical procedures may indirectly indicate the hypothetical and anatomical site of OCD. A review by Flor-Henry (1975) on psychosurgery may be helpful to those interested in this aspect.

Long ago, Schilder (1938) and Schwab, Fabing, and Pritchard (1951) reported the presence of obsessive-compulsive symptoms in Parkinsonian patients. Also, soft neurological symptoms appeared to be present in many OCD patients. Thus, it may be possible that these entities may be histochemically related, suggesting the presence of syndromes that may go unnoticed, may be incorrectly classified, or simply overlapped. For instance, the findings on perceptual changes (Neziroglu and Yaryura-Tobias, 1977) in a subgroup of 29 OCD patients may clinically indicate a link with the physiopathology of schizophrenia since 5-HT has been implicated as a factor in the biochemistry of schizophrenia by Wooley and Shaw (1954) and Smythies (1967) among others. Likewise, the same could be said by biochemical theories of psychoaffective disorders such as in the subgroup of OCD with manic depressive illness.

Should we link our postulates and findings to those theories?

Chlorimipramine and/or L-Trp has been used in depression and manic depressive illness with considerable good results (Wilson and Prange, 1972; Prange and others, 1974; Murphy, 1975; Roos and others, 1975). The pharmacotherapeutic use of these drugs may indicate common elements with OCD. In depression, a combination of Trp and a MAOI was used by Coppen, Shaw, and Farrell (1963), Trp and a pyrrolase inhibitor (nicotinamide, allopurinol, or glucose) by Badawy and Evans (1975); whereas Trp with nicotinamide has been used by Chouinard and others (1977).

Some of the side effects of prolonged therapy with L-Trp are worth mentioning, since those side effects may indicate target zones of a pharmacological action that can be useful to support our hypothesis of work. For instance, drowsiness, calming effect, hypnotic effect, sexual arousal, aggressive behavior, hypomanic state, worsening of psychosis, and increased activity in the slow wave bands of the EEG had been reported (Greenwood and others, 1975; Shopsin, 1976; Morgan, 1977; Yaryura-Tobias, 1978).

The clinical observations made by Neziroglu (1977) in regard to perceptual changes in OCD and her recent findings that therapeutic responses may not be identical in those patients who have prominent symptoms of hand washing and double-checking as compared to other OCD symptoms suggested further studies to determine whether biological differences were present.

True obsessive-compulsive patients were divided in four groups as follows: (a) true OCD without perceptual changes; (b) true OCD with perceptual changes; (c) true OCD with hand washing and double-checking symptoms; (d) true OCD with other symptoms (symmetry, tapping, touching, etc.). Base levels of whole blood 5-HT were obtained in all of them, and intergroup differences were studied. Significant differences were found in whole blood 5-HT between controls and OCD (see Table 8), washers and checkers (see Table 9), and ideational and motor (see Table 10). Contrariwise, 5-HIAA and plasma free and total Trp did not show significant differences between groups. Therefore, it may be assumed that the indolamine defect lies between the conversion of Trp into 5-HT.

TABLE 8 Blood 5-HT, Urinary 5-HIAA, and Plasma Total and Free Tryptophan in OCD Patients and Controls

	Blood 5-HT (μg/ml)	Urinary 5-HIAA (mg/24 hrs)	Total Tryptophan (μg/ml)	Free Tryptophan (μg/ml)
Patients	$\bar{x}$=0.17(19)*	$\bar{x}$=3.36(8)*	$\bar{x}$=10.55(8)*	$\bar{x}$=1.06(8)*
	$\bar{x}$=0.14(71)	$\bar{x}$=3.70(55)	$\bar{x}$= 9.90(28)	$\bar{x}$=1.04(28)
Controls	$\bar{x}$=0.18(19)	$\bar{x}$=4.60(8)	$\bar{x}$=10.11(8)	$\bar{x}$=1.08(8)
T-Test	T(36)=2.0299 $p < .05$			
	T(88)=3.7813 $p < .05$			

*Randomly selected out of the total.

TABLE 9 Blood 5-HT, Urinary 5-HIAA, and Plasma Total and Free Tryptophan in Combined Group of Washer and Checker vs. Other OCD

	Blood 5-HT (μg/ml)	Urinary 5-HIAA (mg/24 hrs)	Total Tryptophan (μg/ml)	Free Tryptophan (μg/ml)
Washers + Checkers	$\bar{x}$=0.14(27)	$\bar{x}$=3.84(33)	$\bar{x}$=10.36(13)	$\bar{x}$=1.01(13)
Other OC Patients	$\bar{x}$=0.16(27)	$\bar{x}$=4.23(21)	$\bar{x}$= 9.60(14)	$\bar{x}$=1.04(14)
T-Test	T(52)=2.5974 $p < .05$	$p > .05$	$p > .05$	$p > .05$

TABLE 10 Blood 5-HT, Urinary 5-HIAA, and Plasma Total and Free Tryptophan in Ideational and Motor OCD

	Blood 5-HT (µg/ml)	Urinary 5-HIAA (mg/24 hrs)	Total Tryptophan (µg/ml)	Free Tryptophan (µg/ml)
Ideational	x=0.17(12)	x=4.21(11)	x=10.41(3)	x=1.08(3)
Motor	x=0.13(12)	x=3.23(11)	x= 9.79(24)	x=1.02(24)
T-Test	t(22)=4.14 $p < .01$	$p > .01$		

The lower 5-HT levels in motor compulsions as compared to ideational symptomatology is not yet fully understood. We are currently investigating these aspects of OCD.

REFERENCES

Ananth, J. and Van Den Stenn, N. (1977). Systematic studies in the treatment of obsessive-compulsive neurosis with tricyclic antidepressants. Curr. Ther. Res., 21, 495-501.

Badawy, A. B. -B. and Evans, M. (1975). Tryptophan plus a pyrrolase inhibitor for depression. Lancet, II, 869.

Bridges, P. K. and Goktepe, E. O. (1973). A review of patients with obsessional symptoms treated by psychosurgery. In L. V. Laitinen and K. E. Livingston (Eds.), Surgical Approaches in Psychiatry. Proceedings of the Third Internatinal Congress of Psychosurgery. University Park Press, Baltimore. pp. 96-100.

Capstick, N. (1975). Depressive reactions in the course of chlorimipramine therapy used in the treatment of obsessional conditions. Scot. Med. J., 20, 45-48.

Chouinard, G., Young, S. N., Annable, L, and Sourkes, T. L. (1977). Tryptophan-nicotinamide combination in depression. Lancet, I, 249.

Coppen, A., Shaw, D. M., Farrell, J. P. (1963). Potentiation of the antidepressive effect of a monoamine-oxidase inhibitor by tryptophan. Lancet, I, 79-81.

Fernández, C. E. and López-Ibor, J. S. (1967). Monochlorimipramine in the treatment of psychiatric patients resistant to other therapies. Act. Iuso Exp. Neurol., 26, 119-147.

Fernstrom, J. A. and Wurtman, R. J. (1971). Brain serotonin content: physiological dependence on plasma tryptophan levels. Science, 173, 149-152.

Flor-Henry, P. (1975). Psychiatric surgery-1935-1973. Evolution and current perspectives. Canad. Psychiat. Assoc. J., 20, 157-167.

Foa, E. B. and Goldstein, A. (in press). Continuous exposure and complete response prevention in the treatment of obsessive-compulsive neurosis. Behavior Therapy.

Greenwood, M. H., Lader, M. H., Kantameneni, B. D., and Curzon, G. (1975). The acute effects of oral (—)-Tryptophan in human subjects. Br. J. Clin. Pharmac., 2, 165-172.

Hassler, R. and Dieckmann, G. (1970). Traitement of stereotaxique des tics et cris inarticules ou coprolaliques consideres comme phenomene d'obsession. Motrice au cours de la maladie de Gilles De La Tourette. Revue Neurologique, 2, 89-100.

Kleist, K. (1921). Autochthonous psychoses of degeneration. Z. ges. Neurol. Psychiat., 69, 215-298.

Laitinen, L. V. and Livingston, K. E. (1973). Surgical Approaches in Psychiatry. Proceedings of the Third International Congress in Psychosurgery. University Park Press, Baltimore.

Marks, I. M., Rachman, S., and Hodgson, R. (1975). Treatment of obsessive-compulsive neurosis: Two year follow-up. Br. J. Psychiat., 127, 349-364.

Moir, A. T. B. and Eccleston, D. (1968). The effects of precursor loading in the cerebral metabolism of 5-hydroxyindoles. J. Neurochem., 15, 1093-1108.

Morgan, R. (1977). Tryptophan overdosage. Br. J. Psychiat., 131, 548.

Murphy, J. (1975). A comparative clinical trial of Org. GB 94 and imipramine in the treatment of depression in general practice. J. Int. Med. Res., 3, 251-260.

Nadvornik, P., Sramka, M., Lisy, L., and Svicka, I. (1972). Experiences with dentatotomy. Confin. Neurol., 34, 320-324.

Neziroglu, F. (1976). Unpublished data.

Neziroglu, F. (1977). Personal communication.

Neziroglu, F. and Yaryura-Tobias, J. A. (1977). Usage of behavior therapy and chlorimipramine in the treatment of obsessive-compulsive and phobic behavior. Presented at the 11th Meeting of Association for Advancement of Behavior Therapy, Atlanta, Georgia, December 9-11, 1977.

Post, F. and Schurr, P. H. (1977). Changes in the pattern of diagnosis of patients subjected to psychosurgical procedures with comments on their use in the treatment of self-mutilation and anorexia nervosa. In W. H. Sweet, S. Obrador, and J. G. Martin-Rodriguez (Eds.), Neurosurgical Treatment in Psychiatry, Pain, and Epilepsy. University Park Press, Baltimore, pp. 261-266.

Prange, A. J., Wilson, I. C., Lynn, C. W., Alltop, L. B., and Stikeleather, R. A. (1974). L-tryptophan in mania. Arch. Gen. Psychiat., 30, 56-62.

Rabavilas, A. D., Boulougouris, J. C., and Stefanis, C. (1976). Duration of flooding sessions in the treatment of obsessive-compulsive patients. Behav. Res. and Therapy, 14, 349-355.

Rack, P. H. (1970). Experience with intravenous Clomipramine. In Obsessional States and their Treatment with Anafranil. Geigy, pp. 10-13.

Roos, B. E., Beskow, J., Carlsson, A., Gottfries, C. G., Skott, A., Winblad, B., Walinder, J., and Ohman, E. (1975). Tryptophane 5-HTP and tricyclic antidepressants in the treatment of depressions. Agents and Actions, 5, 503-504.

Sano, K. (1960). Sedative stereoencephalotomy: fornicotomy, upper mesencephalic reticulotomy and postero-medial hypothalotomy. In T. Tokisane and J. P. Shade (Eds.), Progress in Brain Research. Part B. Clinical Studies. Elsevier, Amsterdam 21B.

Scherer, B. and Kramer, W. (1972). Influence of niacinamide administration on brain 5-HT and a possible mode of action. Life Sci., 11, 189-195.

Schilder, P. (1938). The organic background of obsessions and compulsions. Amer. J. Psychiat., 94, 1397-1416.

Schwab, R. S., Fabing, H. D., and Pritchard, J. S. (1951). Psychiatric symptoms and syndromes in Parkinson's Disease. Amer. J. Psychiat., 107, 901-907.

Shopsin, B. (1976). Tryptophan and Allopurinol in the treatment of depression. Lancet, I, 1189.

Smythies, F. F., Radley, R. F., Johnston, V. S., and Leanard, F. (1967). The behavioral effects of some derivatives of mescaline and N,N-dimethyltryptamine in the rat. Life Sci., 6, 1887.

Solyom. L. (1969). A case of obsessive neurosis treated by aversion relief. Canad. Psychiat. Assoc. J., 14, 623-626.

Solyom, L. and Sookman, D. (1977). A comparison of Clomipramine Hydrochloride (Anafranil) and behaviour therapy in the treatment of obsessive neurosis. J. Int. Med. Res., 5, 49-61.

Spitzer, R. L., Endicott, J., and Robins, E. (1977). Research diagnostic criteria: rationale and reliability. Presented at the Annual Meeting of the American Psychiatric Association, Toronto, Canada, May.

Walinder, J., Skott, A., Carlsson, A., Nagy, A., and Roos, B. E. (1976). Potentiation of the antidepressant action of clomipramine by tryptophan. Arch. Gen. Psychiat., 33, 1384-1389.

Wilson, I. C. and Prange, A. J. Jr. (1972). Tryptophan in mania: Theory of affective disorders, abstracted. Psychopharmacologia, Suppl., 26, 76.

Wolpe, J. (1958). Psychotherapy by Reciprocal Inhibition. Stanford University Press, California.

Wooley, D. W. and Shaw, E. (1954). A biochemical and pharmacological suggestion about certain mental disorders. Proc. Natl. Acad. Sci., 4, 228-231.

Yaryura-Tobias, J. A. (1976). Obsessive-compulsive disorders: A serotonergic hypothesis? Presented at the Society of Biological Psychiatry, San Francisco.

Yaryura-Tobias, J. A. (1978). Brain Monoamines and Vitamins. Presented at the 1978 Scientific Symposium of the Academy of Orthomolecular Psychiatry, May 6-7.

Yaryura-Tobias, J. A., Bebirian, R. J., Neziroglu, F., and Bhagavan, H. N. (1977). Obsessive-compulsive disorders as a serotonergic defect. Res. Commun. Psychol. Psychiat. Behav., 2, 279-286.

Yaryura-Tobias, J. A. and Bhagavan, H. N. (1977). L-tryptophan in obsessive-compulsive disorders. Amer. J. Psychiat., 134, 1298-1299.

Yaryura-Tobias, J. A. and Neziroglu, F. (1975). The action of chlorimipramine in obsessive-compulsive neurosis: A pilot study. Curr. Ther. Res., 17, 111-116.

Yaryura-Tobias, J. A. and Neziroglu, F. (1978). Compulsions, aggression and self-mutilation: a hypothalamic disorder? J. Orthomol. Psychiat., 7, 114-117.

Yaryura-Tobias, J. A., Neziroglu, F., and Bergman, L. (1976). Chlorimipramine, for obsessive-compulsive neurosis: An organic approach. Curr. Ther. Res., 20, 541-548.

Noradrenergic Function in Affective Illness

F. K. GOODWIN and W. Z. POTTER

Clinical Psychobiology Branch, National Institute of Mental Health, Bethesda, Maryland 20014

ABSTRACT

The original formulation of the "norepinephrine hypothesis" of affective illness continues to undergo reevaluation. The purpose of this chapter is to review the current status of this hypothesis, emphasizing the impact of newer drugs and of direct clinical measures of amine function. Taken together, the pharmacological evidence is consistent with the hypothesis associating increased norepinephrine (NE) function with the onset of mania; however, with regard to depression, the pharmacological evidence is not as consistent in supporting a primary etiologic role for decreased norepinephrine. On the other hand, the results of amine metabolite studies are suggestive of decreased functional norepinephrine in some forms of depression, whereas, in mania the metabolite results are not as clear. Further clarification of this paradox may come from studies that reflect the functional status of certain norepinephrine receptors, such as in the hypothalamus (i.e., the neuroendocrine strategies), and in the pineal gland (melatonin studies). The indirect and direct evidence that other neurotransmitter systems are involved in major affective illness raises the two important questions of specificity and of biochemical subgroups.

KEYWORDS

Norepinephrine, catecholamine hypothesis, MHPG, depression, mania, metabolites, neuroendocrine, receptors.

The "Pharmacological Bridge"

Norepinephrine (NE) is established as an important monoamine transmitter both in the peripheral and central nervous systems. A series of findings with drugs which altered NE in animals and affected mood in man were the foundation for the "pharmacological bridge" connecting NE and affective illness. The most straightforward connection proposed was that decreased NE is central to the pathophysiology of depression while increased NE is causally involved in mania; this was the catecholamine hypothesis (Prange, 1964; Schildkraut, 1965; Bunney & Davis, 1965). This paper will review recent attempts to evaluate the role of NE in affective illness.

The "pharmacological bridge" model generated a large number of increasingly sophisticated studies designed to test the extent to which drugs which were known to alter central NE in animals could produce mood changes in man (Table 1). In some instances, the order is reversed with drugs known to alter mood having been evaluated for their effects on NE. One important problem in this area of research is the relative lack of biochemical specificity of many of the drugs. In addition, with only a few recent exceptions, most of the animal pharmacology has been done acutely while clinical changes involve considerably longer time frames. .

TABLE 1

Drug	Acute Effects On NE At Receptor	Clinical Effects: Predisposed To Affective Ill.	Clinical Effects: Depressed Patients	Clinical Effects: Manic Patients
MAOI	↑	Can Precip. Mania	Some Anti-Dep. Activity	?
Tricyclic	↑	Can Precip. Mania	Antidep.	Antimanic (?)
Amphetamine	↑	Can Precip. Mania (?)	Poor Antidep.	Antimanic (?)
Cocaine	↑	Can Precip. Mania	Poor Antidep.	?
L-DOPA	↑ (?)	Can Precip. Hypomania	Activation-No Antidep. Effect	?
Reserpine	↓	Can Precip. Dep.	?	Partial Anti-Manic
Lithium	↓	Does Not Precip. Dep.	Antidepressant (Some Pts.)	Antimanic
CPZ;Haloperidol	↓	?	?	Partial Anti-Manic
AMPT	↓	?	Does Not Reverse IMIP Antidep. Effects	Antimanic
Fusaric Acid (DBH Inhibitor)	↓	?	No Effect	Not Antimanic Psychosis Increased
Pimozide	?	?	?	Partial Antimanic
Iprindole	Minimal	?	Antidep. (?)	?
Mianserin	Moderate	Can Precip. Mania (?)	Antidep. (?)	?
ET-495	None	Can Precip. Mania (?)	Antidep. (?)	Antimanic (?) (Low Doses)

One of the most striking effects of drugs is found in individuals who are predisposed to affective illness (Table 1*, third column). Although space does not allow a detailed review of these studies here, the evidence is convincing that a group of drugs which have in common the acute effect of increasing norepinephrine at its postsynaptic receptor can precipitate mania. Of interest is the fact that only two

*The literature review from which this table is derived is available from the author

of the compounds capable of precipitating mania are established antidepressants, and their antidepressant effect only become apparent following chronic treatment. If antidepressant effects were simply a reflection of immediate increase of NE at the synapse, effects should be rapid as is the case with the precipitation of mania.

A further aspect of the action of these drugs should be noted. Contrary to what would be predicted from the catecholamine hypothesis, the tricyclics and amphetamines have been reported to decrease rather than increase mania once it is established (Akimoto & others, 1961; Kulcsar, 1966). Although these studies were not controlled, contrary data have not been brought forth.

Alternatively one can focus on drugs which decrease amines at the receptor. According to the straightforward theory of norepinephrine deficit, drugs which decrease central NE should be depressants. Reserpine, in fact, seems to fit this description, but lithium, α-methyl-para-tyrosine (AMPT), and fusaric acid (a dopamine-β-hydroxylase inhibitor which decreases NE synthesis) do not (Table 1). Lithium is more specifically antimanic and lacks the acute sedating properties of phenothiazines. Moreover, it is an effective antidepressant in some bipolar patients. The relationship between AMPT administration and depression is not well established; AMPT fails to reverse the antidepressant effects of imipramine while parachlorphenylalanine (a serotonin synthesis inhibitor) does (Shopsin & others, 1975). If replicated, this finding could suggest that serotonin function is more important in the mechanism of action of tricyclics than is NE. Fusaric acid, although proposed as a treatment for mania, not only has failed to be effective, but also has been found to worsen psychosis in manic patients (Sack & Goodwin, 1974). Pimozide, a "specific" dopamine antagonist, which presumably has little effect on NE has been shown to have antimanic properties (Post & others, 1976).

At the bottom of Table 1 are listed three drugs which have been cited as undermining the "pharmacological bridge" in that they are "antidepressants" without major effects on NE or 5HT. However, although iprindole is a relatively weak reuptake inhibitor for both NE and 5HT, mianserin does possess at least modest potency as a NE uptake inhibitor. More critical is the fact that the evidence is as yet insufficient for the superiority of iprindole over placebo in the treatment of those depressions characterized by endogenous symptoms (reviewed in Zis & Goodwin, in press). Finally, ET-495 (a dopamine agonist) has no known direct noradrenergic effect, but preliminary trials in hospitalized depressed patients indicate some antidepressant effect (Post & others, 1978). These latter findings are consistent with present postulating of the involvement of other neurotransmitters (especially dopamine) in mania and depression (Randrup & Braestrup, 1977; Antelman & Caggiula, 1977).

Conclusions based on the "pharmacological bridge" model can only be tentative. Drugs which can acutely increase NE consistently precipitate mania in predisposed individuals; this supports the suggestion that excess NE may play a major role in the etiology or expression of mania. On the other hand, using pharmacological evidence the pathophysiology of mania cannot involve excess NE alone since not all drugs which decrease NE are antimanic and paradoxically, some drugs which increase NE or dopamine may actually abbreviate mania (Akimoto & others, 1961). Statements about the relationship between NE and antidepressant effect are even more difficult to make. Drugs firmly established as effective in non-bipolar depression do have the ability to increase NE in the synapse, although the ability to increase NE does not guarantee that a compound will be an antidepressant.

It is, of course, impossible not to consider the numerous lines of evidence that implicate altered serotonin (5HT) function in at least some patients with affective illness--an area which is reviewed elsewhere in this volume by Dr. Asberg.

Analogous to the catecholamine hypothesis, an early version of the "serotonin hypothesis" (Lapin & Oxenkrug, 1969) suggested a serotonin deficit in depression and an excess in mania. More recently, it has been suggested that both NE and 5HT may be involved in depression, each related to different aspects of the syndrome. Thus, the elevation of mood following tricyclics has been suggested to be related to increased serotonin function while the increase in drive may be associated with elevated NE. Consistent with this is the recent evidence that the potentiation of the antidepressant action of chlorimipramine by concomitant administration of tryptophan involves predominantly elevation of mood rather than improvement in psychomotor state (Walinder & others, 1976). On the other hand, earlier studies of the catecholamine precursor, L-DOPA, in depression indicated that its effects on depression were limited to improvement in psychomotor retardation (Goodwin & others, 1970). In this paper we will limit our discussion of alterations of serotonin function to areas in which questions of the specificity of NE arise. It should already be clear, however, that the evidence for antidepressant efficacy of "serotonergic" drugs argues against a specific NE deficiency in depresssion.

Clinical Studies of Norepinephrine Metabolites

Whatever its limitations, the "pharmacological bridge" model has generated a number of direct clinical studies of NE and its metabolites. Rather than simply listing the studies we will critically review findings in light of current knowledge on the neuropharmacology of NE. Many basic and clinical studies have attempted to elucidate whether the turnover of physiologically "significant" NE could be determined by measurement of NE or its metabolites in cerebrospinal fluid (CSF), plasma or urine. Implicit in the concept of physiological significance is a quantitative relationship whereby some alteration in a substance can at least be correlated with measurable physiological, biochemical or behavioral parameters. Ideally, one would like to demonstrate a causal relationship. Many assumptions have been made concerning the physiological significance of measures of NE or its metabolites; assumptions are also made concerning which sources of NE are most relevant for psychiatric illnesses. For instance, in clinical studies designed to clarify the role of NE in affective illness, it was long assumed that only alterations in NE formed in the CNS would be meaningful. Retrospectively, this may be viewed as an artificial distinction since some structures involved in the central modulation of peripheral synaptic impulses are themselves catecholaminergic (Dahlstrom & Fuxe, 1965; Scriabine & others, 1976). Conversely, it has been shown recently that stimulation of peripheral nerves (saphenous, sural or sciatic) in the rat activates locus coeruleus noradrenergic neurons in the central nervous system (Cedarbaum & Aghajanian,1977). Central modulation has been demonstrated in rats by direct electrical stimulation of the locus coeruleus which produced a two to three fold increase in plasma MHPG (a major metabolite of NE), presumably related, at least in part, to the peripheral release of NE (Crowley & others, 1978). Thus, increased noradrenergic activity in either the central or peripheral nervous system can be a manifestation of events originating either centrally or peripherally. Understanding the importance of reciprocal noradrenergic influences means that so-called positive or negative findings from clinical studies can only be interpreted to the extent that factors which influence either central or peripheral noradrenergic function have been taken into account.

Many of those known factors, or sources of variance, have been discussed in detail elsewhere (Goodwin & others, 1978). What is particularly important here is that it may not be possible to separate extraneous sources of variance from actual characteristics of affective illness. For example, what noradrenergic state of an individual with an "agitated depression" would be most consistent with the hypothesis that NE is involved in the etiology of the syndrome? If one could "control" the agitation, would NE and/or its metabolite be low because the person is basically depressed? Or, are motor activity or anxiety, symptoms reported to be associated with increased NE activity (Ebert & others, 1972; Sweeney & others, 1977) an essential part of the illness.

The problems of interpretation may prove to be much more subtle. For instance, we have found increased urinary MHPG in depressed patients but not normal volunteers when switched from a low to a high monoamine diet (Muscettola & others, 1977). This finding could reflect unrecognized differences in the behavioral response of volunteers and depressed patients when placed on a research protocol involving changes in diet. In any event, it is very difficult to decide whether or not it is appropriate to attempt to "control" a given clinical variable.

With these theoretical and methodological limitations in mind, we will proceed to consider actual clinical studies of MHPG in affective illness. The rationale for measuring MHPG, the principal metabolite of NE in human brain (greater than 90%) is reviewed elsewhere (Goodwin & Potter, 1978). A study on monkeys has demonstrated a dissociation of NE turnover and MHPG concentration, at least in the CSF (Perlow & others, 1978). If a similar situation exists in man this finding may help explain why the determinations of MHPG in the CSF from persons with affective illness have not indicated any consistent differences between patients (either manic, depressed or euthymic) and controls. Earlier reports of statistically significant differences between groups in studies with adequate sample size have not been replicated even in the same center (for review see Goodwin & Potter, 1978). Some of the failure to replicate findings is probably related to differences in the so-called "controls." In one instance, neurological patients were used as controls (Post & others, 1973), and in another, young male volunteers with no identified illness were used (Goodwin & Post, unpublished). In one study, when age was taken into account, differences between depressed patients and controls disappears (Asberg & others, 1977). Thus, measurements of concentrations of MHPG in the CSF do not support (or refute) the hypothesis that alterations in NE play a role in depression.

Much more emphasis has been placed on measurements of urinary MHPG as being relevant to the catecholamine hypothesis. Clinical studies of urinary MHPG have been extensive. The proportion of urinary MHPG that originates in the CNS of man has been estimated to be as high as 70% (Ebert & Kopin, 1975; Maas & others, in press) or as low as 25-30% (Karoum & others, 1978; Kopin, 1978). The methodologies employed (isotope dilution, peripheral perturbation and arterio-venous metabolite differences) each rests on different assumptions, so that some variability in the resultant esimates is to be expected. As previously discussed, the extent to which MHPG in urine originates in the CNS may not be critical in order for alterations to be meaningful. Therefore, in reviewing studies of urinary MHPG, the initial question is whether consistent differences can be found. Interpretation of results is a separate issue.

Table 2 summarizes findings from several groups, most of which have used similar analytical methods (gas chromatography [GC] with an electron capture detector), although at least one has used combined gas chromatography-mass spectrometry (GC-MS) (Goodwin & others, 1978). This methodological point is important, since as shown in the last column of values from "normals," 24-hour urinary MHPG shows a cross-study variation from 1029 μg to 2740 μg. Even in repeated studies from the same groups, normal values vary to a substantial degree. There is no evidence that these differences can be accounted for by factors such as age, sex, diet, activity or anxiety (all of which may influence MHPG in some situations). Since the GC method involves an elaborate calculation of recovery following extraction and enzymatic hydrolysis (Dekirmenjian & Maas, 1970; Bond & Howlett, 1974), the explanation for differences in "absolute" levels in normals may in part be an artifact of variable recovery factors. In our lab direct comparisons of determinations using a reliable GC assay with determinations using GC-MS reveal an excellent correlation (r=0.9) but a systematic difference whereby the GC-MS values are only 0.83 of the GC values. It would, therefore, appear that although absolute values across studies are not directly comparable, relative values within any study (assuming assays were run under identical conditions) may be reliable.

TABLE 2

	All Dep	Major or Primary Dep All	UP	BP	Secondary Minor or Other Dep	Schizo-Affect.	Normal
Maas '68 (F=9; M=7)	1087 (16)						1516 (11)
Shaw '73	1401 (22)	1401 (22)	1401 (22)				
Bond, Howlett '74 (F=7; M=6)							2006 (13)
Goodwin, Beckmann '75 (F=34; M=12)	1351 (44)	1402 (30)	1623 (19)	1020 (11)	1440 (9)	880 (5)	1330 (15)
Deleon-Jones, Mass ;75 (F=33)	1137 (33)	1032 (21)	1069 (16)	911 (5)	1321 (12)		1348 (21)
Joseph '76 (M=13)							2740 (13)
Schildkraut '76 (F=18; M=19)	1544 (37)	1435 (20)	1709 (9)	1211 (11)	1814 (13)	1211 (4)	
Sacchetti '76 (M=5)	845 (5)	845 (5)	845 (5)				
Sharpless '77 (F=10; M=10)	1628 (20)						1884 (11)
Garfinckel '77 (F=3; M=5)	1320 (8)	1320 (8)		1320 (8)			1600 (10)
Hollister '78 (F=6; M=11)							1924 (17)
Sweeney, Maas, '78 (F=24)	902 (24)	902 (22)					
Taube, Maas, '78 (F=14)	791 (14)	791 (14)	803 (10)		759 (4)		1029 (10)
Dekirmenjian, Kinard, Davis '78 (F=62)	1138 (62)	1112 (41)	1158 (29)		1002 (12)		1461 (34)
Goodwin '78 (F=14; M=13)	1658 (27)	1682 (23)	1930 (13)	1360 (10)		1520 (4)	1830 (18)
Mean MHPG	1275 (312)	1229 (206)	1342 (123)	1149 (49)	1400 (46)	1179 (13)	1670 (173)

In spite of the inter-study variation in absolute values, the overall mean for all depressed subjects is 25% lower than normal controls ($p < .02$). The subgroups of bipolar depressed patients consistently have lower urinary MHPG than controls, a finding which has been emphasized previously. In contrast, unipolar depressives in different studies have MHPG that is higher, lower or not different than controls.

The consistent findings in depressed bipolar patients may reflect the relative diagnostic homogeneity of persons with clearcut manic-depressive illness. One might speculate that bipolar depressed patients show the most truly "organic" depressions manifested by profound psychomotor retardation such that both anxiety and activity are particularly low with this group. Attempts to assess the relationship between activity and excretion of MHPG has resulted in conflicting reports (Ebert & others, 1972; Sweeney & others; 1977). Recent studies using a far more precise method of quantifying 24-hour activity show that there is a relationship in any one individual between activity and urinary MHPG (Wehr & others, 1978). A relationship between activity and MHPG across individuals, however, has so far not been demonstrated using the same methodology. Two groups have found an association between anxiety in depressed patients and MHPG (Beckmann & Goodwin, 1975; Sweeney & others, 1977). Despite the fact that quantitation of anxiety is not as precise as direct monitoring of activity, a positive association between anxiety and MHPG is consistent with both human and animal experiments on the effects of stress on plasma NE and MHPG. It may be that depressions which involve considerable anxiety will not be associated with low MHPG and these will be distinct from bipolar depressions in other respects. The finding of low MHPG in bipolar and some "unipolar" patients does not necessarily mean, of course, that decreased NE <u>causes</u> depression. Still, MHPG could prove useful in a difficult differential diagnosis or in the prediction of drug response (see below).

The issue of specificity has other aspects. Not only can alterations of amine metabolites be secondary to variables which may be related to an illness (e.g., anxiety and activity) or to state variables (e.g., age and diet) but to so-called "normal" variance. For instance, taking an example from work with 5HIAA (the metabolite of serotonin) in the CSF, an association between low 5HIAA and suicidality has been noted (Asberg & others, 1977). In a separate study of a population without major psychiatric diagnoses, an association between low 5HIAA and impulsivity and "aggression" was found (Brown & others, 1976). Thus, the connection between low 5HIAA and suicidality in depressed individuals could result from the simultaneous presence of impulsivity and depression. On the basis of this reasoning, low 5HIAA in the depressed patient might be a clinical prognosticator of possible behaviors but it would not necessarily indicate that there was a depressive syndrome caused by low 5HIAA.

Our emphasis on the limitations of clinical research with regard to establishing causality between a biochemical response and a clinical state should not obscure the fact that findings do indicate some decrease of total NE function or turnover in some depressed patients. These metabolite findings can be buttressed by the consistent observation that manias can be precipitated in susceptible individuals by a diverse group of drugs which share the property of at least transiently increasing NE in the synapse.

Alternative Approaches to the Clinical Study of Norepinephrine Function

In attempting to evaluate NE function in depression some investigators have recently utilized the fact that secretion of pituitary hormones by hypothalamic releasing factors is at least partly under the control of monoaminergic systems. Growth hormone (GH) has been the major pituitary hormone explored as a "window" to NE systems in the hypothalamus. This is based largely on pharmacological studies in animals and in man which link decreased NE function to blunted GH release (reviewed by Sachar, 1975).

Several groups have reported a decreased GH response to insulin-induced hypoglycemia in depressed patients (reviewed by Carrol & Mendels, 1976). Similarly, others have found a blunted GH response to amphetamine (Langer & others, 1976), and to clonidine, a direct receptor agonist (Matussek, this volume), in depressed patients.

In an interesting study, Garver & others (1975) demonstrated a positive correlation between hypoglycemia-induced GH release and urinary MHPG excretion in depressed patients, further suggesting that decreased GH responses in depression can all be interpreted as secondary to reduced NE function.

A relatively direct measure of "central" NE receptor function has been made possible by the development of an extremely sensitive GC-MS assay for melatonin which permits the accurate quantitation of picogram amounts in 1 ml or less of plasma (Lewy & Markey, 1978). Melatonin secretion by the pineal gland appears to be primarily under the control of a β-adrenergic receptor (Deguchi & Axelrod, 1972). We find that the area under the 24-hour melatonin curve is increased in patients who are manic as compared to controls. Furthermore, drugs which effect β-receptor function in man alter melatonin in the predicted direction (Wetterberg, personal communication; Lewy & Goodwin, unpublished data). Clinical and animal studies of α- and β-noradrenergic receptor function are also being applied to elucidate the role of NE in affective illness. In general, one looks for supersensitivity (increased 'receptors') or subsensitivity (decreased 'receptors') which may be either a cause or an effect of altered neurotransmitter turnover.

Peripheral approaches in which the pressor effects of tyramine, NE and/or phenylephrine are measured in patients, most consistently show an increased response (supersensitivity) during depression, which would be consistent with a chronic decrease in NE turnover (Ghose & others, 1975; Friedman, 1978). At least one study, however, found a decreased NE pressor response during the depressed as compared to the 'recovered' state (Prange & others, 1967). Peripheral tissues studied *in vitro* (platelets and leukocytes) do not show any α-adrenergic receptor alterations in association with mood disorders (Murphy & others, 1974). One *in vitro* study of β-adrenergic receptor on leucocytes noted decreased sensitivity (cyclic AMP generation) to NE (Pandey & others, 1978). Investigations of the chronic effects of tricyclic antidepressants in animals have shown "subsensitivity" to NE stimulation (Vetulani & Schultz, 1975; Frazer & Mendels, 1977), as well as a reduced number of post-synaptic β-receptors (Banerjee & Kung, 1975). It is of interest that the latter report also showed decreased receptors following iprindole, a drug which has only a very weak effect on the reuptake of NE. Using a different system, it has been shown that chronic administration of reuptake inhibitors for both NE and 5HT results in increased post-synaptic 5HT receptor sensitivity (presumably increased number of receptors) without altering NE receptors (de Montigny & Aghajanian, 1977). These chronic effects of antidepressants on various receptors demonstrate that there are a number of ways in which the drugs can influence NE and/or 5HT. In general, they support the hypothesis that alterations in monoamine function are relevant to the expression and treatment of depression.

CONCLUSIONS

The bulk of the evidence, both direct and indirect, points to an involvement of central NE systems in the pathophysiology of at least some forms of major affective illness. However, the "too little - too much" formulations, derived from models based on the inborn errors of metabolism, are now yielding to more complex multidimensional models which focus on the interrelationships between different neurotransmitters systems; furthermore, recent formulations are giving more attention to the possibility that the pathophysiology of affective illness involves disturbances in adaptative and regulatory mechanisms for the monoamine neurotransmitters. Future clinical studies should include the assessment of alterations in neurotransmitter systems to various perturbations.

REFERENCES

Akimoto, M., Takakuki, Y., Honda, Y., Takahashi, J., Toyoda, K., Sasaki, Y. and Machiyama, Y. (1961). Clinical evaluation of the effects of central stimulants, MAO inhibitors, and imipramine in the treatment of affective disorders. Proceedings of the Third World Congress of Psychiatry, Vol. II, McGill University Press, Montreal, Canada.

Antelman, S.M., and Caggiula, A.R. (1977). Norepinephrine-dopamine interactions and behavior. Science, 195, 646-653.

Asberg, M., Bertilsson, L., Thoren, P. and Traskman, L. (1977). CSF monoamine metabolites in depressive illness. In S. Garattini (Ed.), Depressive Disorders. F.K. Schattauer-Verlag, Stuttgart. pp. 293-305.

Banerjee, S.P., and Kung, L.S. (1977). Development of β-adrenergic receptor subsensitivity by antidepressants. Nature, 268, 455-456.

Beckmann, H., and Goodwin, F.K. (1975). Antidepressant response to tricyclics and urinary MHPG in unipolar patients. Arch. Gen. Psychiat., 32, 17-21.

Bond, P.A., and Howlett, D.K. (1974). Measurement of the two conjugates of 3-methoxy-4-hydroxyphenylglycol in urine. Biochem. Med., 10, 219-228.

Brown, G.L., Goodwin, F.K., Ballenger, J.C. and Goyer, P.F. (1978). CSF amine metabolites in human aggression. Sci. Proc. Am. Psychiat. Ass., 131, 88.

Bunney, W.E., Jr., and Davis, J.M. (1965). Norepinephrine in depressive reactions: a review. Arch. Gen. Psychiat., 13, 483-494.

Carroll, B.J., and Mendels, J. (1976). Neuroendocrine regulation in affective disorders. In E.J. Sachar (Ed.), Hormones, Behavior, and Psychopathology. Raven Press, New York. pp. 193-224.

Cedarbaum, J.M., and Aghajanian, G.K. (1977). Activation of locus coeruleus noradrenergic neurons by peripheral nerve stimulation. Presented at the 7th Annual Meeting for Society of Neuroscience, Anaheim, California.

Crowley, J.N., Hattox, J.W., Maas, J.W. and Roth, R.H. (1978). 3-Methoxy-4-hydroxyphenyl ethylene glycol increase in plasma after stimulation of the nucleus locus coeruleus. Brain Res., 141, 380-384.

Dahlstrom, A., and Fuxe, K. (1965). Evidence for the existence of monoamine neurons in the central nervous system. II. Experimentally induced changes in the intraneuronal amine levels of bulbospinal neuron systems. Acta Physiol. Scand., 64, 1-36.

Deguchi, T., and Axelrod, J. (1972). Control of circadian change of serotonin N-acetyltransferase activity in the pineal organ by the β-adrenergic receptor. Proc. Nat'l. Acad. Sci., 69, 2547-2550.

Dekirmenjian, H., and Maas, J.W. (1970). An improved procedure of 3-methoxy-4-hydroxyphenyl-ethylene glycol determination by gas-liquid chromatography. Anal. Biochem., 35, 113-122.

Deleon-Jones, F., Maas, J.W., Dekirmenjian, H. and Saucher, J. (1975). Diagnostic subgroups of affective disorders and their urinary excretion of catecholamine metabolites. Am. J. Psychiat., 132, 1141-1148.

Ebert, M.H., Post, R.M., and Goodwin, F.K. (1972). The effect of physical activity on urinary MHPG excretion in depressed patients. Lancet, ii, 766.

Ebert, M.H., and Kopin, I.J. (1975). Origins of urinary catecholamine metabolites: differential labeling by dopamine C^{14}. Trans. Ass. Am. Physicians, 28, 256-264.

Frazer, A., and Mendels, J. (1977). Do tricyclic antidepressants enhance adrenergic transmission? Am. J. Psychiat., 134, 1040-1041.

Friedman, M.J. (1978). Does receptor supersensitivity accompany depressive illness? Am. J. Psychiat., 135, 107-108.

Garfinkel, P.E., Warsh, J.J., Stancer, H.C. and Godse, D.D. (1977). CNS monoamine metabolism in bipolar affective disorder. Arch. Gen. Psychiat., 34, 735-739.

Garver, D.L., Pandey, G.N., Dekirmenjian, H. and Deleon-Jones, F. (1975). Growth hormone catecholamines in affective disease. Am. J. Psychiat., 132, 1149-1154.

Ghose, K., Turner, P., and Coppen, A. (1975). Intravenous tyramine pressor response in depression. Lancet, i, 1317-1318.

Goodwin, F.K., Brodie, H.K.H., Murphy, D.L. and Bunney, W.E., Jr. (1970). L-DOPA, catecholamines and behavior: a clinical and biochemical study in depressed patients. Biol. Psychiat., 2, 341-366.

Goodwin, F.K., and Beckmann, H. (1975). Urinary MHPG in unipolar and bipolar affective disorders. Sci. Proc. Am. Psychiat. Ass., 128, 96-97.

Goodwin, F.K., Cowdry, R.W., and Webster, M.H. (1978). Predictions of drug response in the affective disorders: toward an integrated approach. In M. Lipton, A. DiMascio, and K. Killam (Eds.), Psychopharmacology - A Generation of Progress. Raven Press, New York. pp. 1277-1288.

Goodwin, F.K., and Potter, W.Z. (1978). The biology of affective illness: amine neurotransmitters and drug response. In Cole, Frazier, and Schatzberg (Eds.), Depression: Biology, Dynamics and Treatment. Plenum Press, New York. pp. 41-73.

Joseph, M.H., Baker, H.F., Johnstone, E.C. and Crow, T.J. (1976). Determination of 3-methoxy-4-hydroxyphenylglycol conjugates in urine. Application to the study of central noradrenaline metabolism in unmedicated chronic schizophrenic patients. Psychopharmacology, 51, 47-51.

Karoum, F., Rauscher, F., and Wyatt, R.J. (1978). MHPG excretion to determine peripheral and central contributions. Presented at the Annual Meeting of the American Society for Neurochemistry, Washington, D.C., Abstract #308, p. 196.

Kopin, I.J. (1978). Noradrenergic neurotransmission. In M.A. Lipton, A. DiMascio, and K.F. Killam (Eds.), Psychopharmacology: A Generation of Progress. Raven Press, New York. pp. 217-220.

Kulcsar, J.S. (1966). Amphetamine sulphate in mania. Lancet, i, 1164.

Langer, G., Heinze, G., Reim, B. and Matussek, N. (1976). Reduced growth hormone responses to amphetamine in "endogenous" depressive patients. Arch. Gen. Psychiat., 33, 1471-1475.

Lapin, I.P., and Oxenkrug, G.F. (1969). Intensification of the central serotonergic processes as a possible determinant of the thymoleptic effect. Lancet, i, 132-136.

Lewy, A.J., and Markey, S.P. (1978). Analysis of melatonin in human plasma by gas chromatography negative chemical ionization mass spectrometry. Science, 201, 741-743.

Maas, J.W., Fawcett, J., and Dekirmenjian, H. (1968). 3-Methoxy-4-hydroxy phenylglycol (MHPH) excretion in depressive states. Arch. Gen. Psychiat., 19, 129-134.

Maas, J.W., Greene, N.M., Hattox, S.E. and Landis, H. (in press). Neurotransmitter metabolite production by human brain. Catecholamines; Basic and Chemical Frontiers. Pergamon Press, Oxford.

de Montigny, C., and Aghajanian, G.K. (1977). Sensitization of postsynaptic serotonin receptors by chronic pretreatment with tricyclic antidepressants. Presented at the 7th Annual Meeting for Society of Neuroscience, Anaheim, California, Abstract #775, p. 248.

Murphy, D.L., Donnelly, C., and Moskowitz, J. (1974). Catecholamine receptor function in depressed patients. Am. J. Psychiat., 131, 1389-1391.

Muscettola, G., Wehr, T.A., and Goodwin, F.K. (1977). Effect of diet in urinary MHPG excretion in depressed patients and normal control subjects. Am. J. Psychiat., 134, 914-916.

Pandey, G.H., Dysken, M.W., Garver, D.L. and Davis, J.M. (1978). Beta-adrenergic receptor function in affective illness. APA New Res. Abstracts, #9.

Perlow, M., Ebert, M.H., Goodwin, F.K., Ziegler, M.G., Lake, C.R. and Chase, T.N. (1978). The circadian variation of catecholamine metabolism in the subhuman primate. Brain Res., 139, 101-113.

Post, R.M., Gerner, R.H., Carman, J.F., Gillin, J.C., Jimerson, D.C., Goodwin, F.K. and Bunney, W.E., Jr. (1978). Effects of a dopamine agonist piribedil in depressed patients. Arch. Gen. Psychiat., 35, 609-615.

Post, R.M., Gordon, E.K., Goodwin, F.K. and Bunney, W.E., Jr. (1973). Central norepinephrine metabolism in depressed patients: 3-methoxy-4-hydroxyphenylglycol in the cerebrospinal fluid. Science, 179, 1002-1003.

Post, R.M., Jimerson, D.C., and Goodwin, F.K. (1976). Time-related biochemical effects on neuroleptics. Sci. Proc. Am. Psychiat., 129, 309-310.

Prange, A.J., Jr. (1964). The pharmacology and biochemistry of depression. Dis. Nerv. Syst., 25, 217-221.

Prange, A.J., Jr., McCurdy, R.L., and Cochrane, C.M. (1967). The systolic blood pressure response of depressed patients to infused norepinephrine. J. Psychiat. Res., 5, 1-13.

Randrup, A., and Braestrup, C. (1977). Uptake inhibition of biogenic amines by newer antidepressant drugs: relevance to the dopamine hypothesis of depression. Psychopharmacology, 53, 309-314.

Sacchetti, E., Smenaldi, E., Caguasso, M., Biondi, P.A. and Bellodi, L. (1976). MHPG, amitriptyline and affective disorders. Int. Pharmacopsychiat., 11, 157-162.

Sachar, E.J. (1975). Evidence for neuroendocrine abnormalities in the major mental illnesses. In D. Freedman (Ed.), The Biology of the Major Psychoses, Vol. 54, Raven Press, New York. pp. 347-358.

Sack, R.L., and Goodwin, F.K. (1974). Inhibition of dopamine-beta-hydroxylase in manic patients: a clinical trial with fusaric acid. Arch. Gen. Psychiat., 31, 649-654.

Schildkraut, J.J. (1965). The catecholamine hypothesis of affective disorders: a review of supporting evidence. Am. J. Psychiat., 122, 509-522.

Schildkraut, J.J., Orsulak, P.J., Gudeman, J.E., Schatzberg, A.F., Rohde, W.A., LaBrie, R.A., Cahill, J.F., Cole, J.O. and Frazier, S.H. (1978). Norepinephrine metabolism in depressive disorders: implications for a biochemical classification of depressions. In J.O. Cole, S.H. Frazier, and A.F. Schatzberg (Eds.), Depression: Biology, Psychodynamics and Treatment. Plenum Press, New York. pp. 75-102.

Scriabine, A., Clineschmidt, B.V., and Sweet, C.S. (1976). Central noradrenergic control of blood pressure. Ann. Rev. Pharmacol. Toxicol., 16, 113-123.

Sharpless, N.S. (1977). Determination of 3-methoxy-4-hydroxyphenyl glycol in urine and the effect of diet on its excretion. Res. Comm. Chem. Pathol. Pharmacol., 18, 257-273.

Shaw, D.M., O'Keefe, R., MacSweeney, D.A., Brooksbank, B.W.L., Noguera, R. and Coppen, A. (1973). 3-Methoxy-4-hydroxyphenyl glycol in depression. Psychol. Med., 3, 333-336.

Shopsin, B., Friedman, E., Goldstein, M. and Gershon, S. (1975). The use of synthesis inhibitors in defining a role for biogenic amines during imipramine treatment in depressed patients. Psychopharmacol. Comm., 1, 239-249.

Sweeney, D.R., Maas, J.W., and Heninger, G.R. (1977). Anxiety, physical activity and urinary MHPG. Sci. Proc. Am. Psychiat. Ass., #289. p. 173.

Taube, S.L., Kirstein, L.S., Sweeney, D.R., Heninger, G.R. and Maas, J.W. (1978). Urinary 3-methoxy-4-hydroxyphenyl glycol and psychiatric diagnosis. Am. J. Psychiat., 135, 78-82.

Vetulani, J., and Sulser, F. (1975). Action of various antidepressant treatments reduces reactivity of noradrenergic cyclic AMP-generating system in limbic forebrain. Nature, 257, 495-496.

Walinder, J., Skott, A., Carlsson, A., Nagy, A. and Roos, B.-E. (1976). Potentiation of the antidepressant action of clomipramine by tryptophan. Arch. Gen. Psychiat., 33, 1384-1389.

Wehr, T.A., Muscettola, G., and Goodwin, F.K. (in press). Diurnal pattern of urinary 3-methoxy-4-hydroxy phenylglycol (MHPG) excretion: comparison of mania and depressed patients to normal controls. Arch. Gen. Psychiat.

Zis, A.P., and Goodwin, F.K. (1978 - in press). Novel antidepressants in the biogenic amine hypothesis of depression: the case for iprindole and mianserin. Arch. Gen. Psychiat.

The Case for Involvement of Dopamine in Depression and Mania

A. RANDRUP*, I. MUNKVAD*, R. FOG*, C. BRAESTRUP* and L. MOLANDER**

*St. Hans Mental Hospital, Department E, Roskilde, Denmark
**AB Ferrosan, Malmö, Sweden

ABSTRACT

While the dopamine hypothesis for schizophrenia became quite readily accepted, opinions have been more divided about its extension to depression and mania. New evidence in support of this extension has, however, appeared lately, and is reviewed in the present paper. This evidence comprises: new antidepressant drugs with outstanding dopaminergic activity (notably nomifensine), confirmation of the dopaminergic mediation of the euphoric effect of amphetamines, further studies of the antimanic effect of neuroleptics, involvement of dopamine in new more sophisticated animal models of depression and mania, and additional experiments showing dopaminergic effects of thymoleptics, lithium and ECT.

New evidence about interaction among various transmitter systems in the brain is taken into account, and dual, apparently paradoxical effects of dopaminergic drugs are discussed.

KEYWORDS: Depression, mania, schizophrenia, euphoria, dopamine, amphetamines, neuroleptics, nomifensine, antidepressives.

INTRODUCTION

We originally suggested the dopamine hypothesis only for schizophrenia (Fog, Randrup and Pakkeberg, 1966; Randrup and Munkvad, 1968, p. 24; Munkvad and Randrup, 1970) and when we later extended it to encompass also the affective psychoses (Randrup and co-workers, 1973; Randrup, Munkvad and Scheel-Krüger, 1973) it could be argued, that this was asking too much from the dopamine. The extension of the hypothesis is, however, in good agreement with animal experiments with amphetamine and neuroleptics, which indicate that many types of behaviour, including emotional and social behaviours, are affected by manipulation of brain dopamine (Lewander, 1977; Ljungberg and Ungerstedt, 1976; Marshall and Ungerstedt, 1976; Michanek and Meyerson, 1977; Miczek and O'Donnell, 1978; Randrup, Munkvad and Scheel-Krüger, 1973; Schiørring, 1977; van Kammen and Murphy, 1975, p. 222).

Further, we shall see the dopamine hypothesis or "the case for dopamine" in a conceptual frame of reference, which acknowledges interaction between various functional systems and various transmitters in the brain. The dopamine hypothesis will then suggest, that brain dopamine has an important role in this interaction, when psychoses are elicited or antagonized.

The case for involvement of dopamine in the affective psychoses rests on evidence from large fields of clinical, pharmacological and biochemical investigation. In a review written four years ago (Randrup and co-workers, 1975) we tried to present a discussion of all this comprehensive, relevant evidence, including such topics as antimanic, antidepressant and depressogenic actions of neuroleptics; effects of amphetamines and l-DOPA on mood; schizoaffective and manic-depressive types of amphetamine psychosis; mechanisms of action of the various types of antidepressants; animal experiments; biochemical measurements of amine metabolites in patients (discussed in this symposium by Vestergaard and co-workers and Goodwin and Åsberg) and communality of mental diseases and neurological disorders of the basal ganglia (including depression in Parkinson's disease). In this paper we shall mainly discuss selective topics to supplement the former review and particularly refer to new important evidence that has been published during the latest four years.

CLINICAL EVIDENCE. ANTIMANIC EFFECTS OF NEUROLEPTICS

In our 1975-review we emphasized that the antimanic effects of neuroleptics was an especially important piece of evidence, since from the beginning this effect was regarded as one of the most characteristic effects of neuroleptics, while on the biochemical side, action on dopamine so far seems to be the only common and characteristic effect of these drugs.

Shortly after the completion of our review, Shopsin and co-workers (1975) published an important and critical paper on this topic. They found by means of rating scales substantial improvement in characteristic manic sysmptoms including "euphoria" and "grandiosity" (in accord with Prien and co-workers, 1972 and Takahaski and co-workers, 1975), but also emphasized that some remnants of manic symptoms were recognized by additional clinical observation, and that the normalization was not complete. These observations appear similar to experiences with schizophrenia, and also in amphetamine-treated animals we found partial but not complete normalization with neuroleptics (Randrup and co-workers, 1976).

Similar results emerge from the extensive work of Bobon and co-workers (1972, 1974). These authors took care to distinguish the antimanic effect from other neuroleptic effects, e.g. reduction of agitation and psychomotor activity, emphasizing the thymic component (Bobon and Gottfries, 1974, see pp. 451 and 538; Bobon and co-workers, 1972). On this background they report antimanic effect of many neuroleptics, including several that are now regarded as the most specific dopamine antagonists: pimozide, penfluridol, fluspirilene (Bobon and Gottfries, 1974, p. 458).The antimanic effect of pimozide was recently confirmed by an independent group (Post, 1978). Bobon and co-workers (1972) also report differences among the individual neuroleptics; with respect to antimanic effect droperidol (mainly inhibition of psychomotor activity), and clothiapine (strong effect on the thymic component) are seen as extremes (Bobon and Collard, 1972). The differences between the individual neuroleptics may depend on differences in their mode of action on brain dopamine (e.g. differences with respect to balance between action on various dopamine areas in the brain, between pre- and postsynaptic effects, etc.) and/or their individual non-dopaminergic effects.

Also Angyal (1967) distinguishes between the action of haloperidol on psychomotor agitation and its "hypothymizing" effect and states, that the latter requires long term medication to become manifest (p. 156). Similar observations were made by Walcher (1970) with buronil. This time lag seems to be common for all antipsychotic effects, antimanic, antischizophrenic and antidepressive alike, and may be another cue to a common factor in these effects.

EUPHORIC, ANTIDEPRESSANT AND ANTIMANIC EFFECTS OF DRUGS THAT ACTIVATE DOPAMINE

The work of Gunne and co-workers on the mood responses to amphetamine was another important issue in our 1975-review (p. 218 with references). These workers found that the euphoric response of former addicts to intravenous amphetamine (assessed by a self-rating scale in an experimental setting) was significantly reduced (to about 50%) by pimozide, and blocked by α-methylparatyrosine, while the noradrenaline α- and β-blockers phenoxybenzamine and propanolol were without effect in the doses used, the former rather increased the euphoria (Gunne, Änggård and Jönsson, 1972; Gunne and Änggård, 1973; Gunne, 1977; Jönsson, 1972; Änggård and Gunne, 1975).

Confirmatory evidence has now been provided by Wald, Ebstein and Belmaker (1978), who found that haloperidol totally blocked the euphoric response to methylphenidate in 7 out of 10 patients and partially blocked it in the remaining three. Also several other authors have recently confirmed the euphoric response to amphetamines in an experimental setting, studying both normal persons, depressed (antidepressive effects reported) and schizophrenic patients. (Brown, Corriveau and Ebert, 1978; Checkley, 1978; Janowski and co-workers, 1973; Kadouch and co-workers, 1977; Smith and Davis, 1977; van Kammen, 1978; van Kammen and Murphy, 1975 and 1978). None of these authors tried to block the response with neuroleptics, but several compared d- and l-amphetamine, and there is now consistent evidence that the d-form is somewhat stronger for eliciting euphoria, exacerbating schizophrenic symptoms, producing stereotypy in animals (Gunne and Änggård, 1973, p. 485; Janowski and Davis, 1976; Lewander, 1977, pp. 72 and 82; Michanek and Meyerson, 1977; Scheel-Krüger, 1972; Segal, 1975; Smith and Davis, 1977, review; Svensson, 1971; van Kammen and Murphy, 1975) and exerting various effects on brain dopamine (Bunney and co-workers, 1975; Bræstrup, 1977; Holmes and Rutledge, 1976; Koe, 1976; Scheel-Krüger, 1972). All this is in good agreement with the dopamine hypothesis, but a clear distinction between noradrenergic and dopaminergic effects has so far not been obtained by this approach, because of only moderate differences between the biochemical effects of the d- and l-form (Bunney and co-workers, 1975; Lewander, 1977, p. 82).

Wald, Ebstein and Belmaker (1978) studied manic patients, who were euthymic under lithium treatment, and methylphenidate produced not only euphoria but in four patients it was noted, that their mental state became similar to the past natural mania characteristic for each individual. Also this global response was prevented or reduced by haloperidol (see also Gerner, Post and Bunney, 1976).

Exacerbation of manic symptomatology by methylphenidate was previously reported by Janowsky and co-workers (1973), who however found improvement in some patients. The latter response was recently confirmed by Beckmann and Heinemann (1976) with d-amphetamine and by Corsini and co-workers (1977) with apomorphine.

Similar, opposite and apparently paradoxical results are also reported with depressed (Kiloh, Neilson and Andrews, 1974; Post, 1978; Roberts, 1959) and schizophrenic patients (Belart, 1942; Bett, 1946; Bischoff, 1951; Corsini and co-workers, 1977; Segal and Janowski, 1978, p. 1114; van Kammen and co-workers, 1977; van Kammen, 1978) receiving amphetamines and these "paradoxes" seem to be important for the understanding of the relations between dopamine and psychoses (Bunney and Post, 1977; Randrup and co-workers, 1975). There are for example also reports about antidepressant as well as depressogenic effects of neuroleptics (Ayd, 1975, p. 497; Deniker, Ginestet and Loo, 1975; Kielholz, Pöldinger, Terzani, 1976; Lundbeck, 1976; Nahunek, 1962, 1969; Ostow, 1975; Randrup and co-workers, 1975; Sieberns, 1978) and about alleviation as well as production of depression by l-DOPA in Parkinsonian patients (Asnis, 1977; Barbeau and co-workers, 1971, p. 228; Damasio and Caldos, 1975; Messiha and Kenny, 1977; further references in Randrup and co-workers, 1975;

see also Bunney and Post, 1977, p. 153).

Some cues are now available for explanation of these apparent paradoxes. Thus both stimulant and neuroleptic drugs seem to act presynaptically as well as post-synaptically with opposite behavioural effects, and also receptor types, induction of receptor supersensitivity etc. must be considered here (Post, 1978). Further, there are reports about exacerbations of schizophrenic symptoms under neuroleptic treatment, which can be improved by reduction in dose or by antiparkinson drugs. (Carney and Sheffield, 1973, p. 426; Geleberg and Mandel, 1977; Marsden, Tarsy and Baldessarini, 1975; Rifkin, Quitkin and Klein, 1975; van Putten, Mutalipassi and Malkin, 1974). It seems that in certain cases the same symptoms can occur at both elevated and reduced dopaminergic activity. There is some evidence suggesting that the same can also happen in depression (Ayd, 1975, p. 497; Bunney and Post, 1977, p. 153; Nahunek, 1962, 1969; van Putten and May, in press).

It may also be considered that in animals amphetamines cause increase or reduction of the same item of behaviour depending on dose, time after application, animal individual, environment, etc. For example in rats locomotion is strongly increased by smaller doses of d-amphetamine and reduced by larger doses (Randrup, Munkvad and Scheel-Krüger, 1973a).

In spite of these cues the dual or opposite reactions are far from being fully understood, but they do indicate that if there is a relation between dopamine and psychoses, it cannot be a very simple one.

Besides the rapid and temporary effects of amphetamines on mood described above there are now reports of more delayed and prolonged, imipramine-like antidepressant effects of several amphetamines and other drugs that activate dopaminergic systems.

The most important of these drugs is nomifensine with which there is now a comprehensive clinical material demonstrating its antidepressant effect (Amin, Ban and Lehmann, 1978; Amin, Ban and Pecknold, 1978; Bjørndal, Kristjansen and Wæhrens, 1978; Dencker and co-workers, 1978; Hoechst, 1977, symposium; Nicholson and Turner, 1977, symposium; van Scheyen, 1978). Other drugs are bromocriptine (Agué, 1976, 67 patients; Mihovilovic and Bohacek, 1978) piribedil (Angrist, 1977; Oules and Boscredon, 1978; Post, 1978; Shopsin and Gershon, 1978) p-chloramphetamines (strong serotonergic as well as dopaminergic effects, Scheel-Krüger, 1972; van Praag and Korf, 1977) and bupropion (wellbatrin) (Borison and co-workers, 1977; Ferris and co-workers, 1978; Soroko and co-workers, 1977; Stern, Harto and Cummings, 1978).

In the present symposium this subject is covered mainly be Agnoli, who also gives new evidence showing antidepressive effect of l-DOPA.

The question may be raised if there is any relation between these delayed, prolonged antidepressant effects, which are most useful clinically, and the rapid temporary effects mentioned above. At this congress there is one piece of evidence, which may give us a cue: van Kammen and Murphy (1978, and van Kammen, thesis, 1978, report from studies of 13 patients with "primary affective disorder" a significant correlation between long-term antidepressant responses to imipramine and short-term activating, euphoric and antidepressant responses to amphetamine, thus confirming earlier work by Fawcett and co-workers (1972).

NEW EVIDENCE FROM THE WORK ON ANIMAL MODELS

Animal models of depression used in pharmacological work have usually been very crude, but recently the work of McKinney, Harlow, Suomi and others on separation of monkeys reached a stage, where drugs could be studied (McKinney, 1977). The separation of individual monkeys from a group of peers could be done repetitively, and thus allowed comparison between drugs (incl. placebo). The separation syndrome was shown to be responsive to imipramine but not to placebo (confirmed with desmethylimipramine by Hrdina and von Kulmiz, 1978).

α-Methyltyrosine, which inhibits the synthesis of both dopamine and noradrenaline potentiated the "despair phase" of the response to separation, while fusaric acid, an inhibitor of only noradrenaline synthesis, ameliorated this phase. The results thus indicate roles for both dopamine and noradrenaline, but different roles. The inhibitor of serotonin synthesis, PCPA, had no effect, when given alone, but interfered with the action of α-methyltyrosine.

Control experiments indicate that α-methyltyrosine was acting specifically on the despair phase rather than on general behavioural activity. The limited trials with these synthesis inhibitors in the clinic are, as far as they go, in quite good agreement with the results in the monkey model (Bunney and co-workers, 1972 and 1977, p. 330f; Murphy and co-workers, 1978; Usdin and co-workers, 1977, discussion p. 159). Thus four out of six depressed patients became worse, when given α-methyltyrosine (Bunney and co-workers, 1972). In other experiments with patients receiving antidepressive drugs, this effect was not seen (ref. in Murphy and co-workers, 1978). PCPA on the other hand was not found to have antidepressant effect, when given by itself, but it interfered with the action of antidepressant drugs.

Another new animal model is based on the depression noted in patients as a late effect of amphetamine (Bell, 1965 and 1973; Gunne and Änggård, 1973; van Kammen and Murphy, 1975; Watson and co-workers, 1972). Behavioural depression (low motor activity, unresponsiveness, huddling) was seen in rats 24 h after withdrawal of chronic methamphetamine, and imipramine (10 mg/kg, 23 h after the withdrawal) was found to prevent the behavioural depression as well as various changes in brain amines including dopamine (Seltzer and Tonge, 1975). This work is only in its beginning, but seems interesting.

Acute stimulation of rats and mice by lower doses of amphetamine (given alone or in combination with chlordiazepoxide) has been proposed as a model for mania (Bunney and co-workers, 1977, p. 331f; Murphy, 1977). Lithium reduces the behavioral hyperactivity in this model, and has also been found to antagonize effects of amphetamine on activity and mood in depressed patients (van Kammen and Murphy, 1975).

In the animal experiments, it seems, that lithium only antagonizes smaller doses of amphetamine, and a parallel to clinical reports about less satisfactory effects of lithium in severe mania (Bunney and co-workers, 1977 review, p. 331; Spring, 1971) might be considered.

MECHANISM OF ACTION OF CLASSICAL ANTIDEPRESSANT DRUGS

An important issue for our subject is the mechanism of action of the classical tricyclic antidepressants. Some of these are strong inhibitors of uptake of noradrenaline into neurons, others of serotonin uptake, and for a period it was widely believed, that this was the mechanism of their antidepressant action; newer, non-compatible evidence has, however, led to serious doubts about these views in several quarters (Crow, 1978; Jones and Roberts, 1978; Randrup and Bræstrup, 1977 with references). Inhibition of dopamine uptake is much weaker than the strongest effects on noradrenaline and serotonin, but this does of course not imply, that the tricyclics do not have any effect on brain dopamine. In fact, there have been several reports over the years about such effects (Randrup and co-workers, 1975, pp. 215-216 with 9 references; Randrup and Bræstrup, 1977) now supplied by two important papers, which appeared during the year 1977 (Ghosh and Hrdina, 1977;

Westerink and co-workers, 1977; at this congress: Ögren and co-workers, 1978). A variety of effects on dopaminergic systems have been reported, but their possible relations to the antidepressant effect are presently not clear. The effects of the tricyclics on behaviours associated with brain dopamine (potentiation of apomorphine and l-DOPA, anticataleptic effect, antiparkinson effects in patients) seem more readily associable with the clinical action (Molander and Randrup, 1976, 1976a; Randrup and co-workers, 1975, p. 216).

The monoamineoxidase inhibitors have of course long been known to affect brain dopamine (Randrup and co-workers, 1975, p. 217 and 220) and dopaminergic effects are also reported with lithium (Bunney and Murphy, 1976; Fyrö and co-workers, 1975; Hesketh and co-workers, 1978; Klawans and co-workers, 1977; Leonard, 1975; Pert and co-workers, 1978; Randrup and co-workers, 1975; Stefanini and co-workers, 1976), ECT (Dutov, 1976; Green, 1978; Papeschi and co-workers, 1974, 1974a; Post, 1978; Symposium on ECT in this volume) and several of the newest antidepressant drugs, e.g. mianserin, viloxazin (Matussek and Greil, 1977) and amoxapine (Buck and Morez-Ebinger, 1978; Chermat and co-workers, 1976; Smith, 1975). Some of the new drugs show certain neuroleptic properties and thus give additional support to views about a neuroleptic-thymoleptic continuum of drugs (references in Randrup and Bræstrup, 1977).

CONCLUSIONS

The evidence published during the latest four years has given significant additional support for a role of dopamine in depression and mania.

Dopamine thus seems to be involved in affective as well as schizophrenic psychoses. The evidence indicates, that the relation of dopamine with the psychoses is not a very simple one, and that there is much interaction among the various transmitter systems in the brain.

REFERENCES

Agué, C. (1976). CB 154 (bromocriptine). Anti-Depressant. Clinical Expose on Phase A. Report from Sandoz Ltd.

Amin, M. M., T. A. Ban, and H. E. Lehmann (1978). Nomifensin in the treatment of depression: A report on the Canadian part of a transcultural study. Psychol. Bull., 14, 35-37.

Amin, M. M., T. A. Ban, and J. C. Pecknold (1978a). Nomifensin in the treatment of depression: A standard-controlled study. Psychol. Bull., 14, 37-39.

Angrist, B., G. Sathananta, B. Shopsin, and S. Gershon (1977). In E. H. Ellinwood and M. M. Kilbey (Eds.), Cocaine and Other Stimulants, Plenum Press, New York. pp. 689-704.

Angyal, L. (1967). Clinical experiences with the application of haloperidol. Ther. Hung., 15, 155-162.

Asnis, G. (1977). Parkinson's disease, depression, and ECT: A review and case study. Am. J. Psychiat., 134, 191-195.

Ayd, J. (1975). The depot fluphenazines: A reappraisal after 10 years' clinical experience. Am. J. Psychiat., 132, 491-500.

Barbeau, A., H. Mars, and L. Gillo-Joffroy (1971). Adverse clinical side effects of levodopa therapy. In F. H. McDowell, and C. H. Markham (Eds.), Recent Advances in Parkinson's Disease, F. A. Davis Company, Philadelphia, U.S.A. pp. 204-237.

Beckmann, H. and H. Heinemann (1976). D-Amphetamin beim manischen Syndrom. Arzneim.-Forsch. (Drug Res.), 26, 1185-1186.

Belart, W. (1942). Pathogenetisches und Therapeutisches aus Pervitinversuchen bei Schizophrenie. Schweiz. med. Wschr., 23, 41-46.

Bell, D. S. (1965). Comparison of amphetamine psychosis and schizophrenia. Br. J. Psychiat., 111, 701-707.

Bell, D. S. (1973). The experimental reproduction of amphetamine psychosis. Archs gén. Psychiat., 29, 35-40.

Bett, W. R. (1946). Benzedrine sulphate in clinical medicine: A survey of literature. Post-Grad. Med. J., 22, 205-218.

Bischoff, A. (1951). Über eine therapeutische Verwendung der sogenannten "Weck-Amine" in der Behandlung schizophrener Erregungszustände. Mschr. Psychol. u. Neur., 121, 329-344.

Bjørndal, N., P. Kristjansen, and J. Wæhrens (1978). Clinical investigation of the mode of action of nomifensin. 11th C.I.N.P. Congress. July 9-14, Vienna, Austria. Abstract. p. 210.

Bobon, D. P. and C. G. Gottfries (1974). Clinical physiognomy of thioxanthenes. Acta psychiat. belg., 74, 441-568.

Bobon, J. and J. Collard (1972). Present treatment of manic states. Acta psychiat. belg., 72, 617-632.

Bobon, J., D. P. Bobon, A. Pinchard, J. Collard, T. A. Ban, R. de Buck, H. Hippius and P.-A. Lambert (1972). A new comparative physiognomy of neuroleptics: A collaborative clinical report. Acta psychiat. belg., 72, 542-554.

Borison, R., B. Diamond, H. Havdala, and J. M. Davis (1977). Central pharmacology of a new antidepressant. Pharmacologist, 19, 155.

Braestrup, C. (1977). Biochemical differentiation of amphetamine vs methylphenidate and nomifensine in rats. J. Pharm. Pharmac., 29, 463-470 (1977).

Brown, W., D. P. Corriveau, and M. H. Ebert (1978). Acute psychologic and neuroendocrine effects of dextroamphetamine and methylphenidate. Psychopharmacology, 58, 189-195.

Buck, R. de and V. Morez-Ebinger (1978). Amoxapine and imipramine: A double blind evaluation in hospitalized depressed patients. 11th C.I.N.P. Congress. July 9-14, Vienna, Austria. Abstract. p. 212.

Bunney, B. S., J. R. Walters, M. J. Kihar, R. H. Roth, and G. K. Aghajanian (1975). D & L Amphetamine stereoisomers: Comparative potencies in affecting the firing of central dopaminergic and noradrenergic neurons. Psychopharmac. Comm., 1, 177-190.

Bunney, W. E., E. S. Gershon, D. L. Murphy, and F. K. Goodwin (1972). Psychobiological and pharmacological studies of manic-depressive illness. J. Psychiat. Res., 9, 207-226.

Bunney, W. E. and D. L. Murphy (1976). Neurobiological considerations on the mode of action of lithium carbonate in the treatment of affective disorders? Pharmakopsych., 9, 142-147.

Bunney, W. E. and R. M. Post (1977). Catecholamine agonist and receptor hypothesis of affective illness: Paradoxical drug effects. In E. Usdin, D. Hamburg, and J. D. Barchas (Eds.), Neuroregulators and Psychiatric Disorders, Oxford University Press, New York. pp. 151-159.

Bunney, W. E., T. R. Wehr, J. C. Gillin, R. M. Post, F. K. Goodwin, and D. P. van Kammen (1977). The switch process in manic-depressive psychosis. Annls Int. Med., 87, 319-335.

Carney, M. W. P. and B. F. Sheffield (1973). The long-term maintenance treatment of schizophrenic out-patients with depot flupenthixol. Curr. med. Res. Opn., 1, 423-426.

Checkley, S. s. (1978). A new distinction between the euphoric and anti-depressant effects on methylamphetamine. 11th C.I.N.P. Congress. July 9-14, Vienna, Austria. Abstract. p. 283.

Chermat, R., P. Simon, and J. R. Boissier (1976). Neuroleptique et/ou antidepresseur? Un probleme pose aux pharmacologues par l'amoxapine. In D. Baronet-Lacroix (Ed.), 10th C.I.N.P. Congress. July 4-9, Québec, Canada. Abstract. p. 162.

Corsini, G. U., M. del Zompo, S. Manconi, C. Cianchetti, A. Mangoni, and G. L. Gessa (1977). Sedative, hypnotic, and antipsychotic effects of low doses of apomorphine in man. In E. Costa and G. L. Gessa (Eds.), Advances in Biochemical Psychopharmacology, Vol. 16, Raven Press, New York. pp. 645-648.

Crow, T. J. (1978). Biochemical effects of some new antidepressants: Putative mechanisms of antidepressant effect. In J. Boissier (Ed.), 7th International Congress of Pharmacology, July 16-21. Abstract. p. 102.

Damasio, A. R. and A. C. Caldas (1975). Neuropsychiatric aspect. In G. Stern (Ed.), The Clinical Uses of Levodopa, Med. Techn. Publ. Co., Ltd. England. pp.127-154.

Dencker, S. J., K. Jensen, U.-G. Ahlfors, E. Ose and co-workers (1978). Nomifensine and imipramine in endogenous depression. 11th C.I.N.P. Congress. July 9-14, Vienna, Austria. Abstract. p. 210.

Deniker, P., D. Ginestet, and H. Loo (1975). Médicaments psychotropes et mécanismes de régulation de l'humeur. L'Encéphale, 1, 359-362.

Dutov, A. A. (1976). Effect of electro-shock seizures on function of the caudate nucleus. Physiol. J., U.S.S.R. Sechenov., 62, 1118-1123.

Fawcett, J., J. W. Maas, and H. Dekirmenjian (1972). Depression and MPHP excretion. Response to dextroamphetamine and tricyclic antidepressants. Archs gén. Psychiat., 26, 246-251.

Ferris, R., R. Maxwell, H. White, O. J. Beaman, and A. Russull (1978). Some neurochemical properties of a novel antidepressant: Bupropion hydrochloride. 11th C.I.N.P. Congress. July 9-14, Vienna, Austria. Abstract. p. 33.

Fog, R. L., A. Randrup, and H. Pakkenberg (1966). Amines in the corpus striatum associated with the effects of both amphetamine and antipsychotic drugs. Proceedings of the IV World Congress of Psychiatry, Madrid. Excerpta Medica International Congress Series No. 150, pp. 2580-2582.

Fyrö, B., U. Petterson, and G. Sedvall (1975). The effect of lithium treatment on manic symptoms and levels of monoamine metabolites in cerebrospinal fluid of manic depressive patients. Psychopharmacologia, 44, 99-103.

Gelenberg, A. J. and M. R. Mandel (1977). Catatonic reactions to high-potency neuroleptic drugs. Archs gén. Psychiat., 34, 947-950.

Gerner, R., R. Post, and W. Bunney (1976). A dopaminergic mechanism in mania. Am. J. Psychiat., 133, 1177-1180.

Ghosh, P. K. and P. D. Hrdina (1977). Effects of tricyclic antidepressants on the content and metabolism of dopamine in the rat striatum. Can. J. Physiol. Pharmacol., 55, 383-388.

Green, A. R. (1978). Repeated exposure of rats to the convulsant agent flurothyl enhances 5-hydroxytryptamine- and dopamine-mediated behavioural responses. Br. J. Pharmac., 62, 325-331.

Gunne, L. (1977). Effects of amphetamine in humans. In G. V. R. Born, O. Eichler, A. Farah, H. Herken, A. D. Welch (Eds.), Handbook of Experimental Pharmacology, Vol. 45, Springer-Verlag, Berlin/Heidelberg/New York. pp. 247-275.

Gunne, L., E. Ånggård, and L. N. Jönsson (1972). Clinical trials with amphetamine-blocking drugs. Psychiat. Neurol. Neurochir. (Amst.), 75, 225-226.

Gunne, L. and E. Ånggård (1973). Pharmacokinetic studies with amphetamines - Relationship to neuropsychiatric disorders. J. Pharmacokin. Biopharmac., 1, 481-495.

Hesketh, J. N., N. M. Nicolaou, G. W. Arbuthnott, and A. K. Wright (1978). Psycophamacology, 56, 163-166.

Hoechst (Ed.) Alival(R) (Nomifensin). (1977). Symposium über Ergebnisse der experimentellen und klinischen Prüfung. F. K. Schattauer Verlag - Stuttgart-New York.

Holmes, J. and C. O. Rutledge (1976). Effects of the d- and l-isomers of amphetamine on uptake, release and catabolism of norepinephrine, dopamine and 5-hydroxytryptamine in several regions of rat brain. Biochem. Pharmac., 25, 447-451.

Hrdina, P. D. and P. von Kulmiz. (1978). Pharmacological modification of experimental depression in primates. In J. Boissier (Ed.)., 7th International Congress of Pharmacology, July 16-21. Abstract. p. 627.

Janowsky, D. S., M. Khaled El-Yousef, J. M. Davis, and H. J. Sekerke (1973). Provocation of schizophrenic symptoms by intravenous administration of methylphenidate. Archs. gén. Psychiat., 28, 185-191.

Janowsky, D. and J. M. Davis (1976). Methylphenidate, dextroamphetamine, and levamphetamine. Archs gén. Psychiat., 33, 304-308.

Jones, R. S. G. and M. H. T. Roberts (1978). Do antidepressants potentiate by a postsynaptic action? In J. Boissier (Ed.), 7th International Congress of Pharmacology, July 16-21. Abstract p. 345.

Jönsson, L.-E. (1972). Pharmacological blockade of amphetamine effects in amphetamine dependent subjects. Europ. J. Pharmacol., 4, 206-211.

Kadouch, R., R. H. Belmaker, R. P. Ebstein and L.Peres (1977). The mood response and plasma cyclic-AMPT response to intravenous methylphenidate. Neuropsychobiology, 3, 250-255.

Kielholz, P., W. Põldinger, and S. Terzani (1976). Die Langzeitbehandlung periodischer und cyclischer Depressionen mit Flupenthixol-Decanoat. Symposium for Swiss and Dutch Psychiatrists, Lundbeck, Copenhagen. pp. 61

Kiloh, L. G., M. Neilson, and G. Andrews (1974). Repsonse of depressed patients to methylamphetamine. Brit. J. Psychiat., 125, 496-499.

Klawans, H. L., W. J. Weiner, and P. A. Nausieda (1977). The effect of lithium on an animal model of tardive dyskinesia. Prog. Neuro-Psychopharmac., 1, 53-60.

Koe, B. K. (1976). Molecular geometry of inhibitors of the uptake of catecholamines and serotonin in synaptosomal preparations of rat brain. J. Pharmac. exp. Ther., 199, 649-661.

Leonard, B. E. (1975). Changes in rat brain monoamine metabolism following the acute administration of lithium chloride in combination with antidepressant drugs. Archs int. Pharmacodyn., 215, 202-207.

Lewander, T. (1977). Effects of amphetamine in animals. In G.V.R. Born, O.Eichler, A. Farah, H. Herken, and A. D. Welch (Eds.), Handbook of Experimental Pharmacology, Vol. 45. Springer-Verlag Berlin-Heidelberg-New York. pp.33-246.

Ljungberg, T. and U. Ungerstedt (1976). Reinstatement of eating by dopamine agonists in aphagic dopamine denervated rats. Physiol. Behav., 16, 277-283.

Lundbeck, H. (1976). Papers read at the Anglo-Belgian Symposium for Psychiatrists Copenhagen, May 5.

Marsden, C. D., D. Tarsy, and R. J. Baldessarini (1975). Spontaneous and drug-induced movement disorders in psychotic patients. In D. F. Benson and D. Blumer (Eds.), Psychiatric Aspects of Neurological Disease. Grune & Stratton, New York-San Francisco-London.

Marshall, J. F. and U. Ungerstedt (1976). Apomorphine-induced restoration of drinking to thirst challenges in 6-hydroxydopamine-treated rats. Physiol. Behav., 17, 817-822.

Matussek, N. and W. Greil (1977). New antidepressants. In E. Usdin and I. Forrest (Eds.), Psychoterapeutic Drugs. Marcel Dekker, Inc. New York. pp. 1251-1266.

McKinney, W. T. (1977). Biobehavioral models of depression in monkeys. In I.Hanin and E. Usdin (Eds.), Animal Models in Psychiatry and Neurology, Pergamon Press, Oxford.pp. 117-126.

Messiha, F. S. and A. D. Kenny (Eds.) (1977). Parkinson's disease. Adv. Exp. Med. Biol., 90, Plenum Press.

Michanek, A. and B. J. Meyerson (1977). A comparative study of different amphetamines on copulatory behavior and stereotype activity in the female rat. Psychopharmacology, 53, 175-183.

Miczek, K. A. and J. M. O'Donnell (1978). Intruder-evoked aggression in isolated and nonisolated mice: effects of psychomotor stimulants and l-DOPA. Psychopharmacology, 57, 47-55.

Mihovilović, M. and N. Bohaček (1978). Bromocriptin in depressive states. 11th C.I.N.P. Congress. July 9-14, Vienna, Austria. Abstract. p. 211.

Molander, L. and A. Randrup. (1976). Effects of thymoleptics on behaviour associated with changes in brain dopamine. I. Potentiation of dopa-induced gnawing of mice. Psychopharmacologia, 45, 261-265.

Molander, L. and A. Randrup, (1976a). Effects of thymoleptics on behavior associated with changes in brain dopamine. II. Modification and potentiation of apomorphine-induced stimulation of mice. Psychopharmacologia, 49, 139-144.

Munkvad, I. and A. Randrup (1970). Evidence indicating the role of brain dopamine in the psychopharmacology of schizophrenic psychoses. Psihofarmakologija, 2, 45-47. Medicinska Naklada, Zagreb.

Murphy, D. L. (1977). Animal models for mania. In I. Hanin and E. Usdin (Eds.), Animal Models in Psychiatry and Neurology. Pergamon Press, Oxford. pp. 211-223.

Murphy, D. L., I. C. Campbell, and J. L. Costa (1978). The brain serotonergic system in the affective disorders. Prog. Neuro-Psychopharmac., 2, 1-31.

Náhunek, K. (1962). Die Behandlung endogener Depressionen mit Perphenazin und Trihexyphenidyl. Beziehung zur Extrapyramidalen Symptomatologie. Acta psychiat. scand., 38, 108-116.

Náhunek, K. (1969). Zur Qualität und Quantität der therapeutischen Wirkung von Neuroleptika, trizyklischen Thymoleptika und Konvulsionsmethoden bei endogenen Depression. Int. Pharmacopsychiat., 2, 140-147.

Nicholson, P. A. and P. Turner (Eds.) (1977). Proceedings of a Symposium on Nomifensine. Br. J. Clin. Pharmacol., Vol. 4, suppl. 2, 53S-248S.

Oules, J. and J. Boscredon (1978). Effect of a dopaminergic agonist, the piribedil, in psychiatry. 11th C.I.N.P. Congress. July 9-14, Vienna, Austria, Abstract. p. 284.

Ostow, M. (1975). Treating depression with tranquilizers. N.Y. St. J. Med., April, 693-696.

Papeschi, R., A. Randrup, and S. Lal (1974). Effect of ECT on dopaminergic and noradrenergic mechanisms. I. Effect on the behavioural changes induced by reserpine, α-methyl-p-tyrosine or amphetamine. Psychopharmacologia, 35, 149-158.

Papeschi, R., A. Randrup, and I. Munkvad (1974a). Effect of ECT on dopaminergic and noradrenergic mechanisms. II. Effect on dopamine and noradrenaline concentrations and turnovers. Psychopharmacologia, 35, 159-168.

Pert, A., J. E. Rosenblatt, C. Sivit, C. B. Pert, and W. E. Bunney (1978). Long-term treatment with lithium prevents the development of dopamine receptor supersensitivity. Science, 201, 171-173.

Post, R. (1978). Frontiers in affective disorder research. In M. Lipton, A. DiMascio and K. Killam (Eds.), Psychopharmacology: A Generation of Progress. Raven Press, New York. pp. 1323-1327.

Prien, R., E. M. Caffey, and C. J. Klett (1972). Comparison of lithium carbonate and chlorpromazine in the treatment of mania. Archs gén Psychiat., 26, 146-153.

Randrup, A. and C. Bræstrup (1977). Uptake inhibition of biogenic amines by newer antidepressant drugs: Relevance to the dopamine hypothesis of depression. Psychopharmacology, 53, 309-314.

Randrup, A. and I. Munkvad (1968). Behavioural stereotypies induced by pharmacological agents. Pharmakopsychiat. Neuro-Psychopharmakol., 1, 18-26.

Randrup, A., I. Munkvad, R. Fog, J. Gerlach and L. Molander (1973). Possible role of brain dopamine in mania and depression. In M. Mazur (Ed.). IV Congress of the Pharmacological Society, Lodz, Poland. p. 35.

Randrup, A., I. Munkvad, R. Fog, J. Gerlach, L. Molander, B. Kjellberg and J. Scheel-Krüger (1975). Mania, depression, and brain dopamine. In W. B. Essman and L. Valzelli (Eds.), Current Developments in Psychopharmacology, Vol. 2, Spectrum Publications, Inc., New York. pp. 206-248.

Randrup, A., I. Munkvad, and J. Scheel-Krüger (1973). Mechanisms by which amphetamines produce stereotypy, aggression and other behavioural effects. In T. A. Ban, J. R. Boissier, G. J. Gessa, H. Heimann, L. Hollister, H. E. Lehmann, I. Munkvad, H. Steinberg, F. Sulser, A. Sundwall and O. Vinar (Eds.), Psychopharmacology, Sexual Disorders and Drug Abuse. North-Holland Publishing Company, Amsterdam and Avicenum, Czechoslovak Medical Press, Prague. pp. 659-673.

Rifkin, A., F. Quitkin, and D. F. Klein (1975). Akinesia. A poorly recognized drug-induced extrapyramidal behavioral disorder. Archs gén Psychiat., 32, 672-674.

Roberts, J. M. (1959). Prognostic factors in the electro-schock treatment of depressive states. J. Mental Sci., 105, 703-713.

Scheel-Krüger, J. (1972). Behavioural and biochemical comparison of amphetamine derivatives, cocaine, benztropine and tricyclic anti-depressant drugs. Europ. J. Pharmacol., 18, 63-73.

Schiørring, E. (1977). Changes in individual and social behavior induced by amphetamine and related compounds in monkeys and man. In E. H. Ellinwood and M. M. Kilbey (Eds.), Advances in Behavioral Biology, Vol. 21. Plenum Press, New York. pp. 481-522.

Segal, D. (1975). Behavioral characterization of d- and l-amphetamine: Neurochemical implications. Science, 190, 475-477.

Segal, S. S. and D. S. Janowsky (1978). Psychostimulant-induced behavioral effects: Possible models of schizophrenia. In M. A. Lipton, A. DiMascio, and K. F. Killam (Eds.), Psychopharmacology: A Generation of Progress. Raven Press, New York. pp. 1113-1123.

Seltzer, V. and S. R. Tonge (1975). Methylamphetamine withdrawal as a model for the depressive state: Antagonism of post-amphetamine depression by imipramine. J. Pharm. Pharmacol., 27, 16P.

Shopsin, B. and S. Gershon (1978). Dopamine receptor stimulation in the treatment of depression: Piribedil (ET-495). Neuropsychobiology, 4, 1-14.

Shopsin, B., S. Gershon, H. Thompson and P. Collins (1975). Psychoactive drugs in mania. Archs gén Psychiat., 32, 34-42.

Sieberns, S. (1978). Erfahrungen mit dem Depotneuroleptikum Flupentixoldekanoat. Pharmakospychiat, 11, 186-198.

Smith, R. C. and J. M. Davis (1977). Comparative effects of d-amphetamine, l-amphetamine, and methylphenidate on mood in man. Psychopharmacology, 53, 1-12.

Smith, R. D. (1975). Amoxapine, imipramine and placebo in depressive illness. Curr. ther. Res., 18, 346-353.

Soroko, F. E. and R. A. Maxwell (1978). The pharmacology of bupropion HCl (Wellbatrin (R), a novel antidepressant agent. 11th C.I.N.P. Congress. July 9-14, Vienna, Austria. Abstract. p. 34.

Soroko, F. E., N. B. Mehta, R. A. Maxwell, R. M. Ferris, and D. H. Schroeder (1977). Bupropion hydrochloride (($\pm$) α-t-butylamino-3-chloropropiophenone HCl): a novel antidepressant agent. J. Pharm. Pharmac., 29, 767-770.

Spring, G. K. (1971). Some current thoughts on lithium carbonate in manic-depressive illness based on a double-blind comparison with chlorpromazine. Psychosomatics, 12, 336-340.

Stefanini, E., A. Argiolas, G. L. Gessa and F. Fadda (1976). Effect of lithium on dopamine uptake by brain synaptosomes. J. Neurochem., 27, 1237-1239.

Stern, W. C., N. Harto and W. Cummings (1978). A multi-center clinical trial of Wellbatrin (R) (Bupropion) in the treatment of depression. 11th C.I.N.P. Congress, July 9-14. Vienna, Austria. Abstract. p. 98.

Svensson, T. (1971). Functional and biochemical effects of d- and l-amphetamine on central catecholamine neurons. Naunyn-Schmiedebergs Arch. Pharmak., 271, 170-180.

Takahashi, R., A. Sakuma, K. Itoh, H. Itoh, M. Kurihara, M. Saito and M. Watanabe (1975). Archs gén. Psychiat., 32, 1310-1318.

Usdin, E., D. A. Hamburg, and J. D. Barchas (Eds.) (1977). Neuroregulators and Psychiatric Disorders. Oxford University Press, New York.

Van Kammen, D. P. (1978). Studies with amphetamine in schizophrenia and depression. Thesis. University of Utrecht, Holland.

Van Kammen, D. P., W. E. Bunney, J. P. Docherty, D. C. Jimerson, R. M. Post, S.Siris, M. Eberg, and J. C. Gillin (1977). Amphetamine-induced catecholamine activation in schizophrenia and depression: Behavioral and physiological effects. In E. Costa and G. L. Gessa (Eds.), Advances in Biochemical Psychopharmacology, Vol. 16. Raven Press, New York. pp. 655-659.

Van Kammen, D. P., D. L. Murphy (1975). Attenuation of the euphoriant and activating effects of d- and l-amphetamine by lithium carbonate treatment. Psychopharmacologia, 44, 215-224.

Van Kammen, D. P. and D. L. Murphy (1978). Antidepressant drug response prediction by amphetamine in depressed patients. 11th C.I.N.P. Congress. July 9-14, Vienna, Austria. Abstract. p. 321.

Van Prag, H. N. and J. Korf (1977). Chloramphetamines. In E. Usdin and I. S. Forrest (Eds.), Psychotherapeutic Drugs, Marcel Dekker, Inc., New York/Basel. pp. 1217-1244.

Van Putten, T. and P. R. A. May. "Akinetic depression" in schizophrenia. In press.

Van Putten, T., L. R. Mutalipassi, and M. D. Malkin (1974). Phenothiazine-induced decompensation. Archs gén. Psychiat., 30, 102-105.

Van Sheven, J. D. (1978). Nomifensin (Alival), a dopamine agonist, compared with clomipramin in unipolar depression, using the probenecid technique. 11th C.I.N.P. Congress. July 9-14, Vienna, Austria. Abstract. p. 211.

Walcher, W. (1970). Klinische Untersuchungen mit dem Butyrophenonderivat "Buronil". Int. Pharmacopsychiat., 4, 59-66.

Wald, D., R. P. Ebstein, and R. G. Belmaker (1978). Haloperidol and lithium blocking of the mood response to intravenous methylphenidate. Psychopharmacology, 57, 83-87.

Watson, R., E. Hartmann and J. J. Schildkraut (1972). Amphetamine withdrawal: affective state, sleep patterns, and MHPG excretion. Amer. J. Psychiat., 129, 263-269.

Westerink, B., B. Lejeune, J. Korf and G. van Praag (1977). On the significance of regional dopamine metabolism in the rat brain for the classification of centrally acting drugs. Europ. J. Pharmacol., 42, 179-190.

Änggård, E. and L. M. Gunne (1975). Clinical and pharmacological studies of amphetamine-dependent subjects. In J. R. Boissier, H. Hippius and P. Pichot (Eds.), Neuropsychopharmacology, Vol. 9, Excerpta Medica, Amsterdam. pp.253-261.

Ogren, S-O, K. Fuxe and C. Köhler (1978). The effect of the 5-HT reuptake inhibitor zimelidine on monoaminergic mechanisms in rats and mice. 11th C.I.N.P. Congress. July 9-14, Vienna, Austria. Abstract. p. 94.

Peptides in Affective Disorders: A Review

ARTHUR J. PRANGE, JR.*, PETER T. LOOSEN and IAN C. WILSON****

*Department of Psychiatry, University of North Carolina, Chapel Hill, NC 27514, U.S.A.
**Dorothea Dix Hospital, Raleigh, NC 27611, U.S.A.

ABSTRACT

The behavioral effects of three hypothalamic peptide hormones--thyrotropin releasing hormone (TRH), melanocyte stimulating hormone release inhibiting factor (MIF-I), and luteinizing hormone releasing hormone (LHRH)--have been assessed in depression. The behavioral effects of TRH have been assessed in mania. The behavioral effects of all three hormones have been assessed in a variety of non-affective disorders. In depression, controversy surrounds the effects of TRH. MIF-I has appeared to exert an antidepressant effect in both of two trials. LHRH appears not to exert an antidepressant effect. In mania, TRH showed promise in one preliminary trial.

TRH, but not MIF-I or LHRH, has been used to study endocrine responses in depressed patients. About 25% of these patients showed a blunted thyrotropin response. This event appears often, but not always, to be related to elevated cortisol.

KEYWORDS

Peptides, Depression, Thyrotropin releasing hormone, Melanocyte stimulating hormone release inhibiting factor, Luteinizing hormone releasing hormone

INTRODUCTION

Psychoendocrinology is the study of the role of hormones in mental function, and neuroendocrinology is one of its parent disciplines. Remarkable advances in the latter have prompted corresponding progress in the former. One prominent advance has been the chemical description of certain substances which are secreted by some hypothalamic neurons into the portal venous system and which, upon reaching the anterior pituitary gland, stimulate or inhibit the secretion by that organ of its tropic hormones (Martin, Reichlin and Brown, 1977). These substances, all peptides, are called hypothalamic hypophysiotropic hormones (HHHs).

Studies of the activity of hypothalamic extracts suggest the existence of as many as nine HHHs (Martin, Reichlin and Brown, 1977). Four have been chemically identified: thyrotropin releasing hormone (TRH); melanocyte-stimulating hormone release inhibiting hormone (or factor) (MIF-I); luteinizing hormone releasing hormone (LHRH); and somatotropin release inhibiting hormone (or factor) (SRIF, somatostatin).

Psychoendocrinology employs three broad strategies: hormones are given to mental patients (or normal subjects) and induced mental changes, if any, are observed; endocrine disturbances, in the resting state or in response to stimulation, are described in mental patients; mental changes are described in patients with endocrinopathies. In this brief review we shall concern ourselves mainly with affective disorders and mainly with the strategy of psychoendocrinology listed first above. Three HHHs have been used to induce mental changes in patients with affective disorders--TRH, MIF-I and LHRH. All have been used in other conditions as well and these findings will be briefly mentioned. In addition, TRH, but not MIF-I or LHRH, has been used in patients with affective disorders as an agent to provoke endocrine responses. These findings will also be described.

Many hormones other than HHHs are peptides. These include the anterior pituitary hormones, posterior pituitary hormones, and certain hormones of peripheral origin, calcitonin and insulin, for example. (Some peripheral hormones, of course, are modified amino acids or steroids.) One pituitary hormone, β-endorphin, a peptide consisting of 31 amino acids (Martin, Reichlin and Brown, 1977), has been given to three depressed patients (and to patients in other diagnostic categories) in a preliminary study with promising results (Kline and colleagues, 1977).

THYROTROPIN RELEASING HORMONE (TRH)

TRH is pGlu-His-Pro-NH_2 (Boler and colleagues, 1969; Burgus and others, 1969). It causes release from the anterior pituitary gland of thyroid stimulating hormone (TSH, thyrotropin) (Boler and colleagues, 1969; Burgus and others, 1969), prolactin (PRL) (Vale and Rivier, 1975), and under certain conditions growth hormone (GH) (Kato and others, 1975).

Behavioral Effects

Depression. In a double-blind, crossover study of 10 women with unipolar depression, we found that TRH, 0.6 mg given as an i.v. bolus, exerted a rapid, partial, brief beneficial effect. On observer and self-rating assessments patients were improved within a few hours, reaching maximum improvement the day after treatment. Improvement was about 50% as judged by the Hamilton rating scale, but did not correspond to full remission. About a week after injection the patients had relapsed to pretreatment severity (Prange and Wilson, 1972; Prange and others, 1972).

Since our original report trials of TRH have been performed by many investigators. Generally these have been addressed to the question of whether TRH is a treatment for depression competitive with standard treatments, and generally these trials have been disappointing. Various routes, rates, doses, populations, designs, and statistical assessments have been used. We have summarized these studies in Tables 1 and 2. We have classified studies as positive or negative according to the interpretation of their authors. Sometimes we have classified different aspects of the same study in different ways. For example, the nurses working with Lipton and Goodwin (1976) could not detect TRH-saline differences, but an experienced investigator did.

Trials of oral TRH (Table 1) are mainly negative. Four studies involving 66 patients are negative; two studies involving 5 patients are positive. The study by Turek and Rocha (1974) is classified as negative because of negative findings by doctors and nurses. Patient-self-ratings were positive. Oral administration of TRH may not always produce blood levels sufficient to penetrate the blood-brain barrier. Blood readily destroys the tripeptide; its half-life in blood is about 2 min. (Nair, Redding and Schally, 1971). However, Itil (1975) and Itil and others (1975) have shown that oral doses that have failed to show definitive antidepressant utility in other studies have caused EEG changes in their patients.

TABLE 1 Oral TRH in Depression

Studies	Positive	Negative
Single Blind	1 (1 patient)	0
Double Blind	1 (4 patients)	4 (66 patients)
Total	2 (5 patients)	4 (66 patients)

TABLE 2 Intravenous TRH in Depression

Studies	Positive	Negative
Single Blind	5 (188 patients)	6 (61 patients)
Double Blind	6 (43 patients)	8 (109 patients)
Total	11 (231 patients)	14 (170 patients)

Many more studies have employed the i.v. route of administration (Table 2). Ban and colleagues (1974) performed a strict replication of our original experiment and obtained nearly identical findings. Kastin and others (1972) reported a positive result in their first study but later could not replicate it (Ehrensing and others, 1974). Itil and others (1975) emphasized the action of TRH on "instinctive" behavior. Lipton and Goodwin (1976), ignorant of what treatment had been given, found decrease in tension, increase in energy, and enhanced capacity to cope with feelings. Maggini and others (1974) found a reduction in retardation after TRH. Obiols, Pujol and Obiols-Llandrich (1974) and Chazot and colleagues (1974), after studying large numbers of patients with a single blind technique, concluded that the effect of TRH is comparable to that obtained with standard antidepressant drugs.

Most studies of i.v. TRH in depression have been negative. Slow administration (Chazot and others, 1974; Deniker and others, 1974) with the probable consequence of not achieving blood levels sufficient to penetrate brain may have accounted for a small portion of the negative results, though Chazot and others (1974) found positive results with slow administration in patients with primary depression. Rapid crossover may have confounded results in some instances. Benkert, Gordon and Martschke (1974) performed crossover after two days and Coppen and others (1974) after four days. We had shown earlier that full relapse after TRH may require a week.

Deniker and others (1974) found that TRH produced a beneficial effect in half their bipolar patients. Widerlov and Sjostrom (1975) found a statistical advantage ($p < .05$) for TRH 24 hr after treatment when a one-tailed interpretation was applied to their data. At later times saline-treated patients showed as much improvement as TRH-treated patients. A crossover study of 10 patients was done by van den Burg and colleagues (1975). A statistically reliable advantage for TRH was found early in the course of treatment but not thereafter.

In two studies antidepressant drugs were in use during TRH-saline comparisons (Hall and colleagues, 1975; Sorenson, Svendsen and Schou, 1974). Coppen and others (1974a) performed a systematic study, concluding that the tripeptide does not potentiate the effects of amitriptyline.

Mania. Huey and others (1975) studied five euthyroid manic men, one of whom was later rediagnosed as schizophrenic. In a double-blind procedure patients were injected i.v. with TRH, 0.5 or 1.0 mg, or with saline. All differences favored TRH and some were statistically significant: diminished manic intensity 90 min after injection and diminished anger one hr later.

Other conditions. Recently we have provided extensive reviews of the behavioral effects of peptides in humans and animals (Prange and colleagues, 1978; Prange, Nemeroff and Lipton, 1978; Nemeroff and others, 1978, in press). We recorded the evidence that suggests that TRH exerts at least transient beneficial effects in alcohol withdrawal syndrome (Loosen, Prange and Wilson, 1978, in press) and the hyperkinetic syndrome of children (Tiwary and others, 1975). In normal women it appears to produce an alerting and mild euphoriant effect (Betts and colleagues, 1976; Prange and Wilson, unpublished observations; Wilson and others, 1973). The tripeptide is active in schizophrenic patients. It appears to benefit non-paranoid patients (Prange, Wilson and Loosen, unpublished observations; Wilson, Lara and Prange, 1973) and to aggravate paranoid patients (Davis, Hollister and Berger, 1975), though these findings are controversial. In male sexual impotence it has been found to be inactive (Benkert, 1975). TRH appears not to affect the neurological aspects of Parkinson's disease (Chase and others, 1974; Lakke and others, 1974). It has been noted, however, to elevate the mood of patients who were taking L-DOPA (McCaul, Cassell and Stern, 1974).

Endocrine Effects

Depression. In addition to observing behavioral changes, the investigator may measure endocrine responses after TRH administration. Thus far, we have given TRH, 0.5 mg i.v., to 35 unipolar depressed women and measured their response of TSH secretion. The TRH-induced TSH response was found to be blunted in 10 patients (29%). As the criterion for a blunted TSH response we required an increase from baseline (ΔTSH) of less than 5 μU/ml. In our laboratory in a large group of sex-matched controls the lowest ΔTSH observed was 5.8 μU/ml. The finding of a blunted TSH response to TRH in depression has been widely confirmed (Loosen and others, 1976 and Prange, 1977 for reviews). It is not found in schizophrenic patients (Loosen and others, 1977) but is shared by some alcoholic men, in withdrawal syndrome (Loosen, Prange and Wilson, 1978, in press; Loosen and others, 1976), with secondary depression.

In depression TSH blunting seems not to be related to previous drug intake, sex, age, or severity of illness. In a recent report, Gold and colleagues (1977) found a significantly lower TSH response in unipolar depressed patients than in bipolar depressed patients, though findings on this point are inconsistent (Coppen and others, 1974; Ehrensing and others, 1974; Kirkegaard and others, 1975; Loosen and others, 1977; Maeda and others, 1975; Takahashi and others, 1974). Gold and others (1977) suggested that the blunted response may be related to enhanced central serotonergic activity. The fault may resolve with remission of depression (Gold and others, 1977; Gregoire and colleagues, 1977), though this does not always occur (Coppen and others, 1974; Kirkegaard and others, 1975; Loosen and others, 1977; Maeda and others, 1975).

Factors that might account for a blunted TSH response include hyperthyroidism (Hollander, Mitsumi and Nilhei, 1972), hypothalamic or pituitary dysfunction

TABLE 3 TSH Response to TRH Challenge in Depression

Authors	N	Results and Comments
Diminished response found		
Prange and others, 1972	10	All responses borderline low or absent. Thyroid state normal.
Kastin and others, 1972	5	Four showed diminished responses.
Coppen and others, 1974a	16	Four showed no response. Thyroid state normal.
Chazot and others, 1974	30	Fifteen showed diminished responses.
Kirkegaard and others, 1975	8	Group tended toward diminished responses, with recovery of responses after ECT. Elevated free thyroxine could influence initial diminution.
Ehrensing and others, 1974b	8	Three showed diminished responses.
Hutton, 1974	1	Baseline TSH as well as TSH response diminished.
Takahashi and others, 1974	36	Twelve showed diminished responses.
Ban and others, 1974	6	Diminished in all patients. All patients euthyroid.
Kirkegaard and others, 1975	15	Mean response diminished in depression as compared to recovery.
Widerlov and Sjostrom, 1975	10	Baseline TSH as well as TSH responses lower than in hospitalized, non-depressed controls.
Maeda and others, 1975	13	Mean response diminished as compared to controls.
Loosen and others, 1977	23	Six showed diminished responses. No correlation with age, severity of illness, clinical subtypes or clinical remission.
Gold and others, 1977	23	TSH responses lower in unipolar than in bipolar patients or controls. Negative correlation of CSF-5HIAA and baseline TSH.
Vogel and others, 1977	15	Baseline TSH as well as response to TRH diminished.
Normal response found		
Shopsin and others, 1973	2	Responses normal.
Dimitrikoudi and others, 1974	2	Responses normal.

(Schalch and others, 1972), Klinefelter's syndrome (Ozawa and Shishiba, 1975), 36-hour starvation (Vinik and colleagues, 1975), chronic renal failure (Czernichow and others, 1976) and excess SRIF activity in brain (Siler, Yen and Guillemin, 1974).

Some degree of thyroid activation is sometimes seen in depression (Whybrow and others, 1972). Heightened thyroid state, even within the usual range of normality, might induce the blunting through negative feedback. However, all investigators who have studied the matter in depression have found no consistent relationship between thyroid hormones and the TSH response. In fact, Takahashi and others (1974) showed that patients with <u>low</u> free thyroid indices "paradoxically" showed the most reduced TSH responses.

Another potential explanation for TSH blunting needs to be considered. It has been reported that the administration of glucocorticoids interferes with the TSH response to TRH (Otsuki, Dakoda and Baba, 1973; Re and colleagues, 1976). In seven unipolar depressed women we measured serum cortisol levels immediately before TRH injection and correlated these values with the TSH peak response. Basal cortisol and TSH peak showed a significant inverse relationship in depression as well as in a group of sex and age matched controls (Loosen, Prange and Wilson, 1978). These findings indicate that cortisol elevation, which occurs in some depressed patients (Carroll and Mendels, 1976), may account for some instances of TSH blunting in this condition. Nevertheless, the blunted TSH response sometimes persists after remission, as noted above. In such cases the abnormality probably cannot be attributed to elevated cortisol or to any other aspect of the state of depression.

Mania. Endocrine responses to TRH in manic patients have not been reported.

MELANOCYTE STIMULATING HORMONE RELEASE INHIBITING FACTOR (MIF-I)

MIF-I is Pro-Leu-Gly-NH_2 (Nair, Kastin and Schally, 1971). It inhibits release by the anterior pituitary gland of melanocyte stimulating hormone (MSH, melanotropin) (Nair, Kastin and Schally, 1971). Certain other peptide substances also exert this effect. Pro-Leu-Gly-NH_2 also occurs as the side chain of the oxytocin molecule (Prange and others, 1978).

Behavioral Effects

Depression. In a double-blind study Ehrensing and Kastin (1974) treated 18 depressed women. Six received MIF-I, 60 mg/day p.o.; six received 150 mg; six received placebo capsules. The authors reported a marked prompt improvement from the lower dose of the tripeptide. In a second double-blind, placebo-controlled study, the same authors treated 24 patients who had either bipolar or unipolar depression (Ehrensing and Kastin, 1978). For six days patients received MIF-I p.o., 75 or 750 mg per day, or placebo. As in their first study, these workers found that the smaller, but not the larger, dose of the tripeptide produced a significant antidepressant response.

Mania. We are ignorant of studies of MIF-I in manic patients.

Other conditions. The salutary effects of MIF-I on the neurological aspects of Parkinson's disease are reasonably well established (Barbeau, 1975; Fischer and others, 1974; Kastin and Barbeau, 1972).

Endocrine Effects

MIF-I has not been used as a tool for testing endocrine responses in patients with affective disorders.

LUTEINIZING HORMONE RELEASING HORMONE (LHRH)

LHRH is pGlu-His-Trp-Ser-Tyr-Gly-Leu-Arg-Pro-Gly-NH_2 (Matsuo and others, 1971; Monahan and others, 1971). It stimulates the release from the anterior pituitary gland of both luteinizing hormone (LH) and follicle-stimulating hormone (FSH) (Martin, Reichlin and Brown, 1977). Thus it is sometimes called gonadotropin releasing hormone.

Behavioral Effects

Depression. In a double-blind, crossover procedure Benkert, Gordon and Martschke

(1974) injected LHRH, 0.5 mg i.v., and later TRH and saline. Each substance was given once to each of a small series of depressed patients. Both hormones were slightly more effective than the control substance but differences were statistically insignificant.

Mania. LHRH has not been given to manic patients.

Other conditions. LHRH may exert beneficial effects in certain men with sexual impotence (Benkert, 1975; Mortimer and others, 1974; Schwarzstein and others, 1975), though this possibility has not been extensively studied. In light of animal studies that show that LHRH has sexual stimulating properties and that these do not depend upon endocrine effects (Moss, 1975, Pfaff, 1973 for review), it is interesting to note that a beneficial effect on potency has been observed in hypogonadal men even before androgen levels have been restored (Mortimer and others, 1974).

Endocrine Studies

LHRH has not been used as a tool for testing endocrine responses in patients with affective disorders. It has, however, been used in this fashion in schizophrenic patients (Brambilla and colleagues, 1976).

COMMENT

The concept is now generally accepted that many peptide hormones exert behavioral effects in animals and some of these effects have been shown to be independent of endocrine effects (Prange and others, 1978). The status of this concept is less clear in humans, perhaps due to the inherent difficulties of human investigation. Controversy exists except in those situations in which only a few studies have been performed. Thus all of three studies suggest that TRH causes alerting and mild euphoria in normals; both of two studies suggest that MIF-I exerts an antidepressant effect in depressed patients. LHRH has not been adequately studied to clarify its possible behavioral actions in man. It is clear, however, that no endogenous peptide has yet shown itself to be competitive with standard treatments for any behavioral disorder. The elaboration of congeners that may resist degradation and readily penetrate the blood brain barrier provides promise for the future.

Among the peptide hormones the HHHs appear to hold great promise as tools for psychoendocrine investigation. They connect the nervous and endocrine systems. The nerve cells that secrete them have been likened to transducers (Nemeroff and Prange, 1978 in press); they receive nervous impulses and secrete hormonal messages. Moreover, the anterior pituitary hormones that are influenced by HHHs are now for the most part readily measured in blood, by radioimmune assay techniques. It appears that at least some of these hormones are transported in a retrograde fashion to brain itself (Berglund and Page, 1978). Thus the investigator has the possibility of making strong inferences about the activity of populations of hypothalamic cells in patients with one or another disorder. If, as seems likely, the secretions of these cells, the HHHs, possess not only endocrine properties but behavioral properties as well, then these inferences may have enhanced value for understanding disorders of behavior.

REFERENCES

Ban, T. A., H. E. Lehmann, N. P. V. Nair, J. C. Pecknold and L. Orbach (1974). Clinical studies with TRH. 17th National Meeting of APhA Academy of Pharmaceutical Sciences, November 10-14, New Orleans.

Barbeau, A. (1975). Potentiation of levodopa effect by intravenous L-prolyl-L-leucyl-glycine amide in man. *Lancet*, 2, 683-684.

Benkert, O. (1975). Studies on pituitary hormones and releasing hormones in depression and sexual impotence. In, W. H. Gispen, Tj. B. van Wimersma Greidanus, B. Bohus, and D. De Wied (Eds.), *Progress in Brain Research*, Vol. 42, Elsevier, Amsterdam. pp. 25-36.

Benkert, O., A. Gordon and D. Martschke (1974). The comparison of thyrotropin releasing hormone, luteinizing hormone-releasing hormone and placebo in depressive patients using a double-blind cross-over technique. *Psychopharmacologia*, 40, 191-198.

Berglund, R. M. and R. A. Page (1978). Can pituitary secrete directly to brain: Affirmative anatomical evidence. *Endocrinology*, 102, 1325-1338.

Betts, T. A., J. Smith, S. Pidd, J. Mackintosh and P. Harvey (1976). The effects of thyrotropin releasing hormone on measures of mood in normal women. *Br. J. clin. Pharmac.*, 3, 469-473.

Boler, J., F. Enzmann, K. Folkers, C. Y. Bowers and A. V. Schally (1969). The identity of chemical and hormonal properties of the thyrotropin releasing hormone and pyroglutamyl-histidyl-proline-amide. *Biochem. Biophys. Res. Commun.*, 37, 705.

Brambilla, F., C. Rovere, A. Guastalla, A. Guerrini and F. Riggi (1976). Gonadotropin response to synthetic gonadotropin hormone-releasing hormone (GnRH) in chronic schizophrenia. *Acta Psychiat. Scand.*, 54, 131-145.

Burgus, R., T. F. Dunn, D. Desiderio and R. Guillemin (1969). Structure moleculaire du facteur hypothalamique hypophysiotrope TRF d'origine ovine: Mise en evidence par spectrometrie de masse de la sequence PCA-His-Pro-NH_2. *C. R. Acad. Sci. (Paris)*, 269, 1870-1873.

Carroll, J. B. and J. Mendels (1976). Neuroendocrine regulation in depression. In, E. J. Sachar (Ed.), *Hormones, Behavior, and Psychopathology*. Raven Press, New York. pp. 193-224.

Chase, T. N., A. C. Woods, M. A. Lipton and C. E. Morris (1974). Hypothalamic releasing factors and Parkinson disease. *Arch. Neurol.*, 31, 55-56.

Chazot, G., A. Chalumeau, G. Aimard, R. Mornex, A. Garde, B. Schott and P. F. Girard (1974). Thyrotropin releasing hormone and depressive states: From agroagonines to TRH. *Lyon Med.*, 231, 831-836.

Coppen, A., S. Montgomery, M. Peet and J. Bailey (1974). Thyrotropin-releasing hormone in the treatment of depression. *Lancet*, 2, 433-434.

Czernichow, P., M. C. Dauzet, M. Broyer and R. Rapporport (1976). Abnormal TSH, PRL and GH response to TSH releasing factor in chronic renal failure. *J. Clin. Endocrinol. Metab.*, 43, 630-637.

Davis, K. L., L. E. Hollister and P. A. Berger (1975). Thyrotropin-releasing hormone in schizophrenia. *Am. J. Psychiatry*, 132(9), 951-953.

Deniker, P., D. Ginestet, H. Loo, E. Zaririan and M. J. Cottereau (1974). Preliminary study of the action of hypothalamic thyrostimulin (TRH) in depressive states. *Ann. Med. Psychol.*, 1(2), 249-255.

Dimitrikoudi, M., E. Norty-Hanson and F. A. Jenner (1974). T.R.H. in psychoses. *Lancet*, 2, 456.

Ehrensing, R. H. and A. J. Kastin (1974). Melanocyte-stimulating hormone-release inhibiting hormone as an antidepressant. *Arch. Gen. Psychiatry*, 30, 63-65.

Ehrensing, R. H. and A. J. Kastin (1978). Dose-related biphasic effect of prolyl-leucyl-glycinamide (MIF-I) in depression. *Amer. J. Psychiat.*, 135, 562-566.

Ehrensing, R. H., A. J. Kastin, D. S. Schalch, H. G. Friesen, J. R. Vargas and A. V. Schally (1974). Affective state and thyrotropin-releasing hormone in depressed patients. *Am. J. Psychiatry*, 131(6), 714-718.

Fischer, P. A., E. Schneider, P. Jacobi and H. Maxion (1974). Effect of melanocyte-stimulating hormone-release inhibiting factor (MIF) in Parkinson's syndrome. *Eur. Neurol.*, 12, 360-368.

Gold, P. W., F. K. Goodwin, T. Wehr and R. Rebar (1977). Pituitary thyrotropin response to thyrotropin releasing hormone in affective illness: Relationship to spinal fluid amine metabolites. *Amer. J. Psychiat.*, 131, 714-718.

Gregoire, F., H. Braumann, R. DeBuck and J. Corvilain (1977). Hormone release in depressed patients before and after recovery. *Psychoneuroendocrinology*, 2, 303-312.

Hall, R., P. R. Hunter, J. S. Price and C. Q. Mountjoy (1975). Thyrotropin-releasing hormone in depression. *Lancet*, 2, 162.

Hollander, C. S., T. Mitsumi and N. Nilhei (1972). Clinical and laboratory observations in case of triiodothyronine toxicosis confirmed by radio-immunoassay. *Lancet*, 1, 609.

Huey, L. Y., D. S. Janowsky, A. J. Mandell, L. L. Judd and M. Pendery (1975). Preliminary studies on the use of thyrotropin releasing hormone in manic states, depression, and the dysphoria of alcohol withdrawal. *Psychopharmacol. Bull.*, 11(1), 24-27.

Hutton, W. N. (1974). Thyrotropin releasing hormone in depression. *Lancet*, 2, 53.

Itil, T. M. (1975). Effects of steroid hormones and hypothalamic hormones on human brain function. In, J. R. Boissier, H. Hippius and P. Pichot (Eds.), *Neuropsychopharmacology*, Excerpta Medica, Amsterdam. pp. 672-682.

Itil, T. M., C. D. Patterson, N. Polvan, A. Bigelow and B. Bergey (1975). Clinical and CNS effects of oral and I.V. thyrotropin-releasing hormone in depressed patients. *Dis. Nerv. Syst.*, 36(9), 529-536.

Kastin, A. J. and A. Barbeau (1972). Preliminary clinical studies with l-propyl-l-leucyl-glycine amide in Parkinson's disease. *Can. Med. Assoc. J.*, 107, 1079-1081.

Kastin, A. J., R. H. Ehrensing, D. S. Schalch and M. S. Anderson (1972). Improvement in mental depression with decreased thyrotropin response after administration of thyrotropin-releasing hormone. *Lancet*, 2, 740-742.

Kato, Y., K. Chihara, K. Maeda, S. Ohgo, Y. Okanishi and H. Imura (1975). Plasma growth hormone responses to thyrotropin-releasing hormone in the urethane-anesthetized rat. *Endocrinology*, 96, 1114-1118.

Kirkegaard, C., N. Norlem, U. B. Lauridsen, N. Bjorum and C. Christiansen (1975). Protirelin stimulation test and thyroid function during treatment of depression. *Arch. Gen. Psychiat.*, 32, 1115-1118.

Kline, N. S., C. H. Li, H. E. Lehmann, A. Lajtha, E. Laski and T. Cooper (1977). β-endorphin-induced changes in schizophrenic and depressed patients. *Archives Gen. Psychiat.*, 34, 1111-1113.

Lakke, J. P. W. F., H. M. van Praag, R. van Twisk, H. Doorenbos and F. G. J. Witt (1974). Effects of administration of thyrotropin releasing hormone in Parkinsonism. *Clin. Neurol. Neurosurg.*, 3/4, 1-5.

Lipton, M. A. and F. K. Goodwin (1976). A controlled study of thyrotropin releasing hormone in hospitalized depressed patients. *Psychopharmacol. Bull.*, 11(1), 28-29.

Loosen, P. T., A. J. Prange, Jr. and I. C. Wilson (1978). Influence of cortisol on TRH induced TSH response on depression. *Amer. J. Psychiat.*, 1351, 244-246.

Loosen, P. T., A. J. Prange, Jr. and I. C. Wilson (1978, in press). Thyrotropin releasing hormone (TRH) in depressed alcoholic men: behavioral changes and endocrine responses. *Arch. Gen. Psychiat.*

Loosen, P. T., A. J. Prange, Jr., I. C. Wilson and P. P. Lara (1976). Pituitary responses to thyrotropin releasing hormone in depressed patients: A review. *Pharmacol. Biochem. Behav.*, 5 (Suppl. 1), 95-101.

Loosen, P. T., I. C. Wilson, P. P. Lara, A. J. Prange, Jr. and C. Pettus (1976). Treatment of depressive state in alcohol withdrawal syndromes by thyrotropin releasing hormone. *Arzneimittelforschung*, 26, 1164-1166.

Loosen, P. T., I. C. Wilson, P. P. Lara, A. J. Prange, Jr. and C. Pettus (1977). Thyroid stimulating hormone response after thyrotropin releasing hormone in depressed, schizophrenic and normal women. *Psychoneuroendocrinology*, 2, 137-148.

Maeda, K., Y. Kato, S. Ohgo, K. Chihara, Y. Yoshimoto, N. Yamaguchi, S. Kuromaru and H. Imura (1975). Growth hormone and prolactin release after injection of thyrotropin releasing hormone in patients with depression. *J. Clin. Endocr. Metab.*, 40, 501-505.

Maggini, C., M. Guazzelli, M. Mauri, S. Carrara, P. Fornaro, E. Martino, E. Macchia and L. Baschieri (1974). Sleep, clinical and endocrine studies in depressive patients treated with thyrotropin releasing hormone. In, W. P. Koella, P. Levin and M. Bertini (Eds.), 2nd European Congress on Sleep, Karger, Basel. pp. 1-3.

Martin, J. B., S. Reichlin and G. M. Brown (1977). *Clinical Neuroendocrinology*. F. A. Davis Co., Philadelphia.

Matsuo, H., Y. Baba, R. M. G. Nair, A. Arimura and A. V. Schally (1971). Structure of the porcine LH and FSH-releasing hormone. *Biochem. Biophys. Res. Commun.*, 43, 1334-1339.

McCaul, J. A., K. J. Cassell and G. M. Stern (1974). Intravenous thyrotropin-releasing hormone in Parkinson's disease. *Lancet*, 2, 735.

Monahan, M., J. Rivier, R. Burgus, M. Amoss, R. Blackwell, W. Vale and R. Guillemin (1971). Synthesis totale par phase solide d'un decapeptide qui stimule des gonadotropins hypophysaire LH et FSH. *C. R. Soc. Paris*, 273, 508-510.

Mortimer, C. H., A. S. McNeilly, R. A. Fisher, M. A. F. Murray and G. M. Besser (1974). Gonadotropin-releasing hormone therapy in hypogonadal males with hypothalamic or pituitary dysfunction. *Br. Med. J.*, 4, 617-621.

Moss, R. L. (1975). Relationship between the central regulation of gonadotropin and mating behavior in female rats. In, W. Montagna and W. A. Sadler (Eds.), *Reproductive Behavior*. Plenum Press, New York. pp. 55-76.

Nair, R. M. G., A. J. Kastin and A. V. Schally (1971). Isolation and structure of hypothalamic MSH release-inhibiting hormone. *Biochem. Biophys. Res. Commun.*, 43, 1376-1381.

Nair, R. M. G., T. W. Redding and A. V. Schally (1971). Site of inactivation of thyrotropin-releasing hormone by human plasma. *Biochemistry*, 10, 3621-3624.

Nemeroff, C. B. and A. J. Prange, Jr. (1978, in press). Peptides and psychoneuro-endocrinology: A perspective. *Arch. Gen. Psychiat.*

Nemeroff, C. B., P. T. Loosen, G. Bissette, P. J. Manberg, I. C. Wilson, M. A. Lipton and A. J. Prange, Jr. (1978, in press). Pharmacobehavioral effects of hypothalamic peptides in animals and man: focus on thyrotropin-releasing hormone and neurotensin. *Psychoneuroendocrinology*.

Obiols. J., J. Pujol and J. Obiols-Llandrich (1974). Hormonas hipotalamicas y function tiroidea en los sindromes de presivos. Presented at 1st World Congress of Biological Psychiatry, Buenos Aires, Argentina.

Otsuki, M., M. Dakoda and S. Baba (1973). Influence of glucocorticoids on TRH mediated TSH response in man. *J. Clin. Endocr.*, 36, 95-102.

Ozawa, Y. and Y. Shishiba (1975). Lack of TRH-induced TSH secretion in a patient with Klinefelters syndrome: A case report. *Endocr. Jap.*, 22, 269-273.

Pfaff, D. W. (1973). Luteinizing hormone-releasing factor potentiates lordosis behavior in hypophysectomized ovariectomized female rats. *Science*, 182, 1148-1149.

Prange, A. J., Jr. (1977). Patterns of pituitary responses to thyrotropin releasing hormone in depressed patients: A review. In, W. E. Fann, I. Karacan, A. Pikorny and R. L. Williams (Eds.), *Phenomenology and Treatment of Depression*. Spectrum Publishing Co., New York. pp. 1-15.

Prange, A. J., Jr. and I. C. Wilson (1972). Thyrotropin releasing hormone (TRH) for the immediate relief of depression: A preliminary report. *Psychopharmacologia*, 26, 82.

Prange, A. J., Jr., C. B. Nemeroff and M. A. Lipton (1978). Behavioral effects of peptides: Basic and clinical studies. In, M. A. Lipton, A. DiMascio and K. F. Killam (Eds.), *Pshchopharmacology: A Generation of Progress*. Raven Press, New York. pp. 441-458.

Prange, A. J., Jr., C. B. Nemeroff, M. A. Lipton, G. R. Breese and I. C. Wilson (1978). Peptides and the central nervous system. In, L. L. Iversen, S. D. Iversen and S. H. Snyder (Eds.), *Handbook of Psychopharmacology*, Vol. 13. Plenum Press, New York. pp. 1-107.

Prange, A. J., Jr., I. C. Wilson, P. P. Lara, L. B. Alltop and G. R. Breese (1972). Effects of thyrotropin releasing hormone in depression. *Lancet*, 2, 999-1002.

Prange, A. J., Jr. and I. C. Wilson. Unpublished observations.
Prange, A. J., Jr., I. C. Wilson and P. T. Loosen. Unpublished observations.
Re, R. N., I. A. Kourides, E. C. Ridgway, B. D. Weintraub and F. Maloof (1976). The effect of glucocorticoid administration of human pituitary secretion of thyrotropin and prolactin. *J. Clin. Endocr. Metab.*, 43, 338-346.
Schalch, D. S., D. Gonzales-Barcena, A. J. Kastin, A. V. Schally and L. A. Lee (1972). Abnormalities in the release of TSH in response to TRH in patients with disorders of the pituitary, hypothalamus, and basal ganglia. *J. Clin. Endocrinol. Metab.*, 35, 609-615.
Schwarzstein, L., N. J. Aparico, D. Turner, J. C. Calamera, R. Mancini and A. V. Schally (1975). Use of synthetic luteinizing hormone-releasing hormone in treatment of oligospermic men: A preliminary report. *Fertil. Steril.*, 26(4), 331-336.
Shopsin, B., L. Shenkman, M. Blum and C. Hollander. T3 and TSH response to TRH: newer aspects of lithium-induced thyroid disturbance in man. *Psychopharmacology Bulletin*, 9, 29.
Siler, T. B., S. S. C. Yen and R. Gullemin (1974). Inhibition of somatostatin on the release of TSH induced in man by thyrotropin-releasing factor. *J. Clin. Endocr. Metab.*, 38, 742-745.
Sorensen, R., K. Svendsen and M. Schou (1974). T.R.H. in depression. *Lancet*, 2, 865-866.
Takahashi, S., H. Kondo, M. Yoshimura and Y. Ochi (1974). Thyrotropin responses to TRH in depressive illness: Relation to clinical subtypes and prolonged duration of depressive episode. *Folia Psychiat. Neurol. Jap.*, 28, 335-365.
Tiwary, C. M., A. L. Rosenbloom, M. F. Robertson and J. C. Parker (1975). Effects of thyrotropin-releasing hormone in minimal brain dysfunction. *Pediatrics*, 56(1), 119-121.
Turek, I. S. and J. Rocha (1974). Oral thyrotropin-releasing hormone (TRH) in depressive illness. *J. Clin. Pharmacol.*, 14, 612-616.
Vale, W. and C. Rivier (1975). Hypothalamic hypophysiotropic hormones. In, L. L. Iversen, S. D. Iversen and S. H. Snyder (Eds.), *Handbook of Psychopharmacology*, Vol. 5. Plenum Press, New York. pp. 195-238.
van den Burg, W., H. M. van Praag, E. R. H. Bos, A. K. van Zanten, D. A. Piers and H. Doorenbos (1975). TRH as a possible quick-acting but short-lasting antidepressant. In, W. H. Gispen, Tj. B. van Wimersma Greidanus, B. Bohus and D. DeWied (Eds.), *Hormones, Homeostasis and the Brain. Progress in Brain Research*, Vol. 42. Elsevier, Amsterdam. pp. 68-69.
Vinik, A. I., W. J. Kalk, H. McLaren, S. Hendricks and B. L. Primstone (1975). Fasting blunts the TSH response to synthetic thyrotropin releasing hormone (TRH). *J. Clin. Endocrinol. Metab.*, 40, 509-511.
Vogel, H. P., O. Benkert, R. Illig, B. Muller-Oerlinghausen and A. Poppenberg (1977). *Acta psychiat. scand.*, 56, 223-232.
Whybrow, P. C., A. Coppen, A. J. Prange, Jr., R. Noguera and J. E. Bailey (1972). Thyroid function and the response of L-liothyromine in depression. *Arch. Gen. Psychiatry*, 26, 242-245.
Widerlov, E. and R. Sjostrom (1975). Effects of thyrotropin releasing hormone on endogenous depression. *Nord. Psykiatr. Tidsskr.*, 29, 503-512.
Wilson, I. C., P. P. Lara and A. J. Prange, Jr. (1973). Thyrotropin releasing hormone in schizophrenia. *Lancet*, 2, 43-44.
Wilson, I. C., A. J. Prange, Jr., P. O. Lara, L. B. Alltop, R. A. Stikeleather and M. A. Lipton (1973). TRH (lopremone): Psychobiological responses of normal women. I. Subjective experiences. *Arch. Gen. Psychiatry*, 29, 15-21.

Biogenic Amine Metabolites in Cerebrospinal Fluid of Patients with Affective Disorders

P. VESTERGAARD*, T. SØRENSEN*, E. HOPPE, O. J. RAFAELSEN*, C. M. YATES*** and N. NICOLAOU*****

*Psychochemistry Institute, University Department of Psychiatry, Rigshospitalet, Copenhagen, Denmark
**University Department of Neurology, Rigshospitalet, Copenhagen, Denmark
***MRC Brain Metabolism Unit, University Department of Pharmacology, Edinburgh, Scotland

ABSTRACT

The concentrations of homovanillic acid (HVA), 5-hydroxyindoleacetic acid (5-HIAA) and 3-methoxy-4-hydroxyphenylglycol (MHPG) were measured in lumbar CSF from 33 patients with affective illness and from 23 neurological controls. The group of patients with affective illness comprised 29 depressed and four manic patients. During illness, the concentration of HVA was higher in the depressed patients ($P < 0.001$) than in the controls. Both unipolar and bipolar depressed patients had increased HVA levels ($P < 0.001$ and $P < 0.05$, respectively). The concentration of MHPG was greater than control values in the unipolar ($P < 0.01$) and bipolar ($P < 0.02$) subgroups but did not differ from control values in the depressed group as a whole. The concentration of 5-HIAA in the depressed patients as a whole and in the unipolar and bipolar subgroups did not differ from control concentrations. During illness the manic patients had increased levels of HVA ($P < 0.01$) and normal levels of 5-HIAA and MHPG. Sixteen of the 29 depressed patients had a second lumbar puncture after they had recovered. Compared with the pre-recovery values, the concentration of HVA was reduced in the unipolar depressives ($P < 0.01$) and the concentration of 5-HIAA lowered in the depressed group as a whole ($P < 0.02$).

The present findings suggest involvement of catecholamines in affective disorders.

KEY WORDS

Homovanillic acid - 5-hydroxyindoleacetic acid - 3-methoxy-4-hydroxy-phenylglycol - cerebrospinal fluid - affective disorders.

INTRODUCTION

In recent years many studies have reported on cerebrospinal fluid (CSF) levels of biogenic amine metabolites in patients with affective disorders; the aim of the studies was to assess the validity of the amine hypotheses of affective disorders. The main assumptions of these hypotheses, which are based on therapeutic evidence and animal experimental work, are that amine transmitter activity at important receptor sites is low in depression and high in mania (Bunney and Davis, 1965; Coppen, 1967; Schildkraut, 1965). The results of the studies have, however, been conflicting. In depression, the concentrations of 5-hydroxyindoleacetic acid (5-HIAA), homovanillic acid (HVA) and 3-methoxy-4-hydroxyphenylglycol (MHPG), metabolites of serotonin, dopamine and noradrenaline, respectively, have been found low or unaltered (Murphy et al., 1978; Schildkraut, 1978). In mania, the concentrations of the metabolites have been found low, unaltered or elevated (Murphy et al., 1978; Schildkraut, 1978). Several modified hypotheses have attempted to explain the inconsistent findings (Maas, 1975; Medical Research Council Brain Metabolism Unit, 1972; Prange et al., 1974; Åsberg et al., 1976).

The purpose of the present study has been to test some of the inferences of the amine hypotheses:

1) That there is a decrease in the concentration of HVA and/or 5-HIAA and/or MHPG in lumbar CSF in depressed patients during their illness;
2) that lumbar CSF amine metabolite concentrations, if abnormal, remain so after recovery (Ashcroft, 1973)
3) that unipolar and bipolar depressive patients have different lumbar CSF amine metabolite concentrations (Ashcroft, 1973).

METHODS

Affective Illness Patients

Twenty-nine depressed and four manic patients were studied. The depressed patients were divided into three groups: 1) unipolar depressive illness (14 patients) defined as two or more depressive episodes and no manic episodes; 2) bipolar depressive illness (six patients), defined as a present depressive episode and previous hypomanic or manic episodes; and 3) nine patients who had only the present depressive episode and for whom polarity was not determined. The four manic patients all had previous depressive episodes. The diagnostic criteria of Feighner et al.(1972) were used in this study.

The symptoms of depressive illness were rated with the Hamilton Depression Scale (HDS) before treatment was commenced and again after recovery following treatment with ECT (14 patients), tricyclic antidepressants (10 patients), or tricyclic antidepressants followed by ECT (5 patients). The four manic patients were treated with antipsychotic drugs of the phenothiazine or butyrophenone type. Informed consent for lumbar puncture was obtained from the patients. No medication was given during the five days prior to lumbar puncture.

Control Patients

The control group comprised 23 patients from the Department of Neurology of Rigshospitalet who had a lumbar puncture as part of their diagnostic procedure. These patients had no signs of psychiatric involvement, nor did they receive drugs known to influence the CSF amine metabolite levels.

Lumbar Puncture Procedure and CSF Samples

The patients were rested in bed overnight and no food or fluid intake permitted during the 12 hours prior to lumbar puncture between 8 and 9 a.m. A standardized procedure was adopted for the removal of 12 ml CSF from patients in the lateral decubitus position. The first 6 ml CSF were used for routine diagnostic tests, the next 4 ml collected for the analysis of the amine metabolites, and the last 2 ml stored for other purposes. The 4 ml sample was frozen immediately after collection and stored at -20°C or in solid carbon dioxide until assayed in Edinburgh by persons who were unaware of the identity of the sample.

The duration of storage of the CSF samples from the depressed patients was 6.4 ± 3.4 months (n = 50) and from the neurological controls, 6.4 ± 2.2 months (n = 23). For patients where CSF samples were obtained before and after recovery, the samples were stored for the same period of time, which varied from 1 to 13 months between individuals.

Biochemical Estimations

HVA. To 0.5 ml CSF was added 0.4 ml 1 N HCl and sufficient KCl to saturate the solution. The sample was mixed and centrifuged at 12,000 g for 1 min. The supernatant was transferred into a 1.5 ml Eppendorf tube, 0.5 ml toluene added and the tube agitated and centrifuged. The toluene layer was discarded and the extraction repeated with a second 0.5 ml toluene which was also discarded. The aqueous layer was then extracted twice with 0.5 ml ethyl acetate and HVA measured in the pooled ethyl layer by the gas liquid chromatographic method of Pearson and Sharman (1975). The mean recovery of 10-50 ng HVA added to 0.5 ml samples of CSF was 76 %. The results are expressed as ng/ml CSF, corrected for recovery.

5-HIAA and MHPG. 5-HIAA was assayed fluorometrically and total MHPG by gas liquid chromatography after incubation with a sulphatase preparation to hydrolyse MHPG sulphate (Davidson et al., 1977).

RESULTS

The age and sex of the patients with affective illness and the neurological controls are given in Table 1. There was no significant difference between the ages of the depressed and the control patients but the manic patients were older than the control patients.

TABLE 1. Age and Sex of Patients Studied

	Female	Male	Total	Age ± s.d.
Depressed patients	17	12	29	47 ± 15
Manic Patients	3	1	4	63 (53-81)
Controls	7	16	23	39 ± 12

CSF Metabolites and Hamilton Depression Scale (HDS) During Illness

The concentrations of 5-HIAA in the entire depressed group and in the unipolar and bipolar subgroups did not differ from control concentrations (Fig. 1). The concentrations of MHPG were greater than the control levels in the unipolar ($P < 0.01$) and bipolar ($P < 0.05$) subgroups but did not differ from control values in the de-

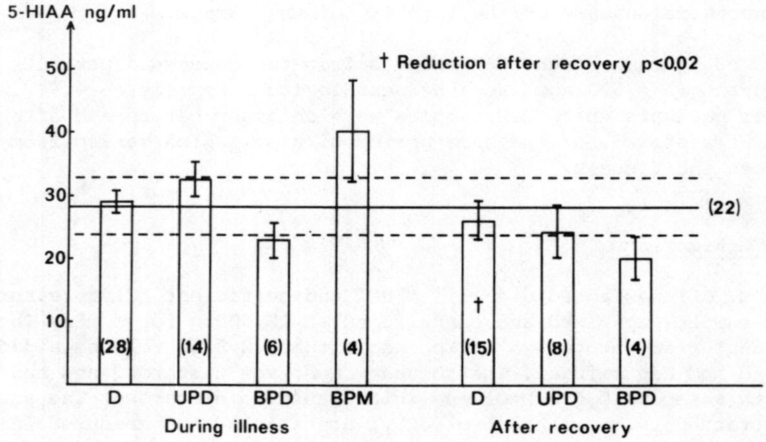

Fig. 1. Lumbar CSF 5-HIAA: Mean values ng/ml ± s.e.m. of all depressed (D), unipolar (UPD), bipolar depressed (BPD) and bipolar manic (BPM) patients during illness and after recovery compared with a control group of neurological patients.

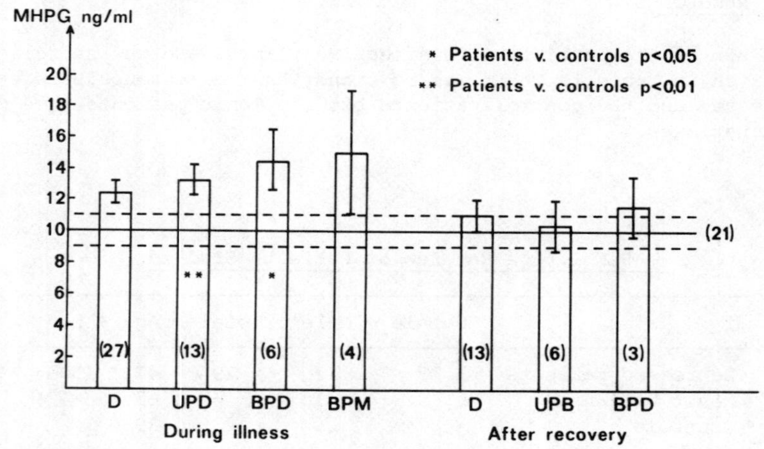

Fig. 2. Lumbar CSF MHPG: Mean values ng/ml ± s.e.m. of all depressed (D), unipolar (UPD), bipolar depressed (BPD) and bipolar manic (BPM) patients during illness and after recovery compared with a control group of neurological patients.

pressed group as a whole (Fig. 2). The level of HVA was higher (P < 0.001) in the entire depressed group and in the unipolar (P < 0.001) and bipolar (P < 0.05) subgroups than in the control group (Fig. 3). There was no significant difference between the concentrations of the three metabolites in the unipolar and bipolar subgroups.

The concentrations of all three metabolites were higher in the manic than in the control patients. These differences only reached significance for HVA (P < 0.01), possibly due to the small number (four) of manic patients (Figs. 1, 2 and 3).

The HDS scores for the entire depressed group for the unipolar and bipolar subgroups are given in Table 2. The "agitation" item on the HDS was not related to the concentrations of HVA, 5-HIAA or MHPG in lumbar CSF (Fig. 4).

CSF Metabolites and Hamilton Depression Scale after Recovery

The metabolite concentrations were lower after than before recovery (Table 2), but this reduction was significant only for 5-HIAA in the entire depressed group (P < 0.02) and for HVA in the unipolar depressed group (P < 0.01)(Figs. 1, 2 and 3).

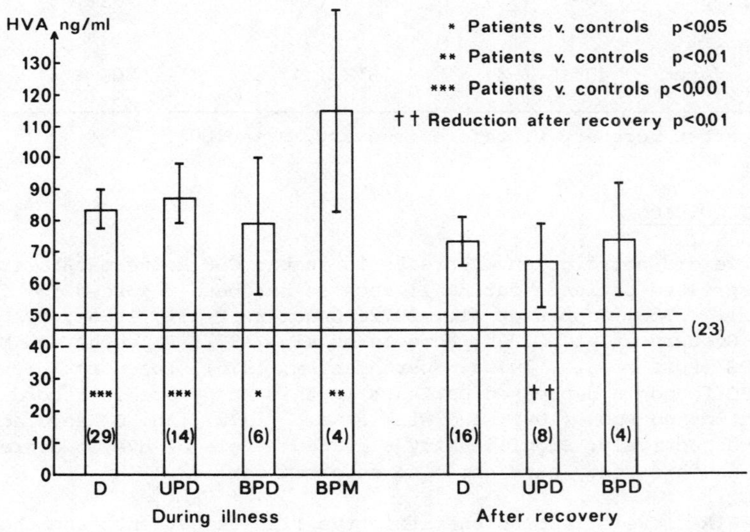

Fig. 3. Lumbar CSF HVA: Mean values ng/ml ± s.e.m. of all depressed (D), unipolar (UPD), bipolar depressed (BPD) and bipolar manic (BPM) patients during illness and after recovery compared with a control group of neurological patients.

Within individuals, the concentrations of 5-HIAA in the two CSF samples were positively correlated (P < 0.001). There was no significant correlation of the concentrations of HVA and MHPG between the two samples of CSF.

The HDS scores were significantly decreased after recovery (P < 0.001)(Table 2).

One-way analysis of variance and t-test for paired and unpaired samples were used for statistical analyses and P-values of $\leq$ 0.05 were taken to indicate a significant difference.

TABLE 2. Lumbar CSF Amine Metabolites and Hamilton Depression Score (HDS) in Patients with Affective Illness

Mean $\pm$ s.d. - Number of Patients in Parentheses

	5-HIAA ng/mg	MHPG ng/ml	HVA ng/ml	HDS
Controls	28±28 (22)	10±4 (21)	45±26 (23)	
Depressed patients				
before recovery	29±12 (28)	12±4 (27)	83±37 (29)	24±4
Unipolar group	32±12 (14)	14±4 (13)	88±37 (14)	24±5
Bipolar group	23± 7 (6)	15±5 (6)	78±54 (6)	25±5
Depressed patients				
after recovery	24±15 (15)	11±4 (13)	73±32 (16)	3±2*
Unipolar group	21±13 (8)	10±4 (6)	66±38 (8)	3±2*
Bipolar group	20± 7 (4)	12±4 (3)	75±38 (4)	4±3*
Manic patients				
before recovery	40±16 (4)	15±8 (4)	115±66 (4)	

* Patients after recovery v. before recovery, $P < 0.001$.

DISCUSSION

In this study we did not find any decrease in lumbar CSF amine metabolite concentrations in depressed patients during illness as has been reported for 5-HIAA (Ashcroft et al., 1966; Coppen et al., 1972; Dencker et al., 1966), HVA (Bowers et al., 1969; Goodwin et al., 1973; Mendels et al., 1972; Papeschi and McClure, 1971), and MHPG (Post et al., 1973a; Subrahmanyam, 1975). The normal levels of 5-HIAA and MHPG found in depressed patients in this study are in accord with reports by Sjöström and Roos (1972) and Wilk et al. (1972), and O'Keefe and Brooksbank (1973), respectively. Significantly elevated levels of HVA in depressed patients as found in this study have not been reported earlier.

The HVA and 5-HIAA levels in both the affective illness patients and the neurological controls were higher in the present than in past studies involving the same diagnostic groups estimated in the MRC Brain Metabolism Unit (Ashcroft et al., 1973; Davidson et al., 1977). The difference may be related to the fact that in the present study, the 7th to 10th ml lumbar CSF was measured, compared with the 1st to 5th ml in earlier studies Jakupčević et al. (1977) have shown that the concentrations of HVA and 5-HIAA increase logarithmically in consecutive 1-2 ml samples of lumbar CSF. It is, however, difficult to explain the elevated HVA levels which we found in the entire group of depressed patients and the elevated MHPG levels in the unipolar and bipolar subgroups (the sum of patients in the two subgroups is less than the number of patients in the entire group of depressed patients due to the number of patients (nine) in which polarity could not be determined). Since psychomotor and physical activity have been reported to increase the concentrations of amine metabolites in CSF and urine (Ebert et al., 1972; Maas et al., 1971; Post et al., 1973b), the patients' scores on the "agitation" item of the HDS were analysed (Fig. 4). Only low to moderate scores were obtained, indi-

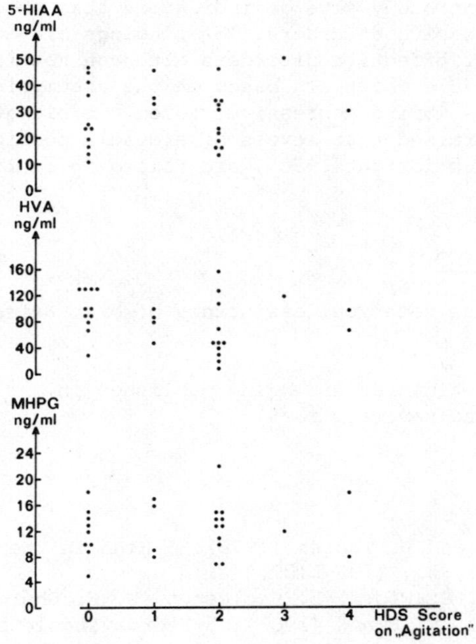

Fig. 4. Score levels on Hamilton Depression Scale item "Agitation" in relation to CSF amine metabolite levels.

cating that the activity of our depressed patients probably was no more pronounced than the activities of depressed patients in earlier investigations. Furthermore, we found no correlation between the agitation item on the HDS and CSF amine metabolite levels (Fig. 4).

The possibility of dividing depressed patients into a unipolar and a bipolar group based on CSF amine metabolite concentrations, as suggested by Ashcroft et al. (1973), was not substantiated in this investigation. No significant differences were found between amine metabolite concentrations in unipolar and bipolar patients (Figs. 1, 2, 3). We were unable to confirm the observations by Åsberg et al. (1976) of a negative correlation between low 5-HIAA values and severity of depression as measured by the HDS. Nor did we find that the 5-HIAA values of depressed patients were distributed differently from the values of the neurological control patients, which weakens the assumption that a subgroup of depressed patients exists, characterized by low 5-HIAA values (Åsberg et al., 1976). Unlike Åsberg et al. we did not find that attempted suicide occurred more frequently in patients with low 5-HIAA values. In our group of depressed patients attempted suicide occurred equally frequently in patients with low and high 5-HIAA values.

The significant reduction in HVA in the unipolar depressed patients after recovery and the tendency for all CSF amine metabolite concentrations to normalize after recovery are contrary to the observation by Ashcroft et al. (1973) that there was no change in the levels of HVA and 5-HIAA in these patients after recovery. Our findings suggest that the elevated amine metabolite levels during illness are related to the presence of depressive episodes and not to a disposition to affective illness.

The results of the present study give no indication that serotonin is involved in the pathogenesis of depressive disorders. The findings are compatible with a catecholamine hypothesis of affective disorders although not in the forms presented by Schildkraut (1965, 1978), which are based on the assumption of low levels of catecholamine metabolites during depressive states and elevated levels during manic states. It may be surmised that levels of arousal, possibly mediated by catecholaminergic systems (Schildkraut 1978), are raised in manic as well as in depressive states.

ACKNOWLEDGEMENT

We acknowledge the careful technical assistance of Mrs. Helen Wilson and Miss Lorraine Lamont.

The results of this investigation are being published in a slightly different form in Acta Psychiatrica Scandinavica.

REFERENCES

Åsberg, M., L. Träskman, and P. Thorén (1976). 5-HIAA in the cerebrospinal fluid. Arch. gen. Psychiat., 33, 1193-1197.

Ashcroft, G. W., T. B. B. Crawford, D. Eccleston, D. F. Sharman, E. J. MacDougall, J. B. Stanton, and J. K. Binns (1966). 5-Hydroxyindole compounds in the cerebrospinal fluid of patients with psychiatric or neurological diseases. Lancet, ii, 1049-1052.

Ashcroft, G. W., I. M. Blackburn, D. Eccleston, A. I. M. Glen, W. Hartley, N. E. Kinloch, M. Lonergan, L. C. Murray, and I. A. Pullar (1973). Changes on recovery in the concentrations of tryptophan and the biogenic amine metabolites in the cerebrospinal fluid of patients with affective illness. Psychol. Med., 3, 319-325.

Bowers, Jr., M. B., G. R. Heninger, and F. Gerbode (1969). Cerebrospinal fluid 5-hydroxyindoleacetic acid and homovanillic acid in psychiatric patients. Int. J. Neuropharmacol., 8, 255-262.

Bunney, W. E., and J. M. Davis (1965). Norepinephrine in depressive reactions. Arch. gen. Psychiat., 13, 483-493.

Coppen, A. (1967). The biochemistry of affective disorders. Brit. J. Psychiat., 113, 1237-1252.

Coppen, A., A. J. Prange, Jr., P. C. Whybrow, and R. Noguera (1972). Abnormalities of indoleamines in affective disorders. Arch. gen. Psychiat., 26, 474-478.

Davidson, D., I. A. Pullar, C. Mawdsley, N. Kinloch, and C. M. Yates (1977). Monoamine metabolites in CSF in multiple sclerosis. J. Neurol. Neurosurg. Psychiat., 40, 741-745.

Dencker, S. J., U. Malm, B.-E. Roos, and B. Werdinius (1966). Acid monoamine metabolites of cerebrospinal fluid in mental depression and mania. J. Neurochem., 13, 1545-1548.

Ebert, M. H., R. M. Post, and F. K. Goodwin (1972). Effect of physical activity on urinary excretion in depressed patients. Lancet, ii, 766.

Feighner, J. P., E. Robins, S. B. Guze, R. A. Woodruff, Jr., G. Winokur, and R. R. Munoz (1972). Diagnostic criteria for use in psychiatric research. Arch. gen. Psychiat., 26, 57-63.

Goodwin, F. K., R. M. Post., D. L. Dunner, and E. K. Gordon (1973). Cerebrospinal fluid amine metabolites in affective illness: The probenecid technique. Amer. J. Psychiat., 130, 73-79.

Jakupčević, M., Z. Lacković, D. Stefoski, and M. Bulat (1977). Non-homogenous distribution of 5-hydroxyindoleacetic acid and homovanillic acid in the lumbar

CSF of man. J. neurol. Sci., 31, 165-171.
Maas, J. W., H. Dekirmenjian, and J. Fawcett (1971). Catecholamine metabolism, depression and stress. Nature (Lond.), 230, 330-331.
Maas, J. W. (1975). Biogenic amines and depression. Arch. gen. Psychiat., 32, 1357-1361.
Medical Research Council Brain Metabolism Unit (1972). Modified amine hypothesis for the aetiology of affective illness. Lancet, ii, 573-577.
Mendels, J., A. Frazer, R. G. Fitzgerald, T. A. Ramsey, and J. W. Stokes (1972). Biogenic amine metabolites in cerebrospinal fluid of depressed and manic patients. Science, 175, 1380-1382.
Murphy, D. L., I. Campbell, and J. L. Costa (1978). Current status of the indoleamine hypothesis of the affective disorders. In M. A. Lipton, A. Dimascio, and K. F. Killam (Eds.), Psychopharmacology: A generation of progress, Raven Press, New York. pp. 1235-1248.
O'Keefe, R., and B. W. L. Brooksbank (1973). Determination of MOPEG, a glycol metabolite, in CSF and urine. Clin. Chem., 19, 1031-1035.
Papeschi, R., and D. J. McClure (1971). Homovanillic and 5-hydroxyindoleacetic acid in cerebrospinal fluid of depressed patients. Arch. gen. Psychiat., 25, 354-358.
Pearson, J. D. M., and D. F. Sharman (1975). The estimation of 3,4-dihydroxyphenyl acetic acid, homovanillic acid and homoisovanillic acid in nervous tissue by gasliquid chromatography and electron capture detection. Brit. J. Pharmacol., 53, 143-148.
Post, R. M., E. K. Gordon, F. K. Goodwin, and W. E. Bunney, Jr. (1973a). Central norepinephrine metabolism in affective illness: MHPG in the cerebrospinal fluid. Science, 179, 1002-1003.
Post, R. M., J. Kotin, F. K. Goodwin, and E. K. Gordon (1973b). Psychomotor activity and cerebrospinal fluid amine metabolites in affective illness. Amer. J. Psychiat., 130, 67-72.
Prange, Jr., A. J., I. C. Wilson, C. W. Lynn, L. B. Alltop, and R. A. Stikeleather (1974). L-Tryptophan in mania. Contribution to a permissive hypothesis of affective disorders. Arch. gen. Psychiat., 30, 56-62.
Schildkraut, J. J. (1965). The catecholamine hypothesis of affective disorders: A review of supporting evidence. Amer. J. Psychiat., 122, 509-522.
Schildkraut, J. J. (1978). Current status of the catecholamine hypothesis of affective disorders. In M. A. Lipton, A. Dimascio, and K. F. Killam (Eds.), Psychopharmacology: A generation of progress, Raven Press, New York, pp. 1223-1234.
Sjöström, R., and B.-E. Roos (1972). 5-Hydroxyindoleacetic acid and homovanillic acid in cerebrospinal fluid in manic-depressive psychosis. Europ. J. clin. Pharmacol., 4, 170-176.
Subrahmanyam, S. (1975). Role of biogenic amines in certain pathological conditions. Brain Res., 87, 355-362.
Wilk, S., B. Shopsin, S. Gershon, and M. Suhl (1972). Cerebrospinal fluid levels of MHPG in affective disorders. Nature (Lond.), 235, 440-441.

Adenylate Cyclase and the Mechanism of Lithium Action

R. H. BELMAKER and R. P. EBSTEIN

Jerusalem Mental Health Center-Ezrath Nashim, POB 140, Jerusalem, Israel

ABSTRACT

Few reports of lithium (Li) inhibition of adenylate cyclases meet criterion of 1) occurring at therapeutically-equivalent lithium concentrations and 2) continuing after chronic in vivo Li administration in a manner parallel to Li's clinical effect. The noradrenaline-sensitive cyclic AMP accumulation in rat brain is shown to remain inhibited after 21-28 days of chronic in vivo Li pre-treatment, at therapeutically-equivalent serum Li levels. Moreover, Li is shown to raise basal adenylate cyclase activity in rat cortical slices while reducing the noradrenaline-induced accumulation, suggesting a unique biphasic action. In humans receiving Li chronically the plasma cyclic AMP rise in response to epinephrine is inhibited. Parallel to this effect, the plasma cyclic GMP response is also inhibited, suggesting balanced presynaptic and postsynaptic actions of Li.

Keywords: Lithium, Adenylate cyclase, Cyclic AMP, Cyclic GMP, Noradrenaline

INTRODUCTION

A variety of experiments in several tissues have led to a concept of lithium (Li) as a general inhibitor of adenylate cyclases (Forn, 1975). However, Li has a remarkably narrow therapeutic index. Plasma levels less than 0.5mM are considered clinically ineffective whereas levels above 2.0mM are associated with severe toxic effects. Some Li experiments in animals have used highly toxic Li concentrations in order to demonstrate effects on adenylate cyclase. Thus it has not been clear whether Li's effect on adenylate cyclases explains its generalized toxicity above 2.0mM or whether a Li effect on a specific adenylate cyclase in brain might be related to Li's mode of action at therapeutic concentrations. Pharmacological research must attempt to carefully separate Li effects on adenylate cyclase into effects at therapeutic concentrations and effects at toxic concentrations. Li's clinical specificity and its relatively small number of side effects (polyuria, hypothyroidism, tremor) at therapeutic doses suggest that Li at therapeutic concentrations may inhibit some but not all adenylate cyclases. In addition, pharmacological research on adenylate cyclase and the mechanism of Li action must prove that effects demonstrated are long-lasting and parallel to Li's clinical effects, rather than short-term in vitro effects of the drug.

Ebstein and colleagues (1976) demonstrated that chronic Li treatment in therapeutic concentrations (serum levels 0.32 to 1.15mM) blocks the epinephrine-stimulated rise in plasma cyclic AMP in man (Fig. 1). It had been previously shown that the epinephrine-induced rise in plasma cyclic AMP is due to stimulation of a peripheral β-adrenergic adenylate cyclase (Ball and colleagues, 1972). The inhibitory effect of Li appeared to be somewhat specific since another antimanic drug, haloperidol, failed to affect the epinephrine-stimulated rise in plasma cyclic AMP (Belmaker and colleagues, 1976; Ebstein and Belmaker, 1977). The Li effect also seemed somewhat specific to the epinephrine-induced rise in plasma cyclic AMP, since Li did not inhibit the glucagon-induced rise in plasma cyclic AMP in humans (Ebstein, Kara and Belmaker, 1977). Kadouch and colleagues (1977) provided evidence that the epinephrine-induced rise in plasma cyclic AMP in man derives from non-neuronal β-adrenergic receptors, such as those in the muscle vascular bed. Thus the effect of Li on the epine-

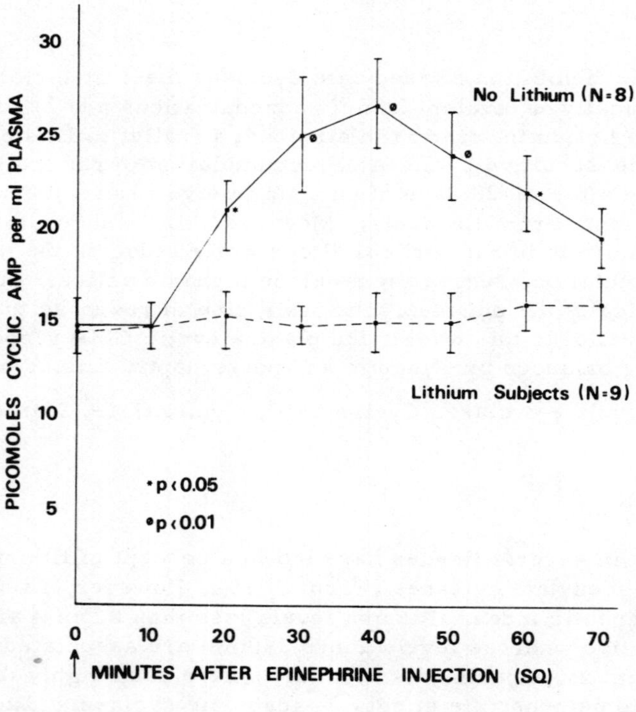

Fig. 1. Inhibition by Li of the plasma cyclic AMP response to adrenaline in man. Subjects received 0.5mg adrenaline subcutaneously at time 0 and blood was drawn every 10 minutes thereafter for cyclic AMP determination. All subjects were physically healthy consenting adults. Li subjects were 6 males, 3 females, mean age 38 $\pm$ 3.7, mean plasma Li level 0.71mM and the drug-free control subjects were 7 males, 1 female, mean age 34 $\pm$ 3.6.

phrine-induced rise in plasma cyclic AMP must be considered an effect of Li on a non-neuronal β -adrenergic adenylate cyclase. Additional evidence that Li can inhibit the peripheral β -adrenergic adenylate cyclase is provided by the in vitro animal experiments of Frazer and colleagues (1975). Incubation of rat hemidiaphragms in epinephrine-containing medium results in a rise in cyclic AMP levels which was significantly inhibited by pre-incubation with Li when intracellular levels of 4mM were attained.

Beck and Kim (1975) reported that the isoproterenol-induced rise in cyclic AMP in dog kidney medullary slices is significantly reduced by Li pretreatment (for 3 days, reaching serum levels of 1.1mM). While this experiment is notable as a demonstration of a Li effect on a possibly autonomically-innervated β -adrenergic adenylate cyclase in vivo at therapeutically-equivalent concentrations, the short (3-day) length of Li treatment is a methodological drawback. Such early effects need to be critically evaluated for possible development of tolerance after continued administration of Li. However, the reports of Ebstein and colleagues (1976) on epinephrine-induced rises in plasma cyclic AMP and of Murphy and colleagues (1973) on human platelet adenylate cyclase stand out as clear demonstrations of the inhibitory effect of Li on specific adenylate cyclases, in therapeutic concentrations in man after chronic administration. The report of Ebstein and colleagues (1976) that Li treatment inhibits the epinephrine-stimulated rise in plasma cyclic AMP has recently been confirmed (Friedman and colleagues, 1978). The study of Geisler, Wraae and Olesen (1972) on the ADH-sensitive adenylate cyclase is the only animal study that meets equivalent criteria of chronic in vivo treatment and therapeutically-equivalent doses.

In a key study Forn and Valdecasas (1971) demonstrated that in vitro Li at 2mM inhibited the noradrenaline (NA)-induced accumulation of cyclic AMP in rat cortical slices. Geisler and Klysner (1977) reported inhibition by Li in vitro of the dopamine (DA)-sensitive adenylate cyclase in a cell-free rat caudate homogenate. However, 10mM Li was used, thus making direct relevance to Li's clinical effects unlikely. Ebstein and Belmaker (1978) found similar results in a cell-free caudate homogenate, a dose-response curve showing that Li inhibition of the DA-sensitive cyclase does not become significant until 10-25mM. On the other hand, Schorderet (1977) reported that 2mM Li inhibited by 27% DA-stimulated cyclic AMP accumulation in intact rabbit retinas.

Reches, Ebstein and Belmaker (1978) examined the possible differential effect of Li on DA- and NA-induced accumulation of cyclic AMP in a resuspended P2 pellet (containing intact synaptosomes) obtained from guinea pig brain. This preparation exhibits properties of a true NA-sensitive adenylate cyclase (from the cortex) and a true DA-sensitive adenylate cyclase (from the caudate). The results (Fig. 2) suggest that therapeutic concentrations of Li which inhibit the NA-induced accumulation of cyclic AMP in the cortex may stimulate DA-sensitive accumulation of cyclic AMP in the caudate nucleus. At 1.0mM Li the difference between the NA-induced accumulation of cyclic AMP and the DA-induced accumulation of cyclic AMP is 54%, $p < .01$. These experiments used a compromise preparation (a resuspended P2 pellet containing intact synaptosomes) in order to achieve a DA and NA response in the same system, since a DA response has been difficult to demonstrate in tissue slices (Blumberg, Taylor and Sulser, 1975; Harris, 1976; Vetulani, Stawarz and Sulser, 1976) and a NA response difficult to demonstrate in true homogenates. Only by examining the effect of Li on DA- and NA-induced accumulations of cyclic AMP in the same preparation can the two responses accurately be compared. Small differences in Li's effects in different preparations may be crucial in understanding Li's effects, but if different preparations are used the concentration-dependent differences may be merely artifacts. The data presented in Fig. 2, while suggesting a true differential effect of Li on the caudate DA-induced cyclic AMP accumulation versus the cortex NA-induced cyclic AMP accumulation, must be tempered by our lack of detailed knowledge of brain Li concentrations (Bond, 1978). However, brain Li levels do not appear to be concentrated markedly above plasma levels in any part of the brain, though subcellular concentrations at synapses or other sites of action are not presently possible to determine (Bond, 1978). Of the two neurotransmitter-related adenylate cyclases presented in Fig. 2, the NA-stimulated cyclase would seem far more likely to be inhibited at therapeutic concentrations.

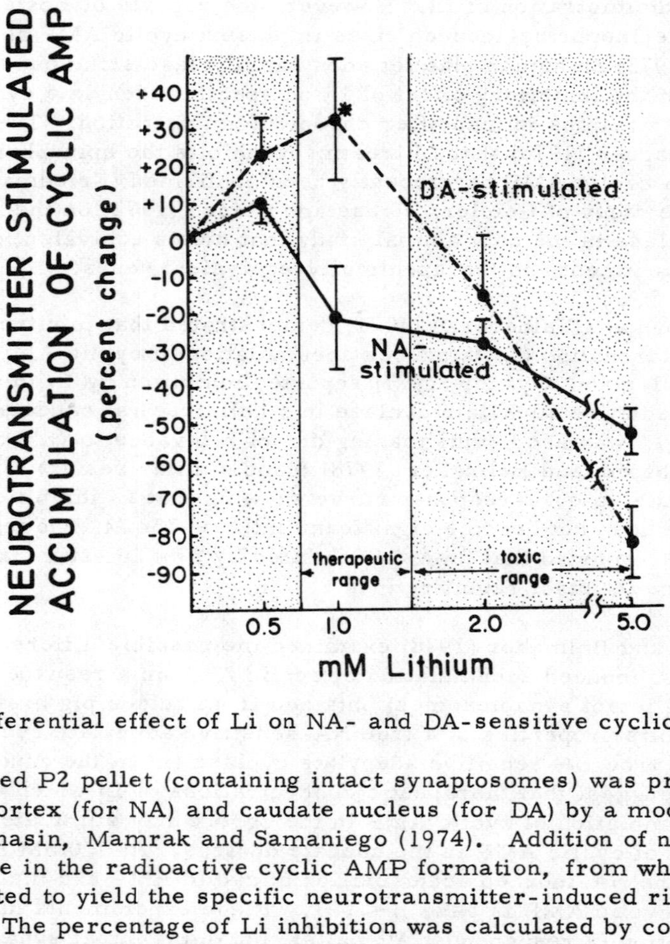

Fig. 2. Differential effect of Li on NA- and DA-sensitive cyclic AMP accumulation.
A resuspended P2 pellet (containing intact synaptosomes) was prepared from guinea pig cortex (for NA) and caudate nucleus (for DA) by a modification of the method of Chasin, Mamrak and Samaniego (1974). Addition of neurotransmitter caused a rise in the radioactive cyclic AMP formation, from which basal activity was subtracted to yield the specific neurotransmitter-induced rise in cyclic AMP formation. The percentage of Li inhibition was calculated by comparing the rise in cyclic AMP formation with neurotransmitter alone to the rises with neurotransmitter in the presence of various Li concentrations.
* $p < 0.01$ paired t-test.

These results prompted an examination in detail of the inhibitory action of Li on the NA-stimulated accumulation of cyclic AMP in rat brain. In cortical slice preparations it was found that at low concentrations Li inhibited the NA-induced accumulation of cyclic AMP (Fig. 3). In the presence of RO20-1724 (phosphodiesterase inhibitor) Li still inhibits accumulation of cyclic AMP in the cortical slices.

THE EFFECT OF IN VIVO LITHIUM

Only three studies (Ebstein and colleagues, 1976; Geisler, Wraae and Olesen, 1972; Murphy, Donnelly and Moskowitz, 1973) have demonstrated Li inhibition of an adenylate cyclase after chronic in vivo treatment. Demonstration of a Li effect after chronic treatment is important as many of Li's biochemical effects disappear after short periods (Schildkraut and colleagues, 1976) and thus cannot be related to Li's continuing therapeutic mode of action. None of the chronic Li and adenylate cyclase studies involved a brain adenylate cyclase, although one (Ebstein and colleagues, 1976) involved a peripheral β -adrenergic cyclase similar to the brain adrenergic adenylate cyclase.

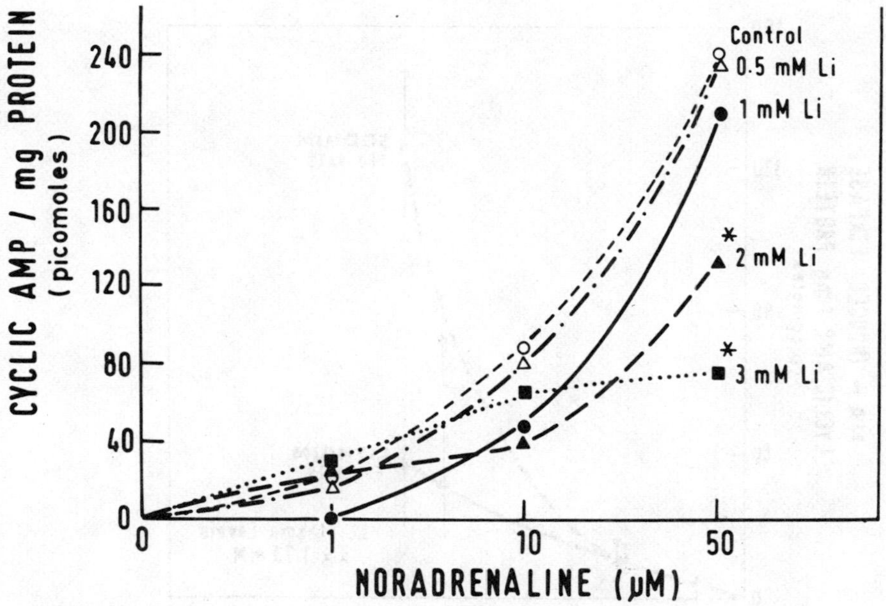

Fig. 3. Inhibition by Li of the NA-stimulated increase in cyclic AMP accumulation in rat cortical slices.
Cortical tissue slices were prepared as described by Kakiuchi and Rall (1968). After a 40 minute pre-incubation the Ringer solution was changed and the tissue incubated for an additional 30 minutes in medium with and without LiCl. NA was then added for an additional 6 minutes.
* $p < .05$, paired t-test.

An experiment was conducted to examine the effect of chronic in vivo Li pretreatment on the NA-induced accumulation of cyclic AMP. After 21-28 days of chronic Li pretreatment the NA-induced accumulation of cyclic AMP was examined (Fig. 4) in rat cortical slices. At 50uM NA the NA-induced accumulation of cyclic AMP in cortical slices obtained from Li-fed rats was significantly reduced compared to the control group. The mean serum levels of the Li pretreated rats on the morning of sacrifice was 1.73mM. While showing poor growth from a starting weight of 75-100 g during the 21-28 days of Li treatment, none of the rats used in the experiment of Fig. 4 died during Li therapy, and all were observed to engage in normal feeding and social behavior up to the day of sacrifice. Figure 4 suggests that inhibition of brain NA-sensitive adenylate cyclase is a continuing effect of Li treatment at therapeutic concentrations, and thus may be involved in Li's mechanism of action. It is of considerable interest that 1.73mM plasma Li levels caused 70% inhibition of the cyclic AMP response to 50uM NA (Fig. 4), whereas 3mM Li was required to achieve an equivalent degree of inhibition with in vitro experiments (Fig. 3). Murphy, Donnelly and Moskowitz (1973) reported a similar greater inhibition of human platelet adenylate cyclase after in vivo as opposed to in vitro Li treatment.

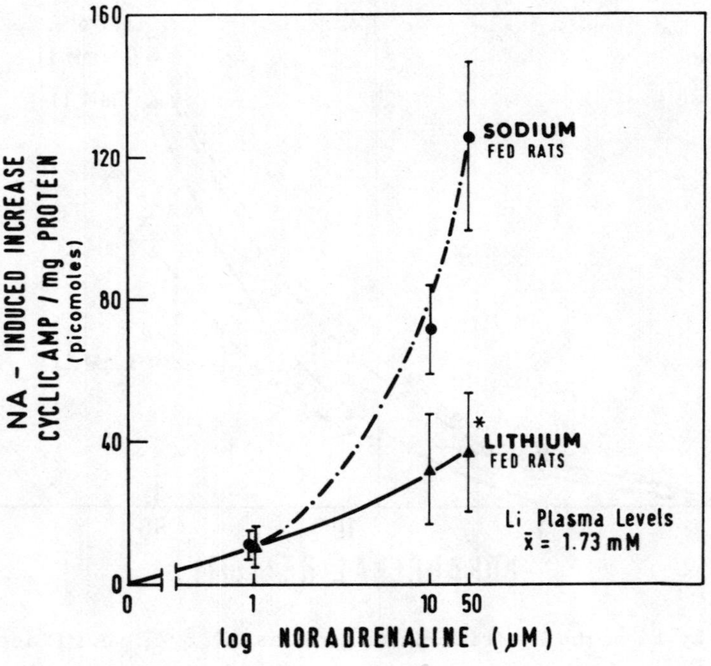

Fig. 4. Inhibition by 21-28 days of Li pretreatment in vivo of the NA-stimulated accumulation of cyclic AMP in rat cortical slices.
Rats were given LiCl or NaCl (both 0.212%) in food for 21-28 days before sacrifice. Cortical slices were prepared as in Fig. 3 and cyclic AMP increases over basal activity calculated after varying NA concentrations.
* $p < .01$, N = 10, paired t-test.

The above discussion concentrated on Li effects on hormone-stimulated adenylate cyclase activity. Adenylate cyclase activity can also be measured in tissue preparations without addition of hormone or neurotransmitter, but the biochemical meaning of this basal activity is unclear. It may represent a sum response to several endogenous stimulators in the tissue or it may represent some baseline functional level of the enzyme. Various experiments have reported conflicting results on the effect of Li on basal adenylate cyclase activity. Li has no effect on basal adenylate cyclase activity in the human renal medulla (Dousa and Hechter, 1970), in the dog kidney (Beck and Kim, 1975), in the thyroid (Wolff, Berens and Jones, 1970), in rat diaphragm (Frazer and colleagues, 1975), in brain homogenates from various regions (Ebstein, Reches and Belmaker, 1978; Geisler and Klysner, 1977; Reches, Ebstein and Belmaker, 1978; Walker, 1974), or in the retina (Schorderet, 1977). Li has been reported to raise to a small degree the plasma cyclic AMP levels in chronically-treated rats (Christensen and colleagues, 1977), to raise basal cyclic AMP accumulation in brain-stem slices (Palmer and colleagues, 1972), and to raise basal adenylate cyclase activity in glial cells in tissue culture (Schimmer, 1971). In the experiment (Fig. 1) involving the human adrenaline-stimulated rise in plasma cyclic AMP, Li did not seem to affect basal plasma cyclic AMP levels in humans. In the resuspended P2 pellet (containing intact synaptosomes) from guinea pig cortex (Fig. 2), Li (up to 5.0mM) had no effect on basal adenylate cyclase activity. These results, in a rough and highly speculative manner, seemed to parallel Li's ability to

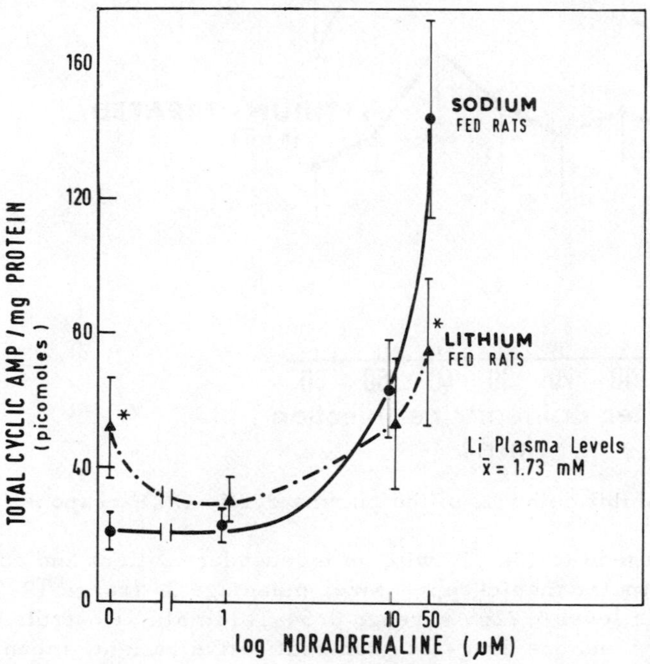

Fig. 5. Biphasic effect of 21-28 days of Li pretreatment in vivo on rat cortical cyclic AMP levels in the presence or absence of NA.
Data taken from the experiments presented in Fig. 4.
* $p < .05$, N = 10, paired t-test.

quiet overactive manic behavior without sedating normal or basal activity. However, rat cortical slice experiments have surprisingly revealed a different picture. Figure 5 shows the total cyclic AMP accumulation in the in vivo Li-treated animals of Fig. 4, where the NA-induced rise above basal activity is shown. Li significantly stimulates basal adenylate cyclase activity (NA concentration zero) while significantly inhibiting the NA-induced rise at 50uM NA. This phenomenon also occurs in acute experiments such as those of Fig. 3, where Li is added to tissue slices. The phenomenon does not occur, however, in the resuspended P2 pellet (containing intact synaptosomes) (Ebstein, Reches and Belmaker, 1978; Reches, Ebstein and Belmaker, 1978) or in caudate homogenates (Ebstein and Belmaker, 1978). Since Li has been reported to stimulate (Schimmer, 1971) basal as well as epinephrine-sensitive adenylate cyclase activity in glia cells in tissue culture, the tissue slice results may represent a complex summation of several effects in a multicellular system. However, propranolol, another potent

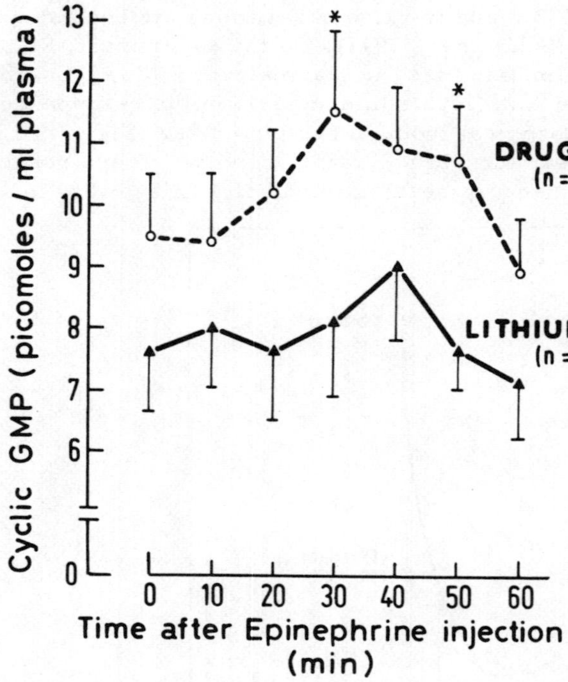

Fig. 6. Partial inhibition by Li of the plasma cyclic GMP response to adrenaline in man.
Method as in the legend to Fig. 1, with an independent patient and control group. Li patients were bipolar manic-depressive, mean age 34 (range 19-56), 5 males, 3 females, mean Li level 0.72mM (range 0.54-1.38mM). Controls were 9 hospital staff members and one drug-free schizoaffective patient, mean age 29 (range 22-40), 7 males and 3 females. The rise of plasma cyclic GMP over baseline is significant in the drug-free subjects at 30 and 40 minutes but is not significant for the Li subjects. The difference in plasma cyclic GMP between the two groups is not significant at baseline but is significant at 30 minutes and 50 minutes after epinephrine.

blocker of β-adrenergic-stimulated rises in cyclic AMP, was found not to affect basal cyclic AMP accumulation in rat cortical slices. The Li effect on basal levels of cyclic AMP accumulation is therefore probably not a secondary effect of β-adrenergic adenylate cyclase inhibition at some other site in the rat cortical slice preparation.

Clinically-motivated research on Li has long sought to demonstrate biphasic or balanced actions of this drug. One possible mechanism of balanced action has been investigated in a preliminary and indirect fashion, using the model of epinephrine-induced rises in plasma cyclic GMP in man. While epinephrine injection raises both plasma cyclic AMP and plasma cyclic GMP, the former effect has been shown to be due to stimulation of a peripheral β-adrenergic receptor and the latter to stimulation of a peripheral α-adrenergic receptor (Ball and colleagues, 1972). In animal brain cyclic GMP may be the product of stimulation of a presynaptic α-adrenergic receptor (Zatz and O'Dea, 1977) whereas cyclic AMP is the product of a postsynaptic β-adrenergic receptor. Figure 6 shows the effect of Li pretreatment on the epinephrine-induced rise in plasma cyclic GMP. In this new group of patients and control subjects the results of Fig. 1 on plasma cyclic AMP were confirmed (results not shown), and a less marked but noticeable inhibition by Li of the α-adrenergic rise in plasma cyclic GMP was shown. The rise in plasma cyclic GMP in controls is less than that of plasma cyclic AMP (Ball and colleagues, 1972) and so pharmacological inhibition is more difficult to demonstrate. Further experiments must be done in animal brain to explore the phenomenon of Li effects on cyclic GMP accumulation.

DISCUSSION

The inhibitory action of therapeutic concentrations of the Li ion has been demonstrated in vivo after chronic treatment for the vasopressin-sensitive adenylate cyclase from rat kidney (Geisler, Wraae and Olesen, 1972), the PGE1-sensitive adenylate cyclase from human platelets (Murphy, Donnelly and Moskowitz, 1973), the peripheral β-adrenergic-sensitive adenylate cyclase in humans (Ebstein and colleagues, 1976) and the NA-induced accumulation of cyclic AMP in rat cortical slices. In contrast to those adenylate cyclases which Li does inhibit, data both in guinea pig resuspended P2 pellet (containing intact synaptosomes) and in rat brain caudate homogenates suggest that Li at therapeutic concentrations does not inhibit the DA-sensitive adenylate cyclase. This is consistent with recent reports that Li does not affect human prolactin (Gruen and colleagues, 1978; Huey, Janowsky and Judd, 1977) or growth hormone levels (Huey, Janowsky and Judd, 1977) or the prolactin or growth hormone response to methylphenidate in humans (Huey, Janowsky and Judd, 1977). In this Li contrasts with all the neuroleptic drugs. Since Li has no neuroleptic properties, its failure to inhibit the DA-sensitive accumulation of cyclic AMP (Fig. 2) agrees with the fact that in contrast to Li all known neuroleptic drugs inhibit the DA-sensitive enzyme (Clement Cormier, Kebabian and Petzold, 1974). The increase of DA-sensitive cyclic AMP accumulation in the presence of low concentrations of Li (Fig. 2) may relate to reported exacerbations caused by this drug in schizophrenic patients (Johnson, Gershon and Hekimian, 1968; Shopsin, Kim and Gershon, 1971). At clinically toxic concentrations (above 2mM), Li loses this specificity and inhibits the DA-sensitive cyclic AMP accumulation as well as the NA-sensitive one. This finding offers a possible biochemical explanation for the Parkinsonian symptoms that have been reported in Li toxicity (Vacaflor, 1975), since Parkinsonian symptoms are thought to be related to reduction in DA neurotransmission.

Chronic Li treatment in rats inhibits the NA-induced accumulation of cyclic AMP in cortical slices. This effect is one of few in Li pharmacology that continues with chronic treatment at therapeutically-equivalent concentrations. The effect of Li treatment may be biphasic since cortical slices obtained from Li-fed rats show significantly higher levels of basal cyclic AMP accumulation than slices obtained from control rats, as well as significant inhibition of the NA-induced rise in cyclic AMP accumulation. This dual aspect of Li's pharmacology may have clinical implications. Although evidence is strongest that Li is an effective treatment in mania (Schou, 1973) this ion also appears to have a prophylactic or even therapeutic (Baron and colleagues, 1975) action against the depressive phase of manic-depressive illness. We may thus be observing in the rat cortical adenylate cyclase preparation a hint to the understanding of Li's unique biphasic and continuing prophylactic clinical action. The effect of Li on epinephrine-induced cyclic GMP accumulation in human plasma needs exploration in animal brain models and may also provide a clue to Li's balanced psychoactive effects and its clinical distinctness from β-receptor blockers like propranolol that also inhibit the β-receptor coupled adenylate cyclase.

REFERENCES

Ball, J.H., N.I. Kaminsky, J.G. Hardman, A.E. Broadus, E.W. Sutherland, and G.W. Liddle (1972). Effects of catecholamines and adrenergic-blocking agents on plasma and urinary cyclic nucleotides in man. J. clin Invest., 51, 2124-2129.

Baron, M., E.S. Gershon, V. Rudy, W.Z. Jonas and M. Buchsbaum (1975). Lithium carbonate response in depression. Arch. Gen. Psychiat., 32, 1107-1111.

Beck, N., and K.S. Kim (1975). Effect of lithium on catecholamine-induced antidiuresis and cyclic AMP in dog kidneys. Endocrinology, 96, 744-748.

Belmaker, R.H., R.P. Ebstein, H. Schoenfeld, and R. Rimon (1976). The effect of haloperidol on epinephrine-stimulated adenylate cyclase in humans. Psychopharmacology, 49, 215-217.

Blumberg, J.B., R.E. Taylor, and F. Sulser (1975). Blockade by pimozide of a noradrenaline-sensitive adenylate cyclase in the limbic forebrain: Possible role of limbic noradrenergic mechanisms in the mode of action of antipsychotics. J. Pharm. Pharmac., 27, 125-128.

Bond, P.A. (1978). Techniques for analysing lithium distribution in brain. In F.N. Johnson and S. Johnson (Eds.), Lithium in Medical Practice, MTP Press, Lancaster. pp. 215-223.

Christensen, S., A. Geisler, I. Bodani et al (1977). Plasma and urinary cAMP levels in normal and lithium-treated rats. Acta pharmacol. toxicol., 40, 455-461.

Clement-Cormier, Y.C., J.W. Kebabian, and G.L. Petzold (1974). Dopamine-sensitive adenylate cyclase in mammalian brain: A possible site of action of antipsychotic drugs. Proc. Natl. Acad. Sci. USA, 71, 1113-1117.

Dousa, T., and O. Hechter (1970). The effect of NaCl and LiCl on vasopressin-sensitive adenyl cyclase. Life Sci., 9, 765-770.

Ebstein, R.P., R.H. Belmaker, L. Grunhaus, and R. Rimon (1976). Lithium inhibition of adrenaline-stimulated adenylate cyclase in humans. Nature, 259, 411-413.

Ebstein, R.P., T. Kara, and R.H. Belmaker (1977). The effect of Li on the glucagon-sensitive adenylate cyclase in vivo in man. Acta pharmacol. toxicol., 41, 80-83.

Ebstein, R.P., and R.H. Belmaker (1977). A comparison of the effect of lithium and haloperidol on human peripheral β -adrenergic adenylate cyclase. In E. Gershon, R.H. Belmaker, M. Rosenbaum, and S. Kety (Eds.), The Impact of Biology on Modern Psychiatry, Plenum Press, New York. pp. 27-40.

Ebstein, R.P., and R.H. Belmaker (1978). Lithium and brain adenylate cyclase. Symposium Volume of the First International Lithium Congress, New York, in press.

Ebstein, R.P., A. Reches, and R.H. Belmaker (1978). Lithium inhibition of the adenosine-induced increase of adenylate cyclase activity. J. Pharm. Pharmac., 30, 122-123.

Forn, J., and F.G. Valdecasas (1971). Effects of lithium on brain adenyl cyclase activity. Biochem. Pharmacol., 20, 2773-2779.

Forn, J. (1975). Lithium and cyclic AMP. In F.N. Johnson (Ed.), Lithium Research and Therapy, Academic Press, London. pp. 485-497.

Frazer, A., E.S. Haugaard, J. Mendels, and N. Haugaard (1975). Effects of intracellular lithium on epinephrine-induced accumulation of cyclic AMP in skeletal muscle. Biochem. Pharmacol., 24, 2273-2277.

Friedman, E., M.A. Oleshansky, P. Moy, and S. Gershon (1978). Lithium and catecholamine-induced plasma cyclic AMP elevation. Symposium Volume of the First International Lithium Congress, New York, in press.

Geisler, A., O. Wraae, and O.V. Olesen (1972). Adenyl cyclase activity in kidneys of rats with lithium-induced polyuria. Acta pharmacol. toxicol., 31, 203-208.

Geisler, A., and R. Klysner (1977). Combined effect of lithium and flupenthixol on striatal adenylate cyclase. Lancet, 1, 430-431.

Gruen, P.H., E.J. Sachar, G. Langer, N. Altman, M. Leifer, A. Frantz, and F. S. Halpern (1978). Prolactin responses to neuroleptics in normal and schizophrenic subjects. Arch. Gen. Psychiat., 35, 108-116.

Harris, J.E. (1976). Beta-adrenergic receptor-mediated adenosine cyclic 3', 5'- monophosphate accumulation in the rat corpus striatum. Molec. Pharmacol., 12, 546-558.

Huey, L., D.S. Janowsky, and L.L. Judd (1977). Methylphenidate antagonism by lithium. APA New Research Abstracts, annual meeting Toronto.

Johnson, G., S. Gershon, and L. Hekimian (1978). Controlled evaluation of lithium and chlorpromazine in the treatment of manic states: An interim report. Com. Psychiat., 9, 563-573.

Kadouch, R., R.H. Belmaker, R.P. Ebstein, and L. Perez (1977). The mood response and plasma cyclic AMP response to intravenous methylphenidate. Neuropsychobiology, 3, 250-255.

Kakiuchi, S., and T.W. Rall (1968). The influence of chemical agents on the accumulation of adenosine 3', 5'- phosphate in slices of rabbit cerebellum. Molec. Pharmacol., 4, 367-378.

Murphy, D.L., C. Donnelly, and J. Moskowitz (1973). Inhibition by lithium of prostaglandin E1 and norepinephrine effects on cyclic adenosine monophosphate production in human platelets. Clin. Pharmacol. Ther., 14, 810-814.

Palmer, G.C., G.A. Robison, A.A. Manian, and F. Sulser (1972). Modification by psychotropic drugs of the cyclic AMP response to norepinephrine in the rat brain in vitro. Psychopharmacologia (Berl.), 23, 201-211.

Reches, A., R.P. Ebstein, and R.H. Belmaker (1978). Differential effect of lithium on noradrenaline- and dopamine-sensitive accumulation of cyclic AMP in guinea pig brain. Psychopharmacology, 58, 213-216.

Schildkraut, J.J., M. Roffman, P.J. Orsulak, A.F. Schatzberg, M.A. Kling, and Th. G. Reigle (1976). Effects of short- and long-term administration of tricyclic antidepressants and lithium on norepinephrine turnover in brain. Pharmakopsych., 9, 193-202.

Schimmer, B.P. (1971). Effects of catecholamines and monovalent cations on adenylate cyclase activity in cultured glial tumor cells. Biochim. Biophys. Acta, 252, 567-573.

Schorderet, M. (1977). Pharmacological characterization of the dopamine-mediated accumulation of cyclic AMP in intact retina of rabbit. Life Sci., 20, 1741-1748.

Schou, M. (1973). Prophylactive lithium maintenance treatment in recurrent endogenous affective disorders. In S. Gershon and B. Shopsin (Eds.), Lithium Its Role in Psychiatric Research and Treatment, Plenum Press, New York. pp. 269-294.

Shopsin, B., S.S. Kim, and S. Gershon (1971). A controlled study of lithium vs chlorpromazine in acute schizophrenics. Brit. J. Psychiat., 119, 435-440.

Vacaflor, L. (1975). Lithium side effects and toxicity: The clinical picture. In F.N. Johnson (Ed.), Lithium Research and Therapy, Academic Press, London. pp. 211-225.

Vetulani, J., R.J. Stawarz, and F. Sulser (1976). Adaptive mechanisms of the noradrenergic cyclic AMP generating system in the limbic forebrain of the rat: Adaptation to persistent changes in the availability of norepinephrine. J. Neurochem., 27, 661-666.

Walker, J.B. (1974). The effect of lithium on hormone-sensitive adenylate cyclase from various regions of the rat brain. Biol. Psychiat., 8, 245-251.

Wolff, J., S.C. Berens, and A.B. Jones (1970). Inhibition of thyrotropin-stimulated adenyl cyclase activity of beef thyroid by low concentration of lithium ion. Biochem. Biophys. Res. Comm., 39, 77-83.

Zatz, M., and R.F. O'Dea (1977). Efflux of cyclic nucleotides from rat pineal: Release of guanosine 3', 5'- monophosphate from sympathetic nerve endings. Science, 197, 174-176.

An Appraisal of Clinical Studies on the Dopaminergic Hypothesis of Depression

A. AGNOLI and S. RUGGIERI

Department of Neurology, School of Medicine, University of L'Aquila, L'Aquila, Italy

ABSTRACT

Although the dopaminergic hypothesis of depression is supported by experimental data it is not closely evidenced clinically with the use of dopaminergic drugs. To verify this disagreement between experimental and clinical data, a group of endogenous depressive patients has been treated with four different dopaminergic drugs:apomorphine, bromocryptine, piribedil and nomiphensine and evaluated using Self Rating Scales, Hamilton Rating Scale for Depression, Side Effects Rating Scales. The Circadian rhythm of prolactin and growth hormone and the central cerebral turnover of DA and 5HT were also studied in some patients using an acute probenecid technique and the evaluation of CSF acid metabolites. Bromocryptine and nomiphensine were particularly active in treatment of the inhibiting forms of depression but good results were also obtained in the agitated forms. The effects for apomorphine and piribedil were inconclusive.

GENERAL ASPECTS

Historical Background

A relation has been proposed between depression, mania and the content of the catecholamines of the central nervous system. The catecholamine hypothesis of depression holds that noradrenaline is the most important agent involved. However, neither the hypothesis nor the pharmacological agents upon which the hypothesis has been based clearly differentiate the relative roles of DA compounds with NE. In fact, the role of DA has not been conclusively defined, although its importance in motility and mood is well-known.

The first casual observation which opened discussion on the dopaminergic theory of depressionwas that in Parkinson's disease akinesia (and rigidity) are correlated to a reduction of DA at the cerebral level.

Hypokinesia is a symptom which is also present in depression. Using the technique of the dosage of the CSF HVA after probenecid to study the cerebral turnover of DA, Van Praag and Korf (1971) showed that while the accumulation of the CSF HVA was the same for depression and control subjects, it was different for retarded and non-retarded depression.

More recently, Birkmayer and Rieder (1975) have shown that the content of DA in the brain of depressed subjects compared to normal subjects is clearly reduced (this is not so for tyrosine). On the contrary, the NE is reduced only at the level of the red nucleus, while there is a general reduction of the 5 HT. The Authors concluded that the reduction of the DA is responsible for the loss of drive and emotional activity, the reduction of the NE is responsible for the characteristic posture of depressive patients and the reduction of the 5 HT is responsible for the insomnia.

The vital listlessness (vital depression), the main symptom of depression, is an expression of the loss of balance.

Even though this data is interesting it has been criticised taking into account that a reduction of cerebral DA and of the central turnover of its main metabolite (HVA) cannot be related to a state of illness (e. g. depression) but only to a symptom: hypokinesia or motor retardation (fig. 1).

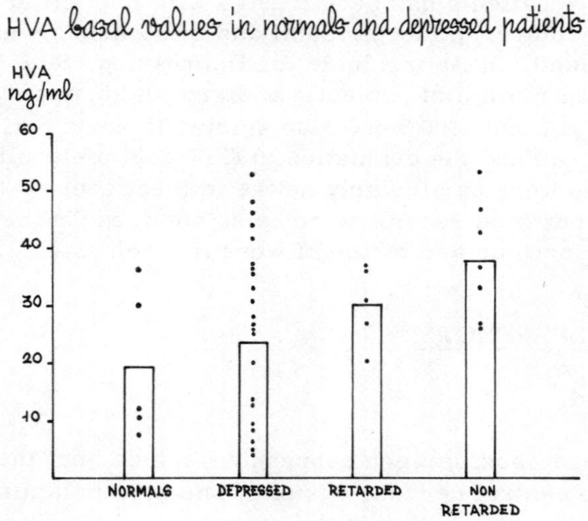

Fig. 1. Basal CSF levels of HVA have been evaluated in normal and depressive patients (retarded and non-retarded). No difference was found between the two groups. However, among the depressive patients the retarded have shown a significant decrease in HVA levels in respect of the non-retarded.

We feel that this aspect can be questioned. Another aspect to be underlined, in a heuristic sense, is the following: a relation between DA and schizophrenia is sufficiently evidenced. However, it is also known that both schizophrenia and mania are treated with the same drugs. During the course of this therapy depressive episodes are observed which are very similar to endogenous depression. The same is so for the other beneficial effects of the neuroleptic drugs on retarded depression or on the motor retardation symptom (Randrup and colleagues, 1975). In this regard we want to recall the intensity and the constancy of the depressive syndrome, listless - retarded, which is observed during the use of long-acting neuroleptics (Agnoli and colleagues, 1976).

There are, therefore, basic data, behavioral and biochemical observations which are stimulating in supposing the role of DA in affective disturbances.

Arbuthnott and Murray (1975) would have us consider another aspect: the controlling influence on mood is the level of effective activation on the postsynaptic receptor for amines rather than the amount of their presynaptic release. The sensitivity of the neuronal system at the mediator should be considered rather than just the quantity of the neuromediator. Consequently, there can be depressed subjects with normal levels of mediators (and of turnover and of metabolites) who have receptors which are less sensitive to treatment.

However, these findings did not definitely confirm a role of DA in the affective disorders, they only imply that other pathways, possibly acting in concert with DA, may be involved.

The Dopa Studies in Man

The scarcity of studies in this field, completely reviewed in the following section, is due mainly to the difficulty of using both L-Dopa and L-Dopa + ID. This difficulty is caused by the quantity of the aminoacid and, therefore, by the inevitable depletion of cerebral serotonin due to the activity of the common enzyme, aromatic decarboxylase. The studies conducted with L-Dopa in subjects with Parkinson's disease have suggested a role of the aminoacids in the control of affectivity, essentially by observing the side effects during the course of therapy:hyperactivity and agitation, delirium and paranoia, changes in the sleep pattern, increased anger, depression or less depression, improved memory function and intelligence quotient.

Further on,we will examine the data obtained in studies with L-Dopa, for now we want to say that any positive result will be criticised in the light of Von Praag's statement: the observed improvement is only secondary to disappearance of motor retardation and the depression does not improve or disappear. We will evaluate this statement later on.

Pharmacological Strategies

Because of these biological findings the clinical results obtained have been extremely contradictory. However, the inhibition of catecholamine synthesis with AMPT or the more selective inhibition of NE synthesis with fusaric acid have shown that the catecholamines, and particularly the DA, may be involved in the modulation of emotional symptoms.

Nevertheless, we must consider that in the clinical studies with AMPT, it was not possible to evaluate the relative contribution of DA versus NE depletion. The inhibition of the DBH with fusaric acid is certainly more selective. However, the accumulated DA can act as a false mediator interfering with the NE receptorial function. We want to point out that the reduction of DA, rather than the reduction of NE, is strongly related to the improvement of mania; whereas, after the use of fusaric acid the patients were no longer meniscal, they were more psychotic.

The findings of Bunney and colleagues (1977) should be mentioned. They underline the problem of the alteration of the receptorial sensitivity even in these clinical situations. In fact, after a short treatment with AMPT, once it is suspended, there are clinical signs which suggest receptorial hypersensitivity.

The data in literature shows that the depletion of a single monoamine is not, in itself, sufficient to justify a clinical depressive syndrome. At most, there are some behavioral modifications which are permanent in time and they are compatible with a depressive symptomatology (Mendels and Frazer, 1974).

Consequently, it is opportune to discuss and consider the necessity of a disorder of the different monoaminergic (or peptidergic) systems as a possible cause of the depressive syndrome (e. g. Parkinson) (Agnoli and colleagues, 1977).

DA Receptors, Agonist or Blockers

The use of DA receptor stimulants would be able to overcome the difficulties observed with the drugs used so far, and thus to better define the role of DA in emotional dysfunction and, in particular, in depression.

Results show that some of these drugs have marked anti-depressive effects. This data, together with the induction of recurrent maniacal episodes and the aggravation of psychogenic symptoms, confirm the current theories on the role of the DA mechanism responsible for the modulation of the emotional and cognitive behavior, as well as the hyperactivity and stereotypes observed in several animal models.

CLINICAL STUDIES

L-Dopa

Beside the problems already described which question the effects studied, we would like to undertake a more detailed discussion. There are controlled and non-controlled studies. The dosage of many of these is questionable; it is my opinion that only that of Matussek using Dopa + ID (750 mg + 75 mg) is a probable therapeutic dosage. We must remember that here we are still in the times when the Dopa had no function in Parkinson's disease. In spite of the basic criticisms, there are results (Frazer and Mendels, 1977). The more recent data of Harvey and colleagues show that in association with the behavioral variations there is a clear modification of the average evoked response and of learning.

Another study, that of Dunner and Pieve (1975),has given conclusive results;by associating L-Dopa with L-Triptophane this study proposed to overcome the problem of the clearing of serotonin.

Reconsidering the interpretation of Van Praag (resumed by Frazer and Mendels) the problem is whether the motor activation and the improvement of motor activity, which certainly are the consequence of the increase of cerebral DA, can trigger the improvement of the other aspects of depression. The data of Van Praag would demonstrate that motor retardation disappears whereas the mood is unchanged.

We would like to discuss this aspect of presenting the results we obtained using three drugs (pyribedil, bromocryptine, nomiphensine) in subjects with Parkinson's disease and depression (Fig. 2).

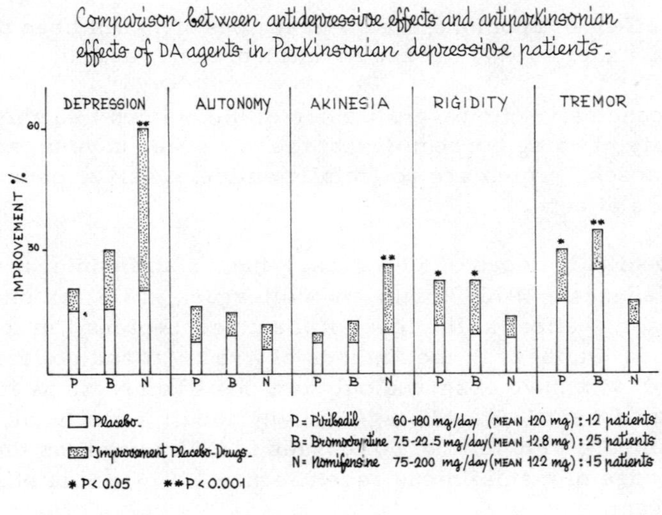

Fig. 2. The figure shows that dopaminergic agonist (pyribedil and bromocryptine) and inhibitors of the DA-re-uptake (nomiphensine)act in different ways on Parkinson's symptoms and on depression. Taking autonomy disturbances as the main symptom of Parkinsonism, it is easy to see that the dopaminergic drugs have a very poor effect while, on the contrary, they have a noticeable effect on depression. In our view this means that improving parkinsonian motor retardation is not improving depression.

The data reveals a dissociation between the effect on motor retardation and on depression. In fact, for bromocryptine and piribedil there is an accordance between the improvement, not significant however, of the motor retardation (deduced from the autonomy and the bradykinesia) and the depression. This is not so for nomophensine: with this drug the motor retardation improves significantly (25%) but depression improves up to 60%.

We accept this data, coming from a controlled study, as preliminary. Nevertheless, we are of the opinion that they cast a doubt on the fact that it is only the improvement of motor retardation that stimulates an improvement of the depressive state.

The Receptorial Agonist Studies in Man

Apomorphine . It has been stated in a non-controlled study (Teserova and Moleano, 1966, 1968, 1972), that apomorphine (0.5 - 1 mg s.c., three times a day for 11 - 14 days) can induce a depressive state which resembles melancholia in 64% of neurotic subjects and in 37.2% of normal subjects. Corsini and colleagues (1977) using acute doses of 20 /kg have observed in at least 30% of the subjects (normal, neurotic, schizophrenic) symptoms of depression which last from 20' to 40'. This data has not been confirmed by Lal and De La Vega (1975).

An antimaniacal effect of apomorphine (3 cases out of 7) has been demonstrated (Corsini and colleagues, 1977) but not an antidepressive effect.

This data is not conclusive. However, we are of the opinion that this is secondary to the impossibility of using correct doses: the low doses have an antimaniacal effect. The high doses, which are potentially antidepressive, cannot be used because of the side effects.

Pyribedil. Pyribedil (in doses of 60 mg/day) has an antimaniacal effect (Spitzer and colleagues , 1975; Porter and colleagues, 1976) which is probably due to its presynaptic effect at the level of the autoreceptors (in low doses). This data does not coincide with the findings of Arbutnott and colleagues (1975) and Murray (1975) who have observed only two positive reactions in 7 maniac patients. In higher doses (180 - 240 mg/day), pyribedil reveals an antidepressive effect in some subjects (Porter and colleagues, 1975) as well as the activation of recurrent episodes of mania in one case (Gerner, 1976). Side effects are always heavily present.

Also a reduction of prolactin in the CSF of depressed patients has been observed (Yemerson and colleagues, 1976) which indicates a stimulating receptorial DA effect.

Bromocryptine . The antimaniacal effect of low doses of bromocryptine (7.5 - 15 mg/day) has been demonstrated by Saren and Achareya (1977) and by Durr and Sathamantha (1977). An antidepressive action with higher doses (20 -30 mg/day) has been demonstrated by Agnoli and colleagues (1976, 1977), by Roccatagliata and colleagues (1976) and by Colonna (1977).

The results we obtained demonstrate that acute doses of bromocryptine (10 mg) do not modify the contents of HVA and 5 HIAA in the CSF after probenecid. The percentage increase for the HVA is not different from the normal; dividing the patients into subjects with a high and subjects with a low content of acid metabolites there is a greater increase for those with a low content.

The clinical cases were subdivided into two large groups: retarded and non-retarded depression. It was observed that in patients with retarded depression there was an increase in HVA after the use of bromocryptine, in the non-retarded depression the increase was in 5 HIAA.

The clinical results demonstrate that bromocryptine is active not only on the total score of the HRSD, but also on different clusters of the HRSD and not only on the cluster which expresses retarded depression.

<u>The Inhibitors of Re-Uptake</u>

<u>Amphetamine</u>. Dextroamphetamine is able to produce euphoria or a mood elevation in patients but it does not have a long-term therapeutic value in the treatment of depression.

Amphetamine elicits stereotyped behavior in man and other mammals (Randrop and Munkvad, 1967 ; Ellinwood and colleagues, 1973). It seems reasonable to assume that in man also the stereotyped behavior is mediated by DA. That the mood elevation and the stereotyped behavior be mediated by DA is confirmed by the data of Gunne and colleagues (1970, 1972). By intravenous injection of amphetamine they elicited euphoria, as assessed by patient self-rating, which they found would be inhibited by AMPT.

Euphoria was reduced by pre-treatment of the specific DA blockers: pimozide, while alpha or beta blockers were without effect (Jonsonn, 1971; Anjerd, 1971).

This data demonstrates that the mood-elevating effect of amphetamine is a consequence of the effect of the DA and not of the NE. This data coincides with that of transitory improvements observed when using amantadine (300 mg i. v.) in depressed subjects (Agnoli and colleagues, in preparation).

<u>Nomiphensine</u>. Nomiphensine is a drug which has an intense inhibiting action on re-uptake of DA and also of NE. There is much clinical data which demonstrates its strong antidepressive effect similar to that of the tricyclic drugs (Hoechst Symposia, Rome and Alval).

Our experience showed an increase of the HVA (after probenecid) more than with bromocryptine. The percentage increase was greater for subjects with a low HVA.

The clinical results have shown that nomiphensine is a strong antidepressive agent not only on the total score of the HRSD but also on the different clusters (Agnoli and colleagues, 1976)

WHY IS IT THAT THE EFFECT ON NORADRENALINE RE-UPTAKE COULD NOT BE RESPONSIBLE FOR THE ANTI-DEPRESSIVE EFFECT?

This problem can be as follows:it is necessary to consider drugs with a central NE action, alpha or beta. Tha data available today is scarce but interesting.

The Alpha Central Stimulants

Of the various alpha central stimulants, only clonidine can be used clinically. There is no data or literature relative to its effects on mood. Our clinical experience is negative.

Considering hypotension, it is impossible to reach sufficient dosages.

The Beta Central Stimulants

On the contrary, there is evidence that these drugs have caused hallucinatory reactions in chronic deliriants (Feline and colleagues, 1975, 1977) and psychic dependence of asthmatic patients (Gauthier, 1976).

A marked and rapid antidepressive action has been attributed to salbutamole in cases of endogenous depression (Lecutier and colleagues, 1977; Widlocher and colleagues, 1977; Jeuvert and colleagues, 1977).

Of these results, we could discuss the action of the mixed inhibitors of re-uptake (NE and DA) such as amphetamine and nomiphensine which could show an anti-depressive action even for an NE effect.

CONCLUSION

Within the catecholamine theory of depression, the role of the NE is extremely contradictory, whereas the role of the DA always has greater experimental and clinical backing.(Fig. 3).

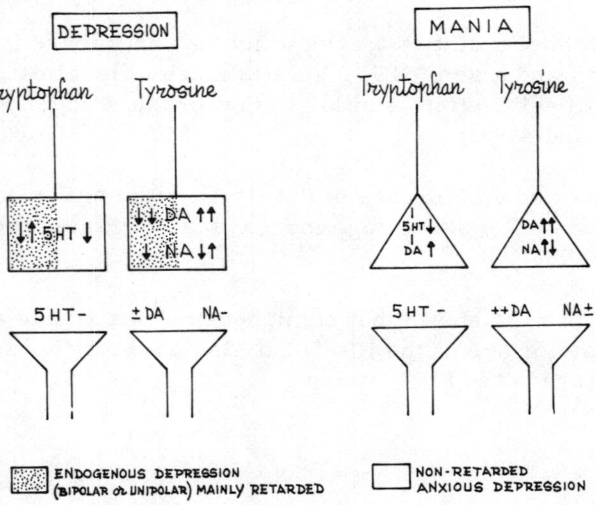

Fig. 3. The biochemical hypothesis in depression and mania can be represented by two different models:
1. The retarded endogenous depression seems to be mainly related to a normal content in 5 HT and a lower content in DA and in less extent in NA.
2. The non-retarded anxious depression is mainly characterized by a clear decrease in 5 HT and a normal content in NA and DA.
Regarding mania there is again decrease in 5 HT and a definite decrease in DA and NA.

REFERENCES

Agnoli, A., Casacchia, M., Zamponi, A., Pirro, R., Martucci, N. (1977a). Assessing the efficacy of long-acting neuroleptics. In Evaluation of New Drugs in Clinical Psychopharmacology. Edited by Bertelli, A., Cassano, G.B., Castrogiovanni, P., Levine, J. Wittenborn, J.R. Published by Prous, J.R. Vol. I, April 1977, pp. 443-446.

Agnoli, A., Ruggieri, S., Cerone, C., Aloisi, P., Baldassarre, M., Stramentinoli, G. (1977b). The Dopamine hypothesis of depression: results of treatment with dopaminergic drugs. In Depressive Disorders Ed. Hoechst, F.K., Schattauer Verlag, Stuttgart, New York. Rome 1977.

Agnoli, A., Polleri, A., Cerone, C., Ruggieri, S., Denaro, A., Fazio, C. (1976) The dopamine hypothesis of depression effect of a dopamine stimulant. C.I.N.P.

ALIVAL - (Nomifensin). Symposium über Ergebnisseder Experimentellen und Klinischen Prufung (1976). F.K. Schattauer Verlag. Publ. by Stuttgart-New York.

Arbuthnott, G.W., Murray, L.G. (1975) Dopamine receptor agonists in psychiatric disease. In D.B. Caine, Chase, T.N. and Barbeu, A. (Ed.), Advances in Neurology, Vol. 9, Raven Press, New York.

Birkmayer, W., Riederer, P. (1975) Biochemical post-mortem finding in depressed patients. J. of Neural Transmission., 37, pp. 95-109.

Bunney, W.E., Kopanda, R.T., Murphy, D.L. (1977) Sleep and behavioral changes possibly reflecting central receptor hypersensitivity following catecholamine synthesis inhibition in man. Acta Psychiatr. Scand., 56, pp. 189-203.

Corsini and colleagues (1977), Personal communication.

Corsini, G.U., Del Zompo, M., Manconi, S., Cianchetti, C., Mangoni, A., Gessa, G.L. (1977) Sedative, hypnotic and antipsychotic effects of low doses of apomorphine in man. In G.L. Gessa (Ed.), Advances in Biochemical Psychopharmacology, Vol. 16, Raven Press, New York.

Deniker, P. (1971). Clinical trials of a new anti-depressive amphetamine: d-I chloro N methyl amphetamine. Therapy, 26, 1, pp. 219-226.

Dorr, C., Satanan Than, K. (1976) Treatment of mania with bromocryptine. British Medical Journal, 29 May 1976.

Dunner, D.L., Fieve, R.R. (1975). Affective disorder: studies with amine precursors. Am. J. Psychiatry, 132, 2.

Dunner, D.L., Fieve, R.R. (1975). Affective disorders and studies with amine precursors. Am. J. Psychiatry, 133, pp. 180-183.

Ellinwood, E.H., Sudilovsky, A., Nelson, L.M. (1973). Am. J. Psychiatry, 130, pp. 1088-1093.

Fawcett, J. (1971a). Depression and MHPG excretion. Response to dextro amphetamine and tricyclic antidepressants. Arch. Gen. Psychiatr., 25, 3, pp. 247 - 255.

Fawcett, J. (1971b). Dextroamphetamine response as a possible predictor of improvement with tricyclic therapy in depression. Arch. Gen. Psychiatr. 25, 3, pp. 243-255.

Feline, A., Quetin, A.M. Effet indesirable de derives beta-stimulants? Emergence d'une symptomatologie psychiatrique aigue chez des malades mentaux. Nouv. Pres. Med. (1975) Vol. 4, pp. 39-41.

Feline, A., Jouvent, R. (1977). Manifestation psycho-sensorielles observees chez des psychotiques soumises a des medication beta-mimetiques. Encephale, 3, pp. 149-158.

Frazer, A., Mendels, J. Use of L-dopa in depression. In E. Costa and G. L. Gessa (Ed.). Advances in Biochemical Psychopharmacology, Vol. 16, Raven Press, New York.

Gaultier, M., Gervais, P., Lagier, G., Danan, L. (1977). Pharmacodependance psychique ai salbutamol en areosol chez una asmatique. Therapie, 31, pp. 149 - 158.

Gerner, R.H., Post, R.M., Bunney, W.E. (1976). A Dopaminergic mechanism in mania. Am. J. Psychiatry, 133, 10.

Gunne, L.M., Anggard, E., Jonsson, L.E. (1970) Blockade of amphetamine effects in human subjects. In A. Tongue and E. Tongue (Ed.), International Institute of the Prevention and Treatment of Drug Dependence, I.C.A.A. pp. 249 - 255, Lausanne, Switzerland.

Gunne, L.M., Anggard, E., Jonsson, L.E. (1972) Clinical trials with amphetamine-blocking drugs, Psychiatr., Neurol., Neurochir., 75, 225.

Henry, G.M., Buchsbaum, M., Murphy, D.L. (1976). Intravenous L-dopa plus carbidopa in depressed patients: average evoked response, learning and behavioral changes. Psychosomatic Medicine, 38, 2.

Jonsson, L.E., Anggard, E., Gunne, L.M. (1971) Blockade of intravenous amphetamine euphoria in man. Clin. Pharmacol. Therap., 12, 889.

Klerman, G.L. (1972). Drug therapy of clinical depression: current status and implication for research on neuropharmacology of the affective disorders. J. Psychiatry Res., 9, 3, pp. 253-270.

Lall, S., De La Vega, C.S. (1975). Apomorphine and psychopathology. J. Neurol. Neurosurg. and Psychiatry, 38, pp. 722-726.

Lecrubier, Y., Jouvent, R., Puech, A., Simon, P., Widlocher, D. (1977). Effet antidepresseur d'un stimolant beta-adrenergique. Nouv. Press. Med., 6, 2786.

Mendels, J., Stern, S., Frazer, A. Biological concepts of depression. In D. M. Gallant and G. M. Simpson (Ed.). Depression: behavioral, biochemical, diagnostic and treatment concepts, Spectrum, New York.

Mendels, J., Frazer, A. (1974). Brain biogenic amine depletion and mood. Arch. Gen. Psychiatry, 30.

Post, R.M., Gerner, R.H., Carman, J.S., Bunney, W.E., Jr. (1976). Effect of low doses of a dopamine-receptor stimulator in mania. The Lancet, pp. 203-204. Jan. 24.

Randrup, A., Munkvad, J., Fog, R., Ayhan, L.E. (1975). Catecholamines in activation stereotypy and level of mood. In A. J. Friedhoff (Ed.). Catecholamines and behaviour, Vol. I, Plenum Press, New York.

Randrup, A., Munkvad, I. (1967). Stereotyped activities produced by amphetamine in several animal species and man. Psicofarmacologia, 2, 30.

Roccatagliata and colleagues, Trattamento delle depressioni endogene con bromoergocriptina. Studio preliminare.

Saran, B.J., Acharya, S. (1977). Bromocryptine in treating mania. Am. J. Psychiatry, 134, Letters to the editor, 6 June.

Tesarova, O. (1972a). Sledovanie mecanizmov thimoleleptikeho ucinku, farmak ma modeli apomorfinovery deprèsie, Activitas Nervosa Superior (Praha), 10, pp. 287-288.

Tesarova, O. (1972b). Experiemntal depression caused by apomorphine and plenoharmane. Pharmakopsychiatrie, Neuropsychopharmacologie, 5, pp. 13 - 19.

Tesarova, O., Molcan, J. (1966). A contribution to the problem of experimental depression. Activitas Nervosa Superior (Praha), pp. 551-552.

Van Praag, H. M., Korf, J. (1971). Retarded depression and the dopamine metabolism. Psychofarmacologia, 19, pp. 199-203.

Van Praag, H. M., Korf, J. (1973) Cerebral monamines and depression. An investigation with the probenecid technique. Arch. Gen. Psychiatry, 28 .

Van Praag, H. M., Korf, J., Lakke, J. P. W. F., Schut, T. (1975). Dopamine metabolism in depressions, psychoses and parkinson's disease: the problem of specificity of biological variables in behaviour disorders. Psychological medicine, 5, 2, pp. 138 - 146.

Widlocher, D., Lecrubier, Y., Jouvent, R., Puech, A., Simon, P. (1977) Antidepressant effect of salbutamol. Lancet, 8 Oct. pp. 767 - 768.

HLA Antigens in Affective Disorders

J. MENDLEWICZ, P. VERBANCK, P. LINKOWSKI and A. GOVAERTS

ABSTRACT

The distribution of HLA antigen frequencies has been studied in patients with affective disorders. There was no significant difference between bipolar and unipolar patients as compared to controls. Preliminary data on HLA antigen distribution in schizophrenic patients are reported. Our negative results in affective disorders are discussed in relation to HLA studies reported from other laboratories, with special reference to some potential methodological problems.

INTRUDUCTION

Recently, a number of investigators have been studying the possible association between some diseases and the major histocompatibility complex (MHC). The HLA complex is on the short arm of chromosome 6 about 20 centimorgans (cM) from the centromere (McKusick and Ruddle, 1977). The HLA system is highly polymorphic, with 27 alleles known up today. It is inherited in a codominant fashion, which makes it possible to apply Mendelian segregation analysis. The membrane structures controlled by these loci are able to induce immune reactions to allografts, but other possible roles, including cell membrane functions are as yet unclear. An association between the HLA system and diseases of autoimmune kind like ankylosing spondylarthritis or Reiter's syndrome has been demonstrated (Brewerton and others, 1973; Morris and others, 1974). Recently studies have been performed to investigate possible associations between the major histocompatibility complex (MHC) and psychiatric disorders, mainly schizophrenia and manic-depressive illness. Despite the big number of papers published so far, definitive conclusions are not available. On the contrary, the interpretation of results is uneasy, as illustrated by Table I and Table II which summarize the results of some studies on the association between HLA system, manic-depressive illness and schizophrenia.

TABLE I: HLA Studies In Affective Illness

Authors	HLA Antigens excess in	deficit in
Bennahum and others (1976)	BW 17	
Stember and Fieve (1977)	B 5 B 13	B 12
Beckman and others (in press)	A 10	B 7
Shapiro and others (1976)¨	BW 16	
Shapiro and others (1977)¨		
Govaerts and others (1977)¨	-	-
Temple and others (in press)¨		CW 3
James and others (in press)¨	-	-

¨P Correction for number of antigens

TABLE II: HLA Studies in Schizophrenia

Authors	HLA Antigens excess in	deficit in
Cazullo and others (1974)	A 1	
Eberhard and others (1975)¨	A 9	
Bennahum and others (1976)	A 2	A 1
Smeraldi and others (1976)¨		A 10
Ivanyi and others (1976)¨	A 28	
Ivanyi and others (1977)¨	CW 4 (only in paranoid patients)	
Mercier and others (1977)	A 9 B 5 (only in paranoid patients)	
Perris and others (in press)		

¨P Correction for number of antigens

The most provocative study to date is the study of Shapiro and others (1976) on 47 affectively ill patients. The antigen BW 16 was present in 40 % of bipolar patients. In a subsequent report, Shapiro and others (1977) have confirmed the finding of a relative excess of BW 16 among affectively ill patients as compared to controls. These results are more reliable because they were adjusted for the number of tests performed and were replicated on a larger series. The conflicting results of all these studies may indicate that there are methodological problems in the design of such studies and in the interpretation of the results.

In this paper, we want to discuss the design and the interpretation of this kind of experiment on the basis of a new study on manic-depressive illness.

Material and Methods

To investigate the existence of an association between HLA system and manic-depressive illness, the best method, we feel, is to retest the previously reported associations on a new sample of patients originating from the same population. In our first study (1977) on 118 affectively ill patients, we reported the possible existence of two associations between the HLA system and affective illness. There was a relative excess in HLA B 5 (P=0.05) and a relative deficit in HLA BW 15 (P=0.02) in the affective group versus the controls (Govaerts and others, 1977). However, statistical associations were no more present when the P error was corrected for the number of antigens tested as suggested by Bodmer (1973). This correction is justified by the fact that the risk for observing a false positive association increases with the number of antigens studied (error type 1). This may very well be the case, but this method of correction may not be best justified. This type of correcting factor does not take into account the size of the sample studied, which is an important variable for the precision and reliability of the results. Moreover, this type of correction is even more dubious when more than one association is reported. Some investigators have attempted to confirm their results by enlarging their series (Shapiro and others, 1976, 1977 for affective illness; Cazullo and others, 1974; Smeraldi and others, 1976; Ivanyi and others, 1976, 1977 for schizophrenia). There is no doubt that larger sampling provides better estimation, but error type 1 can not be satisfactorily estimated. This makes it impossible to determine the expected sample's size, which would unable us to draw valid interpretations for the observed data. The best and simple method for testing the validity of apparently significant results, we feel, is to reassess the first experiment by investigating with the same design new samples, independently from the first ones. The new samples, however, have to originate from the same patients' and controls' populations as in the first study. One can then reassess the significance of the previously observed associations between some antigens and bipolar manic-depressive illness. A new sample of 47 bipolar manic-depressive patients consecutively admitted to the Psychiatric Institute of the University of Brussels was ascertained between October 1976 and September 1977. A new control sample of 74 blood donors or potential kidney donors was also constituted during the same period. Only the antigens which appeared to be associated with manic-depressive illness (HLA B 5 and HLA BW 15) in our first study were investigated, (Govaerts and others, 1977).
All patients and controls were white caucasians of belgian origin. The statistical methods were those of Woolf (1955) for the estimation of the relative risk and its significance, as used in our first study. All manic-depressive patients had experienced several primary affective episodes according to Feighner's criteria (1972). They were subdivided into unipolar depressive (N=23) and bipolar manic-depressive (N=24) patients.

HLA typing was performed on peripheral blood lymphocytes according to the NIH (NIAID) cytotoxicity test (1976) using 120 antisera (neurotransplant and local sera).

Results

TABLE III: Distribution of HLA B 5 and HLA BW 15 in Affective Illness Versus Controls

Antigens	Controls (N=74)		Patients: Unipolar (N=23)		Patients: Bipolar (N=24)		Total (N=47)	
	N	%	N	%	N	%	N	%
HLA B 5	10	9	1	4	6	25	7	15
HLA BW 15	24	21	4	17	2	8	6	13

Table III illustrates the distribution of the HLA B 5 and HLA BW 15 antigens in bipolar and unipolar affectively ill patients. As seen in our first study,there is no difference in the distribution of those antigens in bipolar as compared to unipolar patients, which allows to compare all affective patients to controls, in terms of relative risks. (Table IV)

TABLE IV: Relative Risks for HLA B 5 and HLA BW 15 in Affective Illness Versus Controls

Unipolar Versus Bipolar: X	Unipolar Versus Bipolar: X_W^2	All Affective Versus Controls: X	All Affective Versus Controls: X_W^2
0.13	3.39 (N.S.)	0.75	0.32 (N.S.)
2.32	0.84 (N.S.)	1.06	0.00 (N.S.)

X= Relative Risk

$X_W^2 = X^2$ According to Woolf

N.S.= Non Significant

No more associations can be found between HLA B 5, HLA BW 15 and affective illness. In our sample, there is thus no association between HLA antigens and manic-depressive illness, an observation confirming our previous negative results (Govaerts and others, 1977) with the correction for the number of antigens. These negative findings along with others (James and others, in press; Temple and others, in press), the absence of duplication of previously published associations, as well as conflicting results, indicate that positive or negative HLA association studies in mental disorders may be due to methodological artefacts. To illustrate the possibility of fictive associations between the HLA system and subsamples, we have compared the distribution of HLA antigens in the control sample used in our first study (control I = 113 subjects) to the controls used in the present investigation (control II = 74 subjects).

TABLE V: Comparison of HLA Antigens in Two Control Samples

Antigen HLA	Controls I (N=113)		Controls II (N=74)		Controls I versus Controls II	
	N	%	N	%	X	X^2_W
A1	32	28	18	24	1,23	0,37
A2	60	53	38	51	1,07	0,00
A3	30	26	26	35	0,67	1,56
A9	28	25	15	20	1,30	0,51
A10	9	8	1	1	6,32	3,00
A11	11	10	7	9	1,80	1,35
A28	8	7	4	5	1,33	0,72
A29	6	5	4	5	0,98	0,00
AW23	5/112	4	4	5	0,81	0,09
AW24	22/112	20	13	17	1,15	0,13
AW25	1/112	1	1	1	0,66	0,09
AW26	7/112	6	7	9	0,64	0,65
AW30	3	3	2	3	0,99	0,00
AW31	1	1	1	1	0,66	0,09
AW32	7	6	5	7	0,91	0,02
AW33	4	3	3	4	0,87	0,03
B5	10	9	14	19	0,42	3,89*
B7	30	26	18	24	1,12	0,12
B8	19	17	10	13	1,29	0,37
B12	25	22	15	20	1,12	0,09
B13	2	2	1	1	1,43	0,08
B14	8	7	3	4	1,80	0,18
B18	10	9	7	9	0,93	0,02
B27	11	10	7	9	1,03	0,00
BW15	24	21	9	12	1,95	2,48
BW16	5	4	1	1	3,38	1,21
BW17	9	8	7	9	0,83	0,13
BW21	10	9	3	4	2,30	1,51
BW22	4	3	3	4	0,87	0,03
BW35	25	22	18	24	0,88	0,12
BW39	3	3	3	4	0,65	0,28
BW40	11	10	15	20	0,42	3,99*

X = Relative Risk

$X^2_W = X^2$ According to Wolf

* = Significant ($p < 0,05$)

The two subsamples are originating from the same population of blood donors and potential kidney donors, and the samples are homogenous with regard to ethnic and cultural background. Suprisingly, there was an excess in HLA B5 and HLA BW 40 antigens in the second control sample as compared to the first one. This difference in HLA distribution among control samples has obviously no biologic or genetic significance, but it should be considered as a fictive observation mainly due to methodological artefacts. It does illustrate the potential abuse of interpretation of the studies on the association between some HLA antigens and mental disorders.

Discussion

There are several conflicting studies on the association between the HLA system and major psychoses. These studies may present some methodological problems related to sampling procedures as well as statistical evaluation. As shown in our present investigation, fictive associations should be discarded by careful reevaluation of the results obtained in preliminary studies. We propose the following experimental design to test the validity of HLA association studies. First, one should investigate in a preliminary controlled study the presence or absence of HLA association according to the method of Woolf (1955), which provides an estimation of the value of relative risks for each antigen. Second, if one suspects the presence of positive or negative associations with some antigens, these results should be retested using new samples of patients and controls, independently from the first samples, but originating from the same populations. We have applied this methodology to the search of associations between the major histocompatibility complex (MHC) and affective illness, with negative findings.

Our results therefore do not support the presence of any association between the HLA system and affective disorders of the bipolar or unipolar type. Compared to the number of antigens tested, the samples collected in most studies remain small (in our studies: total number of affectively ill patients= 165), thus limiting the level of sensitivity of the results.

References

Beckman, L., Perris, C., Strandman, E. and Wahlby, L. (in press). HLA antigens and affective disorders. Human Heredity.

Bennahum, D.A., Troup, G.M., Rada, R.T., Kellner, R. and Kyner, T. (1976). HLA antigens in schizophrenic and manic-depressive mental disorders. HLA and disease. (Abstract). Paris: Inserm.

Bodmer, W.F. (1973). Genetic factors in Hodgkin's Disease: Association with a disease-susceptibility locus in the HLA region. National Cancer Institute Monographs, 36, 127-134.

Brewerton, D.A., Caffrey, M., Hart, F.D., James, D.C.O., Nicholls, A. and Sturrock, R.D. (1973). Ankylosing Spondylitis and HLA-27. Lancet, ii, 904.

Cazullo, C.L., Smeraldi, E., Penati, G. (1974). The leucocyte antigenic system HL-A as a possible genetic marker of schizophrenia. British Journal of Psychiatry, 125, 25-27.

Eberhard, G., Frazen, G. and Low, B. (1975). Schizophrenia susceptibility and HL-A antigen. Neuropsychobiology, 1, 211.

Feighner, J.P., Robins, E., Guze, S.B. and Woodruff, R.A. (1972). Diagnostic criteria for use in psychiatric research. Archives of General Psychiatry, 26, 24-26.

Govaerts, A., Mendlewicz, J. and Verbanck, P. (1977). Manic-depressive illness and HLA. Tissue Antigens, 10, 60-62.

Ivanyi, D., Zemek, P. and Ivanyi, P. (1976). HLA antigens in schizophrenia. Tissue Antigens, 8, 217.

Ivanyi, P., Ivanyi, D. and Zemek, P. (1977). HLA-CW4 in Paranoid Schizophrenia. Tissue Antigens, 9, 41-44.

James, N., Caroll, B.J., Haines, R.F. and Smouse, P.E. Genetic markers in affective disorders: ABO and HLA. In press in Genetic of Affective Illness: Current Concepts (eds.) J. Mendlewicz and B. Shopsin. New York: Spectrum Publications.

McKusick, V.R. and Ruddle, F.H. (1977). The status of the gene map of the human chromosomes. Science , 196, 390.

Mercier, R., Sutter, J.M., Julien, R.A. and Kieffer, N. (1977). Schizophrénie: Association de la forme paranoide aux antigènes HLA-A9 et B5. Encéphale, III, 49.

Morris, R., Metzger, A.L., Bluestone, R. and Terasaki, P.L. (1974). HLA-W27, a clue to the diagnosis and pathogenesis of Reiter's syndrome. New England Journal of Medicine, 290, 554.

NIAID. (1976). Manual of Tissue Typing Techniques. US Department of Health, Education and Welfare. pp. 22-24.

Perris, C., Roman, G. and Wahlberg, L. (in press). HLA antigens in patients with schizophrenic syndromes. Neuropsychobiology.

Shapiro, R.W., Bode, E., Rafaelsen, O.J., Ryder, L.P. and Svejgaard, A. (1976). Histocompatibility antigens and manic-depressive disorders. Archives of General Psychiatry, 33, 823-825.

Shapiro, R.W., Ryder, L.P., Svejgaard, A. and Rafaelsen, O.J. (1977). HLA antigens and manic-depressive disorders: further evidence of an association. Psychological Medicine, 7, 387-396.

Smeraldi, E., Bellodi, L. and Cazullo, C.L. (1976). Further studies on the major histocompatibility complex as a genetic marker for schizophrenia. Biological Psychiatry, 11, 655-661.

Stember, R.H. and Fieve, R.R. (1977). Histocompatibility antigens in affective disorders. Clinical Immunology and Immunopathology, 7, 10-14.

Temple, H., Dupont, B. and Shopsin, B. HLA antigen and affective disorders: a report and critical assessment of histocompatibility studies. In press. In Genetics of Affective Illness: Current Concepts, (eds.) J. Mendlewicz and B. Shopsin. New York, Spectrum Publications.

Woolf, B. (1955). On estimating the relation between blood group and disease. Annals of Human Genetics, London, 19, 251.

J. MENDLEWICZ, M.D., PhD. Department of Psychiatry. Erasme Hospital, University of Brussels.
P. VERBANCK, M.D. Resident in Medicine.
P. LINKOWSKI, M.D. Resident in Psychiatry.
A. GOVAERTS, M.D. Department of Immunology. Saint-Pierre Hospital. University of Brussels.

HLA Antigens in Affective Disorders and Cycloid Psychoses

C. PERRIS*, E. STRANDMAN* and L. WÄHLBY**

*Department of Psychiatry, Umeå University, Umeå, Sweden
**Blood Center, Umeå University, Umeå, Sweden

ABSTRACT

A total of 168 patients with different types of affective disorders, and 40 patients with cycloid psychosis were examined with respect to their HLA antigens. The frequency of the A10 antigen was found to be increased in the patients with affective disorders particularly in those with the unipolar type of disease. The frequency of the A1 antigen was decreased among unipolar patients. A decreased frequency of the B7 antigen was found in the total series of patients with affective disorders, and in particular in those with a bipolar type of disease. The cycloid patients showed no significant differences from bipolar patients or controls. As to affective disorders the results in our patients were in disagreement with findings by other investigators.

Key words: HLA antigens, depressive disorders, cycloid psychosis, genetic markers, bipolar/unipolar.

Genetic studies of psychiatric disorders, and of affective illnesses in particular, have acquired a new dimension with the recognition of the relevance of a possible association or linkage with known genetic markers. Since the early studies by Winokur and his co-workers at the end of the sixties (Winokur and Tanna, 1969) much spade work has been done in many quarters and several reports have been published. Several research workers have focused their attention on the possible importance of the histocompatibility antigens (HLA) in contributing to a clarification of genetic issues in the field of psychiatry. Investigations of the HLA antigens distribution in psychiatric disorders have originally been published in Italy by Cazullo and his co-workers (Cazzullo and Smeraldi, 1977; Cazzullo and co-workers, 1976) and in Sweden by Eberhard and co-workers (1975), who attempted to detect a possible association between some of the HLA antigens and schizophrenia. Soon afterwards several research workers, our group among them, became concerned with studies of this genetic system in the field of affective disorders. Besides the investigations carried out by Gowaerts and co-workers (1977) and that by Shapiro and co-workers (1976, 1977), which are discussed in this symposium, a few other studies have been reported by Bennahum and co-workers (1976) and by Smeraldi and co-workers (1978). The most recent among these studies, one carried out in Czechoslovakia by Zvolsky and co-workers (1978), has just appeared in the press.

As will be seen in one of the Tables (Table 3) almost all the investigators have found some significant association with one or another of the HLA-antigens. Results, however, have been inconsistent so far.

However, I do not want to go into a discussion of the different results reported in the literature before having presented our own study. It is a little different from the others so far published, in that it takes into account not only patients who have suffered from the major bipolar and unipolar affective psychoses, but also patients who have suffered from other kinds of depressive illnesses, and also from cycloid psyshoses (for details see Beckman and co-workers, 1978a, 1978b).

Our series in composed of 168 patients suffering from affective disorders, and of 40 patients who had suffered from cycloid psychosis according to our definition. As a control group we have used the results obtained in 449 healthy individuals recruited from the same catchment area as our patients, and collected at the Blood Center of the General Hospital. 22 HLA antigens belonging to the first and second series were tested (by LW) by means of the microtoxicity test. The over all results or our study are presented in Tables 1 and 2.

TABLE 1 HLA Antigens: Per cent Distribution

	Group					
Antigen	Bipolar N=38	Unipolar N=50	Reactive N=50	Unclassified N=30	Cycloid N=40	Controls N=449
→ A1	26.3	6.0	26.0	20.0	22.5	20.7
A2	52.6	52.0	54.0	56.7	55.0	61.5
A3	15.8	30.0	18.0	33.3	15.0	29.6
A9	21.1	20.0	14.0	20.0	17.5	17.4
→ A10	18.4	22.0	16.0	16.7	10.0	10.7
A11	13.2	20.0	14.0	10.0	7.5	11.6
Aw19	7.9	14.0	12.0	10.0	2.5	13.4
A28	10.5	8.0	14.0	10.0	2.5	9.6

TABLE 2 HLA Antigens: Per cent Distribution

	Group					
Antigen	Bipolar N=38	Unipolar N=50	Reactive N=50	Unclassified N=30	Cycloid N=40	Controls N=449
→ B5	13.2	4.0	20.0	23.3	5.0	11.8
→ B7	18.4	40.0	26.0	33.3	22.5	39.0
B8	21.1	14.0	18.0	13.3	15.0	22.1
B12	34.2	36.0	30.0	26.7	30.0	29.2
B13	2.6	0.0	2.0	0.0	0.0	1.1
Bw15	28.9	20.0	22.0	16.7	22.5	23.8
Bw17	5.3	2.0	0.0	0.0	2.5	2.2
B18	2.6	6.0	6.0	3.3	0.0	4.7
Bw22	2.6	0.0	6.0	3.3	0.0	2.4
B27	18.4	26.0	20.0	30.0	17.5	16.7
Bw35	5.3	8.0	2.0	3.3	10.0	8.9
Bw40	21.1	24.0	16.0	30.0	15.0	17.4

As far as patients suffering from affective disorders are concerned a few statistically significant differences emerged. For example, there was a significant increase in the frequency of the A10 antigen in the patients, and in particular in the unipolar group, and a decrease of the A1 antigen in the same group. On the other hand a significant decrease of the B7 antigen was found in the total series of patients, and in particular in those with a bipolar type of disorder. There was also a significant heterogeneity between the four patient groups for the B5 antigen. The lowest frequency (4%) was found in the unipolar, and the highest (23%) in the unclassified group. None of these groups, however, differed significantly from the healthy controls.

The results concerning the cycloid psychotic patients have been completely negative. No differences whatsoever were found in a comparison with the healthy controls, nor could evidence of any difference be found in a comparison with the bipolar group.

Incidentally I would like to mention that there were also no differences found in the distribution of HLA antigens in a comparison between cycloid psychotics and schizophrenic patients carried out on another occasion and reported elsewhere (Perris and co-workers, 1978)

TABLE 3 Significant Associations with HLA Antigens in Patients as Compared with Controls

	Patients				
	Bipolar		Unipolar		
Author	N	Antigens		N	Antigens
Shapiro and co-workers	20	Bw16↗		14	–
Gowaerts and co-workers	50	B5↗	Bw15↘	68	Bw15↘
Bennahum and co-workers	16	Bw17↗		–	–
Smeraldi and co-workers	51	A10↘ A29↘ A30↗ Bw22↗		41	A10↘ A29↘ A30↗ Bw22↗
Zvolsky and co-workers	77	Cw3↘		24	Bw40↗ Cw4↗
Present study	38	B7↘		50	A1↘ A10↗

Table 3 shows an overview of the results reported in the literature with regard to the major affective psychoses. As can be seen, the different studies have given results which are not only inconsistent but even, in some instances, quite contradictory. Apparently the only consistent finding so far is that by Shapiro and co-workers (1976, 1977) concerning a positive association between bipolar manic depressive disorders and HLA Bw16. Unfortunately, at the time of our investigation we lacked the Bw16 in our panel, but we have got it now, and are carrying out a new study. It should be mentioned, however, that Bennahum and co-workers (1976) found an association not with the Bw16 but with the Bw17, whereas Zvolsky and co-workers (1978) report an association with the Bw15. Smeraldi and co-workers (1978) who compared 50 bipolar patients and 646 controls, found no difference in the Bw 16 between the two groups. At least two explanations may account for the discrepancy in the results concerning HLA and affective disorders. The first and most obvious is that all the associations reported so far are spurious and due to chance. This simplistic interpretation seems however to be contradicted by the results by Shapiro and co-workers (1976, 1977) who were able to verify their findings in two apparently independent series. The other explanation is that the populations investigated are, in fact, heterogeneous, even the bipolar group for which a good diagnostic agreement can be reached in different centers. If this is so, then the findings concerning HLA open a challenging perspective for further studies of this very important patient group. Some further hints about these new perspectives will be found in studies concerning the therapeutic response to, for example, lithium, which will be commented upon in another session of this congress.

REFERENCES

Beckman, G., L. Beckman, B. Cedergren, C. Perris, E. Strandman, and L. Wählby (1978a). Genetic markers in cycloid psychosis. Neuropsychobiology, 4, 276-282.

Beckman, L., C. Perris, E. Strandman, and L. Wählby (1978b). HLA antigens and affective disorders. Hum. Hered., 28, 96-99.

Bennahum, D.A., G.M. Troup, R.T. Rada, R. Kellner, and T. Kyner (1976). HLA antigens in schizophrenic and manic depressive mental disorders. HLA and disease. Abstract, Inserm, Paris.

Cazzullo, C.L., and E. Smeraldi (1977). HLA system, psychiatry and psychopharmacology. Prog. Neuro-Psychopharmacol., in press.

Cazzullo, C.L., E. Smeraldi, and G. Penati (1974). The leucocyte antigenic system HLA as a possible genetic marker of schizophrenia. Brit. J. Psychiat., 125, 25-27.

Eberhard, G., G. Franzén, and B. Löw (1975). Schizophrenia, susceptibility and HLA antigen. Neuropsychobiology, 1, 211-217.

Govaerts, A., J. Mendlewicz, and P. Verbanck (1977). Manic-depressive illness and HLA. Tissue Antigens, 10, 60-62.

Perris, C., G. Román, and L. Wählby (1978). HLA antigens in patients with schizophrenic syndromes. Neuropsychobiology, in press.

Shapiro, R.W., E. Bock, O.J. Rafaelsen, L.P. Ryder, and A. Svejgaard (1976). Histocompatibility (HLA) antigens, and susceptibility to manic-depressive disorders. Arch. gen. Psychiat. 33, 823-827.

Shapiro, R.W., L.P. Ryder, A. Svejgaard, and O. Rafaelsen (1977). HLA antigens and manic-depressive disorders: further evidence of an association. Psychological Med., 7, 387-396.

Smeraldi, E., F. Negri, A.M. Melica, R. Scorza-Smeraldi, G. Fabio, P. Bonara, L. Bellodi, E. Sacchetti, M.G. Sabbadini, C.L. Cazzullo, and C. Zanussi (1978). HLA typing and affective disorders: a study in the Italian population. Neuropsychobiology, in press.

Winokur, G., and V.L. Tanna (1969). Possible role of X-linked dominant factor in manic depressive disease. Dis. Nerv. Syst., 30, 89.

Zvolský, P., M. Dvaráková, A. Májský, and K. Soucek (1978). Histocompatibility antigens in primary affective disorders. Arch. Psychiat. Nervenkr., 225, 159-162.

Supported in part by a grant from the Torsten and Ragnar Söderberg's Fund.

HLA-Antigens in Manic-Melancholic Disorders

O. J. RAFAELSEN*, P. KRAMP*, L. P. RYDER, R. W. SHAPIRO*** and A. SVEJGAARD****

*Psychochemistry Institute, Dept., Psychiatry, Rigshospitalet, 9 Blegdamsvej, DK-2100 Copenhagen O, Denmark
**The Tissue-Typing Lab., Blood-Grouping Dept., Rigshospitalet, 9 Blegdamsvej, DK-2100 Copenhagen O, Denmark
***Massachusetts Mental Health Center, Boston, Mass., U.S.A.

ABSTRACT

HLA-antigens have been studied in affective disorders by several research groups with very different results, some of which totally negative. We have in two studies found an increased frequency of BW16. A number of research problems may explain the different results obtained: 1. Diagnostic criteria. 2. Complexity of HLA-typing. 3. Ethnic differences making suitable and sufficient large control material essential. 4. Statistical problems when testing a large number of variables. It is suggested that family studies may help to solve the present confusion within this field.

KEYWORDS

HLA-antigens - affective disorders - manic-melancholic mode - manic-depressive psychosis.

INTRODUCTION

HLA-antigens constitute the major histocompatibility system in man and have shown characteristic deviations in a number of clinical disorders. Most of these diseases have had obvious or possible immunological pathogenetic factors and/or have been known to have genetic components. Both in schizophrenia and affective disorder research, several groups have tried their luck with HLA-antigens. Table 1 shows the very conflicting results in affective disorders.

We cannot provide a synthesis at present, but we may discuss some of the inherent problems and difficulties.

DISCUSSION OF GERNERAL PROBLEMS

Diagnostic Criteria

Here as everywhere in psychiatry this is an ever present problem. To obtain reliability within one's own institution may be difficult enough in itself, but to obtain reliability between institutions and countries is more than difficult.

It is evident that the diagnostic criteria used in the various studies have been widely different, some being more strict than others. The MULTI-CLAD[1]-system developed in Copenhagen is perhaps the most restrictive of them all.

Furthermore the criteria for classifying patients as unipolar and bipolar are not consistent from one investigation to another. Again the MULTI-CLAD system demands three definite (or 2 definite + one or more possible) depressive episodes for assigning a patient to the unipolar groups, where some other researchers have been satisfied when a patient has had two or even one depressive episode as long as the patient had had no manias. Under such liberal classification policies all patients can be assigned to one or the other of the two polarity groups, whereas the more restrictive systems may lead to a third category: definite affective disorder, but polarity uncertain. In the Copenhagen studies 3o-5o per cent of the patients could not be polarized in spite of the fact that the patients had attended for years the Psychochemistry Out-Patient Clinic, which specializes in affective disorders.

Complexity of HLA-Typing

Whereas ABO-typing is a simple routine, HLA-typing is still a complicated undertaking for a limited number of specialized laboratories. In addition, even the best equipped laboratories will from time to time be without one or more of the many antisera needed for a complete investigation, and thus not two of the reports in the literature deal with exactly the same selection of HLA-antigens.

Control Material and Ethnic Differencies

Each of us has three loci for HLA-antigens on chromosome number 6. The combinations are indeed many and the ethnic variations must always be taken into account.

Each laboratory must collect its own control material carefully matching the patient material to be investigated. The background material should have considerable size, at least 5oo and preferably more than one thousand individuals. Some of the studies do not fulfil this criterion. The ethnic differences in the HLA-profiles are very great. Even in the relatively homogenous European populations marked trends are found from one country to another and even within the countries. For obvious reasons these problems are even more complicated in the American and Australian populations.

Statistical Problems

The more variables analysed, the greater the risk of false positive results. With a 5 per cent confidence limit, when 2o variables are investigated, it is likely that there will be a false positive result. This phenomenon of mass significance is an obvious problem with the many HLA-antigens included in these analyses. The statisticians may advise to multiply the "crude" P-values obtained with the number of variables analysed. This is a stringent test which may, however, change the risk of obtaining false positive results to that of obtaining false negative results. This makes it particularly important to confirm previous results on a new patient material.

---

[1]A Multi-axial Classification of Affective Disorders with strict symptomatic and course criteria.

DISCUSSION OF ACTUAL PROBLEMS

It is clearly seen from Table 1 that some of the studies do not yield sufficient information to satisfy some of the criteria outlined above - or to make comparisons easy with the other studies in this field.

The diagnostic criteria has probably varied considerably between studies. In those studies where patients have been divided into unipolar and bipolar, again the criteria are often poorly described and not uniform. A special point is which percentage of patients it has been impossible to asign to any of the two polarity groups. In our own studies some 3o per cent received the diagnosis: Definitely manic-depressive, but polarity uncertain (Shapiro, 1976, 1977).

The complexity of HLA-typing represents another inherent difficulty. Not two of the published studies have analyzed exactly the same selection of HLA-types; some authors directly state that not every patient in their own material has been studied with all the antigens applied in their study due to temporary non-availability of one or more antibodies. Some authors have chosen the strategy in their second material only to analyse for those antigens which showed increased or decreased frequency in their first series (e.g. Mendlewicz and co-workers, 1978). A further difficulty is the considerabel ethnic differences in HLA-profiles. It is mandatory that control materials should be composed of individuals with a similar ethnic and geographic background - and of sufficient size. It is suggested that the control material should be no less than 500, preferable 1,000 individuals; not many control materials are of such a size. When smaller control materials are used, one control material may be different from the next collected by the same researchers (Mendlewicz and co-workers, 1978).

Besides the here-mentioned problems of adequate control materials, the number of HLA-antigens analyzed in itself creates special statistical problems. This may lead both to false positive and negative results. Some have tried to compensate for the risk of committing type 1 errors (false positive results) by multiplying P-values obtained by the number of HLA-antigens analyzed. Only if the values so obtained were still statistically significant, the authors would accept the results as indicative of an HLA-profile different from the normal (Shapiro and co-workers, 1976, 1977; Govaerts and co-workers, 1977, Temple and co-workers, 1978; James and co-workers, 1978). This way of counterattacking the risk of mass significance is a very stringent test, perhaps too stringent.

FUTURE STRATEGY

What shall we then due to settle the issue? There is not much hope that new series by the various research groups involved will bring more light, and at least very little hope that it will bring a final solution.

In the somewhat simpler problem of ABO-blood groups and duodenal ulcer the situation lo-2o years ago was also quite unclear. In the end the problem of an association between blood-groups 0 and duodenal ulcer was solved by family studies (Roberts, 1965). We will suggest that this approach, e.g. the sib-pair method may also be of use in the elucidation of HLA-types and affective disorders.

TABLE 1 HLA-Antigens in Affective Disorders

	N	UP+BP	N	UP	N	BP	CONTROLS
Johnson (1978)		N.I.		N.I.	36	—	780
Govaerts and co-workers (1977)	118	B5↑ BW15↓		N.R.		N.R.	113
Mendlewicz and co-workers (1978)	47	—	23	—	24	—	74
James and co-workers (1978)	114	—	37	—	77	—	439
Beckman and co-workers (1978)	168	A10↑ B7↓		A10↑ A1↓		B7↓	
Bennahum and co-workers (1975)	12	—		N.R.		N.R.	
Stember and Fieve (1977)	50	B5↑ B12↓ B13↑ BW35↑					
Temple and co-workers (1978)	38	CW3↓		N.R.		N.R.	211
Shapiro and co-workers (1976)	47	A3↑ B7↑ B8↓ BW16↑	14	A3↑ B7↑ B8↓	20	B7↑ B8↓ BW16↑	1967
Shapiro and co-workers (1977)	1o7	BW16↑		—		—	1967

N.I.: Not Investigated
N.R.: Not Reported

REFERENCES

Beckman, L., B. Cedergren, C. Perris, and E. Strandman (1978). Blood groups and affective disorders. Hum. Hered., 28, 48-55.

Bennahum, D.A., G.M. Troup, R.T. Rada, R. Kellner, and T. Kyner (1976). HLA antigens in schizophrenic and manic-depressive mental disorders. HLA and disease. (Abstract). Inserm, Paris.

Fraser Roberts, J.A. (1965). ABO blood groups, secretor status, and susceptibility to chronic diseases: An example of a genetic basis for family predispositions. In Neel, Shaw and Schuff (Eds.), Genetics of the Epidemiology of Chronic Diseases. US Dept. of Public Health. pp. 77-86.

Govaerts, A., J. Mendlewicz, and P. Verbanck (1977). Manic-depressive illness and HLA. Tissue Antigens, 1o, 6o-62.

James, N.M., P.E. Smouse, B.J. Carroll, and R.F. Haines (1978). Affective illness and HLA frequencies. To be published.

Johnson, G.F.S. (1977). HLA antigens and manic-depressive disorders. Biol. Psychiat., 13, 4o9-412.

Mendlewicz, J., P. Verbanck, P. Linowski, and A. Govaerts (1978). HLA antigens in affective disorders. Symp. Biol. Res. Depr. Man. (CINP) Vienna.

Shapiro, R.W., Bock, E., Rafaelsen, O.J., L.P. Ryder, and A. Svejgaard (1976). Histocompatibility antigens and manic-depressive disorders. Arch. Gen. Psychiatry, 33, 823-825.

Shapiro, R.W., L.P. Ryder, A. Svejgaard, and O.J. Rafaelsen (1977). HLA antigens and manic-depressive disorders: Further evidence of an association. Psychol. Med., 7, 387-396.

Smeraldi, E. (1978). The HLA system as a possible marker for psychiatric disorders. Symp. Biol. Res. Depr. Man. (CINP) Vienna.

Stember, R.H. and R.R. Fieve (1977). Histocompatibility antigens in affective disorders. Clin. Immunol. Immunopathol., 7, 1o-14.

Temple, H., B. Dupont, and B. Shopsin. HLA antigen and affective disorders: A report and critical assessment of histocompatibility studies. Neuropsychobiol.: In press.

The HLA System as a Possible Marker for Psychiatric Disorders

E. SMERALDI, R. SCORZA-SMERALDI*, L. BELLODI, G. FABIO*, F. NERGI and P. BONARA*

Institute of Clinical Psychiatry, University of Milano, Medical School
*Institute of Internal Medicine IV, Laboratory of Cellular Immunology

ABSTRACT

HLA antigens have been determined in Italian patients with affective disorders and their families, in the hope of obtaining a valid indicator of subjects at risk among the as-yet normal relatives. In addition, an attempt has been made to identify a biological or functional role of the membrane structures which might be correlated with the mental disorder. We have studied Li^+ uptake into RBC in pairs of sibs with different degrees of HLA similarities.

In this presentation we would like to stress some points which seem to be of some importance when dealing with HLA and psychiatric disorders. In previous papers (Smeraldi et al., 1976: Smeraldi et al., 1978) we reported that the associations between HLA antigens and psychiatric disorders are weak. Often the results obtained in one population are not confirmed in samples of different ethnic origin. Many of these are probably false negative or false positive associations, for different and already discussed reasons (Cazzullo and Smeraldi, 1978).

More recent studies which have investigated the relationships between HLA antigens and psychiatric diseases, have obtained interesting findings mainly when the clinical subgroups were considered. Associations were found which, although low and often not significant, were confirmed by later studies in the same population and even in patient groups of different ethnic origin. Therefore it is probable that the employment of common and well-standardized diagnostic criteria might increase the discriminatory power of such studies by allowing comparison of more homogeneous groups.

An example can be drawn from the HLA studies in different schizophrenic populations. When we take into consideration the subtypes, not just the schizophrenic condition per se, it appears that in 3 different populations one particular antigen occurs with significantly increased frequency. In Italian (Smeraldi et al.,1976), English (McGuffin et al., 1978) and Czech (Ivanyi, 1976) schizophenics an increased frequency of the antigen HLA-A 1 is observed in those patients defined as "hebephrenic", "first-rank symptoms" or "non-paranoid". This observation deserves careful consideration, both with regard to the extent of the coincidence of such defined groups and to the influence that the respective definitions have on the genetic interpretation. Furthermore, when the paranoid subtype in patients of different ethnic origin is considered, there is found a suggestive and often very significant increase in the antigens A 9 and B 5. An even more striking increase in some of the haplotypes carrying these artigens is observed, namely the haplotypes A 9, B 5 and A 9, B 35, Cw 4 (Julien et al., 1978). At this point, it must be stressed that the data presented so far do not necessarily imply a dichotomy between the two schizophrenic subtypes. More sophisticated and informative studies, such as the family segregation studies that also consider the main clinical variables of the disorder, might reveal a more complex relationship between HLA loci and a specific genetic liability to the disorder, that is to say a partially common genetic background can be hypothesized.

With regard to affective disorders, 19 additional patients have been added to our previous data (Smeraldi et al., 1978a). Table 1 summarizes the findings in the final group of 110 affective subjects. The deviances in the antigenic frequencies between our sample and a corresponding control population that were previously seen have been largely confirmed, with a significant decrease in A 10 and A 9 and an increase in A 29 and B 22. However, at this time some deranged frequencies previously reported in other populations and not confirmed in our first study are now emerging although still not significantly. This includes a decrease in B 7, as reported for the Swedish (Perris et al., 1978) and Danish (Rafaelsen and Shapiro, in press) populations, and an increase in Bw 16 (Danish population). The frequency of Bw 16 was not assessed in the Swedish population. However, in the swedish bipolar subgroup an important increase in the frequency of the Aw 26 was observed. Since this last displays a strong linkage disequilibrium with Bw 16, it is possible that its increased frequency is partially dependent on the increase in the frequency of Bw 16.

Nevertheless, at the present time family studies must be undertaken to confirm the existence of a linkage between HLA genes and those determining the susceptibility to psychiatric disorders, or in any case to some of their subtypes.In fact, if such a linkage be confirmed, HLA typing can be used to detect the subjects at risk in affected families. Independently of the antigens involved, HLA segregation analysis would mark the simultaneous transmission of the linked disease gene in that family. One of the possible

TABLE 1 Frequencies of HLA antigens in Italian Patients with Affective Disorders

Antigens	Controls (n= 646) %	Affective Patients (n= 110) %	x-value	2 Woolf
A 1	.263	.254	.956	.036
A 2	.464	.414	.828	.807
A 3	.234	.190	.773	.978
A 9	.260	.227	.836	.530
A 10	.249	.081	.268	13.38 **
A 11	.093	.090	.976	.004
A 28	.057	.045	.783	.248
A 29	.034	.109	3.473	11.021**
Aw 30	.080	.018	.211	4.54 *
Aw 31	.023	0.		
Aw 32	.076	.063	.828	.203
B 5	.243	.300	1.334	1.610
B 7	.135	.081	.572	2.060
B 8	.122	.109	.878	.153
B 12	.196	.245	1.32	1.375
B 13	.100	.063	.607	1.464
B 14	.049	.036	.724	.356
B 18	.034	.072	2.224	3.51
B 27	.079	.036	.440	2.39
Bw 15	.083	.027	.307	3.834
Bw 16	.073	.127	1.858	3.665
Bw 17	.063	.045	.702	.528
Bw 21	.023	.045	2.003	1.737
Bw 22	.034	.090	2.836	6.919*
Bw 35	.167	.109	.609	2.334
Bw 40	.039	.045	1.182	.112

* p .05
** p .01

examples for such a study is our study of the zygotic assortment of parental haplotypes in families with multiple cases of Affective Disorders and in sibling pairs discordant for the disease (Smeraldi et al., 1978).

According to the hypothesis of a linkage between the HLA loci and a hypothetical major locus for susceptibility to the disease, zygotic assortment should not be completely random as in unselected families, so that HLA haplotype repeats should significantly increase when two or more affected siblings are compared, and decrease in siblings discordant for the disease. Our findings in 21 multiple-case families evidenced a significantly higher frequency of haplotype repeats than expected (p= .046).

However, the fact that a random distribution of haplotypes was found among the 19 pairs of siblings discordant for the disease, rather than the expected decrease in the repeats, raises many theoretical and practical problems, such as the prolonged period of risk of Affective Disorders, the effect of penetrance and the mode of inheritance. In the case of reduced penetrance, the absebce of the disease does not exclude specific inheritance of the disorder or, of course, of the HLA linked genes. The possibility of carriers for the disease susceptibility genes among phenotypically unaffected siblings was not considered in the discordant pairs investigation.

Studies of the association between HLA and psychiatric disorders are not limited to the search for a pure genetic marker, but raise the question of the biological and functional roles of these membrane structures.

In a recent study on the correlation between HLA antigens and the response to long-term Li^+ treatment, Perris et al. (1978) reported that 5 of the 6 Bw 35 positive patients had high RBC/plasma Li^+ ratios. Contemporaneously, this in vivo finding was confirmed by an in vitro investigation which was carried out by our group (Smeraldi et al., 1978b). In fact, it was found that 79% of the individuals whose intracellular Li^+ concentrations were higher than the discriminant value of 0.25 mEq/l after 24 hr in vitro incubation of their RBC in the presence of a fixed extracellular concentration (1.5 mEq/l), had the antigen Bw 35 on their membrane surfaces. It seems that the presence of Bw 35 may facilitate in vitro a high RBC Li^+ uptake, which is a rather stable and reproducible individual characteristic, genetically controlled. We must remember that in this case we are not interested in the pharmacological effects of Li^+, but in the distribution of ions across the cell membranes, mainly of Na^+, for which Li^+ serves as an indicator system, allowing us to speak about the role of the HLA system as a real functional role. However, the idea that just one antigen may be involved in the relationship between the HLA system and Li^+ transport across the membrane may be an oversimplification. In fact, it is possible that all the HLA antigens, or at least those of the B locus, have effects on the Li^+ transport system, though varying quantitatively according to the structure of each antigen.

We have tested this hypothesis by evaluating the differences between pairs of sibs in in vitro RBC uptake of Li^+, the sibs were classified according to whether they shared 0, 1 or 2 HLA haplotypes. It is evident that, according to our hypothesis, the differences between sibs in the in vitro Li^+ uptake would be expected to be inversely, related to the degree of intrapair closeness with regard to HLA type, independent of the individual antigen present on the membrane and of the absolute value of intracellular Li^+ incorporation.

Fifteen pairs of sibs were thus investigated with regard to the intrapair differences in Li^+ uptake; 5 pairs had no haplotypes in common, 7 pairs had 1 and 3 pairs had 2. Table 2 reports the results of the analysis of variance for our data: the comparison of pairs with no shared haplotypes with those pairs with one or two is highly significant (p .01), indicating that the differences in Li^+ uptake between sibs completely dissimilar for HLA are significantly greater than in those cases where some antigens are shared by both sibs .

TABLE 2 Analysis of variance of differences in Li^+ uptake *in vitro* in pairs of sibs grouped according to the HLA haplotype repeats

Source of variation	Sum of squares	d.f.	Mean square	F	p
Among groups	62.01	2	31.01	5.67	
0 vs. 1+2	58.80	1	58.8	10.7	.01
1 vs. 2	3.21	1	3.21	n.s.	
Error	65.59	12	5.47		

These are very preliminary data which may indicate a new perspective from which to considering the HLA system, but which need to be tested by means of more informative methods, such as link age and segregation studies. Moreover, we must remember that ion transport across membranes is a very complex system, in which 3 different functional mechanisms have been identified: passive diffusion, ouabain-sensitive Li^+ uptake and phloretin-sensitive Li^+/Na^+ transport. What we can see in our *in vitro* system is the resu ltant effect of all three activities, so that at this moment we cannot establish to which of these the HLA system may be related. Since the phloretin-sensitive transport seems to represent the most important mechanism in control of the intracellular Li^+ concentration *in vitro*, the estimation of the relationship between this activity and HLA system may turnout to be a more informative approach.

REFERENCES

Cazzullo, C.L., and Smeraldi, E. (1978). HLA system and psychiatry. Paper read at the II World Congress of Biological Psychiatry, Barcelona.

Ivanyi, D. (1976). HLA antigens in schizophrenia. In HLA and disease. Inserm, Paris

Julien, R.A., Mercier, P., Chouraqui, P. and Sutter, J.M. (1978). Schizophrénies et antigènes d'histocompatibilité. Encephale IV, 99-113.

McGuffin, P., Farmer, A.E. and Rajah, S.M. (1978). Histocompatibility antigens and schizophrenia. Br. J. Psychiat. 132, 149-51.

Perris, C., Strandman, E.and Wahlby, L. (1978). HLA antigens in affective disorders and cycloid psychoses. Paper read at the 11 CINP Congress, Vienna.

Rafaelsen, O.J. and Shapiro, R.W. Psychopharmacological studies in genetically determined subgroups of psychiatric patients. In press

Smeraldi, E., Bellodi, L., Scorza-Smeraldi, R., Fabio, G. and Sacchetti, E. (1976). HLA-SD antigens and schizophrenia: statistical genetical considerations. Tissue Antigens 8, 191-96.

Sme raldi, E., Negri, F., Melica, A.M. and Scorza-Smeraldi, R. (1978). HLA system and affective disorders: a sibship genetic study. Tissue Antigens 12, 270-74.

Smeraldi, E., Negri, F., Melica, A.M., Scorza-Smeraldi, R., Fabio, G., Bonara, P., Bellodi, L., Sacchetti, E., Sabbadini-Villa, M.G., Cazzullo, C.L. and Zanussi, C. (1978a). HLA typing and Affective Disorders: a study in the Italian population. Neuropsychobiology 4, 344-52.

Smeraldi, E., Scorza-Smeraldi, R. and Cazzullo, C.L. (1978b). HLA system and psychopharmacology. Paper read at the II World congress of Biological Psychiatry, Barcelona.

Diurnal Rhythms in Manic-Depressive Disorders

H. GIEDKE and B. PFLUG

Psychiatric Clinic, University of Tübingen, D-7400 Tübingen, Germany

ABSTRACT

A short review of experimental findings is presented relevant to the hypothesis that manic-depressive disorders are linked to disturbances of internal synchronization of bodily functions in the circadian frequency range. So far, there is no conclusive evidence that such disturbances play a considerable role in depression, since true desynchronization is suggested by no more than two long-term, single-case studies. However, divergent and/or more variable phase relations of various functions could be demonstrated in several cross-sectional studies. Mainly bipolar depressed patients seem to be affected.

KEY WORDS: Manic depressive disorder, diurnal system, circadian rhythms, desynchronization

The observation of temporal aspects of mental illness has led to terms such as "folie circulaire" (Falret, 1854), "periodische Geistesstörung" (Hitzig, 1898; Pilcz, 1901), and "Zyklothymie" (Kraepelin, 1913). All these terms, as well as the concept of depressed and schizophrenic phases, imply a chronobiological model of the disease which, in the case of depression, today refers mainly to the diurnal rhythms.

The hypothesis that depression and diurnal rhythms are connected was first expressed by Halberg in 1967, and can be formulated as follows: Depression is accompanied by a disturbance of the synchronization between external "Zeitgeber" or synchronizer (Aschoff, Klotter, Wever, 1965), and the diurnal variation of one or several bodily functions.

If this were so, we should be able to observe disturbances some of which are shown in Fig. 1. Horizontally, the local time is indicated, which is the most important Zeitgeber in human beings. It has a period of 24 hours. Given vertically are the daily phasic reference points of a measured variable. The normal is a more or less stable phase relation over a long period of time (case a, Fig. 1). When synchronization is disturbed, the phase may show a greater variation (case b, Fig. 1) or a new phase relationship may be built up (case c, Fig. 1).

In the case of desynchronization (case d, Fig. 1), the measured variable shows a different length of period than the Zeitgeber.

"External desynchronization" means different period lengths of Zeitgeber (T), and the organism as a whole (τ): $T \neq \tau$. The term "internal desynchronization" refers to single bodily functions differing in their period lengths, always implying partial external desynchronization. Desynchronization can only be verified if the measurement covers enough periods to rule out that only a new phase relation becomes established. If the period lengths of the free running period and the synchronizer do not deviate too much from each other, beat phenomena can emerge (possibly corresponding to the phasic course of diseases, e.g. manic depression (cf. Halberg, 1968; Papousek, 1975).

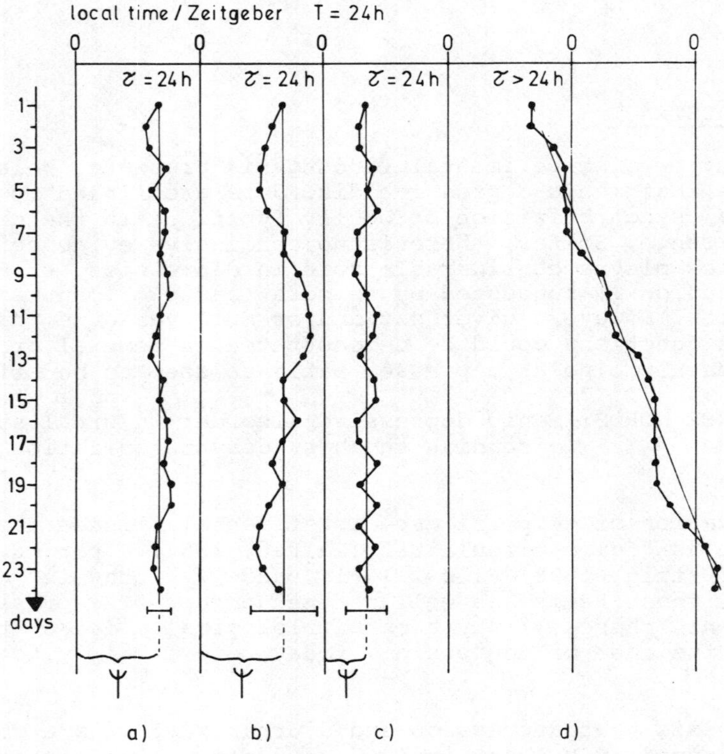

Fig. 1 Schematic presentation of some possibilities for the phase relationship between Zeitgeber and a physiological variable in the case of weakened synchronizing mechanisms.

Cases (b), (c), and (d) of Fig. 1 could appear successively in one variable and simultaneously in different variables. Only (d) corroborates the hypothesis directly. Not shown are more complicated conditions such as courses with several peaks.

From Fig. 1, it is evident that in order to verify the hypothesis, longitudinal studies over many days are necessary. They allow, moreover, a direct comparison of the different stages of the illness (depression, manic phase, interval) for each individual patient. However, only indirect indications can be expected from cross-sectional or transverse studies of only one or two days.
What results do we have up to date and how far do they corroborate or refute the hypothesis?

As far as psychopathology is concerned, the daily fluctuations in mood with depression in the morning and brightening up towards the evening were one of the reasons that led to the chronobiological hypothesis of the origin of depression. What is essential is the observation that the presence, as well as the intensity of diurnal ups and downs, change with the severity of the depression (Waldmann, 1972; Stallone and co-workers, 1973; Supprian, 1975), and that diurnal deviations in the manic phase are, if present at all, only slight. These findings can be explained by a diurnal oscillation model but do not necessitate the supposition of a defective synchronization mechanism (Waldmann, 1972). Some depressed patients, however, have reported a morning deep progressively extending into the forenoon, or a brightening up of the mood beginning progressively earlier in the evening during the time of remission (Middelhoff, 1967). This observation could apply to cases (b) or (d) of Fig. 1, but it is in contradiction to Waldmann's (1972, p. 86) notion. We are not aware of systematic studies of these phenomena.

It is to be noted that, while diurnal oscillations in mood are particularly frequent with depessed patients (v. Knorring and co-workers, 1977), they can also frequently be found in healthy subjects (Hampp, 1961), and in patients suffering from other mental illnesses (v. Knorring and co-workers, 1977). Therefore, they cannot be considered specific for depression.

Another indication of a disturbed diurnal rhythm is the sleep disturbance in depressives. It consists mainly in frequent changes of sleep stages, in frequent intermediary and excessively early waking up, in a decrease of sleep stages III and IV, increased variability of several REM parameters, and a decreased REM latency (Papousek, 1975; Kupfer, 1976; Mendelson, Gillin, Wyatt, 1977). All these findings are not specific for depression. In the sense of a desynchronization hypothesis, the decreased REM latency could be interpreted as a phase shift of the diurnal rhythm of REM periods (case c, Fig. 1). To date, no studies of the sleep of depressed patients over whole 24-hour periods have been published, as has been done for healthy subjects. Furthermore, there is a lack of investigations of the diurnal course of tiredness and readiness for sleep, which seem often to be dissociated in the clinical picture of depressives.

As far as biochemical parameters are concerned, the concentration of cortisol in blood and its elimination in urine respectively have best been investigated. The higher cortisol level during depression has been proven. However, consistent phase angle differences between

healthy and depressed subjects, supporting the hypothesis of desynchronization, could not be found (Durell, 1968; Sachar and co-workers, 1973). Aschoff (1977) has given a summary of the findings till 1977. We do, however, only know of two long-term studies: One was carried out by Jenner and co-workers (1968) on a manic-depressed patient with a persisting 48-hour cycle; the other on several depressed patients is currently being carried out at the Max-Planck-Institut für Psychiatrie in Munich by v. Zerssen and co-workers (1978). In neither case disturbances of the phase relations could be found.
Cross-sectional studies have been carried out on the diurnal course of electrolytes (Lobban and co-workers, 1963; Moody and Allsopp, 1969; Pflug, 1976a), and biogenic amines, their precursors and metabolites in the plasma or in the urine (Birkmayer and Linauer, 1970; Klempel, 1972; Riederer and co-workers, 1974; Kishimoto, 1977; Wirz-Justice and Pühringer, 1978). The results of these studies are not consistent and are difficult to interpret due to differences and imperfections in methodology, e.g. lack of control groups, small samples, too few measurements across the day.
In a study by Niskanen and co-workers (1976), the diurnal course of the free tryptophan in serum showed in the depressed group a 12-hour component. Similar 12-hour components have been reported by Waldmann (1972) on the diurnal course of mood; and by Nikitopoulou and Crammer (1976) in a longitudinal study on axillary temperatures of six depressed patients. On the contrary, in the manic phase of these six patients, inconspicuous one-peak temperature courses were found.
Mendlewicz (1977) found a large interindividual distribution of TSH acrophases in a cross-sectional study of bipolar depressed patients compared to a healthy control sample. Van Cauter and Mendlewicz (1978) in a 24-hour study with sampling intervals of 30 - 60 minutes reported a more irregular and sometimes polycyclic diurnal pattern of plasma dopamine-beta-hydroxylase (DBH) levels in unipolar and especially in bipolar depressed patients, compared to healthy controls. In addition, maxima of DBH concentration were found somewhat earlier in the afternoon in the patients' group (combination of cases (b) and (c), Fig. 1).
In cross-sectional investigations, no differences in the course of pulse frequency and systolic blood pressure could be found by Rudolf and Tölle (1977). Kripke and co-workers (1977), however, observed a higher inter-individual variation (corresponding to case (b) of Fig. 1 of the acrophases of physical activity, oral temperature, urine volume and natrium-chloride excretion, but only in their bipolar depressed group.

Palmai and Blackwell (1965) in a cross-sectional study reported an inversion of the normal 24-hour rhythm of salivary flow in 20 depressed women.
During a 21-day investigation of manic-depressed twins, one of whom was going through a hypomanic phase, Trapp and co-workers (1977) found no definite disturbance of phase relations.

So far, only two longitudinal studies have been published which show directly a partial or entire free-running of physiological parameters in depressed patients.
One of these studies, in which free-running of oral temperature and pulse was shown for one manic-depressed patient, was done by Atkinson, Kripke and Wolf (1975). Fig. 2 shows at the horizontal axis the days of investigation, vertically the local time is marked. The acrophases for pulse and temperature shift at earlier times each day between September 15 and October 3 corresponding to a mean period of τ=22.2 h.

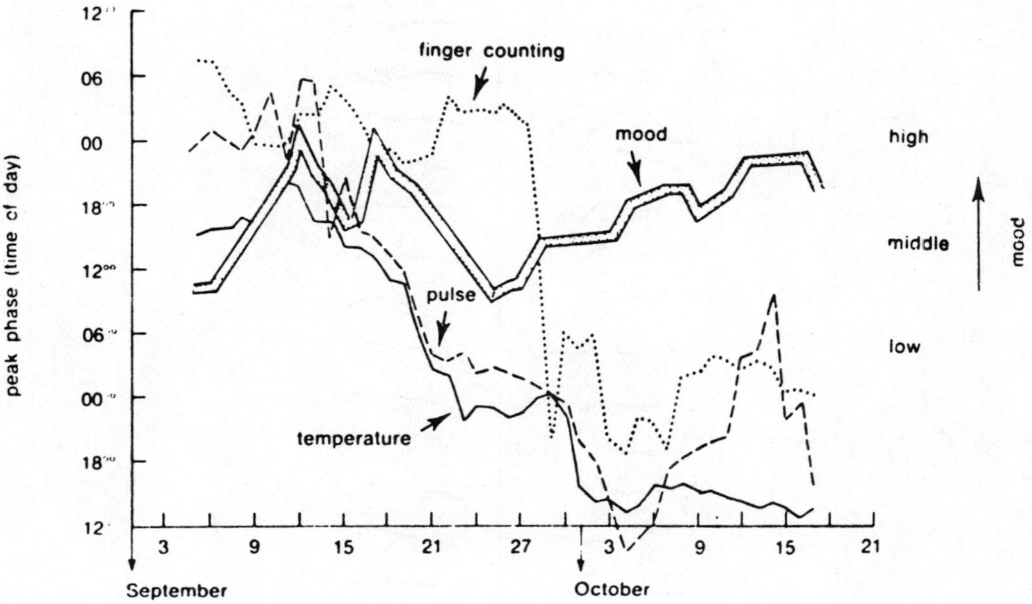

Fig. 2 Daily acrophases of pulse rate, oral temperature, finger counting frequency, and mood, in a bipolar depressed patient, depressive phase.

(By permission, from: Atkinson and co-workers, 1975)

Figure 3 is from the second study which was done by Pflug and co-workers (1976). On the left, the course of oral temperature of a manic-depressed woman during a depressive phase measured only during wakefulness is shown. The temperature curves are irregular compared to the curves in the depression-free interval on the right.

Figure 4 shows the power spectrum of the very temperature curves. In depression, a peak can be found at a τ-value of 22.5 h besides the main peak at $\tau=24$ h.

In both studies mentioned, the patients themselves have measured their temperatures, which is not unproblematic, and in both cases, the oral temperature was measured, which is less reliable than the rectal temperature. On the other hand, it is noteworthy that both patients suffered from bipolar depression, and that in both cases the free-running rhythm or free-running component respectively show a frequency which is higher than one cycle per day ($\tau<24$ h).

In this point, they differ from the few non-depressed patients free-running under normal conditions, who were reported so far. These

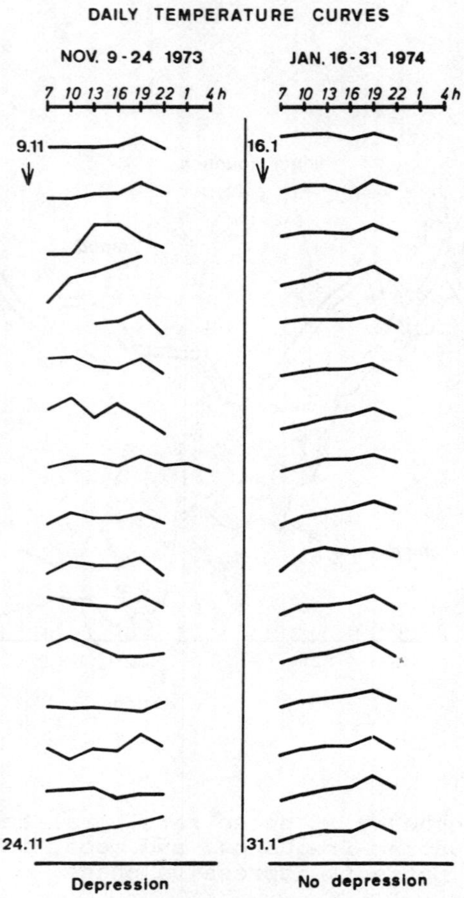

Fig. 3 Daily courses of oral temperature in a bipolar depressed patient, depressive phase (left) and interval (right).

(By permission, from: Pflug and co-workers, 1976)

controls showed periods of more than 24 hours as measured e.g. in sleep-wakefulness and rectal temperature (Miles and co-workers, 1977; Weitzman and co-workers, 1977). Healthy subjects in isolated chambers also do not show activity periods shorter than 24 hours, unless there is internal desynchronization between activity rhythm and vegetative functions (Wever, 1975). On the other hand, results obtained by Mills and co-workers (1977) suggest that there may be rhythms of temperature and sleep-wakefulness with $\tau < 24$ h in chronic schizophrenic patients held in isolation.

The two other bipolar cases reported by Atkinson, Kripke and Wolf did not reveal such clear-cut findings. Also Pflug observed temperature courses in both unipolar and bipolar depressed patients which were normal over long periods. In the longitudinal study carried out at the Max-Planck-Institut für Psychiatrie in Munich, inconspicuous, as well as shifted and more scattered phases, but no free-running temperature curves were found (v. Zerssen and co-workers, 1978).

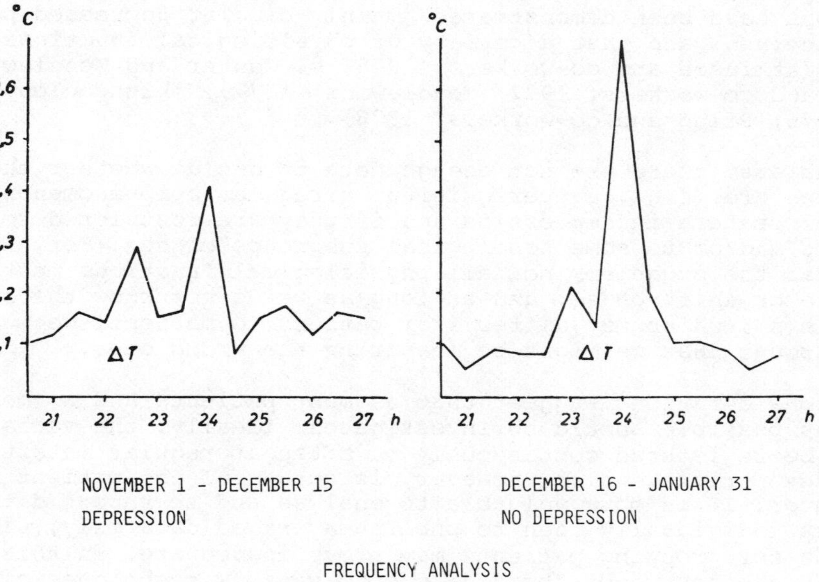

Fig. 4 Frequency analysis of the curves shown in Fig. 3. (By permission, from: Pflug and co-workers, 1976)

Lithium improved the patient mentioned by Atkinson, Kripke and Wolf (1975). But, contrary to expectations, Lithium did not improve the patient of Pflug and co-workers (1976).

Lithium has proved to have a significant lengthening effect on free-running endogenous periodicities in investigations with plants and more recently also with animals (Engelmann, 1973; Engelmann and co-workers, 1976; Hofman and co-workers, 1978). The prophylactic, anti-manic, and partly anti-depressive effect of Lithium on the one hand, and its slowing down effect on the diurnal system - which still has to be proved in man - on the other hand, is one of the findings which might be in favour of the hypothesis formulated at the beginning. Another support is the effect of therapeutic sleep deprivation, which could consist in a facilitation of the restitution of physiological phase relationships (Pflug, Tölle, 1971; Pflug, 1976b). No experimental results on depressed patients are known to date. Some studies with healthy subjects, however, have shown a slightly retarding effect of sleep deprivation on diurnal rhythms (Ringer, 1972). The effect of electro-convulsive therapy may be due to a similar mechanism. Also tri-cyclic antidepressives have proved favourably to influence re-synchronization in animals after experimental phase-shifts (Baltzer and Weisskrantz, 1975).

To summarize: Up to date, there are some indications that internal, as well as external phase relations of the diurnal system might be disturbed in depression, but conclusive evidence is still lacking. It is conspicuous that in the few cases in which disturbances of phase relations have been demonstrated, mainly bipolar depressed patients are concerned, and that a variety of physiological functions are affected (Atkinson and co-workers, 1975; v. Cauter and Mendlewicz, 1978; Kripke and co-workers, 1977; Mendlewicz, 1977; Nikitopoulou and Crammer, 1976; Pflug and co-workers, 1976).

Nevertheless, there are not enough data to decide whether these disturbances are, e.g., a prerequisite, a regular epiphenomenon or just a casual feature in depression and if they are restricted to some patients and/or to some nosological subgroups or not. For, in order to impair the organism, not all physiological functions must desynchronize or shift phase; and as long as we do not know the critical variable(s), which may differ from patient to patient, we must take into account that we might be measuring the wrong ones.

These considerations suggest that as many patients and as many variables as possible should be investigated. Ideally, the variables should be registered continuously or often at regular intervals and over many periods, which, however, is stressful for patient and investigator. It is more valuable to analyse and to report data of patients individually than to publish averaged data only, since our criteria for grouping patients may prove inadequate. In this context, a possible biassing of the data due to various techniques of time series analysis should be considered (Giedke and co-workers, 1974; Pöppel, 1975). Also the superposition of circadian, infradian, and ultradian rhythms must be taken into account.

Temporary desynchronization in the diurnal system can often be observed due to night or shift work, air trips to other time zones, certain experimental circumstances, or even without known reason. It is often accompanied by a decreased feeling of well-being, and decreased efficiency, but, as a rule, not by depression. The disturbance in the synchronization as such is therefore certainly not specific for depression - except - possibly - in cases of disturbances which are longlasting, very intensive and involving special variables. Even then, the question as to the etiological significance for depression would have to be clarified.

REFERENCES

Aschoff, J. (1977). Wie gestört ist der zirkadiane Rhythmus bei Depressiven? In H. Heimann (Ed.), Neue Strategien in der Depressionsforschung. Symposium a. d. Weitenburg/Tübingen. (To be published.)

Aschoff, J., K. Klotter, R. Wever (1965). Circadian vocabulary. A recommended terminology with definitions. In J. Aschoff (Ed.), Circadian clocks. Proc. Feldafing Summer School, Sept. 7-18, 1964, North Holland Publ. Comp., Amsterdam, pp. X-XIX.

Atkinson, M., D. F. Kripke, S.R. Wolf (1975). Autorhythmometry in manic-dpressives. Chronobiologia, 2, 325-335.

Baltzer, V., L. Weiskrantz (1975). Antidepressant agents and reversal of diurnal activity cycles in the rat. Biol. Psychiatry, 10, 199-209.

Birkmayer, W., W. Linauer (1970). Störung des Tyrosin- und Tryptophanmetabolismus bei Depression. Arch. Psych. Nervenkrankh., 213, 377-387.

Cauter, E. van, J. Mendlewicz (1978). 24-hour dopamine-beta-hydroxylase pattern: a possible biological index of manic-depression. Life Sciences, 22, 147-156.

Durell, J. (1968). Biological rhythms and psychiatry: psychoendocrine mechanisms. In J. de Ajuriaguerra (Ed.), Cycles biologiques et psychiatrie. Symposium Bel-Air III, Geneva, September 1967. pp 321-338. Georg + Cie, Geneva. Masson + Cie, Paris.

Engelmann, W. (1973). A slowing down of circadian rhythms by Lithium ions. Z. Naturforsch., 28c, 733-736.

Engelmann, W., I. Bollig, R. Hartmann (1976). Wirkung von Lithium-Ionen auf zirkadiane Rhythmen. Arzneim.-Forsch. (Drug. Res.), 26, 1085-1086.

Falret, J. P. (1854). Mémoire sur la folie circulaire. Bull. de l'académie de médecine.

Giedke, H., M. Fatranska, P. Doerr, E. Hansert, D. Stamm, H. Wisser (1974). Tagesperiodik der Rectaltemperatur sowie der Ausscheidung von Elektrolyten, Katecholaminen und 17-Hydroxycorticosteroiden mit dem Harn beim Menschen mit und ohne Lichtzeitgeber. Int. Arch. Arbeitsmed., 32, 43-66.

Halberg, F. (1968). Physiologic considerations underlying rhythmometry with special reference to emotional illness. In J. de Ajuriaguerra (Ed.), Cycles biologiques et psychiatrie. Symposium Bel-Air III, Geneva, September 1967, pp. 73-126. Georg + Cie, Geneva. Masson + Cie, Paris.

Hampp, H. (1961). Die tagesrhythmischen Schwankungen der Stimmung und des Antriebes beim gesunden Menschen. Arch. Psych. + Z. f. d. ges. Neurol., 201, 355-377.

Hitzig, E. (1898). Über die nosologische Auffassung und über die Therapie der periodischen Geistesstörung. Berl. klin. Wschr., 1, 2, 3.

Hofmann, K., M. Günderoth-Palmowski, G. Wiedenmann, W. Englemann (1978). Further evidence for periodic lengthening effect of Li^+ on circadian rhythms. Z. Naturforsch., 33c, 231-234.

Jenner, F. A., J. C. Goodwin, M. Sheridan, I. J. Tauber, M. C. Lobban (1968). The effect of an altered time regime on biological rhythms in a 48-hour periodic psychosis. Brit. J. Psychiat., 114, 213-224.

Kishimoto, H. (1977). The level and circadian rhythm of plasma tryptophan, tyrosine and cortisol in manic-depressive patients and its clinical significances. Psychiatr. Neurol. Jpn., 79, 375-392.

Klempel, K. (1972). Orientierende Untersuchung des zirkadianen Plasma-Tyrosin-Rhythmus depressiver Syndrome unterschiedlicher Ätiologie. Arch. Psychiat. Nervenkr., 216, 131-152.

Knorring, L. v., C. Perris, E. Strandman (1977). Diurnal variations in intensity of symptoms in patients of different diagnostic groups. Arch. Psychiat. Nervenkr., 224, 295-312.
Kraepelin, E. (1913). Klinische Psychiatrie. 8. Aufl., Barth, Leipzig.
Kripke, D. F., D. Mullaney, M. Atkinson, L. Huey, B. Hubbard (1977). Circadian rhythms phases in affective illnesses. Chronobiologia, 4, 125.
Kupfer, D. J. (1976). REM-Latency: A psychobiologic marker for primary depressive disease. Biol. Psychiat., 11, 159-174.
Lobban, M., B. Tredre, A. Elithorn, P. Bridges (1963). Diurnal rhythms of electrolyte excretion in depressive illness. Nature, 199, 667-669.
Mendelson, W. B., J. C. Gillin, R. J. Wyatt (1977). Human sleep and its disorders. Plenum Press, New York - London.
Mendlewicz, J. (1977). Personal communication.
Middelhoff, H. D. (1967). Tagesrhythmische Schwankungen bei endogen Depressiven im symptomfreien Intervall und während der Phase. Arch. Psychiat. u. Z. f. d. ges. Neurol., 209, 315-339.
Miles, L. E. M., D. M. Raynal, M. A. Wilson (1977). Blind man living in normal society has circadian rhythms of 24.9 hours. Science, 198, 421-423.
Mills. J. N., R. Morgan, D. S. Minors, J. M. Waterhouse (1977). The free-running circadian rhythms of two schizophrenics. Chronobiol., 4, 353-360.
Moody, J. P., M. N. E. Allsopp (1969). Circadian rhythms of water and electrolyte excretion in manic-depressive psychosis. Brit. J. Psychiat., 115, 923-928.
Nikitopoulou, G., J. L. Crammer (1976). Changes in diurnal temperature rhythm in manic depressive illness. Brit. Med. J., 1, 1311-1314.
Niskanen, P., M. Huttunen, T. Tamminen, J. Jääskeläinen (1976). The daily rhythm of plasma tryptophan and tyrosine in depression. Brit. J. Psychiat., 128, 67-73.
Palmai, G., B. Blackwell (1965). The diurnal pattern of salivary flow in normal and depressed patients. Brit. J. Psychiat., 111, 334-338.
Papousek, M. (1975). Chronobiologische Aspekte der Zyklothymie. Fortschr. Neurol. Psychiat., 43, 381-440.
Pflug, B. (1976a). Methodische Probleme der klinischen Rhythmusforschung bei Depressiven. Arzneim.-Forsch. (Drug Res.), 26, 1065-1068.
Pflug, B. (1976b). The effect of sleep deprivation on depressed patients. Acta psychiat. scand., 53, 148-158.
Pflug, B., R. Erikson, A. Johnsson (1976). Depression and daily temperature. Acta psychiat. scand., 54, 254-266.
Pflug, B., R. Tölle (1971). Disturbance of the 24-hour rhythm in endogenous depression and treatment of endogenous depression by sleep deprivation. Int. Pharmacopsychiat., 6, 187-196.
Pilcz, A. (1901). Die periodischen Geistesstörungen. G. Fischer, Jena.
Pöppel, E. (1975). Parameter estimation or hypothesis testing in the statistical analysis of biological rhythms? Bull. Psychonomic. Soc., 6, 511-512.
Riederer, P., W. Birkmayer, E. Neumayer, L. Ambrozi, W. Linauer (1974). The daily rhythm of HVA, VMA, (VA) and 5-HIAA in depressionsyndrom. J. Neur. Transm., 35, 23-45.
Ringer, C. (1972). Circadiane Periodik psychologischer und physiologischer Parameter bei Schlafentzug. Med. Thesis, Munich.
Rudolf, G. A. E., R. Tölle (1977). Circadian rhythm of circulatory functions in depressives and on sleep deprivation. Int. Pharmacopsychiat., 12, 174-183.

Sachar, E. J., L. Hellmann, H. P. Roffwarg, F. Halpern, D. K. Fukushima, T. F. Gallagher (1973). Disrupted 24-hour patterns of cortisol secretion in psychotic depression. Arch. Gen. Psychiat., 28, 19-24.

Stallone, F., G. J. Huba, W. G. Lawlor, R. R. Fieve (1973). Longitudinal studies of diurnal variations in depression: A sample of 643 patient days. Brit. J. Psychiat., 123, 311-318.

Supprian, U. (1975). Zur chronopathologischen Struktur der depressiven Tagesschwankung. Arch. Psychiat. Nervenkr., 220, 9-22.

Trapp, G., E. Eckert, P. Vestergaard (1977). Psychophysiologic circadian rhythmometry on manic-depressive twins. Chronobiologia, 4, 179-180.

Waldmann, H. (1972). Die Tagesschwankung in der Depression als rhytmisches Phänomen. Fortschr. Neurol. Psychiat., 40, 83-104.

Weitzman, G. D., C. Kokkoris, C. P. Pollak, A. Spielman, C. A. Czeisler, H. Bradlow, J. Axel, A. Katoroff, W. Gruen (1977). Development of a long term solid state portable core body temperature recorder ("Solicorder"). Application to a patient with a circadian rhythm sleep-wake disturbance. Paper pres. 13th Intern. Conf. Intern. Soc. Chronobiology, Pavia.

Wever, R. (1975). The circadian multi-oscillator system in man. Int. J. Chronobiology, 3, 19-55.

Wirz-Justice, A., W. Pühringer (1978). Seasonal incidence of an altered diurnal rhythm of platelet serotonin in unipolar depression. J. Neur. Transmission, 42, 45-53.

Zerssen, D. v., R. Lund, H. Schulz, P. Doerr, M. Fischler, H. M. Emrich, D. Ploog (1978). Personal information.

48-Hour-Cycles of Depression and their Biological Concomitants with and without 'Zeitgebers'. A Case Report

D. VON ZERSSEN, R. LUND, P. DOERR, M. FISCHLER, H. M. EMRICH and D. PLOOG

Max-Planck-Institute für Psychiatrie, Munich, FRG

INTRODUCTION

There are several reports in the literature concerning patients with 48-hour-cycles of mental disorders. From the end of the 18th century up to 1960 more than 70 cases have been described (Menninger-Lerchenthal, 1960; Richter, 1960). Since then five other such cases have been recorded (Bunney and Hartmann, 1965; Delay and others, 1961; Gelenberg and others, 1978; Jenner and others, 1967; Kupfer and Heninger, 1972). Whereas formerly more than a quarter of the 48-hour-cycles could be related to organic diseases of the brain (circulatory, tumorous, inflammatory/degenerative) this was not true for those reported after 1930. This may be due to the fact that general paralysis which could be prevented or treated effectively during the last decades had been the most frequent organic brain disease leading to regular cycles of psychopathology (cf. Menninger-Lerchenthal, 1960).

A general feature of 48-hour-cycles in the mental state is that mainly, though not exclusively, general activity and mood are involved, with a dramatic change from either one abnormal extreme (expansion/elation) to the opposite extreme (lethargy/depression) or from one of them to a normal state. Commonly one state lasts for 24 hours so that, in the latter case, 'bad' days and 'good' days run in alternation. In most cases the change takes place during the night while the patients are sleeping so that they awake in the morning with quite a different mental condition compared to the day before. The time of change may vary between patients (usually within the limits of 11 p.m. and 7 a.m.), but for each individual this time may be remarkably stable (Sitaram, Gillin and Bunney, 1978). Very often the change occurs very rapidly, in some instances even within a few seconds (e.g. Moravcsik, 1908). The transition involves a whole spectrum of symptoms in the areas of activity, mood, thought content and others (Arndt, 1930). The resulting syndromes cannot be differentiated from those seen in other organic or functional mental disorders, either general paralysis with excitement and/or affective symptomatology or episodic psychoses of a schizophrenic (catatonic), schizoaffective or purely affective (bipolar manic depressive or unipolar depressive) type. Purely affective disorders may reach the degree of a psychosis or not. In the latter case they were described as 'intermittent neurasthenia' by some authors (e.g. Dunin, 1898; Oddo, 1894/1896; cf. Kraepelin, 1913). Very often the cycle of mental state is accompanied by a cycle of somatic functions. These not only include changes in general motor activity and expressive movement, but also changes in body temperature, carbohydrate metabolism, urine excretion (volume, electrolytes and other compounds, particularly steroids of adrenal origin) and others (Bunney, Hartmann and Mason, 1965; Dubois, 1901; Jenner and others, 1967; Schaefer, 1896).

Even in cases where there is no indication of an organic origin of the disorder hereditability does not seem to play a major role in the etiology of the syndromes and their course of cycling. Only in a few instances could a family history of functional psychoses be found, but - with one exception (Ennen, 1902) - a similar periodic pattern was not recorded in afflicted relatives. Therefore, the strict periodicity of cycles is commonly related to other factors than those underlying the symptom formation as such (Arndt, 1930; Ennen, 1902). Nevertheless, the 48-hour-cycles are of great theoretical importance since they allow the investigation of periodic phenomena which do not follow directly a diurnal (24-hour-)rhythm, though strictly related to it (48 hours = 2 x 24 hours). This kind of rhythm is not found in the environment and must therefore be of an internal origin.

The investigation of the phenomenon is facilitated by the fact that the cycles are short and - at least in patients with no obvious organic brain disease - tend to persist with remarkable regularity for years or even decades. Most afflicted individuals are more than 40 years of age at the beginning of the cycling course of their disorder which may have taken the usual irregular episodic course before. In some cases the periodic disorder does not perish spontaneously once it has started. Therefore, the investigation of the disorder is also of great practical importance for the patient himself and his family. Two such cases with a monopolar depressive and a bipolar manic depressive disorder, respectively, were successfully treated by lithium carbonate after careful investigation from a psychopathological and biological point of view (Gelenberg and Klerman, 1978; Hanna and others, 1972). During the course of the investigation one of them had also been observed in an isolation unit with his psychiatrist under an artificial 22-hour-regimen of daily routines (Jenner and others, 1968). The (bipolar affective) psychopathology then followed only this time schedule, thus changing from a 48- to a 44-hour-cycle, whereas variations of urine excretion and other autonomic functions exhibited 22-, 24- and 44-hour-components, and 17-ketogenic steroid excretion an additional 48-hour-component. Other periods than those mentioned here have not yet been observed in any of the cases in question. From the point of view of Halberg's hypothesis of internal desynchronization of diurnal variations in autonomic functions as the physiological basis of 'periodic' mental disorders - particularly 'periodic' depression (Halberg, 1968) - one would predict that 48-hour-periods of psychopathology resulted from the interference of a free running 16-hour-period with the externally entrained 24-hour-period of variations in biological functions (48 hours = 2 x 24 hours = 3 x 16 hours). One could argue that the 16-hour-period may be masked, though, by the superimposed 24-hour-period (cf. Halberg and others, 1960), but then it should be clearly observable at least in an environment without external 'zeitgebers'.

We had the opportunity to study a patient with a 48-hour-cycle of monopolar depression longitudinally at a psychiatric ward and in an environment devoid of zeitgebers. The latter part of the study was performed in collaboration with Dr. Wever and co-workers at the Max-Planck-Institut für Verhaltensphysiologie at Andechs. The following is a preliminary report of some of our findings. Further details will be dealt with in subsequent papers (e.g. Doerr and others, to be published).

CASE HISTORY

Our patient, a married annuitant, who has one adult married son, was 66 years of age when he was admitted to our hospital. The diagnosis was that of monopolar endogenous depression. There was no evidence of psychiatric disorders in his family. His medical record was unremarkable up to the beginning of his thirties when he first experienced depressive episodes of initially only one and later a few days duration. He then had temporary difficulties in sleeping and spent much time brooding. A few years later these episodes became more frequent and - at the age of 40 - also more prolonged, lasting from about three to four weeks. He became nervous, listless, brooding, short of energy, and finally suicidal. He was admitted to psychiatric hospitals a number of times, mostly because of serious suicidal attempts, and therefore became compulsorily retired in his 42nd year of age. Except for one series of ECT he was only treated with various psychotropic drugs, mainly neuroleptics, tranquilizers and hypnotics but not in a consistent fashion. Antidepressants were administered only on two occasions for a few weeks and apparently without success.

The course of the disease changed to a cycle of alternating 'good' and 'bad' days when he was about 53. He had committed his last suicidal attempt by taking an overdosage of drugs about several months before, so that an organic component in the etiology of the cycles has to be seriously considered. Until the beginning of antidepressant medication in our hospital at the age of 66 the cycles persisted for 13 years with only some irregularity (sequences of two or more good days in intervals of about one to two weeks). The patient had developed drug-dependence (diazepam and hypnotics), but after several years the abuse was successfully interrupted. This was about half a year before he entered our hospital. After the cessation of drug-abuse the cycles became even more pronounced than before. The patient thereafter received only low amounts of tranquilizing drugs which were withdrawn shortly before the beginning of our clinical observation.

After admission, when the patient was free of medication he continued to exhibit rather regular cycles of mood and behaviour. Every morning he woke up early in a gloomy state of mood, having slept for only a few hours. He felt miserable, was restless, short of energy, lacking initiative, his facial expression was unhappy and helpless, and his movements slow and without vigour. On his bad days the state did not change much until he went asleep the following night, but the next day was usually a good one, although the change took place only gradually during the late morning or in the afternoon. Mood and behaviour then became normalized in every respect. The patient could make jokes and laugh, but never seemed elated in a pathological way. He was rather a quiet, friendly, good-humoured old man, with a limited range of interests. Because of a residual L_5/S_1-syndrome of the left leg after disk surgery three years ago he often lay in bed just resting, perhaps listening to the radio, reading a journal or sleeping (for no longer than one hour). The sequence of good and bad days was interrupted on several occasions, but we never observed more than two or three consecutive days of similar behaviour.

Psychological testing revealed an average intelligence (IQ = 97) and gave no indication of an organic brain syndrome. The patient's physical state was that of a man in his late sixties. Except for his vertebragenic disorder no serious somatic abnormalities could be detected. X-ray of the scull, EEG and CT of the brain did not show significant deviations from the normal range for the patient's age group. Our clinical diagnosis was that of monopolar endogenous depression with a 48-hour-cycle. Treatment with antidepressant drugs alone and in combination with lithium was postponed after intensive clinical observation and a psychobiological investigation which will be dealt with in the following section.

TABLE 1 Variables and Measurements*

Variable	Measurement	Author(s)
sleep-waking-cycle (in the isolation unit)	light switched off and on by the patient before and after, respectively, his 'night'-sleep**	Wever (1979)
mood	self-rating 'adjective check list' ('Befindlichkeits-Skala' = Bf-S)	v. Zerssen (1976a/b)
	'visual analogue scale' (line-test)	Luria (1975)
motor activity (at the ward)	wristwatch-actometry of left arm and leg	McFarlain and Hersen (1974), modified by Emrich and others (1977)
body temperature	rectal thermometry	Wever (1979)
salivation rate (at the ward)	measurement of weight increase of 'dental rolls'	Busfield and Wechsler (1961), modified by Emrich (to be published)
urinary free cortisol	competitive protein-binding method	Köbberling and von zur Mühlen (1972)

* only those referred to in this paper are represented in this Table.

** recording of motor activity in the isolation unit by electromechanical transducers on the floor and under the bedsprings (cf. Wever, 1979) could not be evaluated because of the patient's many resting periods in bed during his 'day'-time and because of the constant presence of another person in the isolation room.

METHODS

During two periods of 26 and 9 days, respectively, the patient was observed under controlled conditions at an open ward according to a design for chronobiological investigation of patients with endogenous depression during the depressive episode and the free interval. In his case about every second day and the following morning could be regarded as an episode alternating with a free interval of usually less than 24 hours. Later on the investigation was repeated in an isolation unit at the Max-Planck-Institut für Verhaltensphysiologie at Andechs[1] (cf. Wever, 1979), where the patient spent a fortnight without zeitgebers. He was continuously in the company of one of six students who relieved each other every two to five hours according to a random schedule. They took the measurements immediately after the patient had been to the toilet. This was done in the same order as used at regular intervals during the respective investigation at the psychiatric ward of our institute. The set of variables was, however, reduced whilst the patient was in the isolation unit. This report discusses only some of the measurements in selecting those variables which either show marked differences between good and bad days under ward conditions (mood scales, motor activity, salivation rate and urinary excretion of free cortisol) or are regarded as adequate indicators of internal desynchronization in isolation experiments (sleep-waking-cycle and temperature). These variables are listed in Table 1.

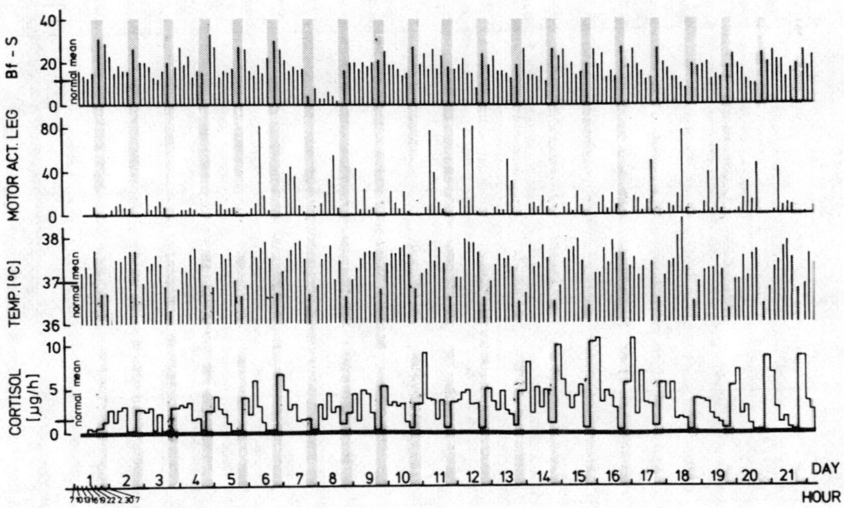

Fig. 1 Diurnal variations in mood and biological variables during a depressive episode in a 33 year old male in-patient.

---

[1]We are indebted to Prof. Aschoff, Dr. Wever and co-workers for their kind support of this part of the study.

At the ward all measurements were taken at regular intervals of three hours while the patient was awake (from 7 a.m. to 10 p.m.) and once each night after waking him at about 2:30 a.m. As mentioned above this time schedule was adapted to the patient's subjective sense of time whilst he was living in the isolation room.

Preliminary data analysis included a visualization of the time course of each variable, the variables being plotted together as functions or real time. For comparison, Fig. 1 shows the time course of mood, motor activity, body temperature, and urinary excretion of free cortisol in a 33 year old male patient during a depressive episode of a bipolar affective disorder. Apparently, there exist 24-hour- (but not longer) cycles of mood (upper section of the Fig.) with mood at its nadir in the night and early morning. There is but one marked exception to this sequence on day 8 when the patient appeared hypomanic for about 24 hours from a clinical point of view (cf. v.Zerssen and Cording, 1978).

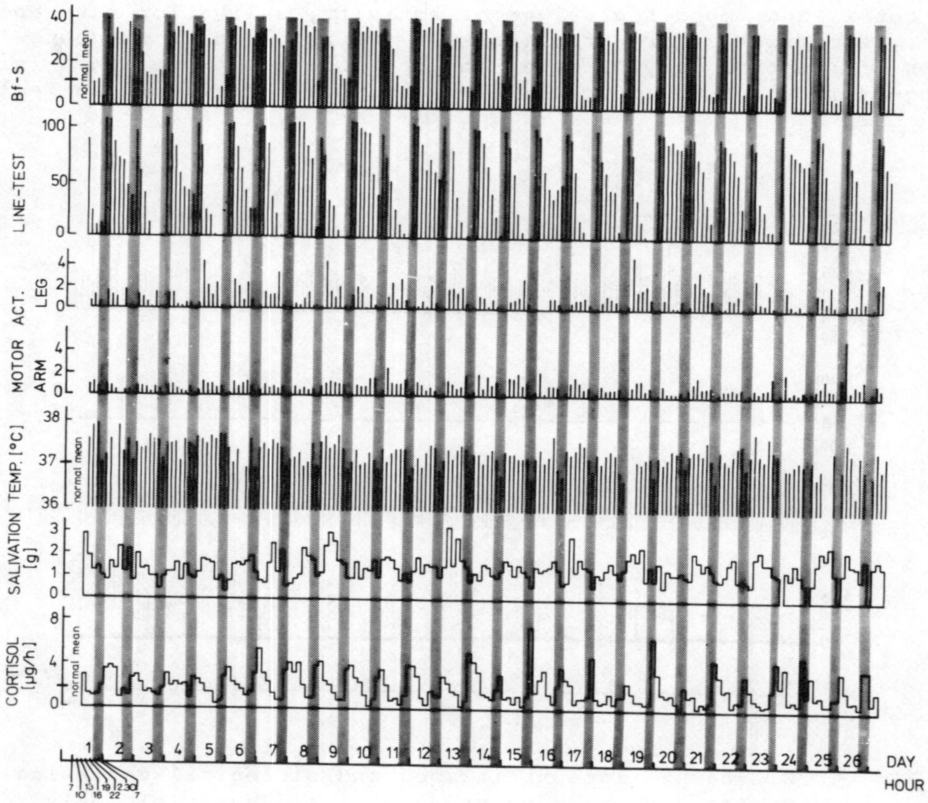

Fig. 2 Diurnal variations in mood and biological variables in a 66 year old male in-patient with a 48-hour-cycle of monopolar depression.
First observation period at an open ward.

RESULTS AND DISCUSSION

Observation With Zeitgebers

In our patient with 48-hour-cycles of depression (Fig. 2) the data of both mood scales used in the study reflects a 48-hour-period of mood changes, but with some exceptions, e.g. the fluctuations in the two mood scales are either not concordant (particularly at day 7) or both of them indicate a sequence of two or three good days (days 13, 14, 15, days 21, 22, 23 and days 25, 26). Diurnal variation is very pronounced on good days with a dispersal of his clouded mood during the late morning or in the afternoon as likewise observed clinically before and during the trial. The 'visual analogue scale' (line-test), moreover, reflects diurnal variation with definite improvement in the afternoon of bad days. This tendency is not obvious in the 'adjective checklist' (Bf-S) and was not very conspicuous from a clinician's point of view.

Obviously, systematic fluctuations in the biological variables are primarily of a diurnal type. At close sight some additional variation can also be detected when comparing good and bad days. Motor activity, body temperature and salivation all tend to be lower, and cortisol excretion tends to be higher on some of the bad days. Relative to the standards known for the variables of Bf-S, rectal temperature and free cortisol in urine there is a deviation to abnormally high values in the depressive mood scale (Bf-S), particularly on bad days, to slightly elevated body temperature - on good days rather than on bad days and in the first part of the trial more than in the second part - and to slightly elevated levels of cortisol on a few of the bad days. For the other two variables (motor activity and salivation) no standard values are as yet available.

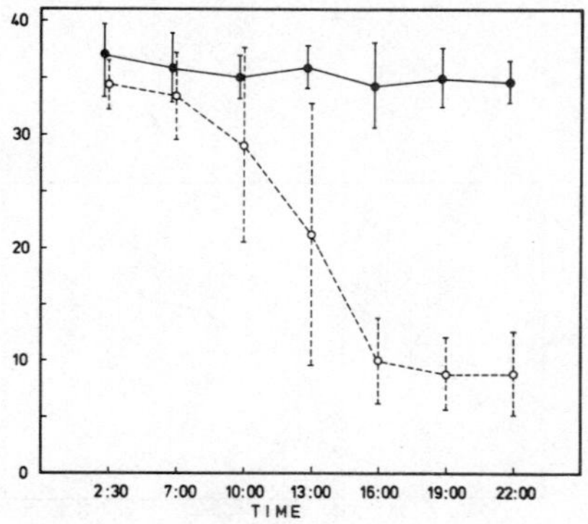

Fig. 3 Average diurnal variation of mood on '<u>good</u>' and '<u>bad</u>' days (means and standard deviations of the 'Befindlichkeits-Skala')

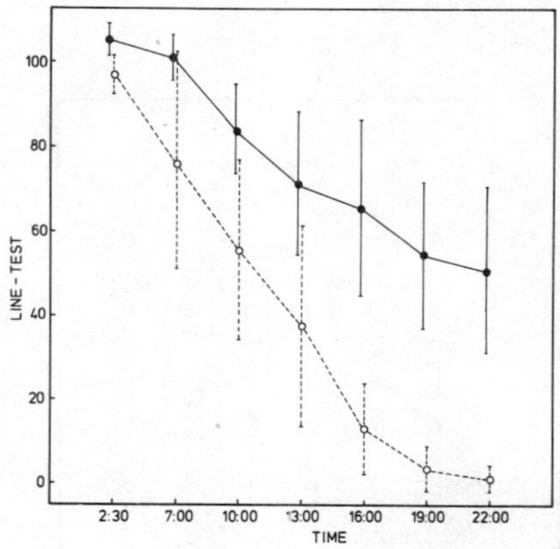

Fig. 4 Average diurnal variation of mood (line-test) on '<u>good</u>' and '<u>bad</u>' days.

Some of these tendencies become more apparent in the next step of the analysis, e.g. the computation of the diurnal variation averaged for good days and bad days separately. For this purpose 12 definitely good days (days 3, 5, 9, 11, 13, 15, 17, 19, 21, 23, 25, and 26) and 8 definitely bad days (days 2, 4, 6, 10, 12, 16, 20, and 24) were selected according to the Bf-S-values for a time period lasting from 2:30 a.m. to 10 p.m. (cf. Fig. 3). As to be expected from the visual analysis of Fig. 2 the analogue scale (line-test) shows some improvement even on bad days (Fig. 4, solid line). This trend, however, is much more pronounced on good days (Fig. 4, dotted line). Motor activity of the leg (Fig. 5) also exhibits a more pronounced diurnal variation on good days, but with two maxima in the morning and the afternoon, respectively, and minimal values in the late evening and at night. The average value is somewhat higher on good days, particularly in the early morning and in the afternoon. Similarly, body temperature (Fig. 6) has two maxima, although they appear somewhat later than the maxima of motor activity, and the mean values during the day time are somewhat higher on good days. Therefore, it seems possible that shape and level of the time course of temperature are partially determined by motor activity. The difference between good and bad days is particularly marked in the salivation rate (Fig. 7) at 10 a.m. where the peak value of good days is missing at bad days. Consequently, during bad days there is a pronounced reduction of the amplitude of the rhythm. In contrast to this finding urinary cortisol excretion (Fig. 8) shows the same pattern of diurnal variation on good and bad days with a maximum at night and a minimum in the evening, but it reaches a higher level throughout the bad days (cf. Doerr and others, to be published).

Altogether the biological differences between good and bad days are in line with findings in similar cases (e.g. Bunney and others, 1965; Jenner and others, 1967).

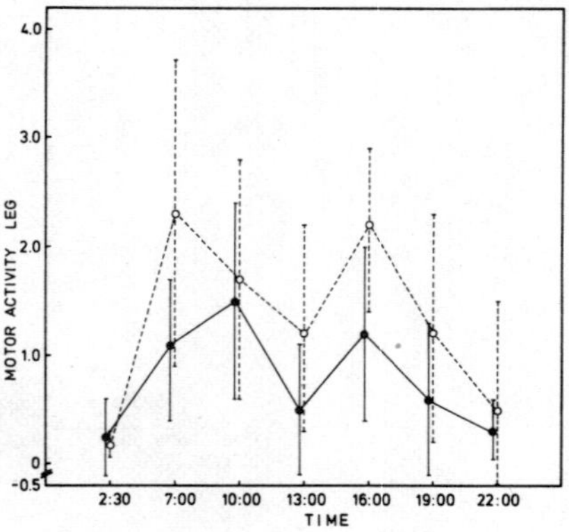

Fig. 5 Average diurnal variation of motor activity on 'good' and 'bad' days.

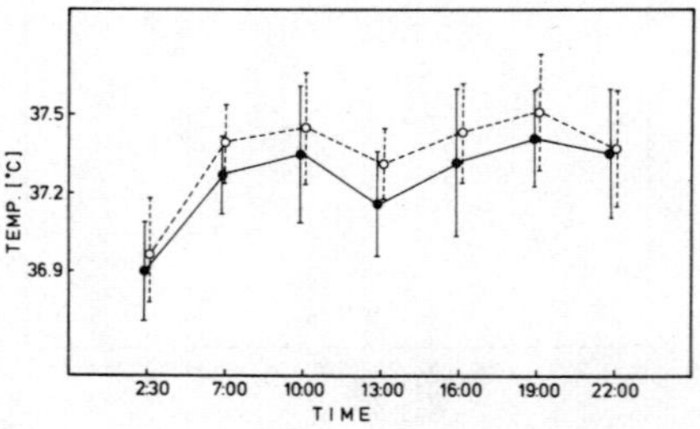

Fig. 6 Average diurnal variation of rectal temperature on 'good' and 'bad' days.

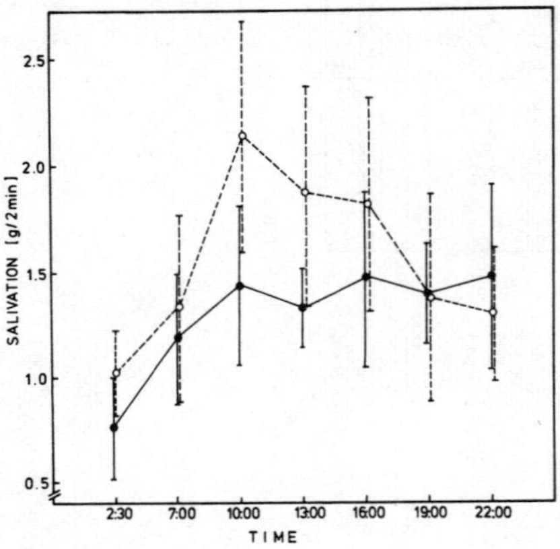

Fig. 7. Average diurnal variation of salivation rate on 'good' and 'bad' days.

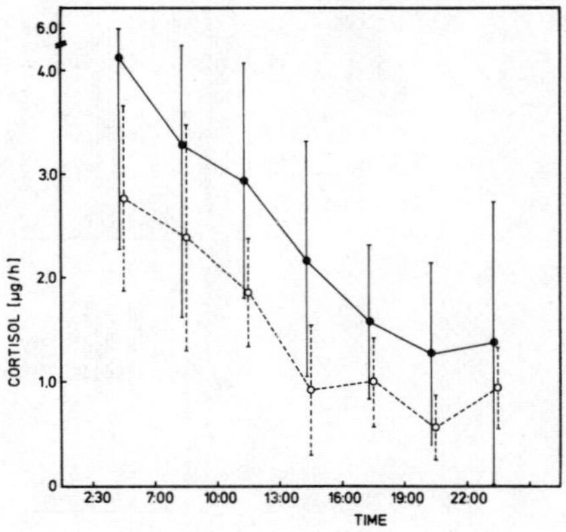

Fig. 8. Average diurnal variation of urinary free cortisol on 'good' and 'bad' days.

Observation Without Zeitgebers

A visualization of the time course of variables in the isolation unit (Fig. 9) - without motor activity and salivation which were not measured for technical reasons - reveals a similar pattern as that found in the hospital. This seems particularly remarkable in view of the fact that the length of the sleep-waking-cycle was reduced and rather irregular as can be seen from the bars above the figure which symbolize the time spent in bed with lights off. According to this measure of the cycle its period averages about 19 hours (according to a regression analysis). Thus there is a desynchronization between the sleep-waking-cycle and autonomic functions. A 16-hour-cycle cannot be found in any of the variables (sleep-waking, mood, temperature, cortisol excretion). In Fig. 10 the time course of variables for the time the patient spent in the isolation unit is plotted (solid lines) against the background of the equivalent time course observed at the psychiatric ward (dotted 'hills'). Apparently, there is a marked concordance in the circadian rhythm of cortisol excretion (lowest section). Fluctuations in body temperature are very irregular under both conditions and, therefore, more difficult to compare. According to a spectral analysis (to be published later in more detail) the main periods of variation in temperature during the patient's stay in the isolation unit are similar to those to be discovered under ward conditions, namely (about) 24 hours and 48 hours.

The mood cycles exhibit a similar pattern with and without zeitgebers. Whereas the main period of mood (at about 48 hours) does not

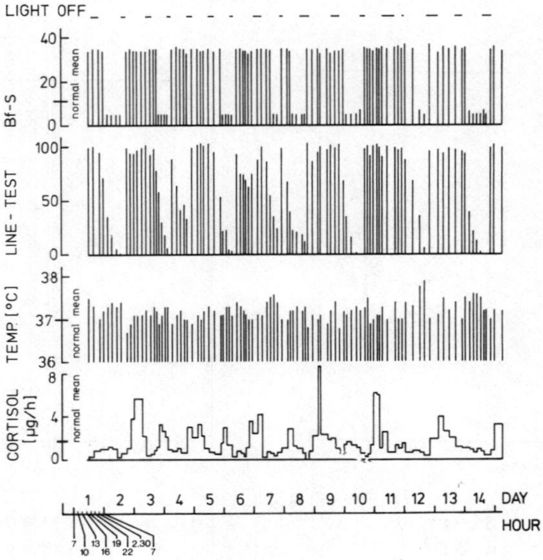

Fig. 9. Diurnal variations in mood and biological variables. observation period in an isolation unit without external zeitgebers.

change a phase shift at the beginning of the patient's stay in the isolation unit can be easily recognized: The minima fall about 9 to 15 hours behind the local time at which they occurred under the conditions of ward routine in our institute. Thus, the cycles are out of phase with those observed earlier. This phase shift may have been triggered by the change in the sleep-waking-cycle since the worsening of mood always fell in a period of the patient's 'night'-sleep (below the black bars in the upper row of the diagram). Hence, the mood cycle seems to be influenced in length by the circadian rhythm of autonomic functions (doubling their 24-hour-periodicity) and in phase by the sleep-waking-cycle. The latter conclusion is well in line with the fact that in almost all cases with 48-hour-cycles reported in the literature the changes in mood and behaviour occurred concurrently during the night (cf. Sitaram, Gillin and Bunney, 1978).

It is not surprising that our 66 years old patient - whilst in the isolation unit - showed internal desynchronization between his sleep-waking-cycle and autonomic rhythms. Furthermore, the period length of about 19 hours for the free running sleep-waking-cycle is not remarkable. These findings are in accordance with observations of elderly people in good physical and mental health living without external zeitgebers (cf. Wever, 1979).

If the periodicity of the patient's affective disorder resulted from internal desynchronization it had to be explained why the period was two days (48 hours). This discrepancy between facts and hypothesis

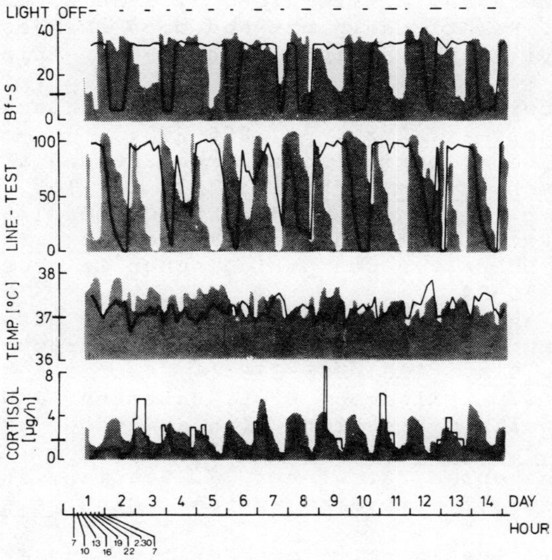

Fig. 10. Diurnal variations in mood and biological variables. Observation period in an isolation unit (line) projected on first part of observation period at an open ward (dotted areas).

could only be solved by the assumption of a mechanism which couples a 19-hour-clock (responsible for the sleep-waking-cycle) and a 24-hour-clock (responsible for circadian rhythms of autonomic functions) in such a way that changes in mood (hypothetically depending on both these clocks; cf. Wever, 1979) are forced into a 48-hour-cycle, at least if there is a predisposition for an affective disorder. If such a mechanism can be ruled out the desynchronization hypothesis does not find support with respect to the 48-hour-cycles of this patient, although this kind of cycling depression is one of the most striking examples of periodicity of mental illness.

REFERENCES

Arndt, M. (1930). Über täglichen (24stündigen) Wechsel psychischer Krankheitszustände. Allg. Z. Psychiat., 92, 128-150.

Bunney, W. E. jr., and E. L. Hartmann (1965). Study of a patient with 48-hour manic-depressive cycles. Part I. Arch. gen. Psychiat., 12, 611-618.

Bunney, W. E. jr., E. L. Hartmann, and J. W. Mason (1965). Study of a patient with 48-hour manic-depressive cycles. Part II. Arch. gen. Psychiat., 12, 619-625.

Busfield, B. L., and H. Wechsler (1961). Studies of salivation in depression. Arch. gen. Psychiat., 4, 10-15.

Delay, J., P. Pichot, P. Deniker, and D. Jousselin (1961). Psychose cyclique avec inversions quotidiennes de l'humeur. Ann. Méd. Psychol., 119, 125-129.

Doerr, P., D. v. Zerssen, M. Fischler, H. Schulz, and R. Wever (to be published). Relationship between mood changes and adrenal cortical activity in a patient with 48-hour unipolar-depressive cycles.

Dubois (1901). Ueber intermittierende psychopathische Zustände. Korresp.-Bl. schweiz. Ärz., 31, 265-270.

Dunin, T. (1898). Ueber periodische, circuläre und alternirende Neurasthenie. Dtsch. Z. Nervenheilk., 13, 147-162.

Emrich, H. M., J. B. Aldenhoff, and D. v. Cramon (1977). Registration of motor activity in postcomatous states. Excerpta med., 427, 33.

Ennen (1902). Zur Lehre von den periodischen Geistesstörungen. Neur. Centrbl., 21, 50-54.

Gelenberg, A. J., and G. L. Klerman (1978). The effects of amitriptyline and lithium on a patient with 48-hour recurrent depressions. J. nerv. ment. Dis., 166, 365-368.

Gelenberg, A. J., G. L. Klerman, E. L. Hartmann, and P. Salt (1978). Recurrent unipolar depressions with a 48-hour cycle: Report of a case. Brit. J. Psychiat., 133, 123-129.

Halberg, F., R. Loewenson, R. Winter, J. Bearman, and G. H. Adkins (1960). Physiologic circadian systems. Minn. Acad. Sci. Proc., 28, 53-75.

Halberg, F. (1968). Physiologic considerations underlying rhythmometry, with special reference to emotional illness. In J. de Ajuriaguerra (Ed.), Cycles Biologiques et Psychiatrie. Symposium Bel-Air III, Genève, Septembre 1967. Georg, Genève and Mason, Paris. pp. 73-126.

Hanna, S. M., F. A. Jenner, I. B. Pearson, G. A. Sampson, and E. A. Thompson (1972). The therapeutic effect of lithium carbonate on a patient with a forty-eight hour periodic psychosis. Brit. J. Psychiat., 121, 271-280.

Jenner, F. A., L. R. Gjessing, J. R. Cox, A. Davies-Jones, R. P. Hullin, and S. M. Hanna (1967). A manic depressive psychotic with a persistent forty-eight hour cycle. Brit. J. Psychiat., 113, 895-910.

Jenner, F. A., J. C. Goodwin, M. Sheridan, I. J. Tauber, and M. C. Labban (1968). The effect of an altered time regime on biological rhythms in a 48-hour periodic psychosis. Brit. J. Psychiat., 114, 215-224.

Köbberling, J., A. von zur Mühlen (1972). Methodische Untersuchungen zur Bestimmung der freien Harn-Corticoide mit der Proteinbindungsmethode. Z. Klin. Chem. Biochem., 10, 495-501.

Kraepelin, E. (1913). Psychiatrie, Vol. 3, part 2, 8th ed. Barth, Leipzig.

Kupfer, D. J., G. R. Heninger (1972). REM activity as a correlate of mood changes throughout the night. Arch. gen. Psychiat., 27, 368-373.

Luria, R. E. (1975). The validity and reliability of the visual analogue mood scale. J. psychiat. Res., 12, 51-57.

McFarlain, R. A., M. Hersen (1974). Continuous measurement of activity level in psychiatric patients. J. Clin. Psychol., 30, 37-39.

Menninger-Lerchenthal, E. (1960). Periodizität in der Psychopathologie. Maudrich, Wien-Bonn-Bern.

Moravcsik, E. E. (1908). Rascher Wechsel expansiver und depressiver Zustandsbilder in einem Falle progressiver Paralyse. Zbl. Nervenheilk. Psychiat., 31, NF 19, 409-411.

Oddo, C. (1896). Neurasthénie circulaire à forme alternante quotidienne. (Revue de Médicine, Juillet 1894). Neur. Centrbl., 15, 177.

Richter, C. P. (1960). Biological clocks in medicine and psychiatry: Shockphase hypothesis. Proc. nat. Acad. Sci. (Wash.), 46, 1506-1530.

Schaefer, A. (1896). Stoffwechselerscheinungen bei einem eigenartigen Falle von circulärem Irresein. Neur. Centrbl., 15, 1067-1072.

Sitaram, N., J. C. Gillin, and W. E. Bunney jr. (1978). Circadian variation in the time of 'switch' of a patient with 48-hour manic-depressive cycles. Biol. Psychiat., 13, 567-574.

Wever, R. A. (1979). The circadian system of man. Springer, New York-Berlin-Heidelberg.

Zerssen, D. v., with the collaboration of D.-M. Koeller (1976). Klinische Selbstbeurteilungs-Skalen (KSb-S) aus dem Münchener Psychiatrischen Informations-System (PSYCHIS München). Beltz, Weinheim.
a) Allgemeiner Teil.
b) Die Befindlichkeits-Skala.

Zerssen, D. v., and C. Cording (1978). The measurement of change in endogenous affective disorders. Arch. Psychiat. Nervenkr., 226, 95-112.

Chronobiological Aspects of Manic-Melancholic Disorders

E. T. MELLERUP, H. DAM, ALICE WIDDING and O. J. RAFAELSEN

Psychochemistry Institute, Rigshospitalet, 9, Blegdamsvej, DK-2100 Copenhagen Ø, Denmark

ABSTRACT

Diurnal rhythms of oral temperature, plasma phosphate, and urinary pH were determined in manic-melancholic patients and control persons. The two groups were compared with respect to the occurrence of maxima and minima values for the variables. Desynchronization of the rhythms would lead to greater variability in the times for maxima and minima values, and according to current theories it was anticipated that relatively more patients would have a diurnal rhythm, which deviated from the mean rhythm. However, in this respect no difference was found between the patients and the control persons.

KEYWORDS

Manic-melancholic disorders - chronobiology - temperature - plasma phosphate - plasma potassium - urinary pH.

INTRODUCTION

Almost every biological system has adapted to the 24 hours of a day and a night, as can be seen from the many biological variables having a rhythm with a period of 24 hours. When the influence of exogenous time markers or synchronizers are reduced, e.g., under experimental conditions or in the arctic, the exact 24 hour rhythm may change into a circadian rhythm with a period slightly different from 24 hour (Halberg and co-workers, 1977). When one rhythm continues with a 24 hour period, while another becomes free running with a shorter or longer period, the two rhythms are said to be desynchronized. As the days are going such two rhythm will deviate more and more from each other until they are 180° out of phase, then deviation gradually decreases until the two rhythms again become synchronized. It has been observed in monkeys that severe stress could lead to desynchronization phenomena (Stroebel, 1969), and it has been suggested that desynchronization of various rhythms may take place during depression (Halberg, 1968; Pflug, 1976). This theory would explain a number of observations related to the course of manic-melancholic episodes and it offers also an explanation for the effect of sleep deprivation on depressive symptoms (Pflug, 1976; Mellerup and Rafaelsen, 1978).

Experimentally the theory has been supported by a number of studies (Pflug, 1976; Atkinson and co-workers, 1975; Nikitopoulou and Crammer, 1976; Kripke and co-workers, 1978), all of which demonstrated changes in the circadian rhythm of body temperature during affective episodes.

The only way to determine the length of a circadian period is to analyze the appropriate variable (e.g., temperature) several times each day, during many consecutive days. If the rhythm deviates clearly from the 24 hour period, a graphic representation of the results may directly show the circadian period. If the rhythm contains components with different periods, these periods may be computed by mathematical methods (Halberg and co-workers, 1972).

When a variable is measured several times during a single 24 hour period, it is possible to determine the maxima and minima and the time of their occurrence.

In the case of desynchronization this time may deviate considerably from the usually observed times for maxima and minima, depending on the magnitude of change in period length and on the number of days since the desynchronization started. This means that although it is impossible to determine the exact length of a circadian period by measurements during 24 hour, it may be possible to get an indication of an eventual desynchronization.

In the present study a large number of manic-melancholic patients and normal control persons have been investigated during a single 24 hour period. The procedure has been described previously (Mellerup and co-workers, 1976).

The original purpose of the study was to compare lithium-treated patients with patients not treated with lithium and with normal controls. However, the data from the two latter groups may also be used to compare the rhythms of various variables in order to see whether there might be any indications of desynchronization.

A number of variables have been selected on the basis of their obvious diurnal rhythms. These were oral temperature, plasma phosphate, urinary pH, and plasma potassium, the mean values of which all showed distinct minimum and maximum values at certain times or time intervals. Most of the individual persons will also have maximum and minimum values at these particularly times. However, in a person where the rhythm of one or more variables for some time has been desynchronized the maximum and minimum may be placed several hours before or after the maximum and minumim times for the mean values. A very simple way to analyze this possibility is to count the number of patients and control persons, who actually have their minima and maxima values at times which are different from the times of minima and maxima of the mean curves.

The temperature curves for the normal controls and the patients not treated with lithium (psychiatric controls) (Fig.1) are very similar. Both have a maximum at 16.oo and a minimum between 23.oo and 8.oo.

Fig. 1

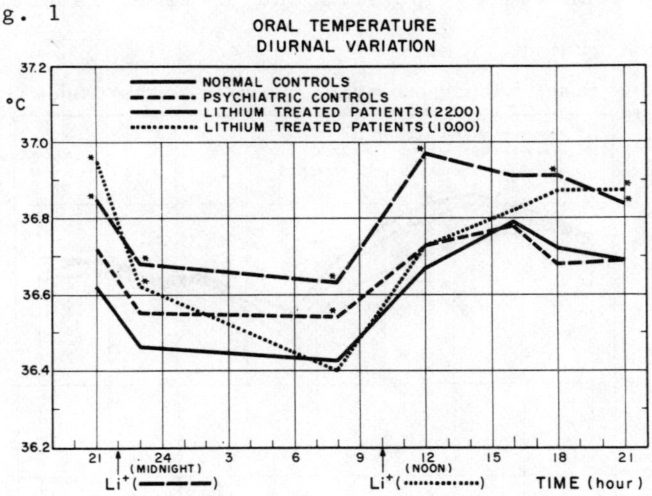

TABLE 1a Oral Temperature - Max. at 16.oo H.	Yes	No	Total
Control Persons	27	49	76
Manic-Melancholic Patients	4o	45	85
Total	67	94	161
χ^2 = 2.6 N.S.			

TABLE 1b Oral Temperature - Max. at 23.oo-o8.oo H.	Yes	No	Total
Control Persons	54	22	76
Manic-Melancholic Patients	53	32	85
Total	1o7	54	161
χ^2 = 1.o1 N.S.			

The temperature of the patients is slightly higher, but the difference is only significant at 8.oo. Table 1a shows the result of a chi-square test, where the control persons and the patients are divided according to the presence or absence of a maximum value at 16.oo.

It is seen that among the manic-melancholic patients (without lithium) relatively more had maximum temperature at 16.oo, but the difference between control persons and patients is not significant.

Fig. 2

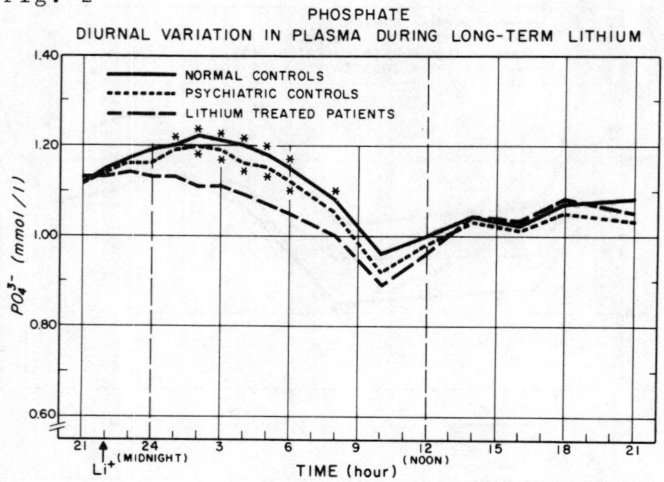

TABLE 2a Plasma Phosphate - Max. at o1.oo-o3.oo H.	Yes	No	Total
Control Persons	58	51	1o9
Manic-Melancholic Patients	55	49	1o4
Total	113	1oo	213
χ^2 = 0 N.S.			

TABLE 2b Plasma Phosphate - Max. at 1o.oo H.	Yes	No	Total
Control Persons	56	53	1o9
Manic-Melancholic Patients	64	4o	1o4
Total	12o	93	213
χ^2 = 1.9 N.S.			

The variation in plasma phosphate is seen in Fig. 2. The mean values for the normal controls and for the psychiatric controls are close to each other with the maximum occurring in the hours after midnight and the minimum sharply at 1o.oo. However, these mean values hides a large inter-individual variability. Thus Table 2a shows the distribution of the maximum values, and it is seen that only half of both control persons and patients had their maximum plasma phosphate in the interval from 1.oo to 3.oo.

It is also seen that the distribution is the same in the two groups. Table 2b shows that despite the pronounced minimum at 1o.oo for the mean values of plasma phosphate only half of the control persons had a minimum at this time, whereas more of the patients had minimum at 1o.oo. The difference between the two groups was, however, not statistical significant.

Figure 3 shows the rhythm of urinary pH, a variable which is strongly affected by the lithium-treatment, but which also displays a difference between the normal controls and the psychiatric controls. It is seen that both groups had a maximum at 17.oo, and again (Table 3a) the distribution in time of the maximum pH-values was the same for both the normal control persons and the manic-melancholic patients. When the normal controls and the psychiatric controls (the patients not in lithium-treatment) are compared with the lithium-treated patients, the two groups differ significantly with respect to the distribution of maximum values for urinary pH (Table 3b).

Fig. 3

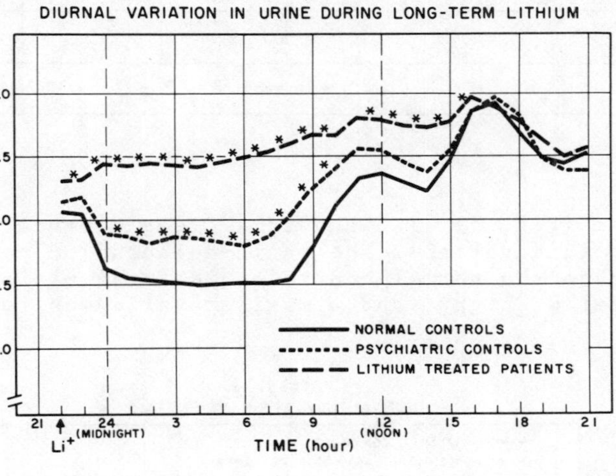

TABLE 3a Urine pH - Max. at 17.oo H.	Yes	No	Total
Control Persons	38	9	47
Manic-Melancholic Patients	3o	1o	4o
Total	68	19	87
χ^2 = o.14 N.S.			

TABLE 3b Urine pH - Max. at 17.oo H.	Yes	No	Total
Control Persons	68	19	87
Li-Treated Manic-Melancholic Patients	22	2o	42
Total	9o	39	129
χ^2 = 8.5 P < o.o1			

Plasma potassium (Fig. 4) also showed a clear diurnal rhythm, and with respect to this variable the manic-melancholic patients had higher values than the normal controls. The mean minimum value occurred shortly after midnight, and a maximum value was found around noon.

Fig. 4

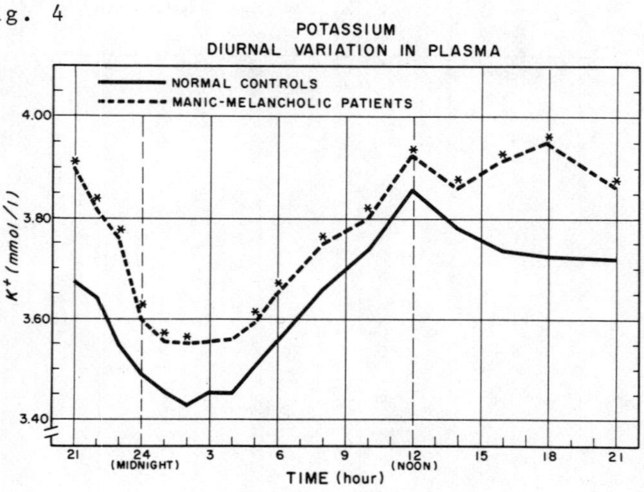

From Table 4a and b is seen that the distribution of maximum and minimum for plasma potassium was about the same for the control persons and the patients.

TABLE 4a Plasma Potassium - Max. at 12.oo-14.oo H.	Yes	No	Total
Control Persons	51	4o	91
Manic-Melancholic Patients	25	36	61
Total	76	76	152
χ^2 = 3.3 N.S.			

TABLE 4b Plasma Potassium - Min. at oo.oo-o2.oo H.	Yes	No	Total
Control Persons	69	22	91
Manic-Melancholic Patients	44	17	61
Total	113	39	152
χ^2 = o.1 N.S.			

Results from more prolonged studies have suggested that desynchronization of various circadian rhythms may occur in depressed patients. For the pertinent functions the times of occurrence for maxima and minima thus should show a larger variability in patients than in normal persons.

We have investigated the distribution in time of the maxima and minima of several variables, and generally the results did not support the idea of desynchronization as a more common phenomena in manic-melancholic patients than in normal controls. When those patients, who had the highest depression scores, were analyzed separately, and compared with the normal controls, still no differences in distribution of maxima and minima were found.

That the method as such could be used to demonstrate a change in time of the occurrence of a peak value, was obvious from the results which could be obtained by comparing the normal or the psychiatric controls with the lithium-treated patients.

One explanation for our negative finding may be that we have analyzed the wrong variables; another explanation may be that even if a function is desynchronized it may still contain elements with a 24 hour periodicity, and in such cases it is obvious that results from one single 24 hour period are not enough to disclose the occurrence of a desynchronization.

REFERENCES

Atkinson, M., D.F. Kripke, and S.R. Wolf (1975). Autorhythmometry in manic-depressives. Chronobiologica, 2, 325-335.

Halberg, F. (1968). Physiolgic considerations underlying rhythmometry with special reference to emotional illness. In J. de Ajuriaguerre (Ed.), Cycles Biologiques et Psychiatrie, Masson & Cie, Paris, pp. 73-126.

Halberg, F., E. Johnson, W. Nelson, W. Runge, and R. Sothern (1972). Autorhythmometry procedures for physiologic self-measurements and their analysis. Phys. Teacher, 1, 1-11.

Kripke, Daniel F., D.J. Mullaney, M. Atkinson, and W. Sanford (1978). Circadian rhythm disorders in manic-depressives. Biol.Psychiat., 13, 335-351.

Mellerup, E.T., B. Lauritsen, H. Dam, and O.J. Rafaelsen (1976): Lithium effects on diurnal rhythm of calcium, magnesium and phosphate metabolism in manic-melancholic disorder. Acta Psychiat. Scand., 53, 36o-37o.

Mellerup, E.T. and O.J. Rafaelsen (1978). Circadian rhythms in manic-melancholic disorders. In W.B. Essman and L. Valzelli (Eds.), Current Developments in Psychopharmacology, Spectrum, New York, pp. 51-66.

Nikitopoulou, G. and J.L. Crammer (1976). Change in diurnal temperature rhythm in manic-depressive illness. Br.Med.J., I:1311-1314.

Pflug, B. (1976). The effect of sleep deprivation on depressed patients. Acta Psychiat. Scand., 53, 148-158.

Stroebel, C.F. (1969). Biologic rhythm correlates of disturbed behavior in the rhesus monkey. In F.H. Roles (Ed.), Circadian Rhythms in Nonhuman Primates, Bibliotheca primatologica, No. 9, Karger, Basel, pp. 91-1o5.

A New Classification of the Affective Disorders

PROFESSOR SIR MARTIN ROTH

Department of Psychiatry, University of Cambridge Clinical School,
New Addenbrooke's Hospital, Hills Road, Cambridge

ABSTRACT

Observations derived from three groups of investigations have been brought together to serve as a basis for a new classification of affective disorders. The investigations were those concerned with (1) the relationship of 'endogenous' and 'neurotic' depression (2) the dividing line between depressive illness and anxiety states and (3) the associations of affective and schizoaffective disorders. The classification takes the form of a logical decision tree entailing distinctions that have to be made at each of 4 hierarchical levels. A fifth subsidiary level depicts the relationships of affective and schizoaffective disorders. A reasonable measure of correlation obtains between the classification and the pattern of treatment response within affective disorders.
(New Classification of Affective Disorders.)

INTRODUCTION

The classification of affective disorders to be described in this paper has been derived from a synthesis of observations undertaken in recent years on different aspects of the problem with older concepts of proven value from which much of our thinking about this subject continues to derive. A new synthesis is needed for three main reasons. The first is the inter-relatedness of the many problems in this field. This appears to have received scant recognition. The nature of the association between 'endogenous' (or 'autonomous', 'psychotic' etc) and 'neurotic' or ('reactive') depression, the differentiation of bipolar and unipolar disorders, the discreteness or confluence of depressive and anxiety states and the existence or otherwise of a clear line of demarcation between affective and 'schizoaffective' disorders have been studied by different investigators as if they constituted independent and unrelated problems. This failure to heed the close inter dependence of the whole range of issues has probably caused some of the inconsistency, disagreement and error in studies of classification. In this paper all these problems of the taxonomy of affective illness are therefore taken together.

The second reason is connected with the re-emergence in recent years of the unipolar-bipolar principle in the classification of depressive illnesses. Leonhard (1957) who originally made the distinction confined it to the endogenous states. But in the decade that has elapsed since the resurgence of interest in the bipolar-unipolar concept following the work of Angst (1966) Perris (1967) Winokur (1967) this limitation has been increasingly ignored. The concept has proved scientifically fruitful in many respects and this has engendered the belief that it would suffice by itself as a clear and parsimonious basis for the sub division of all disorders of affect. This belief has been reinforced by criticisms of the terms 'endogenous' and 'psychotic' as archaic and obsolete. One adverse effect of these developments has been the expansion in the scope of the concept of unipolar depression. In the absence of the stringent criteria both for exclusion as well as for inclusion of patients, which were explicit in Leonhard's original formulation, this syndrome has come to constitute a heterogenous group of disorders of affect liable to differ in composition from one investigator to the next.

A third reason for looking afresh at the taxonomy of this group of disorders is related to the second. During the past decade in particular a poverty of correlation has become evident between diagnosis on the one hand and treatment response on the other. It is possible to adduce evidence from controlled trials that one or other tricyclic compound is effective in the treatment of all forms of depressive illness. As far as prophylaxis is concerned one could advance the claim both for tricyclic substances and lithium carbonate. Yet all clinical psychiatrists are aware that though these treatments constitute significant advances they fail in a substantial proportion of cases. But current classification provides little assistance in the prediction of success or failure.

It may be, of course, that there is no correlation to be found between classification and treatment response. The other possibility is that our present classifications are too crude and too far divorced from systematic clinical observation to yield such correlations.

The present paper presents a brief outline of a classification of disorders of affect which has been described fully together with the relevant evidence in which it is based in two papers (Roth 1977 and In Press). The studies which have provided its factual basis have been concerned with three interrelated problems.

1. The relationship between endogenous and neurotic depression and the bearing of the distinction on treatment response. This was initially studied by Kiloh et al (1962) and Kiloh and Garside (1963) and subsequently by Carney, Roth and Garside (1965) and Kay et al (1970).

2. The relationship of and the line of demarcation between anxiety and phobic states on the one hand and the depressive states on the other. From an early stage this problem proved to share much common ground with the first one. (Roth 1959 and 1960, Roth and Harper 1962, Harper and Roth 1962, Roth et al 1972, Gurney et al 1970, 1972, Kerr et al 1972, 1974, Schapira et al 1972, Mountjoy and Roth 1977.

3. The nature of the association between affective and schizoaffective disorders. In a small proportion of acute phobic anxiety and phobic-depersonalisation states (Roth 1959, 1960) transient psychotic states with mixed features were observed to evolve. The differentiation between 'nuclear' and 'schizophreniform' disorders has also been studied and a brief report of these later investigations has been published (McClelland et al 1966).

Most of the investigations in the last 15 years have been undertaken with the aid of multi variate statistical techniques in an attempt to identify clusters of covarying features in patient groups and to differentiate between them as sharply as possible. Independent validation for the main groupings that have emerged, has been sought through follow-up enquiries to determine course and outcome and in some cases evaluation of their response to treatment.

The diagnostic scheme is a logical decision tree entailing distinctions that have to be made at each of four hierarchical levels. In the sections that follow these levels will be described in sequence from the first to the fourth. Separate consideration will be given to the schizophreniform disorders which have been shown apart of the four main levels because their relationships are not wholly and exclusively confined to the realm of affective disorders.

Figure 1 represents the proposed scheme in diagramatic form. A variety of diagnostic rubrics is represented but as will emerge in the section that follows each group of disorders is to be found within the case material utilised in different enquiries ostensibly concerned with the problems of 'depressive illness' alone. While the main sub divisions at the four hierarchical levels of the diagnostic scheme have been based on such data formal evidence of this character is not available in the case of every one of the sub divisions proposed.

2. THE RELATIONSHIP BETWEEN DEPRESSIVE ILLNESS AND NORMAL AFFECTIVE RESPONSE (FIG. 1)

The rubric affective disorder at level 1 entails a decision that the patient is suffering from an affective disorder that (a) is not secondary to some other psychiatric illness such as an organic or schizophrenic illness and (b) that the emotional state in question can be regarded as beyond the range of normal variation in affective response. The line of demarcation between normal and pathological affective disturbance is to be found in the psychologically understandable short-lived and self-terminating nature of the former and the differences between them in mode of response to a variety of drugs (Goodwin et al 1975). Thus dextro-amphetamine is an effective antidote for everyday despondency but a very weak anti-depressant. In contrast the most powerful anti-depressants cause unpleasant side effects, such as tremor, perspiration and drowsiness in normal subjects without influencing grief and sadness.

3. THE RELATIONSHIP BETWEEN ENDOGENOUS AND NEUROTIC AFFECTIVE DISORDERS (FIG. 2)

The terms used in the heading are generally recognised as being unsatisfactory. 'Endogenous' depressions may be preceded by adverse life events and may arise in 'neurotic' rather than stable individuals while 'neurotic' depressions will at times evolve in well adapted persons exposed to onerous stresses. Such contradictions do not invalidate the total syndromes to which these terms refer. Nor have any wholly satisfactory alternatives to them been proposed.

The main problem at this level is whether a clear categorical distinction can be made between the different forms of endogenous affective illness on the one hand and all other forms of affective disorder on the other. There is little direct evidence bearing on this question for most enquiries have been ostensibly devoted to the relationship between 'psychotic' or 'endogenous' and 'neurotic' depressions. However, as subsequent sections of this paper will show the latter group will almost invariably include a number of distinct forms of neurotic illness unless anxiety, phobic and depersonalisation state and related neuroses have been explicitly excluded. But this step is not taken by most investigators, precedence being arbitrarily given in diagnosis to depressive features.

Some of the most impressive testimony favouring a clear line of demarcation at this level has been derived from data advanced in support of the unitarian view which holds that disorders of affect merge insensibly with one another.

Lewis's influential papers of 40 years' ago (Lewis 1934, 1936) are of particular interest in this connection because he judged affective psychosis, psychogenic depression and anxiety neurosis among other disorders of affect as inseparable diagnostically and considered that his findings upheld this unitarian concept. His material must therefore have been drawn from disorders of affect extending over the entire range of the classification depicted here. His case histories published as an appendix in one of the papers (Lewis 1936) were given in great detail thus enabling Kiloh and Garside (1977) to submit them to independent statistical tests with the aid of principle components and cluster analyses. Each method showed the patients to be separated by their scores on the relevant dimensions into two clearly distinct groups. The authors concluded that there must be at least two qualitatively different affective illnesses. The results were therefore consistent with the separation proposed at this level into those patients with endogenous disorders on the one hand and those with a neurotic illness whether predominantly depressed or anxious on the other.

It should be noted that two of Lewis's cases were considered to be schizophrenic at follow up and Kiloh judged seven others to merit this diagnosis. Their inclusion in Kiloh and Garside's analysis did not affect the results. Lewis's study of 1936 is therefore consistent with other evidence suggesting that the common borderland with the schizophrenic disorders, represented below in the four main levels in Figure 1, cannot be omitted from any scheme for the classification of disorders of affect.

In a recent study also relevant for this level of decision making (Post 1972, Kendell and Post 1973), the distribution of patients' symptom scores on the Newcastle diagnostic index was judged by the authors to substantiate the view that no clear lines of demarcation existed within the depressive disorders. But statistical analysis of this distribution showed it to be significantly non-normal and non-unimodal (Garside 1973, Roth and Garside 1973) both in patients under and patients over the age of 60 years. Moreover, the group of patients in the third mode of the distribution were characterised by Post as showing,(1972) poor sleep and appetite, loss of interest in outside matters and non-delusive preoccupations with unpleasant physical sensations, tension and anxiety.' They were also judged to exhibit "neither over depression nor depressive thought content." It seemed justifiable to conclude (Garside 1973) that these patients were likely to have suffered from anxiety states rather than depressive illnesses in a strict sense.

4. THE BIPOLAR AND UNIPOLAR DISORDERS (FIG. 3)

The diagnosis entailed in the broad differentiation between bipolar and unipolar disorders shown on the left half of level III of the scheme have been studied by many workers. But the criteria proposed by Perris (1974) and Angst (Angst and Perris 1972) for the diagnosis of 'definite' and 'probable' cases, both in the 'bipolar' and 'unipolar' groups have provided a reasonably clear guide for clinical practice and useful operational definitions for scientific purposes. In addition to heredity, age of onset, personality differences and course, certain biochemical and physiological differences are held to separate the bipolar from unipolar disorders (Perris 1974). In the view of Perris (1974) for a diagnosis of bipolar disorder both manic and depressive episodes are required, whereas for certain uipolar disorders at least 3 depressive episodes must have occurred with complete remission after each.

It is the unipolar disorders that have constituted the main source of diagnostic inconsistency and confusion. The fact that Perris's criterion of 3 successive attacks entails some 13% of misclassification (Angst 1974) is not the main source of this. Confusion has stemmed mainly from the wide-ranging connotation given to 'unipolar depressions'. Leonhard (1957) who introduced the bipolar-unipolar concept, as also Angst and Perris (1972) who have been influential in shaping its modern version, confined this dichotomy to the endogenous psychoses. Thus in defining the unipolar disorders Perris sets a relatively unequivocal demarcation line by insisting that depressive attacks must have been endogenous or of 'psychotic' severity to qualify for admission.

But this limitation has been ignored by many workers who have dismissed the terms 'psychotic' and 'endogenous' as imprecise and unscientific. Yet once these concepts have been jettisoned we are left with an indefinite phenomenological characterisation of the unipolar group. These cases are said to have higher anxiety scores, more agitation and more somatic complaints than bipolar cases. But such features are commonplace throughout the far more numerous population of patients to be found on the other side of the central dividing line, namely the depressive and anxiety neuroses.

Now the bipolar cases constitute a small group amounting to less than 10% of the total number of affective disorders reported in most series. Hence when Leonhard's restriction is ignored and differentiation between unipolar and bipolar groups made prior to all other diagnostic judgments, the unipolar concept is at risk of being applied to the majority of patients within the family of affective disorders that remains, so subsuming psychotic and neurotic cases, anxious and retarded depressions and probably also agoraphobic and other neuroses that may exhibit a strong colouring of depression. It has in other words evolved into a portmanteau concept largely defined by prior elimination of a small minority of bipolar cases rather than definitive phenomenological criteria of its own. In such a situation investigators are bound to find it difficult to achieve consistent results.

5. 'ENDOGENOUS' AND 'NEUROTIC' DEPRESSION (FIG. 3)

It will be clear from the foregoing discussion of Level II that the long-standing debate between 'unitarians' and 'pluralists' regarding the classification of depression, and the evidence that bears upon it, are also relevant for the division at Level III between the two groups of psychoses on the left and the depressive neuroses on the right. The long history of this controversy over more than half a century has been reviewed by several authors (Partridge 1949, Kiloh and Garside 1963, Kendell 1968, Klerman 1971) and comments here about the present situation have to be confined to a few points.

Mendels and Cochrane (1971) reviewing seven factor analytic studies (Hamilton and White 1959, Kiloh and Garside 1963, Carney, Roth and Garside 1965, Hordern 1965, Rosenthal and Klerman 1966, Rosenthal and Gudeman 1967, Mendels and Cochrane 1968) concluded that there was a "sufficient concensus" to support the independence of endogenous and neurotic group disorders. Further a number of enquiries have yielded distributions (derived from principle components and discriminant function analysis) in which clear separation between the neurotic and endogenous groups was achieved. (Carney et al 1965, Fahy et al 1969, Garside et al 1971). The fact that unimodal distributions have been reported in other enquiries (Paykel 1971) does not necessarily conflict with the 'pluralistic' view particularly as the data published by those who have supported a psychotic-neurotic continuum have in some instances been shown to be incompatible with such an interpretation of their own findings.

It is therefore a clinical profile with a number of features drawn from the familiar cluster of endogenous features that must set a limit to the unipolar concept. They include unvarying mood disturbance of rapid onset, vital disturbances such as late insomnia, diurnal variation, weight loss, a qualitatively distinct feel in mood and somatic malaise, self critical or reproachful beliefs, ideas of hopelessness and the less common delusions of poverty, nihilism and deserved rejection or persecution.

Some diagnostic decisions within the limited area of overlap are simplified by the fact that a cluster of indubitable 'psychotic' or endogenous features has to be given precedence in diagnosis over associated non specific neurotic features according to a hierarchical principle inherent in the Kraepelinian system of classification. Endogenous depressions prove to have a more favourable outcome and respond better than the neurotic group to most known forms of pharmacological and physical anti-depressive treatment, (Kiloh et al 1962, Carney et al 1965.) As the former are usually more severely depressed this result defies interpretation unless qualitative differences are assumed to exist between the groups.

6. <u>THE RELATIONSHIP OF DEPRESSIVE AND ANXIETY STATES</u> (FIG. 3)

That the affects of anxiety and depression are correlated in some manner with one another has been stressed by biologists all the way from Darwin through Freud to Seligman (1975).

Rating scales for anxiety and depression have been found in numerous studies to exhibit a correlation co-efficient of about 0.5 thus explaining approximately 25 per cent of the common variance. But it is precisely for this reason that the extent of the association between the syndromes in which these affects are predominant has to be investigated by multivariate techniques.

There is some indubitable association between certain anxiety and depressive symptoms. However, anxiety syndromes may be differentiated with reasonable sharpness from those designated as depressive.

The evidence came from four main sources :

(i) Phenomenological analysis in 145 patients has shown that although certain clinical features were common to the two groups the clinical profiles of depressive disorders and anxiety states proved to differ significantly in several respects (Roth et al 1972). With the aid of principal components and discriminant function analyses it was possible to achieve clear separation with relatively little overlap between patient groups with anxiety and phobic states on the one hand and those with depressive illnesses on the other (Gurney et al 1972). The findings were confirmed by an independent cluster analysis of the items which succeeded in assigning about 82% of patients in each category into an appropriate cluster.

    In an investigation by Mountjoy and Roth (Submitted for publication) in which seven rating scales were used in addition to clinical examination an anxiety depression component was extracted. The loadings of the seven measures showed the two types of scale which showed some overlap in their items separated in factor space with some measure of overlap. However the distribution of scores on this component was significantly non-unimodal showing that there were two relatively distinct populations corresponding to the groups of patients who had scored high on anxiety and depressive scales respectively. The same result was obtained in respect of clinical ratings. An enquiry into the relationship between anxiety and depressive states by Prusoff and Klerman (1977) led the authors to the same conclusion.

(ii) As there is a measure of inevitable circularity in phenomenological investigations, validation of these results was attempted by a number of techniques. The most important of these comprised independent follow up studies undertaken over a 45 month period (Kerr et al 1972, 1974, Schapira et al 1972). They showed that depressed patients enjoyed a significantly better prognosis than those with anxiety neurosis.

(iii) There was little cross over in pattern of illness displayed in the course of relapses during the follow up period. Those with anxiety and depressive syndromes tended to exhibit disorders closely similar to those recorded at the time of the initial examination.

(iv) The clinical indices which best predicted outcome in the anxiety states proved to be a different set from those which yielded the best forecast in depression, with relatively little overlap (Schapira et al 1972, Kerr et al 1974), a finding difficult to reconcile with distinct forms of illness that merge insensibly with one another.

It is worthy of note that it is not wholly independent and uncorrelated syndromes that have emerged from this study but negatively correlated ones with some measure of overlap. This point is lent emphasis by the fact that in investigations of patient populations ostensibly suffering from depressive disorders alone, multi-variate analysis has repeatedly brought to light a cluster of anxiety features and of patients in whom such features were prominent (Hordern et al 1965). But in many clinical trials the correlations of these features with treatment response are of opposite sign to that exhibited by typical depressive features.

7. ENDOGENOUS, BIPOLAR AND UNIPOLAR DEPRESSIONS AND NEUROTIC DEPRESSIONS (Figs 1, 4 & 5)

There is relatively little formal evidence from clinical and statistical analysis regarding the sharpness or otherwise of the separation between the different syndromes in each of the groups at level IV. The subdivisions shown are therefore derived to some extent from clinical description. In a few instances they are validated by differences in treatment response and attention will be drawn to any such evidence.

Bipolar Endogenous Depression (Fig. 4)

At this level the bipolar endogenous states are sub divided into four groups. The first on the extreme left manifests both as manic and depressive illness within a relatively short time of the first attack, but endogenous depression is the commonest mode of manifestation. Psychomotor behaviour is more often retarded than agitated; retardation has emerged from many studies with high positive loading on factors and dimensions which differentiate endogenous from other forms of depression. The next group comprises recurrent mania now recognised by most workers as having a familial and genetical kinship with bipolar rather than unipolar cases. A careful history elicits short periods of depression, retardation or diminished drive, prior to the onset of elation in a proportion of cases. The third category refers to patients who exhibit both manic and depressive features in the same attack or have 'mixed' psychoses in the old sense of the term. In the fourth group the mood change may be atypical or inconspicuous, the picture being dominated by irritable, aggressive, overbearing and litigious behaviour together with paranoid delusions of a persecutory kind which may assume bizarre forms such as being spied upon by special apparatus and sometimes symptoms indistinguishable from passivity feelings. Auditory hallucinations are rare and the premorbid setting is distinctive in that the premorbid personality has often been energetic, outgoing, assertive, and well adapted. As Wing (1975) has pointed out solitary Schneiderian features do not warrant a diagnosis of schizophrenia. Yet the blend of affective and schizophrenic-like features makes diagnosis difficult. For this reason the group is represented both as 'paranoid (pseudo schizophrenic) mania' with the bipolar disorders and as atypical manic or 'mixed' psychosis within the schizophreniform group.

Unipolar Endogenous Depression Fig. 5

Agitation is often described as typical of unipolar depression (Angst and Perris 1972, Perris 1974) but it is not specific and retardation may predominate. The first two groups refer to these syndromes. The third group comprises cases of depression with brief sub-clinical upswings of mood after recovery. The status of these cases is uncertain. But where elevation of mood proves self-limiting and not severe enough to require treatment, classification with the unipolar group seems appropriate for the present.

A distinction has been recently drawn by Winokur et al (1971) within the unipolar group between 'pure depressive disease' and 'depressive spectrum disease'. The former commences in middle age mainly in men and there is a family history of depression in both male and female first degree relatives. In 'depressive spectrum disease' the patients are predominantly female. The illness is of relatively early onset, with a family history of alcoholism in male and depression in female relatives. These interesting findings await confirmation.

Depressive Neuroses (Fig 6)

The depressive neuroses at level 4 have been divided into the four distinct sub groups shown because they emerge with impressive consistency from the multivariate analyses of the features of depressed patients undertaken by different workers. Thus a syndrome denoted as 'hostile depression'has been independently identified by Overall et al (1966) Paykel (1971) and Kiloh et al (1972). It appears similar to the hysteroid dysphoria of Klein and Davis (1969) the angry depressives of Grinker et al, the 'self-pitying constellation' of Rosenthal and Gudeman (1967) and the chronic characterologic syndrome' of Schildkraut (1970). It is noteworthy also that almost half a century ago Gillespie (1929) had sub divided reactive depressions into 'psychoneurotic depressions' and 'depressions in constitutional psychopaths.' But the task of defining the syndromes in this group more precisely poses difficult problems.

8. ANXIETY STATES FIG. 8

The anxiety neuroses at level 4 may be divided into (1) simple anxiety states which are predominantly somatic or psychic but often exhibit a blend of both kinds of symptomatology. (2) Agoraphobic and social phobic neuroses. (3) Phobic states with prominent depersonalisation. (4) Anxiety states with isolated specific phobias.

In the first mentioned and commonest group hypochondriacal preoccupations of a shifting kind are relatively common. But special mention is merited by a group of patients often with conspicuous premorbid obsessional traits in whom fears of disease constitue a leading feature. These recurrent fearful preoccupations with disease have been described as 'illness phobias' in the classification of Marks (1970). But whereas the phobic patients experience a fear-laden aversion for some specific situation or object usually with insight these patients fluctuate between doubt and delusions in the belief that they suffer cardiac, venereal, malignant or other life threatening disease. Severe exacerbations of emotional disturbance carry a serious suicidal risk in such patients.

Agoraphobic and social phobic neuroses exhibit some differences including sex incidence (Marks 1970) but as there is much overlap in clinical features they are shown together. In both groups,patients are subject to panic attacks of crippling severity which may limit their movements so as to render them housebound or severely restrict their social activities and relationships.

These groups are not sharply delimited from phobic states with prominent depersonalisation. Depersonalisation and associated phenomena are found in varying severity at different stages of anxiety neuroses and this group refers to those cases in which such symptoms are prominent and persistent. In rare instances the conjunction of anxiety and depersonalisation alters abruptly to become a chronic depersonalisation syndrome. The individual loses capacity for affective response, experiences subjective blunting and distortion of perception and complains of being an empty automaton observing himself as a spectator in an empty and lifeless world. But there are surges of panic in special situations.

Recent investigations have confirmed the specific nature of the association between depersonalisation symptoms and anxiety (Roth 1959, Noyes and Klettie 1977). The former has, for example, been demonstrated in transient form in a high proportion of normal subjects exposed to life threatening danger and among psychiatric patients in times of crisis and imminent panic. Depersonalisation emerges as an adaptive mechanism that combines opposed tendencies; one serving to heighten alertness and the other to dampen emotions that could disorganise behaviour (Roth 1959, Roth and Harper 1962, Noyes and Klettie 1977). Animal and other specific phobias and other isolated phobic symptoms are of limited clinical importance and unlike the other neuroses in this group, can rarely be regarded as true disorders of affect.

9. SCHIZOPHRENIFORM AND SCHIZOAFFECTIVE DISORDERS FIG. 1

Below the four numbered levels a lower level is shown comprising the schizophreniform and related psychoses. The interupted lines drawn between this lower level and level 3 are intended to indicate that the kinship with affective illness is not exclusive; this group would also have to be brought into consideration in any account of the classification of schizophrenic illness. But there is evidence to bring certain groups of cases tentatively into association with the forms of affective disorder on which the interupted lines terminate at level 3. This is summarised here because it opens up clear lines of enquiry into a large group of disorders which is clearly heterogeneous and delineated by a bewildering variety of names such as 'schizoaffective', 'psychogenic', 'schizophreniform', 'cycloid', 'oneiroid' and 'mixed' psychoses and in the French literature as 'bouffee delirante'. If some clarity and order could be imported into the area a number of problems of classification of schizophrenia, affective psychosis and neurosis would be brought closer to resolution.

There are two groups of cases in which evidence is available from observations on premorbid status, antecedent and subsequent pattern of illness, precipitating factors, response to treatment, hereditary factors or all of these - for some relationship with affective disorder. The first of these groups appears to have a kinship with anxiety neuroses and markedly anxious phobic cases in particular.

In our early clinical studies (Roth 1959, 1960) we drew attention to a small minority of agoraphobic patients in whom acute, benign and short-lived schizophreniform illness developed in stepwise fashion following the impact of a new and severely stressful circumstance. Prior to the 'key' events such patients had been anxious, over-sensitive, self-conscious, lacking in self-esteem and handicapped to varying degrees by phobias. The picture returned, after recovery, to the previous pattern of neurotic illness.

In a later Newcastle comparative study of schizophreniform disorders (McClelland et al 1966) it was noteworthy that these patients did not differ from cases of 'nuclear' schizophrenia in terms of 'Schneiderian' symptoms. Precipitating factors, abrupt onset, hysterical symptoms, depersonalisation and a depressive colouring were the features of discriminating value. Anxiety and phobic features commonly figured in the premorbid picture. The link with anxiety neuroses is further substantiated by McCabe's study of psychogenic paranoid psychoses. In his recent monograph (McCabe 1975) 3 of 17 such cases had seemingly suffered from an anxiety neurosis and in the first degree relatives of three other cases a similar diagnosis had been applied. An earlier report from the same department (Welner and Stromgren 1958) showed first degree relatives of schizophreniform patients to have a low prevalence of schizophrenia and manic depressive psychosis while affective and neurotic disorders were common. The 'Emotion' psychoses described by Swiss authors (Rohr 1961, Labhardt 1963) appear to belong to the same groups of schizophreniform disorders in that nuclear schizoprhenic features are common, but illness follows overwehelming psychological stress, the picture is coloured by anxiety, terror, depression and hysterical features together with severe autonomic disturbance. Recovery tends to be swift and complete.

In the second group several lines of evidence favour some kinship with bipolar endogenous disorders. The description of 'cycloid psychosis' by Leonhard (1957) refers to patients with a blend of schizophrenic and affective symptoms who have a tendency to complete the remission between attacks which tend to recur. The low prevalence of precipitating factors (Perris 1974) is in striking contrast with the first group and suggests an endogenous state. The genetic affinities are the subject of controversy (Clayton et al 1968, Perris 1974), some workers favouring the existence of a third group of atypical psychoses. But an affinity of a proportion of cases with bipolar disorders is suggested by (a) the cyclical course (b) the phenomenology of the illness which commonly includes prominent endogenous depressive clinical features (c) a tentative claim by Perris (1974) among others, that lithium significantly reduces the chance of recurrence. That more inconsistent findings that have been reported by other investigators (Schou 1974) is perhaps understandable in view of the heterogeneity of 'atypical' psychosis.

Atypical (pseudo-schizophrenic) mania already referred to above should be classed with this second group. It may be mentioned that auditory hallucinations are uncommon and that the appropriate diagnosis may be futher suggested by the frequently delayed or disappointed response to phenothiazines, even in acute florid forms of this psychosis.

The form in which the disorder presents in this and other syndromes may over long periods of observation shift from schizophreniform to typical affective disorder or vice versa. The direction of the terminal arrows on the interrupted connecting lines in Figure 1 is intended to indicate this.

10. THE RELATIONSHIP BETWEEN CLASSIFICATION AND TREATMENT

Although a classification cannot in our view be created out of predictive indices alone importance has always been attached in medicine to the validation of diagnostic distinctions by the demonstration of parallel differences in course, outcome and response to treatment. The present classification proves to show a promising measure of association with the pattern of treatment response in affective disorders. Commencing on the left of level 4 endogenous depressives have been shown to respond better than neurotic depressives to tricyclic anti-depressant drugs (Kiloh et al 1962; Greenblatt et al 1964) electrical convulsive therapy (Carney et al 1965; Astrup et al 1959) and also to achieve remissions that are more stable and of better quality than neurotic depressions (Kay et al 1970, Paykel et al 1974). Depressives with delusional and other psychotic features very rarely respond to drugs but electrical convulsive therapy is effective.

During attacks of illness, treatment with lithium is effective, both in mania and in a proportion of bipolar cases with a mixture of depressive and manic features. As far as prophylaxis is concerned the efficacy of lithium in bipolar cases is well established. From a recent comprehensive review of prophylaxis Davis (1976) concludes that they are equally effective in unipolar cases. But it remains to be determined whether the effect extends beyond unipolar, endogenous and psychotic states so as to include neurotic depressions and other disorders of affect.

A number of recent investigations have shown tricyclic compounds to be effective prophylactic agents in neurotic as well as endogenous depression (Paykel et al 1975, Mindham et al 1973) as also in unipolar depression (Prien et al 1973). But there is no conflict with the older observation that the results of endogenous cases are superior. There is therefore a gradation in the effects of this form of treatment as one moves from left to right on Level IV. Moreover, prominent anxiety appears to be one conspicuous defining characteristic of depressions that exhibit an adverse response to tricyclic compounds. Thus in the recent studies of Paykel et al (1972, 1976) psychotic depressives showed the most marked improvement while 'anxious depressives' though only a little less severely ill benefited far less than other neurotic depressions and exhibited the most severe residual symptoms of all groups. In fact both in relation to ECT and tricyclic compounds marked anxiety seems to have a prognostic significance of opposite sign to that of severe retardation (Hollister et al 1966, 1967, Kiloh et al 1962, Carney et al 1965, Gurney et al 1970, Kerr et al 1972).

Hence when we reach the depressive neuroses the response to tricyclic compounds becomes uncertain. This group also marks a point of transition in an opposite sense. For much of the existing evidence suggests that all the bipolar and other depressive illnesses shown at level 3 and those deriving from them at level 4 fail to respond to monoamine oxidase inhibitors. Thus the MRC clinical trial of 1965 as also Kay et al (1970) found this group of substance of no value in depressive illness. However, evidence from three independent clinical trials with phenelzine (Tyrer et al 1973, Robinson et al 1973, Mountjoy and Roth (i) 1975, (ii) In Press 1977) suggests a signicant effect in the mitigation of such symptoms as anxiety, hypochondriasis, phobia, fatigue and other somatic complaints. In a recent report of a controlled therapeutic trial (Zitrin et al 1977) describes a favourable response by agoraphobic patients to Imipramine but the effects appear to have been confined to panic attacks.

It needs to be stressed that all the disorders described in this classification manifest depressive symptoms in some stages of the disorder or over its entire duration. The whole range of conditions requires to be investigated with the aid of comparative studies making use of biochemical and physiological measures as well as further therapeutic trials.

As far as neurochemical studies are concerned it has recently been claimed (Asberg et al 1974, 1976 a & b, 1977) that endogenously depressed patients have significantly lower levels of the serotonin metabolite 5 hydroxyindoleacetic acid (5-HIAA) than normal volunteers. The distribution of metabolite levels in this group was shown to be bimodal and patients with low CSF 5-HIAA were found to be more prone to commit suicide than other patients. In the studies of Asberg and her colleagues the level of 3-methoxy-4 hydroxyphenylglycol (MHPG) in the CSF did not differ in endogenous depressions from the levels in normal subjects. However, according to some workers (Beckman and Goodwin 1975) urinary MHPG is lower in bipolar than in unipolar patients and within the latter lower levels are associated with favourable response to Imipramine while high levels of excretion are claimed to correlate with a good response to Amitryptline (Schildkraut 1973). These marked inconsistencies to be found in the published observations regarding biochemical correlates and their predictive value may stem in part from differences in the composition of the relevant patient populations. Such inconsistencies will be likely to become less common when a wider measure of agreement than obtains at present has been reached regarding the classification of the entire group of affective disorders.

Angst, J. (1966) Zur Atiologie und Nosologie endogener depressiver Psychosen. Berlin, Springer Verlag.

Angst, J., Perris, C. (1972) The Nosology of Endogenous Depression: Comparison of the Results of Two Studies. Int. J. Ment. Health Vol. 2, pp. 145-148.

Asberg, M., Thoren, P., Traskman, L., Bertilsson, L., Ringberger, V.-A. (1976) "Serotonin depression" - a biochemical subgroup within the affective disorders. Science 191: 478.

Asberg, M., Traijksman, L., Thoren, P.,(1976) S-HIAA in the cerebrospinal fluid. Arch. Gen. Psychiatry 33: 1193-1197

Asberg, M., Ringberger, V.-A., Sjoqvist, F., Thoren, P., Traskman, L., Tuck, J. R., (1977) Monoamine metabolites in cerebrospinal fluid and serotonin uptake inhibition during treatment with chlorimipramine. Clin.Pharmacol. Ther. 21: 201.

Asberg, M. (1978) Biological Research in Depression and Mania: The Case for Involvement of Serotonin. Paper read at 11th CINP Congress. July 9-14 Vienna.

Astrup. C., Fossum, A., Holmboe, R. (1959) A follow-up study of 270 patients with acute affective psychosis. Acta psychiat. scand. 35 (Suppl.): 1-65.

Beckmann, H., Goodwin, F. K. (1975) Antidepressant response to tricyclics and urinary MHPG in unipolar patients. Arch. Gen. Psychiatry 32: 17-21

Carney, M.W.P., Roth, M., Garside, R.F. (1965) The diagnosis of depressive syndromes and the prediction of ECT response. Brit. J. Psychiat. 111. 659-674.

Clayton, P., Rodin, L., Winokur, G. (1968) Family History Studies; III Schizoaffective Disorder. Clinical and Genetic Factors Including a one to two year follow-up. Comprehens. Psychiat. 9, 31-49.

Davis, J. M. (1976) Overview: Maintenance therapy in psychiatry. II Affective disorders. Amer. J. Psych. 133, 1-13.

Fahy, J. T., Brandon, S., Garside, R. F. (1969) Clinical syndromes in a sample of depressed patients: a general practice material. Proc. R. Soc. Med. 62. 331-335.

Garside, R. F., Kay, D. W. K, Wilson, I. C., Deaton, I. D., Roth, M. (1971) Depressive Syndromes and the Classification of Patients. Psych. Med. 1. 333-338.

Garside, R. F. (1973) Depressive Illness in Late Life (Correspond) Brit. J. Psych. 12. 118-119.

Gillespie, R. D. (1929) The Clinical Differentiation of types of Depression Guy's Hospital Report 2, 306-344.

Goodwin, F. K., Post, R. M., Sack, R. (1975) Clinical evidence for neurochemical adaptation to psychotropic drugs. Neurobiological mechanisms of adaptation and behaviour. Editor A. J. Mendell. Raven Press, New York.

Greenblatt, M., Grosser, S. H., Webster, H. (1964) Differential response of hospitalised depressed patients to somatic therapy. Amer. J. Psychiat.120, 935.

Gurney, C., Roth, M., Garside, R. F., Kerr, T. A., Schapira, K. (1972) Studies in the classification of affective disorders. II. The relationship between anxiety states and depressive illness. Brit. J. Psychiat. 121. 162-166.

Hamilton, M., White, J. M. (1959) Clinical syndromes in depressive states. J. of Ment. Sci. 105, 985-998.

Harper and Roth (1962) Temporal lobe epilepsy and the phobic anxiety depersonalisation syndrome. Part 1: A comparative study. Comprehensive Psychiatry, 3. 129-151. Part II: Practical and theoretical considerations. Comprehensive Psychiatry, 3. 215-226.

Hollister, L. E., Overall, J. E., Pennington, V. (1966) Nosology of depression and differential response to drugs JAMA 195, 946-948.

Hollister, L. E., Overall, J. E., Shelton J. (1967) Amitryptiline, perphenazine, and amitryptiline-perphenazine combination in different depressive syndromes. Arch. Gen. Psychiat. 17: 486-493.

Kay, D. W. K., Fahy, T., Garside, R. F. (1970) A seven month double-blind trial of amitriptyline and diazepam in ECT treated depressed patients. Brit. J. Psychiat. 117, 667-671.

Kendell, R. E. (1968) The Classification of Depressive Illness. Inst. of Psychiat. Maudsley Monograph No. 18 O.U.P. London.

Kendell, R. E., Post, F. (1973) Depressive Illness in Late Life (correspondence) Brit. J. Psychiat. 122, 615-617.

Kerr, T. A., Roth, M., Schapira, K., Gurney, C. (1972) The assessment of prediction of outcome in affective disorders. Brit. J. Psychiat. 121, 167-174.

Kerr, T. A., Roth, M., Schapira, K., (1974) Prediction of Outcome of Anxiety States and Depressive Illness. Brit. J. Psych. 124. 125-133.

Kiloh, L. G., Ball, J. R. B., Garside, R. F. (1962) Prognostic factors in the treatment of depressive states with imipramine. Brit. Med. J. 1. 1225-1227.

Kiloh, L. G., Garside, R. F. (1963) The independence of Neurotic Depression and Endogenous Depression. Brit. J. Psych. 109, 451-463.

Kiloh, L. G., Andrews, G., Neilson, M., Bianchi, G. N. (1972) The Relationship of the Syndromes called Endogenous and Neurotic Depressions. Brit. J. Psychiat. 121. 183-196.

Klerman, G. L. (1971) Clinical research in depression. Arch. Gen. Psychiat. 24. 305-319.

Klein, D., Davis, J. (1969) Diagnosis and Drug Treatment of Psychiatric Disorders. Baltimore, Williams and Wilkins Co. 180-185.

Lewis, A. J. (1934) Melancholia: A Clinical Survey of Depressive States. J. Psych. 109. 451-463.

Lewis, A. J. (1936) Melancholia: Prognostic studies and case-material. Journal of Mental Science 82, 488-550.

MacCabe, M. S. (1975) Reactive Psychoses. A clinical and genetic investigation. Acta Psychiat. Scand. Supplementum 259. Munksgaard.

McClelland, D. H., Roth, M., Neubauer, H., Garside, R. F. (1966) An analysis of psychiatric, physical, personality and social characteristics in 195 patients with 'schizophrenic' symptoms. A study in classification. Proc. Fourth World Congr. of Psychiat. Madrid Sept 1966. Excerpta Medica Internat. Congress Series, No. 117 ed JJ Lopez Ibor, London Excerpta Medica Foundation.

Mendels, J., Cochrane, C. (1968) The Nosology of Depression: the endogenous-reactive concept. Amer. J. Psychiat. 124. Suppl. 1 - 11.

Mindham, R. H. S., Howland, C., Shepherd, M. (1973) An evaluation of continuation therapy with tricyclic antidepressants in depressive illness. Pyschol. Med. 3. 5-17.

Mountjoy, C. Q., Roth, M., Garside, R. F., Leitch, I. M. (1977) A clinical trial of phenelzine in anxiety depressive and phobic neuroses. Brit. J. Psychiat. 131, 486-492.

Overall, J. E., Hollister, L. E., Johnson, M. (1966) Nosology of depression and differential response to drugs. JAMA 195: 946-950.

Partridge, M. (1949) Some reflections on the nature of affective disorders arising from the results of prefrontal leucotomy. J. Ment. Sci. 95. 795.

Paykel, E. S. (1971) Classification of Depressed Patients: A cluster analysis derived grouping. Brit. Psych. 118. 275-288.

Paykel, E. S. (1972) Depressive typologies and response to amitriptyline. Brit. J. Psychiat. 120. 147-156.

Paykel, E. S., Klerman, G. L., Prusoff, B. A. (1974) Prognosis of depression and endogenous-neurotic distinction. Psychol. Med. 4. 57-64.

Paykel, E. S., Damascio, A., Haskell, D., Prusoff, B. A. (1975) Effects on maintenance amitriptyline psychotherapy on symptoms of depression. Psychol. Med. 5. 67-77.

Perris, C., (1973) The heuristic value of a distinction between bipolar and unipolar affective disorders. Classification and Prediction of OUtcome of Depression. (Angst. J. ed.) F. K. Schattauer Verlag, Stuttgard and New York.

Perris, C. (1974) A Study of Cycloid Psychoses. Acta Psychiat. Scand. Supplementum, 253. Munksgward, Copenhagen.

Post, F. (1972) The Management and Nature of Depressive Illness in Late Life: A Follow-through Study. Brit. J. Psychiat. 121. 393-404.

Robinson, D., Nies, A., Ravaris, L. (1973) The monoamine oxidase inhibitor phenelzine in the treatment of depressive-anxiety states; a controlled clinical trial. Arch. Gen. Psychiat. 29. 407-413.

Rosenthal, S. H., Klerman, G. L. (1966) Content and Consistency in the Endogenous Depressive Pattern. Brit. J. Psychiat. 112. 471-484.

Rosenthal, S. H., Gudeman, J. E. (1967) The Endogenous Depressive Pattern; an empirical investigation. Arch. Gen. Psychiat. 16. 241-249.

Roth, M. (1959) The phobic anxiety-depersonalization syndrome.. Proc. Roy. Soc. Med. 52. 587-596.

Roth, M. (1960) The phobic anxiety-depersonalisation syndrome and some general aetiological problems in psychiatry. J. Neuropsychiat. 1. 293-306.

Roth, M., Harper, M. (1962) Temporal lobe epilepsy and the phobic anxiety-depersonalization syndrome. Comp. Psychiat. 3. 215-226.

Schapira, K., Roth, M., Kerr, T., Gurney, C. (1972) The prognosis of affective disorders. The differentiation of anxiety states from Depressive Illness. Brit. J. Psych. 121. 175-181.

Schildkraut, J.J. (1973) Norepinephrine metabolites as biochemical criteria for classifying depressive disorders and predicting responses to treatment. Preliminary findings. Am. J. Psychiat. 130. 695-699.

Winokur, G., Clayton, P. (1967) Family History Studies I. Two Types of Affective Disorders separated according to genetic and clinical factors. Recent advances in biological psychiatry, 9, 35-50.

Winokur, G., Cadoret, R., Dorzab, J. (1971) Depressive Disease. A genetic study. Arch. Gen. Psychiat. 24. 135-144.

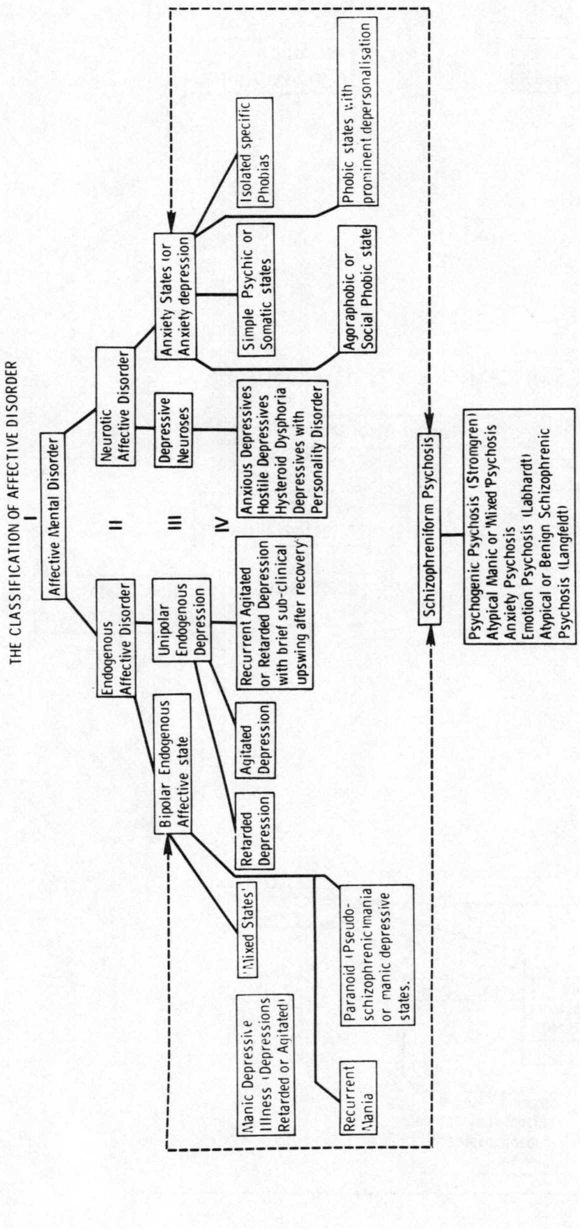

The classification of affective disorder.
Conomitant systemic medical disease,
Endocrine disturbance, Alcoholism or
other addictional dependence, evidence
of CNS lesion need to be specified
separately in each disorder, Rationale
for the procedure is discussed in Roth (1976)

Fig. 1.

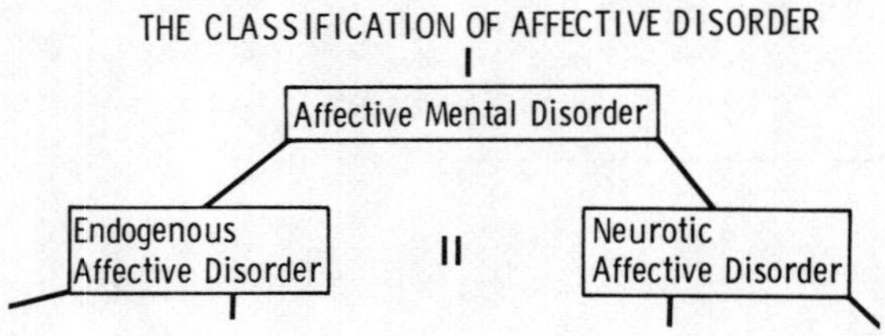

Fig. 2.

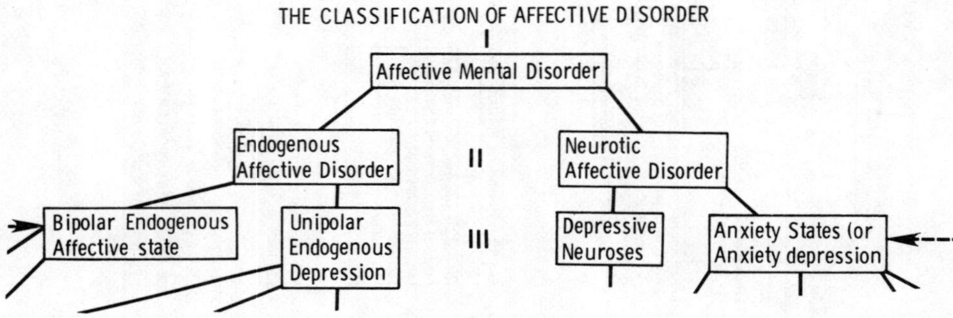

Fig. 3.

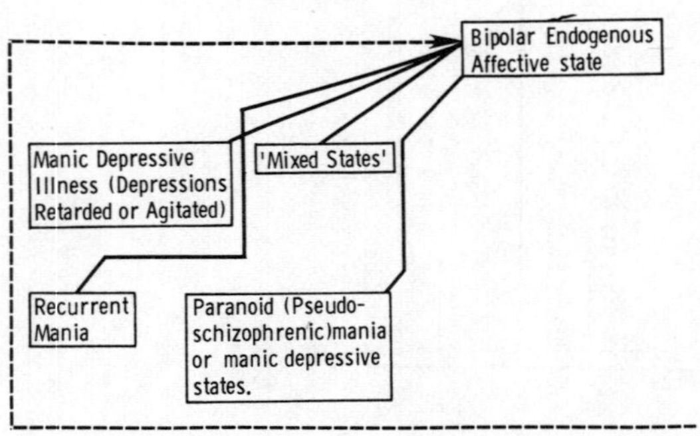

Fig. 4

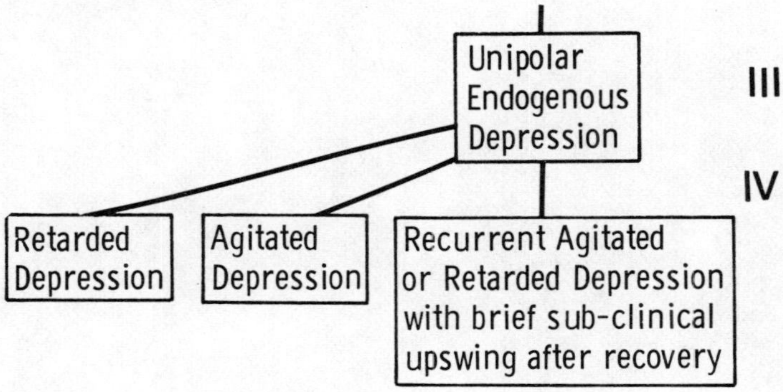

Fig. 5.

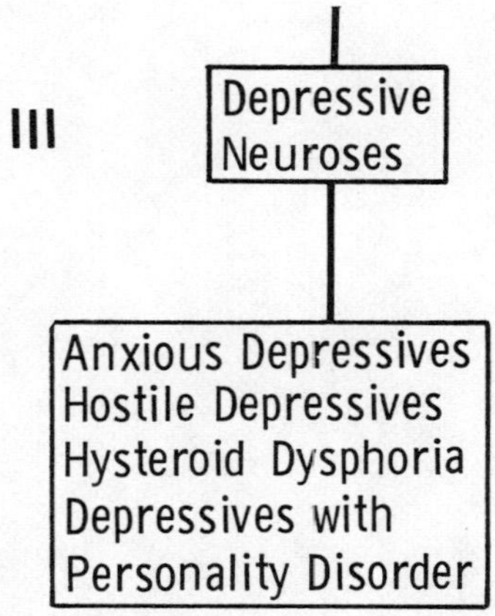

Fig. 6.

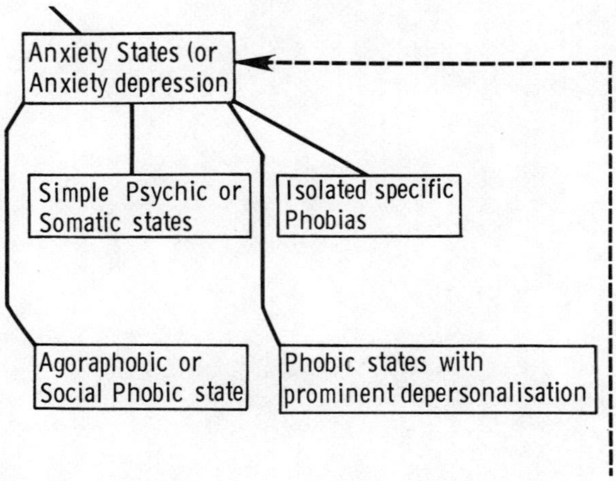

Fig. 7.

Endocrinological and Biochemical Peripheral Markers as an Index of Central Neurochemical Modifications

General Survey of the Possible Correlations Between Psychiatric Disorders and Biological Modifications

E. ZARIFIAN* **and H. LOO*

*Service Hospitalo-Universitaire de Santé Mentale et de Thérapeutique
(Pr. P. Deniker), Hôpital Ste-Anne, Paris, France
**Synthélabo-LERS, Department of Clinical Research, 58, rue de la Glacière,
75013 Paris, France

ABSTRACT

Psychiatry is a branch of medicine where symptoms have no objective evidence and where no demonstrations of organicity have ever been prooved. It is why, for a long time, attempts have been made to correlate psychiatric symptoms with specific biological modifications. The situation of the brain inside the skull allows only peripheral investigations. Different types of biological approaches to psychiatry are critically reviewed and a new way of thinking is proposed. It seems that no consistent correlation is possible between a diagnosis and a biological modification because a diagnosis is a notion too much complex and heterogeneous. On the opposite correlations between basic symptoms and biological modifications are maybe possible and could possibly be more fruitful. Examples are given where psychotropic drugs are used as pharmacological tools in such a perspective.

INTRODUCTION

For a very long time biological alterations have been suspected in various types of psychiatric disorders. This does not mean that biological modifications can explain by themselves or summarize all the factors involved in the origin of psychiatric troubles. But we have good reasons to think that in certain types of abnormal behaviours,social, environmental and psychological factors are not enough to explain the symptomatology. Furthermore the dramatic improvements produced by psychotropic drugs are a good argument in favor of biological modifications in mood swing and schizophrenia.

However, the CNS is localized in regions which are not easily accessible. The brain is out of direct approach, its cells are so highly specialized that they cannot divide and biopsy raises an ethical aspect. Furthermore the brain is totally separated from the periphery by the blood brain barrier which is a selective and active filter between the CNS and the blood stream. It is why, at the present time, the only way to appreciate possible biological modifications in the CNS is limited to dosages in blood, urine and CSF. Many attempts have been made to find a peripheral model able to mimic the central modifications or to give a more or less direct reflection of what happens inside the brain.

Unfortunately most of the substances coming from the CNS into the blood are also produced at the peripheral level and the difference between their origins is sometimes impossible to make. But nevertheless, and in spite of these difficulties, some incontestable correlations have been established between the main psychotic troubles and certain biological modifications. It is important to emphasize that in many cases psychotropic drugs used as pharmacological tools have been of great interest in clarifying these biological changes. We have biochemical and pharmacological arguments to show that psychotic disorders, whatever they are, affective troubles or schizophrenic manifestations, are paralleled with biological modifications. Changes of the symptomatology under drugs interfering with monoamine metabolism and variations of neurotransmitters metabolites are in favor of this hypothesis.

However, it is very difficult to say at the present time if biological modifications are a cause or a consequence of psychiatric disorders. Many biological investigations have been made in psychiatry and various human fluids have been explored (Joseph,1976). We can try to give very schematically a general picture of these investigations. In the CSF different metabolites of the monoamines can be measured GABA and other substances can also be evaluated. But we are aware that it is difficult to say what percentage of these compounds really comes from the CNS (Ebstein,1976; Enna,1977; Goodwin,1975; Gottfries,1976; Griswold,1969; Zohar,1978) Precursors and metabolites of neurotransmitters may also be measured in plasma. But, as it was mentionned for the CSF, only a small percentage of these metabolites comes from the CNS.

Blood platelets which can be easily collected are able to store 5 HT, catecholamines and MAO (Berrettini,1977; Stahl,1977) with certain restrictions they can be considered as a model of a central neuron. The relationship between brain hormones and amine metabolism becomes more clear (Casper,1977) and various psychotropic drugs can modify the secretion of hypothalamic substances. It is why the dosage of various hormones is widely developped and the radio immuno-assay method is used routinely (Ettigi,1977; Meltzer,199; Rotrosen,1976). Different enzymes play a role in the metabolism of brain amines. It was consistent to appreciate their modifications. That is possible in the plasma or in the blood cells (Stefanis,1977). But post mortem studies are also of great interest (Farley,1978; McGeer,1977, Wilk,1978). Unfortunately there are only a small number of studies devoted to brain enzymes and there are many possibilities for error with this type of technique. Some peptides are the latest substances which have been measured in the CSF. The promising development of endorphins is at the origin of new speculations in psychiatry (Kline,1977; Lindström,1978; Meyer,1978).

But biological investigations are not limited to dosages in various human fluids or tissues. Neurophysiological measures have also been developed (De Bonis,1978; Fenton,1978; Holzman,1977; Saletu,1977) Recently, studies using computerized EEG have been published concerning the hemispheric cerebral lateralization in schizophrenia and this field seems to be developing very fast.

We can add also to neurophysiological studies the exploration of the motor activity from an enzymatic, histological and physiological point of view (Crayton,1977; Meltzer,1977) This schematic landscape of biological investigations in psychiatry shows the wide field of possible dosages or measurements. Thousands of papers are published every year on this topic and the interest for biological psychiatry is increasing everywhere. But, finally what can we say if we try to summarize the results from a practical point of view ? The following speakers are going to review in details the main aspects of the biological modifications and our aim is only to present some general considerations.

No specific biological modification has been found in any case. The diagnosis in psychiatry is still based only on clinical considerations even if, sometimes, consistent biological changes were observed. In fact, even in these cases there is no consensus among the authors and some discordant or opposite results have been reported. Furthermore, when the clinical picture has a mirror image, like depressive and manic states it is not possible to demonstrate biological changes which are mutually contradictory.

How can we interpret these rather pessimistic considerations ? Schematically there are three possibilities. The first one is the failure of our diagnosis to represent an homogeneous clinical picture (Cowdry,1977). This is a very important point and we will see it later. The second is that neurotransmitters would not play a role in psychotic disorders. We have strong arguments, coming from the efficacy of drugs modifying amines metabolism to think that this hypothesis is wrong. The precursors of monoamines when given under certain conditions can modify the symptomatology of depression or schizophrenia. Furthermore, neuroleptics and antidepressants whether they are or not MAOI or tricyclics are know as modifying agents of amine transmission. But it would be naïve to think that the modifications of one neurotransmitter or even of two of them can be correlated with an abnormal behavior. And it is maybe because we have tried too often to make a direct relationship between one biological parameter and a complex behaviour that we are so often deceived. The third possibility is the failure of our techniques for assessing neurotransmitter changes. But, with the standardization of the methods of dosages the comparison of the results is now valid.

In fact, the variations of biological data are conditioned by many factors and the role of the pathology is only one of them. When comparing biological results we do not take enough into consideration the numerous factor linked to each subject and able to induce physiological variations, like diet, stress or motor activity. Very often also the control groups are not very well defined and for ethical reasons are made of neurological patients. Al these bias can lead to errors in the appreciation of the results.

But the main difficulty when trying to make correlations between clinical symptomatology and biological modifications is linked to the ambiguity of what is a diagnosis in psychiatry. The comparisons between patients or between different publications are based upon the similarity of the diagnosis and the homogeneity of the symptomatology. Unfortunately in psychiatry the same words do not signify always the same realities. Many factors can play a role in the poor reliability of a diagnosis and the use of rating scales is unable to minimize the consequences of this imprecision. Furthermore, it is possible that some diseases, which are different from a biological point of view have the same unique clinical expression. So, it is maybe exaggerated to speak of <u>the</u> schizophrenia or <u>the</u> depression when it would be better to use the plural.

We must add also that a diagnosis is a complex and heterogeneous entity made of objective symptoms, but also made of the deep-seated conviction of the psychiatrist that the thoughts of his patient are wrong. In consequence of this subjective participation in the diagnosis it is probably illusory to make correlations between psychiatric diagnosis and biological modifications. On the other hand it would be maybe more realistic and more modest to focus our attention on basic behaviours or on symptoms, above all when these symptoms have a mirror image in the different clinical aspects of the same disease. Motor activity, for instance, can be modified without specificity in different diseases. The regulation of motor activity is easier to understand and to study than the psychiatric disease where motor activity is modified.

Furthermore psychotropic drugs are symptomatic drugs and they have the same efficacy on the same symptoms whatever might be the disease. Psychotropic drugs can be used as pharmacological tools in so far as we begin to know their mechanisms of action. It is interesting to see that, if we consider the two opposite aspects of the same disease, the same type of drugs improve or worsen the same type of symptoms. These symptoms belonging to different diseases, but modified in the same way by the same drugs must share something together. It is also interesting to see that psychotropic drugs, in certain conditions, can swing symptoms to their opposite aspects. In these conditions we could try to evaluate if these clinical opposite changes are paralleled with biological opposite changes.

In summary we think that the analysis of a symptom in its biological basis would be easier than the analysis of a diagnosis and that the study of a basic behaviour like the modifications of the motor activity or the mood changes could be a better guideline for biological investigations. It is in this way that Deniker says that psychotropic drugs can be used as analyzers of the symptomatology. The improvment in biological investigations can also be made on certain points like the standardization of the techniques of dosages, the use of more specific psychotropic drugs or the spreading of biochemical post-mortem studies made in good technical conditions. But it is not enough and we need new approaches of the brain functions.

A reasonable hope is raised with the possibility of labelling precursors of neurotransmitters or psychotropic drugs with C_{11}. This isotope has a very short half life and its use is safe in humans. With this technique the mapping and the kinetic studies of psychotropic drugs in the brain are possible in vivo. Furthermore, the study of various receptors could be possible using tracer doses of pharmacological tools. Finally, even if we have to be very critical towards the present results of biological investigations in psychiatry we can consider that biological psychiatry which is at its very beginning is a new science very promising.

REFERENCES

Berretteni,W.H.W.H.Vogel,and R.Clouse (1977).Platelet monoamine oxidase in chronic schizophrenia. Am.J.Psychiatry,134:7,805-806.

Casper,R.C.,J.M.Davis,G.N.Pandey,D.L.Garver,and H.Dekirmenjian (1977). Neuroendocrine and amine studies in affective illness.Psychoneuroendocrinology,2,105-113.

Cowdry,R.W.,and F.K.Goodwin (1977).Amine neurotransmitter studies and psychiatric illness : toward more meaningful diagnostic concepts. In R.Spitzer (Ed.) Current issues in Psychiatric diagnosis. Raven Press,New-York.

Crayton,J.W.,H.Y.Meltzer,and D.J.Goode (1977).Motoneuron excitability in psychiatric patients. Biological Psychiatry,12:4,545-561.

De Bonis,M.,and E.Freixa I Baque (1978). Diphasic electrodermal response,heart rate and moods. Biological Psychology,6,77-91.

Ebstein,R.P.,J.Biederman,R.Rimon,J.Zohar,andR.H.Belmaker (1976).Cyclic GMP in the CSF of patients with schizophrenia before and after neuroleptic treatment. Psychopharmacology,51,71-74

Enna,S.J. (1977).γ-aminobutyric acid (GABA) in human cerebrospinal fluid : radioreceptor assay.Journal of Neurochemistry,28,1121-1124.

Ettigi,P.G.,and G.M.Brown (1977).Psychoneuroendocrinology of affective disorder : an overview. Am.J.Psychiatry,134,493-501.

Farley,I.J.,K.S.Price,E.McCullough,J.H.N.Deck,W.Hordynski,and O.Hornykiewicz (1978) Norepinephrine in chronic paranoïd schizophrenia : above normal levels in limbic forebrain.Science,200,456-457.

Fenton,G.W.,P.B.C.Fenwick,W.Ferguson,and C.T.Lam (1978).The contingent negative variation in antisocial behaviour : a pilot study of broadmoor patients. Brit.J. Psychiatry, 132,368-377.

Goodwin,F.K.,M.H.Webster,and R.M.Post (1975).Cerebrospinal fluid amine metabolites in affective illness and schizophrenia : Clinical and pharmacological studies Presented at the Intra-Science Research Foundation Symposium " New Vistas in the Biochemistry of Mental Disorders " Santa Monica,California.

Gottfries,C.G.,L.Von Knorring,and C.Perris (1976).Neurophysiological measures related to levels of 5-hydroxy-indoleacetic acid,homovanillic acid and tryptophan in cerebrospinal fluid of psychiatric patients.Neuropsychobiology 2,1-8.

Griswold,R.L.,N.Pace,and B.W.Grunbaum (1969).Metabolic concomitants of schizophrenia.Comprehensive Psychiatry,10:1,1-5.

Holzman,P.S.,E.Kringlen,D.L.Levy,L.R.Proctor,S.J.Haberman,andN.J.Yasillo (1977). Abnormal pursuit eye movements in schizophrenia.Arch.Gen.Psychiatry,34,802-805.

Joseph,M.H.,H.F.Baker,E.C.Johnstone,and T.J.Crow (1976). Determination of 3-methoxy-4-hydroxyphenylglycol conjugates in urine. Application to the study of central noradrenaline metabolism in unmedicated chronic schizophrenic patients Psychopharmacology,51,47-51.

Kline,N.S.,C.Haoli,H.E.Lehmann,A.Lajtha,E.Laski,and T.Cooper (1977). β-endorphin-induced changes in schizophrenic and depressed patients. Arch.Gen.Psychiatry. 34,1111-1113.

Lindström,L.H.,E.Widerlöv,L.M.Gunne,A.Wahlström,and L.Terenius.(1978) Endorphins in human cerebrospinal fluid : clinical correlations to some psychotic states Acta Psychiat.Scand.,57,153-164.

McGeer,P.L.,and E.G. McGeer (1977).Possible changes in striatal and limbic cholinergic systems in schizophrenia. Arch.Gen.Psychiatry,34,1319-1322.

Meltzer,H.Y.,S.Piyakalmala,P.Schyve,and V.S.Fang (1977).Lack of effect of tricyclic antidepressants on serum prolactin levels. Psychopharmacology,51,185-187.

Meltzer,H.Y.(1976). Neuromuscular dysfunction in schizophrenia. Schizophrenia Bulletin,2:1,106-135.

Meyer,R.E.,J.J.Schildkraut,S.M.Mirin,P.J.Orsulak,M.Randall,M.McDougle,P.A.Platz,E. Grab,and T.Babor (1978).Opiates, catecholamines,behaviour and mood.Psychopharmacology,56,327-333

Rotrosen,J.,B.M.Angrist,S.Gershon,E.J.Sachar,andF.S.Halpern(1976).Dopamine receptor alteration in schizophrenia : neuroendocrine evidence. Psychopharmacology 51,1-7.

Saletu,B. (1977). The evoked potential in pharmacopsychiatry. Neuropsychobiology, 3,75-104.

Stahl,S.M. (1977). The human platelet.A diagnostic and research tool for the study of biogenic amines in psychiatric and neurologic disorders. Arch.Gen.Psychiatry,34,509-516.

Stefanis,C.N.,E.Likouras,E.Garelis,and E.Varsou (1977). Cyclic AMP in the plasma of chronic schizophrenics, before and after treatment.Prof.Neuro-psychopharmac.,1,323-327.

Wilk,S.,and M.Stanley (1978).Dopamine metabolites in human brain. Psychopharmacology,57,77-81.

Zohar,J.,Biederman,R.Rimon,R.Ebstein,and R.H.Belmaker (1978). Clinical correlates of CSF cyclic nucleotides in schizophrenia. Am.J.Psychiatry,135:2,253-255.

Blood Platelets as a Model for Brain Neurones: Relevance to Psychiatric Disorders and Mental Abnormalities

D. J. BOULLIN

M.R.C. Unit and University Department of Clinical Pharmacology, Radcliffe Infirmary, Oxford, England

ABSTRACT

Platelets are a model for functional activity of central serotoninergic neurones. The model analogy also applies to catecholamines in respect of platelet receptors. Many studies have been made of platelet uptake, storage and metabolism (MAO activity) in psychiatric disorders, but studies have rarely been replicated by other investigators. Only reduced platelet 5-HT in DS has been successfully confirmed. There are now other avenues of platelet function and biochemistry to be explored. Platelet shape change and aggregation may be equated with synaptic events in central neurones. Neuroleptic drugs with activity on 5-HT systems affect platelets, but no studies have been made in psychiatric disorders.

INTRODUCTION

Much experimental evidence indicates that the blood platelet is a model for central monoaminergic function[Δ] (Pletscher, 1978; Paasonen, 1965). However the analogy is only partial. This paper will review most aspects of the platelet model and describe the way it has been used in the past as a guideline to central neuronal function. The text will conclude with an account of aspects of the platelet which have received little or no attention from scientists concerned with the aetiology of psychiatric disorders and mental abnormalities, and will signpost likely directions for future work.

[Δ] To reduce the number of references in this paper, most citations are reviews where further original references can be found.

[ΔΔ] Abbreviations used in this paper:
5-hydroxytryptamine (5-HT); noradrenaline (NA); dopamine (DA); adenosine diphosphate (ADP); chlorpromazine (CPZ); fluphenazine (FPZ); disodium edetate (EDTA); monoamine oxidase (MAO); catechol-ò-methyl transferase (COMT); platelet rich plasma (PRP); Brief Psychiatric Rating Scale (BPRS); 5-methoxy-tryptamine (5-MT); 5,6,dihydroxytryptamine (5-6-DHT); 2-(1-piperazinyl) quinoline maleate, quipazine (QPZ); γ-aminobutyric acid (GABA); 5-hydroxyindolyl acetic acid (5-HIAA); 5-hydroxytryptophol (5-HTOL); thioxidiazine (THR); lysergic acid diethylamide (LSD); Down's Syndrome (DS); 4-hydroxyquinoline (4-OHQ); tryptamine (TRY); octopamine (OCT); m-iodobenzylamine (m-ib); benzylamine (BENZ); tyramine (TYR).

TABLE 1 Aspects of Platelet Function Related to Psychiatric Disorders and Mental Abnormalities Involving Serotonin

Parameter	Neurone/Platelet Comparisons
Storage (endogenous concentration)	Comparable (except chromogranin absent from platelets)
Uptake	Comparable. Uptake inhibitory drugs have comparable potencies
Release and metabolism	5-HT efflux and catabolism <u>versus</u> platelet MAO activity in disrupted platelets
Turnover	Neuronal turnover fast. Platelet 5-HT may also turnover
Physiological function	Trans-synaptic neuronal activity <u>versus</u> platelet aggregation and shape change
Drug-receptor interactions	Ligand binding to receptors Not known whether comparable

Table 1 shows various aspects of platelet physiology which have counterparts in central monoaminergic neurones. The evidence for similarities between platelets and neuronal function particularly applies to 5-HT (serotonin)[ΔΔ]. Human platelets contain only 5-HT of the monoamines but NA and DA are taken up by active transport and DA can be highly concentrated. From the viewpoint of assessing the relevance of platelet uptake mechanisms to neuronal mechanisms in psychiatric disorders, tricyclic antidepressants and other neuroleptic drugs influence both platelet and neuronal uptake and platelet aggregation (Boullin and colleagues, 1978a and b).

Although NA and DA are normally absent from platelets, monoamine receptors are present for 5-HT and for catecholamines. The latter are α-receptors and have been characterised by ligand binding studies and by conventional drug-receptor interactions by inhibiting the physiological responses of platelets to monoamines (platelet aggregation, see below) (Drummond, 1976; Boullin and colleagues, 1977; Boullin, Molyneux and Roach, 1978; Alexander, Cooper and Handin, 1978).

It is unlikely that all platelet receptors have been characterised. Apart from monoamines, platelets actively transport a variety of aminoacids which are putative neurotransmitters including GABA, glycine and taurine (Boullin and Green, 1972).

Investigation of relationships between neuronal and platelet receptors in psychiatric disorders should be a fruitful field for research, particularly now methods for characterising receptors by ligand binding studies are developing.

PLATELET RECEPTORS

Receptors mediate functional activity. The platelet equivalents of transmitter release at the neuronal synaptic junction (i.e. trans-synaptic activity, see below, 5-HT RELEASE) are platelet aggregation and the more rarely studied platelet shape change. There have been few investigations of platelet aggregation in psychiatric disorders, but one study with 5-HT aggregation will be outlined here. It is known that 5-HT aggregation is altered in migraine (Lance, 1978), iron-deficiency anaemia (Woods and colleagues, 1977) and in diabetes (Simpson, Hockaday and Boullin, 1975). Possibly changes in platelet responses to 5-HT may reflect alterations in receptors in central serotoninergic neurones, but this is purely speculative.

In order to consider the platelet model in full, platelet physiology has to be compared to the synthesis, storage, release actions of central monoamine transmitters in neurones and catabolism. It must be emphasised that apart from uptake mechanisms and receptor studies where the platelet may be a model for all monoamines (5-HT, DA and NA), in other aspects the model analogy applies only to 5-HT.

5-HT SYNTHESIS

Platelets do not synthesise any neurotransmitter. Early data suggesting 5-HT synthesis have not been replicated in recent years (Lingjaerde, 1977).

5-HT STORAGE

Platelet and neuronal 5-HT storage mechanisms show close similarities. In both structures 5-HT is stored in complex with ATP in electron-dense organelles. The best evidence for the platelet neuronal model analogy comes from work with Down's syndrome (trisomy 21, mongolism).

In 11 separate investigations carried out over more than a decade an average of 49% reduction in platelet 5-HT was reported (Boullin, 1978).

Furthermore in a recent study brain monoamines were reduced in brain regions in 3 DS children compared to 3 controls of comparable ages, as shown in Table 2. This appears to be the only instance where platelet data have been consistently replicated and related to comparable changes in the brain. However it is interesting that the changes in brain monoamines were not confined to 5-HT. Indeed the depletion of NA and DA in all brain regions but the cortex were greater than for 5-HT. The catecholamine changes could not be compared with endogenous platelet catecholamine concentrations because human platelets do not contain endogenous NA or DA.

TABLE 2 Changes in Brain Monoamines in Down's Syndrome

Region	6-HT	NA	DA
Cortex	0	*	+371.4
Caudate and putamen	-36.3	-60.0	- 89.4
Hypothalamus	-26.7	-68.4	- 28.6
Brain stem	-42.3	-52.6	- 33.3

*NA not detectable (<10 ng/g)

Data obtained from brains of 3 DS children (aged 1, 3 and 5) and 3 normal children (2, 3 and 5). Further details including actual monoamine values (ng/g) given in Boullin (1978).

The aetiology of the generalised reduction in neuronal monoamines was not studied; in DS platelets the reduction appears to be due to a combination of factors: enhanced 5-HT efflux plus a reduction in the platelet ATP pool involved in 5-HT storage (Boullin and O'Brien, 1971a). There are no data on catecholamine uptake in DS, but in infantile autism there were no changes in platelet NA and 5-HT uptake (Boullin and O'Brien, 1971b).

In spite of the difficulties involved, more estimations of brain monoamines should be made in mental abnormalities and patients dying of psychiatric disorders including schizophrenia. Measurements of platelet 5-HT and MAO activity are often made in chronic patients who eventually die. Post mortem brain measurements could be related to the earlier platelet data. This has recently been done in chronic alcoholics (Oreland, 1976). Some years ago there were numerous investigations of brain monoamines in suicides from various causes; also attempts were made to correlate platelet 5-HT and central monoamine turnover by measuring CSF metabolites (Pletscher, 1978; Lingjaerde, 1977; Lott, Murphy and Chase, 1972).

It is clear from Table 1 that there is a direct analogy between platelet and neuronal uptake and storage mechanisms for 5-HT. On the other hand, when we come to a comparison of neuronal and platelet mechanisms for monoamine release and catabolism the situation is extremely complicated.

5-HT RELEASE

Microiontophoretic and histochemical studies indicate that 5-HT is a neurotransmitter in central neuronal pathways but this topic cannot be reviewed here. Transmitter release is presumably in increments (i.e. quanta) and occurs hundreds of times/second. Serotoninergic neurones synapse with dopaminergic neurones and others containing acetylcholine or other neurotransmitters.

The events occurring at the central synapse may be collectively termed trans-synaptic activity. This consists of transmitter release, receptor binding, post-synaptic activation of other neurones plus inactivation of transmitter by catabolism and active uptake (presynaptic neuronal retrieval). The platelet equivalent of trans-synaptic activity is monoamine-induced platelet shape change and aggregation. Platelet aggregation has been extensively studied, but not in mental disorders; there is no information on platelet shape change although both parameters are easy to study. Most work has concentrated on the biochemical aspects of monoamine catabolism and this will be considered below.

TURNOVER

Neuronal 5-HT in animals has a high rate of replacement (turnover). The classical view is that platelets initially obtain 5-HT by uptake from intestinal enterochromaffin cells and thereafter retain it for their life span. However we have evidence that platelet 5-HT is exchangeable in animals. Platelet 5-HT in CPZ treated goats is dramatically reduced during drug treatment but the platelets partly refill with 5-HT. Depletion is maximal 0.5 hrs after CPZ but the cellular content increases considerably in the next 3.5 hrs, suggesting turnover (Fig. 1). If human platelet 5-HT does turnover, then this is an important resemblance between platelets and serotoninergic neurones and this should now be studied.

5-HT CATABOLISM - PLATELET MAO ACTIVITY

Both platelets and neurones contain MAO, which seems to exist in different forms, MAO-A and MAO-B. This distinction is based upon the different substrate specificities of partly purified enzyme preparations and the actions of specific inhibitors as shown.

MAO type	A	B
Preferential substrates	5-HT, NA and OCT	phenylethylamine BENZ TRY
Specific inhibitor	clorgyline	deprenil
Tissue displaying activity	? neurone	? platelet

DA and TYR are substrates for both enzymes.

Originally it was believed that the above tissue specificity for MAO-A and MAO-B was absolute (Woods and colleagues, 1977), but recent work with animals indicates that a clear distinction cannot be made (Youdim, 1977). In any event, platelet MAO has been studied in a wide variety of psychiatric disorders, with confusing and inconclusive results.

Pletscher (1978) refers to the 13 studies on platelet MAO in schizophrenia and manic-depressive illness since the original observations of 1972 showing reduced MAO activity which were reviewed in 1974 (Murphy, Belmaker and Wyatt, 1974). Pletscher mentioned the possibility that there are in fact differences in schizophrenics but only in a small proportion of the population.

Although no conclusion can be drawn, some assessment of the significance of 5-HT release by platelets is essential. My view is that the study of platelet MAO in disrupted platelets is of only biochemical interest and can throw no light whatsoever on physiological release mechanisms. The extent of the problem can be gauged from Table 3. This gives values for platelet MAO activities found by various investigators in control and schizophrenic adults and infantile autistic children in the period 1972-1976 together with our data on catabolism of 5-HT loaded platelets (last data in Table 3; "endogenous content").

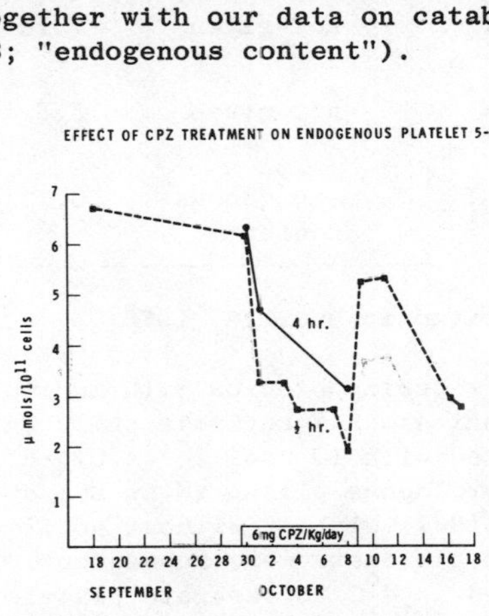

Fig. 1. Effect of CPZ treatment on endogenous goat platelet 5-HT. Platelet 5-HT was measured by spectrophotometry. CPZ was given i.v. daily as indicated. Blood was collected 0.5 and 4 hrs after injection, PRP prepared and platelet 5-HT measured. Note the change in platelet 5-HT values between 0.5 and 4 hours post-CPZ. This may indicate platelet 5-HT turnover (see text).

The values for both control and schizophrenic/infantile autistic groups overlap. This is the case even when the different substrates for MAO-A and MAO-B are utilised. Consequently data of this type are virtually worthless. Similar remarks could be made for other psychiatric disorders and there appears no point in studying platelet MAO activity further in psychiatric disorders unless there is *a priori* evidence for defects in brain MAO.

TABLE 3 Comparative MAO Activities in Controls and Mentally Abnormal Subjects

Author*	Substrate	Conc (nmol ml^{-1})	Metabolism (nmol^{-1}mg^{-1}h^{-1}) Controls	Mentally abnormal	
Benson and Southgate (1971)	4-OHQ	not given	7.48±0.53	1.62±0.08	DS
Wyatt and colleagues (1973)	TRY	200	6.4 ±2.7	3.9 ±2.3	
Meltzer and Stahl (1974)	TRY	1000	3.8 ±1.08	2.04±1.4	
	TRY	1000	4.65±1.29	2.06±0.91	S
	OCT	1000	3.81±1.29	2.22±1.03	
	m-ib	1000	4.92±2.08	1.57±0.62	
Nies and colleagues (1974)	TRY	800	3.6 ±0.4	2.6 ±0.2	S
	BENZ	800	22.1 ±2.8	19.1 ±1.9	S
Friedman and colleagues (1974)	TRY	29	1.91±0.17	1.58±0.19**	S
Shaskan and Becker (1975)	TRY	160	1.6 ±0.34	3.09±0.53	S
Boullin and colleagues (1975)	5-HT	200	6.34±0.72	5.84±0.66	A
	DA	200	7.62±0.28	9.0 ±0.88	A
	TRY	200	12.92±0.76	13.8 ±1.74	A
Carpenter and colleagues (1975)	TRY	not given	5.20±0.20	5.16±0.32	S
				4.94±0.29	CS
Domino and Khanna (1976)	TRY	not given	7.14±0.16	3.38±0.20	S
Schildkraut and colleagues (1976)	TRY	not given	5.8 ±0.4	6.0 ±0.4	S
Present work†	5-HT	endogenous content	0.11±0.02	0.017±0.002	DS

*These references are cited in Boullin, 1978
**Selected data
S = schizophrenic; SA = schizophrenics with auditory hallucinations;
CS = chronic schizophrenics; A = autistic children;
†Platelets were incubated with 10 µmol l^{-1}{^{14}C}5-HT for 90 min and then resuspended in fresh autologous plasma (N or DS) or in Ca^{2+}-free Krebs solution (see Boullin, 1967)* with or without addition of 4 µmol l^{-1} reserpine. Resuspended platelets were subsequently reincubated for 90 min and then centrifuged at 4°C to separate platelets from the incubation solution. 5-HT and 5-HIAA were identified in the efflux medium by paper chromatography (Boullin and O'Brien, 1973).

5-HT CATABOLISM - EFFLUX

Are there other ways of studying 5-HT efflux and catabolism from platelets? One possibility is to load platelets with exogenous 5-HT (commonly radiolabelled) and examine the output of 5-HT and metabolites when the platelets are separated from the original plasma and resuspended in fresh autologous plasma or other incubation media (see legend to Table 3). We devised this procedure some years ago and found enhanced 5-HT efflux in DS children's platelets loaded by incubation with 10^{-5}M 5-HT (see Boullin, 1978; Kamoun and Jerome, 1978). Kamoun and Jerome (1978) have shown that platelet 5-HT storage capacity can be measured by a similar method to ours using 10^{-3}M 5-HT. If 5-HT is separated from 5-HIAA and 5-HTOL then catabolism can be assessed.

Using our method we measured 5-HT efflux and catabolism in DS platelets and controls. The results are given in Table 4.

TABLE 4 5-HT Efflux and Catabolism

Platelet	Medium	% Lost	% Metabolised	nmols 5-HIAA formed*
N	Autologous plasma	1.8±0.1	4.9±0.4	1.94± 0.2
DS	Autologous plasma	12.4±1.1	7.5±0.9	7.8 ± 0.8
N	Saline	12.1±1.1	43.3±5.0	112.6 ±13.2
DS	Saline	13.2±1.4	15.0±1.4	16.6 ± 1.5
N	Saline +	44.4±2.7	10.6±1.0	101 ± 9.4
DS	reserpine	49.3±3.9	5.0±0.7	20.6 ± 2.9

*nmols formed/10^{11}platelets/hr after 2 hours incubation. For further information see Boullin (1978) and Boullin and O'Brien (1973). The platelets were loaded with 5-HT until they contained 2144 nmols (10^{11} cells (normal) or 839 nmols/10^{11} cells (DS) at equilibrium. The discrepancy between N and DS reflected the well-known inability of DS platelets to store 5-HT.

After initial separation from radiolabelled 5-HT and reincubation in fresh plasma only small amounts of 5-HT were lost from the normal platelets. Incubation in saline dramatically increased efflux and catabolism to about 45%. Subsequent addition of reserpine caused no further changes in efflux or catabolism.

In DS platelets efflux was 7 times greater than controls in plasma, but only a small percentage was metabolised. Incubation in saline did enhance release; but catabolism was only doubled. Finally the dramatic increase in efflux with reserpine did not enhance metabolism. We might conclude that DS platelets have defective MAO.

If we take these data, include them in Table 3 and compare them with the other data, it is clear that the rates of formation of 5-HT metabolites are only $\frac{1}{100}$ the rate seen in conventional MAO experiments. It may not be established which technique is most relevant to mental disorders but one is undoubtedly incorrect.

PHYSIOLOGICALLY INDUCED RELEASE

Here platelet physiology is equated with trans-synaptic neuronal activity.

Platelets undergo both shape change and aggregation in response to 5-HT. The methods of study were both devised by Born and a recent paper cites relevant references (Born and colleagues, 1978).

AGGREGATION

Aggregation is more commonly studied and consists of a reversible phase (I) and an irreversible phase (II). The latter undoubtedly involves 5-HT release and the release of other substances. The stimulus-secretion coupling seen in phase II has been equated with catecholamine secretion by the adrenal medulla (MacIntyre, 1976), but this seems wrong because of the irreversible nature of the phase II response. However phase I aggregation (Fig. 2) apparently also involves 5-HT release followed by reuptake (MacIntyre, 1976). This action is not readily repeatable but can be made to be repeatable in the presence of catecholamines (Ball, Boullin and Glenton, 1977).

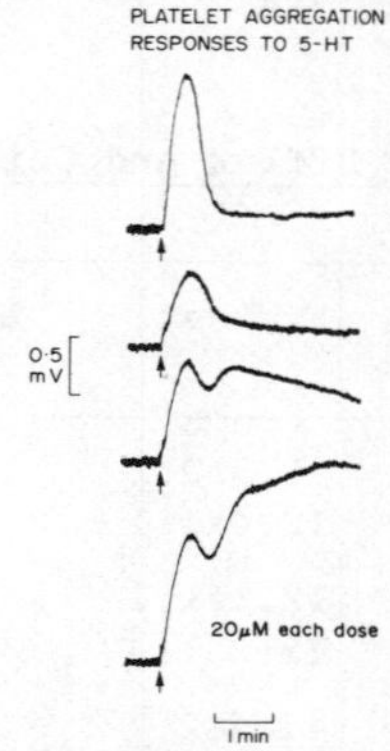

Fig. 2. Normal platelet responses to 5-HT in 4 different volunteers. Top 2 records show phase I responses; 3rd record from top shows phase I and beginnings of phase II; bottom record shows phase I and phase II. In large responses phase I and II may merge (see Figs. 3 and 10).

Changes in biogenic amines in the brain have been implicated in the aetiology of psychiatric disorders including schizophrenia for many years. Therefore it is of interest to know that platelet aggregation responses to 5-HT and DA are changed in schizophrenia (Boullin and Grimes, 1976; Boullin and colleagues, 1978a). The responses are converted from phase I to phase II as in other conditions including migraine and iron deficiency (see above).

We found that in both man and animals CPZ treatment was associated with enhancement of 5-HT aggregation. In CPZ treated schizophrenics responses changed from phase I (top record, Fig. 1) to phase I and II (bottom record, Fig. 2). In many instances phases I and II merged (Fig. 3). Interruption of CPZ therapy in chronic schizophrenics resulted in the disappearance of enhancement and the reappearance of a normal response; after reintroduction of CPZ, enhancement occurred again (Fig. 3).

TABLE 5 Platelet Aggregation Studies in Phenothiazine Treated Patients

Study No.	Date	Drug and Treatment Schedule	No. of Patients	% Incidence of Enhanced 5-HT Aggregation Responses	Psychiatric Assessment
1	1974/5	CPZ chronic	9	78	No
2	1975	FPZ chronic	18	56	Yes*
3	1976	CPZ acute	12	88	Yes
4	1976	CPZ chronic	34	74	Yes
5	1978	CPZ acute	14	7	No

* = Not with BPRS CPZ = Oral Chlorpromazine FPZ = Depot Fluphenazine

The question was considered as to whether there was any relationship between the improvement in clinical condition of the patients and effects on the platelet.

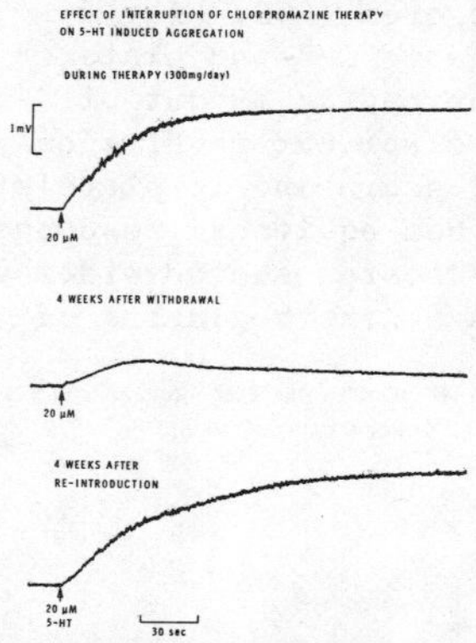

Fig. 3. Platelet aggregation responses in a CPZ treated schizophrenic during therapy (300 mg/day: upper record); 4 weeks after CPZ withdrawal; and 4 weeks after drug reintroduction.

In the period 1974-1978 5 studies were made of the 5-HT aggregation responses in CPZ treated schizophrenics. Aggregation was assessed by measurement of the area of the aggregation curve (total change in PRP optical density) and/or the initial rate of aggregation (V_{max}) and expressed in terms of the maximum response evoked by ADP (5-HT% of ADP). The psychiatric status of the patients in 3 studies (details in Table 2) was determined using the BPRS (full details are given in Boullin and colleagues (1978a and b) and Orr and Boullin (1976). None of the studies was double-blind and in Study 5 the incidence of enhanced aggregation responses was very low, no greater than normal (see Boullin and colleagues, 1978b and c).

Considering Studies 2-4, we found an inverse relationship between platelet aggregation responses and clinical condition. That is, in those patients in good clinical condition with a low score on the BPRS 5-HT aggregation was normal (viz Fig. 2, top record) whereas those with much symptomatology and a high BPRS score, aggregation was enhanced. This was perhaps the opposite to the expected result because one might suppose that drug therapy would be associated with "abnormal" (i.e. enhanced) responses.

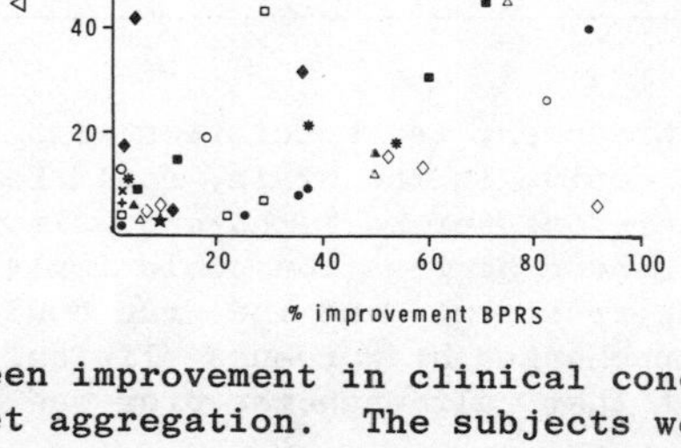

Fig. 4. Relationship between improvement in clinical condition (% improvement BPRS, abscissa) and platelet aggregation. The subjects were 12 acute patients in Study 3; each symbol type refers to a different subject.

Figure 4 shows that in the 12 patients of Study 3 who improved with CPZ therapy, there was a rather weak correlation between improvement in BPRS score and increase in platelet aggregation curve area (ΔOD; Fig. 4). In Study 4 there was also a weaker correlation between plasma CPZ and platelet aggregation (Fig. 5). Four weeks' interruption of CPZ therapy in 29 out of 34 of the chronically treated patients of Study 4 resulted in clear cut results only in patients that relapsed. There was an increase in BPRS score and in platelet aggregation. The majority of patients who did not relapse had equivocal responses (Boullin and colleagues, 1978a and b). Aggregation and BPRS scores showed wider variation; and 8/20 patients did not have enhanced aggregation at the beginning of the investigation.

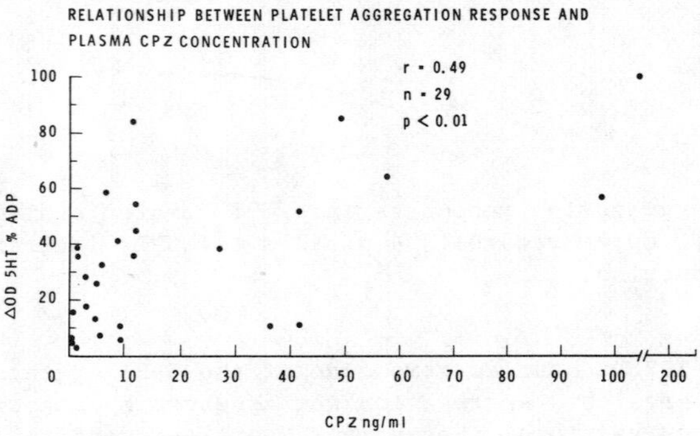

Fig. 5. Relationship between platelet aggregation and plasma CPZ concentration in 29 subjects from Study 4. Each point represents a single measurement in each subject.

On the basis of the clear-cut findings we made the following proposals for guidelines for monitoring and planning treatment (Table 6).

TABLE 6 Implications for Monitoring and Planning of Treatment

Patient	Aggregation	Clinical State	? Drug Acting	Suggest
A	Enhanced	Improved	Yes	Maintain drug
B	Normal	Improved	No	? Withdraw drug
C	Enhanced	Unchanged or worse	Yes	Change drug
D	Normal	Unchanged or worse	No	Increase dose ? Bioavailability

In patient A, clinical improvement in association with enhanced aggregation would suggest that the drug was active in the brain, could have contributed toward improvement and should therefore not be withdrawn. In patient B, clinical improvement in the absence of enhanced aggregation would imply that improvement was due to factors other than drug treatment, and the drug could therefore safely be withdrawn. In patient C, an unchanged or worsened clinical state in spite of enhanced aggregation, would suggest that, although the drug was active in the brain, the patient was not going to respond to it and an alternative treatment might be necessary (e.g. a different drug or E.C.T.). In patient D, an unchanged or worsened clinical state in the absence of enhanced aggregation would imply that the drug was not having the desired pharmacological effect in the brain, perhaps as a result of incorrect dosage or of problems associated with bioavailability, and that this might be corrected by increasing dosage or changing the route of administration.

These predictions were based on the results of the first 4 studies cited in Table 5 which suggested that enhanced 5-HT aggregation in platelets from patients receiving CPZ was a universal phenomenon with an overall incidence of about 56% or more compared to the 8-10% incidence in a normal population (Besterman and Gillett, 1973). However the results of Study 5 show that this is not the case. In the latest investigation 22 tests of 5-HT aggregation were made in the 14 subjects, and enhancement was observed in only 1 test. Plasma CPZ was measured in 8 of the patients and higher values were obtained (mean ± S.E.: 53.1 ± 14 ng/ml). These are comparable to earlier values (Boullin and colleagues, 1975).

Although only time will tell whether there is any value in this type of study and its associated predictions, it does at least represent a new approach to the use of the platelet model and the principles may be applied in other situations.

MECHANISM OF CHANGES IN AGGREGATION PRODUCED BY DRUGS

The changes in 5-HT aggregation described above were associated with therapy with some phenothiazines including CPZ, FPZ and THR but not prochlorperazine. An important point in view of the failure to replicate the results of Studies 1-4 in the latest investigation (Study 5) is that CPZ administration to goats enhances platelet aggregation (Fig. 6). The effect appears slowly after starting the drug and persists for many days after the drug is stopped (Fig. 7).

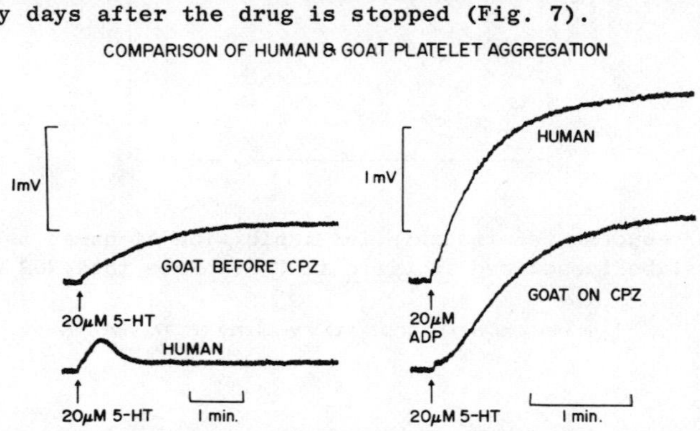

Fig. 6. Human and goat aggregation induced by 5-HT. Left figure shows human and goat aggregation before 5-HT. Right figure shows aggregation 5 days after 6 mg/kg/day CPZ i.v. compared to normal human ADP response. (Human 5-HT responses are shown in Figs. 2 and 3).

Another important point is that aggregation enhancement is almost certainly not a direct effect of CPZ or any of its commonly measured metabolites.

The reasons for this are as follows:

1. CPZ and metabolites added to human PRP produce dose dependent inhibition of 5-HT aggregation (Boullin and colleagues, 1975) (Fig. 8).

2. In goats enhancement of 5-HT aggregation is less at 0.5 hrs than 4 hrs after

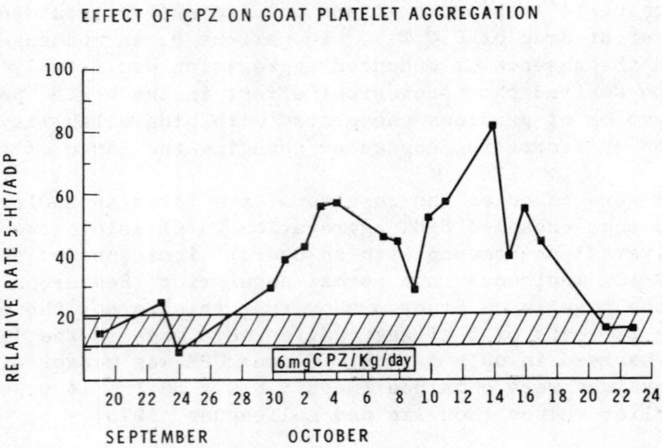

Fig. 7. 5-HT aggregation in a goat before, during and after CPZ (6 mg/kg/day). Hatched area represents mean ± S.E.M. of 5-HT aggregation prior to CPZ; responses of a single animal are shown.

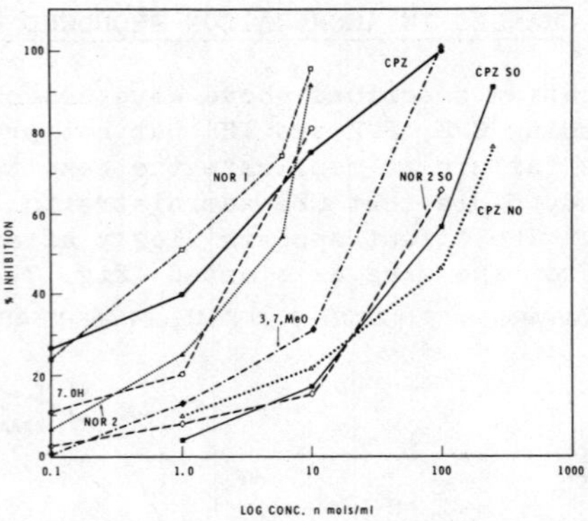

Fig. 8. Log dose/response relationship for inhibition of human 5-HT aggregation by CPZ and various metabolites added in vitro to PRP. Note that NOR CPZ is more potent than CPZ.

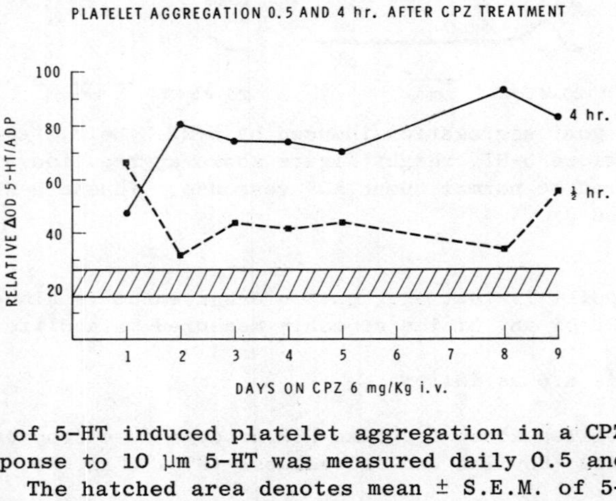

Fig. 9. Inhibition of 5-HT induced platelet aggregation in a CPZ treated goat. The aggregation response to 10 μm 5-HT was measured daily 0.5 and 4 hours after i.v. CPZ (6 mg/kg). The hatched area denotes mean ± S.E.M. of 5-HT aggregation prior to CPZ treatment. Responses were obtained in a single animal.

i.v. administration (Fig. 9) when plasma concentrations are highest. This demonstrates the direct inhibitory effect of CPZ in vivo.

The conclusion drawn is that CPZ inhibits 5-HT aggregation by a direct action but that enhancement occurs by some indirect mechanism, which may involve some primordial change in platelet properties. As the enhancing action is delayed 5 days the change may occur during megakaryocytosis. CPZ may also exert its effect on brain neurones by a similar indirect action. The reason for this is that when hyperactivity syndromes are induced in animals by administration of L-dopa or L-tryptophan plus a MAO inhibitor, CPZ produces inhibition of hyperactivity. On the other hand when CPZ is given for 6 days, stopped for 24 hours and then the hyperactivity challenge given, hyperactivity is enhanced (Heal and colleagues, 1976).

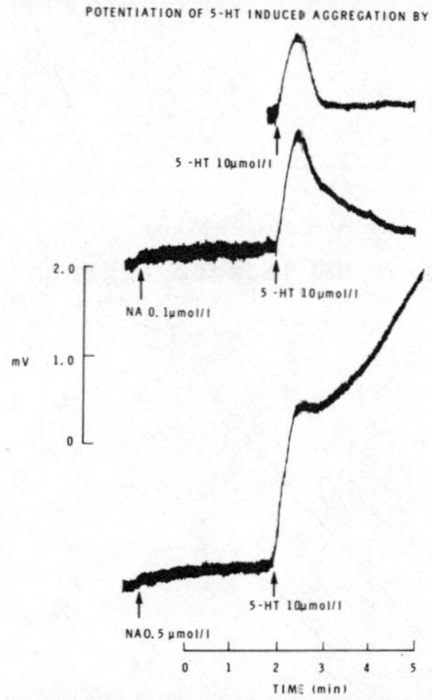

Fig. 10. Potentiation of normal human 5-HT aggregation by NA in vitro. Addition of NA converts a phase I 5-HT response to a phase I and phase II response (compare with Figs. 2 and 3).

Another possible explanation of the CPZ induced changes involves catecholamines. 10^{-8}M NA enhances 5-HT aggregation to convert phase I to phase II responses (Fig. 10). This is in the range of plasma NA concentrations found in stressed subjects (Benedict and Grahame-Smith, 1978) and CPZ treated schizophrenics may be stressed.

It is tempting to believe that neuroleptic drugs may have 2 actions, acute direct effects and chronic indirect actions involving cellular adaptation.

FUTURE AVENUES FOR PLATELET RESEARCH IN PSYCHIATRIC DISORDERS

Receptor Studies and Aggregation

Apart from 5-HT receptors, platelets possess α-adrenergic receptors (Boullin and Glenton, 1978) aggregating to catecholamines as well as 5-HT. This is seen most clearly by studying the inhibitory effects of neuroleptic and other drugs on 5-HT and NA aggregation.

Figure 11 shows that the α-receptor blocker phentolamine is the most potent inhibitor of NA aggregation, but Fig. 12 shows much more interesting results. The spectrum of blockade of 5-HT aggregation is very wide. The most interesting thing is that 1 drug is an even more potent inhibitor than methysergide and LSD; this is spiroperidol. The other butyrophenone haloperidol is 100 times less potent. One

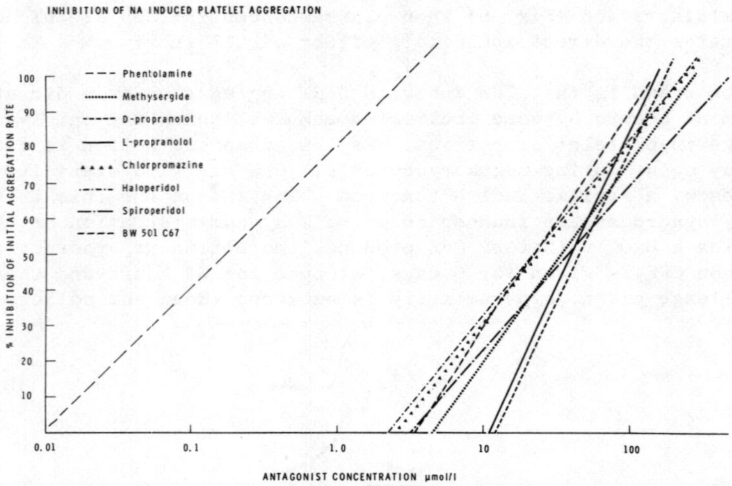

Fig. 11. Drug induced inhibition of NA induced aggregation using normal human PRP <u>in vitro</u>.

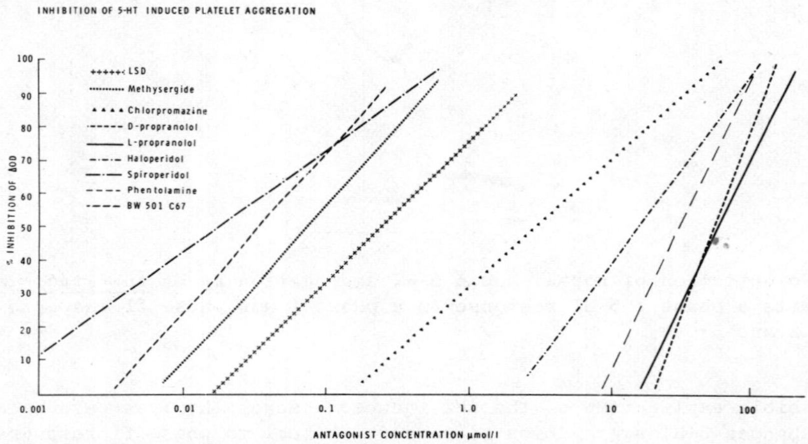

Fig. 12. Drug induced inhibition of 5-HT induced aggregation using normal human PRP <u>in vitro</u>.

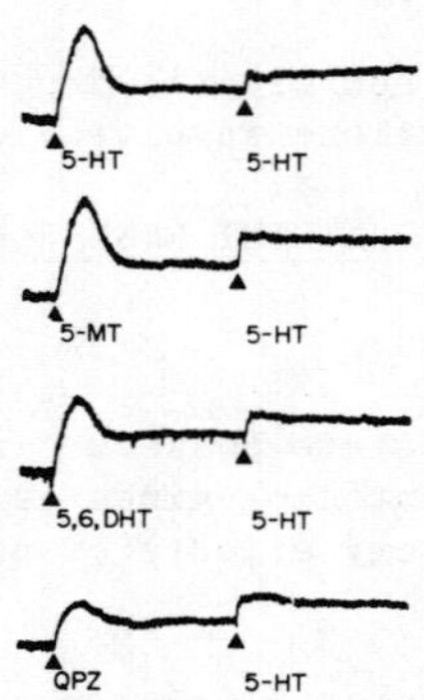

Fig. 13. Normal human platelet aggregation induced by 5-HT and drugs having central 5-HT-like actions. Note that only the first of two drug additions produces aggregation; this is evidence for stimulation of 5-HT receptors (see text).

wonders whether this extreme specificity on platelets is reflected in brain neurones; does spiroperidol in contrast to haloperidol have potent central actions on 5-HT related to therapeutic effects?

The final point is that some drugs are not antagonists of platelet 5-HT effects but agonists. This can be shown by very simple experiments.

5-HT stimulates aggregation but subsequent doses are without effect due to receptor desensitisation. What are the actions of drugs having central 5-HT actions on platelets? Figure 13 shows the responses of drugs known to have 5-HT-like activity in the CNS, which all cause 5-HT-like aggregation only upon the first challenge, and thereafter inhibit 5-HT itself. Thus the platelet aggregation system may be used for assessment of drugs used in psychiatric disorders and having both agonist and antagonist 5-HT-like activity.

Receptor Studies and Platelet Shape Change

Human platelet shape change has been studied in some detail by Born (see Born and colleages, 1978). It can occur in the absence of aggregation. Born studied the effects of 10^{-6}M 5-HT on shape change (Born and colleagues, 1978). We now find that normal human platelets undergo shape change with femtomolar concentrations of 5-HT (10^{-15}M), when aggregation does not occur. When 5-HT is given alone at 10^{-15}M, the shape change effects are small, but they are greatly potentiated by prior administration of NA. In any event the concentrations of 5-HT required are minute and involve specific receptors because shape change is blocked by specific 5-HT antagonists such as methysergide and BW501C67 (Wellcome Laboratories Ltd., Beckenham, Kent) (Fig. 14). Between 10^{-11} and 10^{-8}M 5-HT shape change is variable; in some instances it is maximal and in others it does not appear, but at 10^{-7} to 10^{-5}M shape change occurs and precedes aggregation.

The emphasis of the shape change investigations is that the results are mirrored closely by the kinetics of ^{3}H-5-HT binding to human platelets. In the latter experiments a high affinity site with Ka in the range 10^{-15} to 10^{-13}M, and a low affinity site with Ka in the range 10^{-15} to 10^{-13}M, have been detected. Thus the ligand binding corresponds to platelet shape change and aggregation as far as concentration ranges are concerned. There does not appear to have been any work with platelet shape change in relation to psychiatric disorders, but doubtless such studies will be made soon.

PLATELET SHAPE CHANGE INDUCED BY 10^{-15} to 10^{-11} M 5 HT

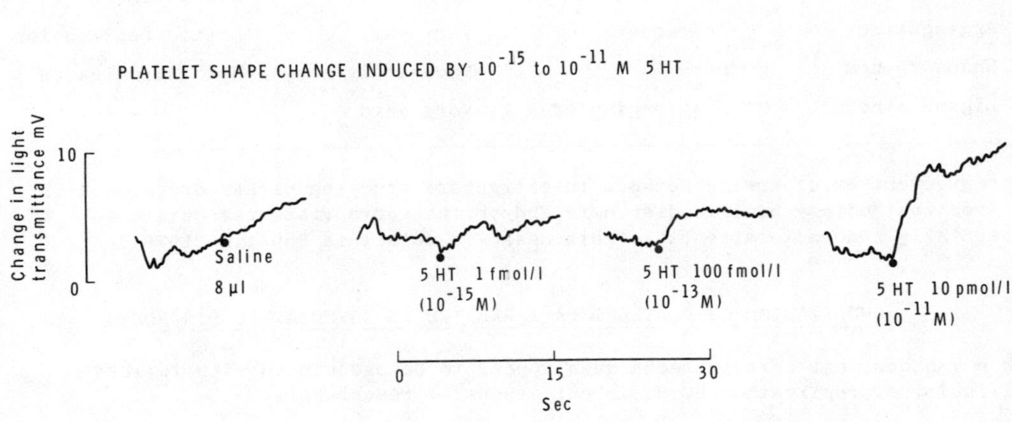

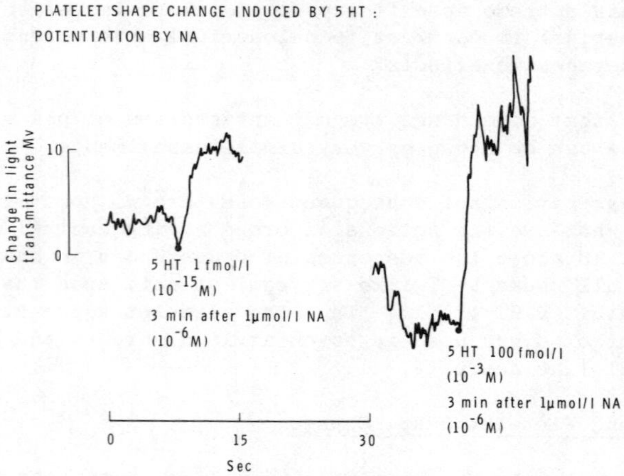

Fig. 14. Shape change of normal human platelets produced by femtomolar concentrations of 5-HT and effects of inhibitors. Upper records: responses to 5-HT alone; lower records: potentiation by NA pretreatment.

Table 7 shows my assessment of the various platelet techniques available to the biological psychiatrist. Clearly there are several areas which may be exploited in the future.

TABLE 7 Platelet Techniques Relevant to Psychiatry

Parameter	Study Frequency	Technique	Data*
Total cell content	Very frequent	Easy	Agreement
Cell storage	Pletscher	Very hard	
Uptake	Frequent	Easy	Agreement
Efflux	Boullin/Yuwiler**	Not easy	Disagreement
MAO activity	Very frequent	Difficult	Disagreement
Aggregation	Infrequent	Very easy	Little replication
Shape change	Born	Moderately easy	Not investigated
Ligand binding	Just beginning	Very hard	-

*Agreement or otherwise between investigators studying either drugs used in treatment of psychiatric disorders and/or the appropriate parameters in mentally abnormal patients. **Discussed in detail in Boullin (1978).

REPLICATION OF PLATELET DATA RELATED TO PSYCHIATRIC DISORDERS

Table 7 shows that certain techniques appear to be associated with failure or difficulty of replication by different groups of researchers.

The worst instance of this is platelet MAO and schizophrenia as mentioned earlier in this article. The 5-HT efflux method also described above has suffered in this regard. We were unable to replicate our original work showing enhanced efflux in autistic children (see Boullin, 1975 and 1978) and more recently Yuwiler's group has failed to do so (Yuwiler and colleagues, 1975). There have been no attempts to replicate the recent work with altered aggregation in schizophrenics by other groups, but we have ourselves had difficulties in our fifth study as described earlier.

On the other hand the platelet data in DS are extremely well replicated.

The reasons for failure to replicate data are likely to be as follows:

1. Difficult methodology.

2. Intrinsic factors: daily variations in response due to diet, sampling time, circadian rhythms etc.

3. Difficulty in diagnosis and characterisation of syndromes.

While platelet data relating to biological psychiatry have little value unless replicated, it may be that subtle differences in biochemical responses may lead psychiatrists to diagnose discrete patient subgroups who are amenable to therapy or require different therapy. Recently certain subjects falling in the 10 percentile range of low platelet MAO activity had greater evidence of psychiatric disorders (Buchsbaum, Coursey and Murphy, 1976).

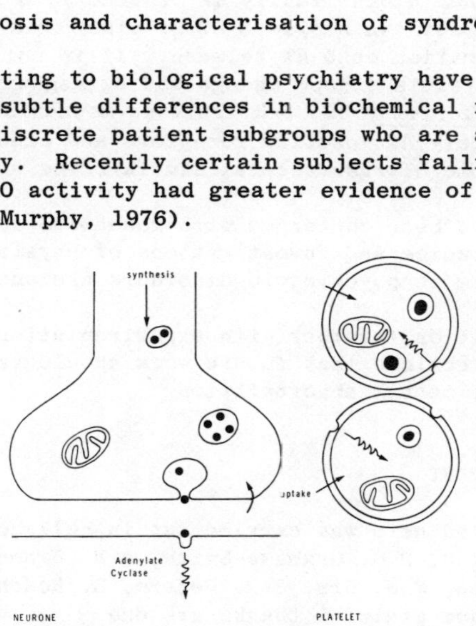

Fig. 15. Platelet neuronal model. Only neurones synthesise transmitter (synthesis). Uptake and storage mechanisms are similar (↑, ●). Adjacent platelets aggregate to monoamines via receptors (⌣) thus mimicking <u>trans-synaptic activity</u>. 5-HT release in both tissues occurs from electron-dense organelles possibly by exocytosis.

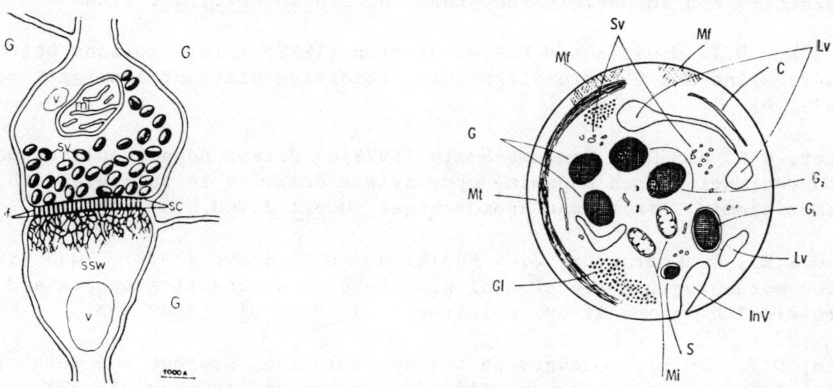

Fig. 16. Diagramatic comparisons of ultra structure of neurone (left) and platelet (right):

Neurone		Platelet	
G	= glial cell	s	= dense-cored vesicle containing 5-HT
SV	= dense-cored vesicle containing neurotransmitter	mf	= microfilaments
sf	= synaptic filament(s)	Sv	= small vacuole
sc	= synaptic cleft	Lv	= large vacuole
SSW	= subsynaptic web	$G_1G_1G_2$	= α-granules
mi	= mitochondrion	InV	= invagination
V	= vacuole	mi	= mitochondria
		gl	= glycogen granules

CONCLUSION

Platelets resemble neurones biochemically in respect to 5-HT uptake and storage (Fig. 15). Platelets do not synthesise 5-HT or other transmitters and there is little comparative information on 5-HT release. It is not known whether physiological responses of platelets (shape change and aggregation) can be equated with trans-synaptic neuronal activity but 5-HT release mechanisms may be different. Platelets possess a variety of specific receptors and others may yet be characterised. They also show some ultrastructural similarities with neurones (Fig. 16).

Most work in the past has been concerned with monoamine uptake, storage and metabolism. Drug-receptor studies and investigations of physiological responses of platelets to drugs of use in psychiatric disorders are unexplored fields.

These types of investigation together with experimentation with new platelet methods signpost the directions that future work should take in relation to the biological psychiatry of mental abnormalities.

ACKNOWLEDGEMENT

Most of the work described here was carried out in collaboration with S.E. Ball, M. Coleman, P.A.M. Glenton, D.G. Grahame-Smith, A.R. Green, R.P.J. Grimes, D. Molyneux, R.A. O'Brien, M.W. Orr, J.R. Peters, B. Roach, D. Wiles, H.F. Woods and M.B.H. Youdim, to whom grateful thanks are due.

REFERENCES

Alexander, R.W., B. Cooper and R.I. Handin (1978). Characterisation of the human platelet and adrenergic receptor. J.Clin.Invest., 61, 1136.

Ball, S.E., D.J. Boullin and P.A.M. Glenton (1977). Interactions between noradrenaline and 5-hydroxytryptamine involving platelet aggregation. J.Physiol., 272, 98.

Benedict, C.R. and D.G. Grahame-Smith (1978). Plasma noradrenaline and adrenaline concentrations and dopamine-hydroxylase activity in patients with shock due to septicaemia, trauma and haemorrhage. Quart.J.Med.N.S., 47, 1.

Born, G.V.R., R. Dearnaley, J.G. Foulks and D.E. Sharp (1978). Quantification of the morphological reaction of platelets to aggregating agents and of its reversal by aggregation inhibitors. J. Physiol., 280, 193.

Boullin, D.J. (1975). Changes in the accumulation, storage and metabolism of serotonin in mental abnormalities. Agents and Actions, 5, 492.

Boullin, D.J. (1978). Biochemical indicators of central serotonin function. In, D.J. Boullin (Ed.), Serotonin in Mental Abnormalities, Wiley, Chichester. pp. 1-40.

Boullin, D.J. and P.A.M. Glenton (1978). Characterisation of receptors mediating 5-hydroxytryptamine and catecholamine-induced platelet aggregation, assessed by the actions of α and β blockers, butyrophenones, 5-HT antagonists and chlorpromazine. Br.J.Pharmac., 62, 537.

Boullin, D.J., P.A.M. Glenton, D. Molyneux, J.R. Peters and B. Roach (1977). Binding of 5-hydroxytryptamine to human blood platelets. Br.J.Pharmac., 61, 453.

Boullin, D.J. and A.R. Green (1972). Mechanisms by which human blood platelets accumulate glycine, gaba and amino acid precursors of putative neurotransmitters. Br.J.Pharmac., 45, 83.

Boullin, D.J. and R.P.J. Grimes (1976). Increased platelet aggregation in patients receiving chlorpromazine: responses to 5-hydroxytryptamine, dopamine and N-dimethyl dopamine. Br.J.Clin.Pharmac., 3, 649.

Boullin, D.J., J.M. Knox, J.R. Peters, M.W. Orr, M.G. Gelder and D.G. Grahame-Smith (1978c). Platelet aggregation and chlorpromazine therapy. Br.J.Clin.Pharmac. (in press).

Boullin, D.J., D. Molyneux and B. Roach (1978). The binding of haloperidol to human blood platelets and interactions with 5-hydroxytryptamine and dopamine. Br.J.Pharmac., 63, 561.

Boullin, D.J. and R.A. O'Brien (1971a). Abnormalities of 5-hydroxytryptamine uptake and binding by blood platelets from children with Down's Syndrome. J.Physiol., 212, 287.

Boullin, D.J. and R.A. O'Brien (1970). Uptake and loss of ^{14}C dopamine by platelets from children with infantile autism. J.Autism.Childh.Schizophr., 2, 47.

Boullin, D.J. and R.A. O'Brien (1973). The metabolism of 5-hydroxytryptamine by blood platelets from children with mongolism. Biochem.Pharmac., 22, 1647.

Boullin, D.J., M.W. Orr and J.R. Peters (1978a). The platelet as a model for investigating the clinical efficacy of centrally acting drugs: relations between platelet aggregation and clinical condition in patients treated with chlorpromazine. In, S.D. de Gaetano and S. Garattini (Eds.), Platelets: A Multidisciplinary Approach, Raven Press, New York (in press).

Boullin, D.J., M.W. Orr, J.R. Peters and J.M. Knox (1978b). Blood platelets as a model for the actions of psychotropic drugs on central serotoninergic neurones. In, P. Le Chat (Ed.), Proceedings of the 7th International Congress of Pharmacology, Pergamon Press, Oxford (in press).

Boullin, D.J., H.F. Woods, R.P.J. Grimes, D.G. Grahame-Smith, D. Wiles, M.G. Gelder and T. Kolakowska (1973). Increased platelet aggregation responses to 5-hydroxytryptamine in patients taking chlorpromazine. Br.J.Clin.Pharmac., 2 29.

Buchsbaum, M.S., R.D. Coursey and D.L. Murphy (1976). The biochemical high risk paridigm: behavioural and familial correlates of low platelet monoamine oxidase activity. Science, 194, 339.

Drummond, A.H. (1976). Interactions of blood platelets with biogenic amines: uptake stimulation and receptor binding. In, J.L. Gordon (Ed.), Platelets in Biology and Pathology, North Holland, Amsterdam. pp. 203-239.

Heal, D.J., A.R. Green, D.J. Boullin and D.G. Grahame-Smith (1976). Single and repeated administration of neuroleptic drugs to rats; effects on striatal dopamine sensitive adenylate cyclase and locomotor activity produced by tranylcypromine and L-tryptophan or L-dopa. Psychopharmacology, 49, 287.

Kamoun, P. and H. Jerome (1978). Changes in blood serotonin in mental abnormalities. In, D.J. Boullin (Ed.), Serotonin in Mental Abnormalities, Wiley, Chichester. pp. 119-154.

Lance, J.W. (1978). Mechanism and Management of Headache, 3rd Ed., Butterworth's London. pp. 159-183.

Lingjaerde, O. (1977). Platelet uptake and storage of serotonin. In, W.B. Essmann (Ed.), Serotonin in Health and Disease, Spectrum, New York. pp. 139-199.

Lott, I.T., D.L. Murphy and T.W. Chase (1972). Down's Syndrome, central monoamine turnover in patients with diminished platelet serotonin. Neurology, 22, 967.

Macintyre, D.E. (1976). The platelet release reaction: association with adhesion and aggregation and comparison with secretory responses in other cells. In, J.L. Gordon (Ed.), Platelets in Biology and Pathology, North Holland, Amsterdam. pp. 61-85.

Murphy, D.L., R. Belmaker and R.J. Wyatt (1974). Monoamine oxidase in schizophrenia and other behavioural disorders. J.Psychiat.Res., 11, 221.

Oreland, L. (1976). Studies on monoamine oxidase activity in relation to ethanol abuse. Acta.Physiol.Scand., Suppl. 440, 46.

Orr, M.W. and D.J. Boullin (1976). The relationship between changes in 5-HT induced platelet aggregation and clinical state in patients treated with fluphenazine. Br.J.Clin.Pharmac., 3, 925.

Paasonen, M.K. (1965). Release of 5-hydroxytryptamine by blood platelets. J.Pharm. Pharmacol., 17, 681.

Pletscher, A. (1978). Platelets as models for monoaminergic neurones. In, M.B.H. Youdim, W. Lovenberg, D.F. Sharman and J.R. Lagnado (Eds.), Essays in Neuropharmacology, Wiley, Chichester. pp. 49-101.

Simpson, R.D., T.D.R. Hockaday and D.J. Boullin (1975). Studies of platelet aggregation in diabetic coma. Clin.Sci.Mol.Med., 49, 19.

Woods, H.F., M.B.H. Youdim, D. Boullin and S. Callender (1977). Monoamine metabolism and platelet function in iron-deficiency anaemia. In, Iron Metabolism, Ciba Foundation Symposium No. 51, Ciba Foundation, London. pp. 227-247.

Youdim, M.B.H. (1977). Factors influencing the deamination and functional activity of biogenic amines. In, E.S. Gershon, R.H. Belmaker, S.S. Kety and M. Rosenbaum (Eds.), The Impact of Biology on Modern Psychiatry, Plenum, New York. pp. 125-136.

Yuwiler, A., E. Ritvo, E. Geller, R. Glousman, G. Schneiderman and D. Matsuno (1975). Uptake and efflux of serotonin from platelets of autistic and nonautistic children. J.Autism.Childh.Schizophr., 5, 83.

Measurement of Neuro-Transmitter Metabolites in Blood, Urine and CSF in Psychiatric Patients

H. BECKMANN

Psychiatric Hospital of the University Munich
Present address: Zentralinstitut für Seelische Gesundheit, Mannheim

Hypotheses that functional abnormalities in neurotransmitter amines may be a biological substrate for various psychopathological states are largely derived from indirect evidence of pharmacological studies in animals.

Therefore attempts have been made by various groups of investigators to evaluate central neurotransmitter function by measuring the levels of their metabolites in blood, urine and cerebrospinal fluid (CSF) of psychiatric patients. However, existence of an effective blood brain barrier and large contributions to the amines and their metabolites from pools outside the CNS render the relevance of many of these measurements questionable.
Another disadvantage is that not all investigators use an uniform system for classifying the psychiatric disorders. Factors shown to modify catecholamine excretion as psychic stress, physical activity, posture, or dietary factors have not always adaquately been controlled. Furthermore, the specificity of the laboratory methods to determine the amines and their metabolites has not always been reliably demonstrated.

This presentation attempts to review recent selected findings on noradrenaline and its metabolites in body fluids and to discuss some of the methodological difficulties coherent with this research strategy.

Noradrenaline and its metabolites in blood and urine.

Noradrenaline (NA), adrenaline (A), normetanephrine (NMN) and vanillymandelic (VMA) acid have been measured by various groups of psychiatric investigators predominantly in manic-depressive patients.
However, since there exists an effective blood brain barrier for noradrenaline, it is questionable whether the peripheral levels are indicative for the metabolism of the catecholamines in the CNS.

In summary, excretion of noradrenaline and its O-methylated metabolite normetanephrine tend to be somewhat decreased in patients with endogenous depressions and increased in patients with mania. Agitated and/or anxious depression seem to have increased levels of NA, NMN and A in urine. NA levels have been found to be elevated in plasma and CSF (Dencker et al., 1966) of anxious-depressed patients.

MHPG in CSF, urine and plasma

Various lines of evidence suggest that 3-methoxy-4-hydroxyphenyl-glycol (MHPG) is the major metabolite of noradrenaline in the CNS of various animals (Mannarino et al., 1963; Rutledge and Jonason, 1967; Maas and Landis, 1968; Schanberg et al., 1968) and in man. Free and conjugated MHPG have been demonstrated in CSF. CSF levels of MHPG are determined by the rate of efflux of MHPG from the CSF, which is not effectively blocked by probenecid in humans. Recent studies have shown that, in the CNS, MHPG is continously lost through capillaries within tissue, and thus only a portion of the MHPG that is produced ever reaches the CSF (Kessler et al., 1976). It has also been demonstrated that MHPG in lumbar CSF reflects NA metabolism in spinal cord as well as in brain.
Studies of lumbar CSF MHPG levels exist which report lower levels in depressed patients as compared to controls, but not all studies agree (Wilk et al., 1971; Shaw et al., 1973). In one study MHPG levels were not different from control values in depressed patients, but manic patients showed markedly elevated levels of MHPG with a decrease to normal values during successful treatment with lithium (Wilk et al., 1972).
Our findings in small but homogenous groups of hypercinetic, catatonic schizophrenics and manic patients as compared to psychiatrically healthy controls and during clozapine therapy are depicted on Fig. 1 (Ackenheil et al., 1974).
In another approach of our group (Athen et al., 1977) neurotransmitter metabolites where measured in patients with alcoholic delirium. Patients with this syndrom exhibited a highly significant elevation of MHPG levels in CSF, however, not of HVA and 5-HIAA as compared to a control period upon recovery and off drugs. This was paralleled by elevated NA and dopamine-beta-hydroxylase levels in plasma and increased urinary catecholamine excretion (Fig. 2).

Based on data from several strategies in man and in different species, it has been estimated that from 30 % to 50 % of the MHPG excreted with urine may have its origin in the metabolism of brain pools of NA (Gitlow et al., 1971; Maas et al., 1973). Ebert and Kopin (1975), using (C^{14}) dopamine infusions in patients and normal controls suggested that the majority of urinary MHPG in man has its origin in brain pools of NA, whereas virtually all of the urinary VMA results from metabolism of peripheral NA.
This metabolite, therefore, may be valuable as an indicator of central NE turnover in brain.

Urinary MHPG has been reported to be significantly decreased in depressed patients when compared with controls (Maas et al., 1968; Maas et al., 1973). Other investigators have shown that urinary MHPG levels in depressed patients increase after recovery

(Greenspan et al., 197o) and that MHPG excretion is higher in patients in the manic than in the depressed phase (Bond et al.,1972; Jones et al., 1973).

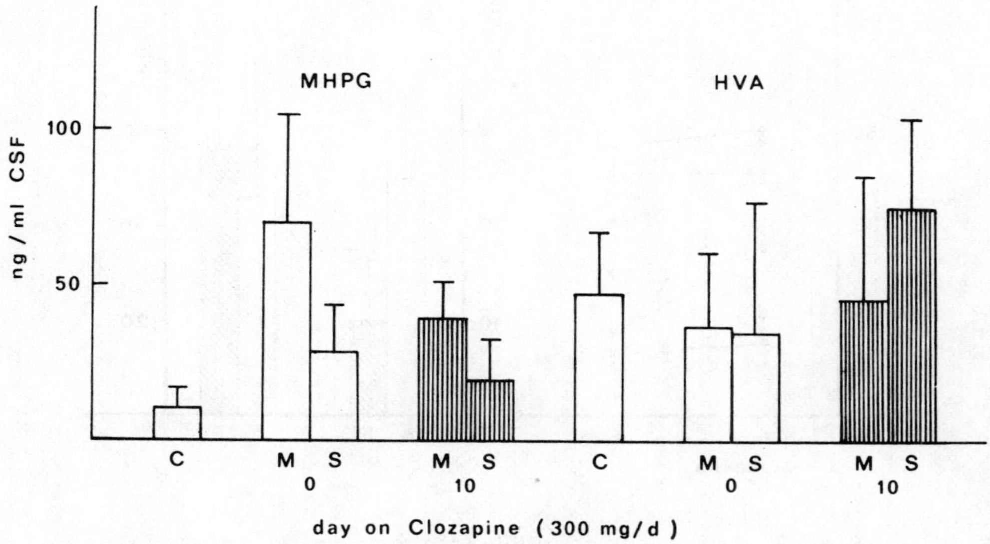

Fig. 1. Lumbar CSF MHPG, HVA and 5-HIAA in manic (M) (n = 3) and schizophrenic (S) (n = 6) patients before and during treatment with clozapine and controls; unshaded bars - untreated; shaded - after 10 days of treatment. Means ± SEM.

Others have confirmed earlier reports that urinary MHPG is significantly elevated in the manic compared to depressed phase. However, a significant increase in MHPG prior to the switch into mania, as reported by Jones et al. (1973), was not found.

Beckmann and Goodwin (1978) studied a large group of hospitalized depressed patients and compared them with controls (patients and methods are described elsewhere.)

Overall, the urinary excretion of MHPG was not significantly different in the total group of depressed patients compared to the normal controls, nor was there any difference between the depressed patients and the normal controls when the males and females were examined separately. However, when the depressed patients were subdivided according to the unipolar-bipolar dichotomy, it can be noted that the bipolar I group excreted about 30 % less MHPG than the controls. The small group of schizoaffective depressed patients had the lowest mean MHPG excretion. Within the depressed population, clear unipolar-bipolar differences in urinary MHPG excretion are apparent.

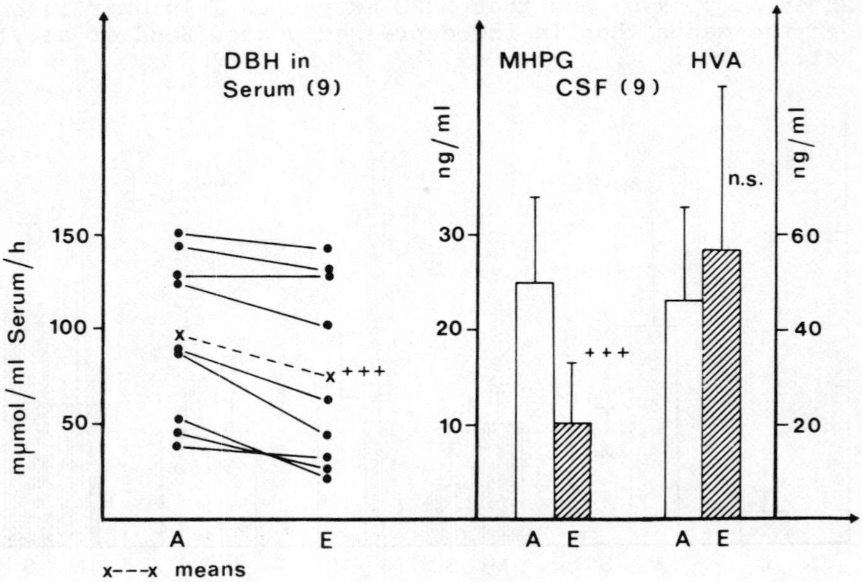

Fig. 2. Left: plasma DBH-activity in delirium (A) and after recovery (E).
Right: lumbar CSF MHPG and HVA in delirium (A) and after recovery (E).
n = in ( )

Significant differences between subgroups are as follows: (1) Bipolar I versus controls ($p < 0.05$); (2) Unipolar (single episode) versus controls ($p < 0.05$); (3) Schizoaffective versus controls ($p < 0.01$); (4) Unipolar (single phase + recurrent) versus bipolar I ($p < 0.001$); (5) Schizoaffective versus unipolar (single phase + recurrent) ($p < 0.001$); (6) Bipolar II versus unipolar (single phase + recurrent) ($p < 0.01$, males only).

These findings are partially concordant with earlier reports from Maas et al. 1973 and from Schildkraut et al. 1973 on significantly lower MHPG excretion in bipolar depressions as compared with unipolar depression or healthy controls. Unfortunately, in both, the study of Maas et al. and our study the research diagnostic criteria for primary affective disorder were applied retrospectively using recorded material.

These findings suggest the possibility that distinctions between depressions with relatively low and high MHPG excretion may provide a reasonable biochemical criterion for classifying depressive disorders.
In another approach baseline MHPG excretion has been used to p r e d i c t the clinical response to antidepressant drugs. Four groups of investigators (Schildkraut et al., 1971; Maas et al., 1972; Beckmann and Goodwin, 1975; Sacchetti et al., 1977) reported that MHPG may be of predictive value for the response to both amitriptyline and imipramine.

These findings are summarized:

Low MHPG excretion	High MHPG excretion
Imipramine response (Maas et al., 1972)	Amitriptyline response (Schildkraut, 1973; Beckmann and Goodwin, 1975; Sacchetti et al., 1977)
Imipramine response in unipolar (Beckmann and Goodwin, 1975)	Imipramine non-response (Maas et al., 1972; Beckmann and Goodwin, 1975)
Amitriptyline non-response (Schildkraut, 1973; Beckmann and Goodwin, 1975)	

Although these are preliminary results from a relatively small number of patients, they show some consistency with animal studies on the differential effects of various tricyclic drugs on different amine neurotransmitter systems in the brain.

Influence of psychoactive drugs on MHPG-excretion

a) Tricyclic antidepressants amitriptyline and imipramine.
There is a highly significant decrease under both antidepressant drugs, which is independent of clinical response. Other tricyclics produce changes in MHPG levels in animal brain that vary with the duration of drug administration and attempts to relate MHPG excretion to changes in clinical state under the drug treatment may be confounded by the direct pharmacological effects of the drugs on noradrenaline metabolism.

b) The expected effect of the MAO inhibiting drug phenelzine on MHPG excretion is a highly significant decrease under daily administration of 60 mg p.o./die. It is to be mentioned that baseline MHPG excretion in depressed patients was not of predictive value for clinical antidepressant response.

c) d-l-amphetamine
D-amphetamine decreased MHPG-excretion in depressed patients significantly, a finding which is in agreement with that of Fawcett et al. (1972) and Shekim et al. (1977) in hyperactive children, but not with Angrist et al. (1972).

d) Lithium
This substance had no unequivocal influence on urinary MHPG-excretion in depressed patients (Beckmann et al., 1975).

Other variables

Evidence suggests that non-specific factors such as physical activity (Ebert et al., 1972) psychic stress (Maas et al., 1971) and diet (Muscettola et al., 1976) can alter the urinary excretion of this metabolite in depressed patients. In this regard it should be noted that we found no significant correlation between MHPG excretion and ratings of agitation, or retardation, or both in depressed patients which is in agreement with the observations of Schildkraut et al. (1973) and of Maas et al. (1973).

However, the known difficulty in the assessment of these behavioral phenomena and the finding previously published that physical activity clearly can alter MHPG excretion (Ebert et al., 1972) suggest that the possible contribution of psychomotor activity state to urinary MHPG in affective disorder is still an open question.

The positive correlation to blood pressure found to exist in our investigation is further of importance which has to be integrated into an adequate evaluation of urinary MHPG excretion in depressed patients (Beckmann and Goodwin, 1978).

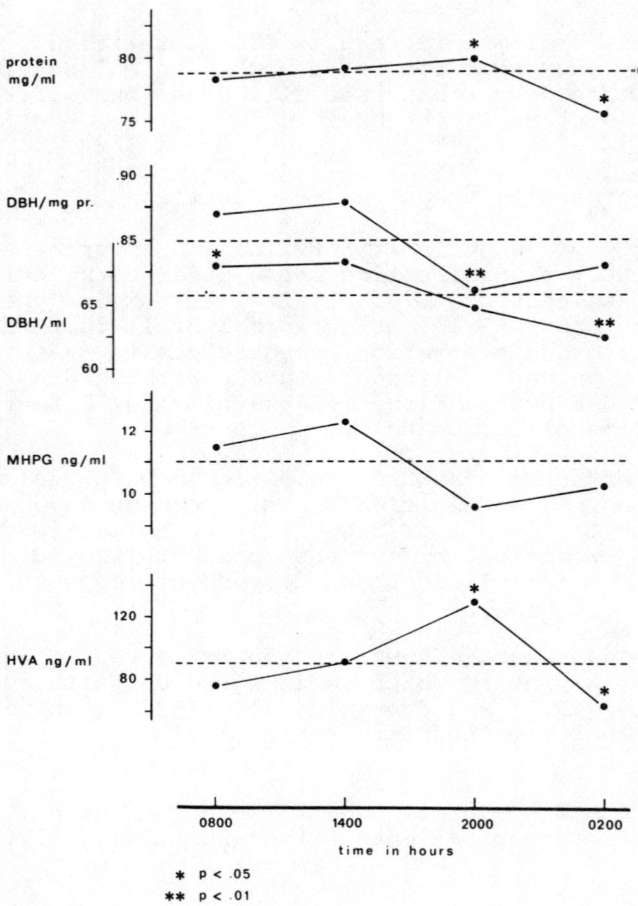

Fig. 3. Diurnal variations of various parameters in serum of 11 male volunteers. Dotted lines represent the mean of the individual means for the four estimations.

Relatively few reports exist on NA-metabolites in blood and serum of psychiatric patients. In the published reports no consistent alterations have been found.
In addition to the notion that probably most of the neurotransmitter metabolites are of peripheral origin, which are influenced by above mentioned factors there are circadian rhythms for several substances, as shown in one of our studies (Markianos and Beckmann,1976; Fig. 3).

Few reports exist on intraindividual correlations between neurotransmitter substances and their metabolites in different body fluids. No correlation has been found between urinary and CSF MHPG. In another study we were unable to detect correlations between platelet and plasma monoamine oxidase and urinary MHPG excretion in depressed patients. Furthermore in monozygote twins discordant for schizophrenia platelet MAO, plasma DBH and 24 hour urinary MHPG did not show significant correlations (Belmaker et al., 1975).

In conlusion, measurement of NA-metabolites i.e. MHPG in body fluids may be one important strategy to evaluate pathological functions in the CNS of man. However, one has to be aware that various physiological and pathophysiological conditions can influence the level of these substances.

Urinary MHPG, measured under well controlled conditions and over longer periods of time seem to indicate to a certain extend NA turnover in the CNS. Its estimation in psychiatric patients is assumed to be valuable to obtain information on one presumably critical neuronal function in psychopathological states.

REFERENCES

Ackenheil, M., H. Beckmann, W. Greil, G. Hoffmann, E. Markianos, and J. Raese (1974): Antipsychotic efficacy of clozapine in correlation to changes in catecholamine metabolism in man. In: J.S. Forrest, C.J. Carr, and E. Usdin (Eds.), The Phenothiazines and Structurally Related Drugs, Raven Press, New York. pp. 647-657.

Angrist, B.M., B. Shopsin, and S. Gershon (1972). Metabolites of monoamines in urine and cerebrospinal fluid, after large dose amphetamine administration. Psychopharmacologia, 26, 1-9.

Athen, D., H. Beckmann, M.Ackenheil, and E. Markianos (1977). Biochemical investigations into the alcoholic delirium. Arch. Psychiat. Nervenkr., 224, 129-14o.

Beckmann, H., F.K. Goodwin (in press). Urinary MHPG in subgroups of depressed patients and normal controls. Neuropsychobiology.

Beckmann, H., F.K. Goodwin (1975). Antidepressant response to tricyclics and urinary MHPG in unipolar patients. Arch. Gen. Psychiat., 32, 17-21.

Beckmann, H., St. Laurent, J. Goodwin, and F.K. Goodwin (1975). The effect of lithium on urinary MHPG in unipolar and bipolar depressed patients. Psychopharmacologia, 42, 277-283.

Belmaker, R., H. Beckmann, F.K. Goodwin, D. Murphy, W. Pollin, M. Buchsbaum, R. Wyatt, R. Ciarnello, and F. Lamprecht (1975). Relationships between platelet and plasma monoamine oxidase, plasma dopamine-beta-hydroxylase, and urinary 3-methoxy-4-hydroxy phenylglycol. Life Sci., 16, 273-28o.

Bond, P.A., F.A. Jenner, and A. Sampson (1972). Daily variations of urine content of 3-methoxy-4-hydroxyphenylglycol in two manic-depressive patients. Psycholog. Med. 2, 81-85.

Dencker, S.J., U. Malm, R.E. Roos, and B. Werdinius (1966). Acid monoamine metabolites of cerebrospinal fluid in mental depression and mania. J. Neurochem. 13, 1545-1548.

Ebert, M., I.J. Kopin (1975). Differential labelling of origins of urinary catecholamine metabolites by dopamine-C^{14}. Trans. Ass. Americ. Phycns., 28, 256-262.

Ebert, M.H., R.M. Post, and F.K. Goodwin (1972). Effect of physical activity on urinary MHPG excretion in depressed patients. Lancet, Vol. II, 766.

Fawcett, J., J.W. Maas, and D. Dekirmenjian (1972). Depression and MHPG excretion. (Response to dextroamphetamine and tricyclic antidepressants.) Arch. Gen. Psychiat., 26, 246-251.

Gitlow, E., M. Mendlowitz, L.M. Bertani, S. Wilk, and E.K. Wilk (1971). Human norepinephrine metabolism. J. Clin. Invest. 5o, 859-865.

Greenspan, K., J.J. Schildkraut, E.K. Gordon, L. Baer, M.S. Aronoff, and J. Durell (197o). Catecholamine metabolism in affective disorders-III. J. Psychiat. Res., 7, 171-183.

Jones, F.D., J.W. Maas, H. Dekirmenjian, and J.A. Fawcett (1973). Urinary catecholamine metabolites during behavioral changes in a patient with manic-depressive cycles. Science, 17o, 3oo-3o2.

Kessler, J.A., J.D. Fenstermacher, and C.S. Patlak (1976). 3-methoxy-4-hydroxyphenylethyleneglycol (MHPG) transport from the spinal cord during spinal subarachnoid perfusion. Brain Res., 1o2, 131-141.

Maas, J.W., and D.H. Landis (1968). In vivo studies of the metabolism of norepinephrine in the central nervous system. J. Pharmacol. Exp. Ther., 163, 147-162.

Maas, J.W., H. Dekirmenjian, and F. Jones (1973). The identification of depressed patients who have a disorder of NE metabolism and/or disposition. In E. Usdin and S. Snyder (Eds.). Frontiers of Catecholamine Research. Pergamon Press, New York. 1o91-1o96.

Maas, J.W., H. Dekirmenjian, D. Garver, D.E. Redmond, and D.H. Landis (1973). Excretion of catecholamine metabolites following intraventricular injection of 6-hydroxydopamine in the macaca speciosa. Europ. J. Pharmacol., 23, 121-13o.

Maas, J.W., J.A. Fawcett, and H. Dekirmenjian (1972). Catecholamine metabolism, depressive illness, and drug response. Arch. Gen. Psychiat., 26, 252-262.

Maas, J.W., H. Dekirmenjian, and J. Fawcett (1971). Catecholamine metabolism, depression and stress. Nature, 23o, 2, 33o-331.

Mannarino, E., N. Kirshner, and B.S. Nashold jr. (1963). The metabolism of (C^{14}) noradrenaline by cat brain in vivo. J. Neurochem., 1o, 373-379.

Markianos, E., and H. Beckmann (1976). Diurnal changes in dopamine-beta-hydroxylase, homovanillic acid and 3-methoxy-4-hydroxyphenylglycol in serum of man. J. Neural. Transm., 39, 79-93.

Muscettola, G., T. Wehr, and F.K. Goodwin (1977). Effect of diet on urinary MHPG excretion in depressed patients and in normal controls. Am. J. Psychiat., 134, 914-916.

Rutledge, O., and J. Jonason (1967). Metabolic pathways of dopamine and norepinephrine in rabbit brain in vitro . J. Pharmac. Exp. Ther., 157, 3, 493-5o2.

Sacchetti, E., E. Smeraldi, E. Allaria, M. Cagnasso, and P.A. Biondi (1977). MHPG, amitriptyline and depression: a collaborative study. In A. Frigerio, and E.L. Ghisalberti (Eds.), Mass Spectrometry in Drug Metabolism. Plenum Publ. Corp., New York, pp. 215-224.

Schanberg, S.M., G.R. Breese, J.J. Schildkraut, E.K. Gordon, and I.J. Kopin (1968). 3-methoxy-4-hydroxyphenylglycol sulfate in brain and cerebrospinal fluid. Biochemical Pharmacology, 17, 2oo6-2oo8.

Schildkraut, J.J. (1973). Norepinephrine metabolites as biochemical criteria for classifying depressive disorders predicting responses to treatment: preliminary findings. Am. J. Psychiat. 13o, 6.

Schildkraut, J.J., P.R. Draskoczy, E.S. Gershon, P. Reich, and E.L. Grab (1971). Effects of tricyclic antidepressants on norepinephrine metabolism: basic and clinical studies. In B.T. Ho, and W.M. McIsaac (Eds.), Brain Chemistry and Mental Disease. Plenum, New York. pp. 215-236.

Schildkraut, J.J., B.A. Keeler, M. Papousek, and E. Hartmann (1973). MHPG excretion in depressive disorders: relation to clinical subtypes and desynchronized sleep. Science, 181, 762-764.

Shaw, D.M., R. O'Keefe, D.A. Mac Sweeney, B.W.L. Brooksbank, R. Noguera, and A. Coppen (1973). 3-methoxy-4-hydroxyphenyl-glycol in depression. Psychol. Med., 3, 333-336.

Shekim, W.O., H. Dekirmenjian, and J.L. Chapel (1977). Urinary catecholamine metabolites in hyperkinetic boys treated with d-amphetamine. Am. J. Psychiat., 134, 11, 1276-1279.

Wilk, S., B. Shopsin, S. Gershon, and M. Suhl (1972). Cerebrospinal fluid levels of MHPG in affective disorders. Nature, 235, 44o-441.

Wilk, S., K.L. Davis, and S.B. Thacker (1971). Determination of 3-methoxy-4-hydroxyphenylethylene glycol (MHPG) in cerebrospinal fluid. Anal. Biochem., 39, 498-5o4.

Endocrinological and Peptide Modifications in Psychiatric Illness

MICHAEL H. SHEARD

Yale University School of Medicine and the Connecticut Mental Health Center, 34 Park Street, New Haven, Connecticut 06508, U.S.A.

ABSTRACT

A review of recent developments relating endocrinological findings to psychiatric conditions is presented. The relevance of endocrinologic changes will be discussed as an index of (1) brain monoamine functions; (2) the intactness of psychologic defenses; (3) response to stress; and (4) as a major patterned output indicative of the response of the nervous system to stimulation. Secondly, a brief review will be presented of recent findings on the role of endogenous brain peptides or endorphins.

INTRODUCTION

One of the most popular hypotheses of a biochemical basis for schizophrenia in recent years derives from observations that phenothiazines and butyrophenones appear to block dopamine receptors in brain. It has been known for many years since the early work of Carlsson (1963) that neuroleptic drugs had an action on central dopaminergic mechanisms. The evidence for this has been mostly indirect but recently it has been reported that long term treatment with haloperidol specifically increases the binding of H^3 haloperidol and H^3 apomorphine (a dopamine receptor agonist) in areas of the striatum and hypothalamus (Muller and Seeman, 1977). The most direct test of the possibility that there is an increased release of dopamine in schizophrenia was not confirmed by the finding that the major metabolite of dopamine, homovanillic acid, is not elevated in cerebrospinal fluid (Persson and Roos, 1969; Bowers, 1973). It is to be noted, however, that this metabolite comes predominantly from the caudate and is related to activity in the nigro striatal dopamine pathway. Also, thioridazine and clozapine have a lower incidence of extrapyramidal side effects and a weaker effect on dopamine turnover than is warranted by their therapeutic efficacy. This may be accounted for by the finding that thioridazine has a much stronger anticholinergic action than other phenothiazines, and anticholerinergic agents antagonize the dopamine turnover enhancing effects of drugs in the striatum more than in the limbic system. Clozapine causes a greater increase in dopamine turnover in the limbic system than in the caudate. Thus, attention turned to the tuberoinfundibular dopamine system. Since it had been shown that the dopamine tubero-infundibular system inhibited prolactin secretion (Fuxe and others, 1969), blood levels of prolactin could be used as a peripheral index of central dopamine activity.

Prolactin secretion is under both inhibitory and facilitatory control. While it appears probable that inhibition is mediated by dopamine, there is less certainty about stimulation. It may be in part serotonergic since L-tryptophane increases serum prolactin and this is partially blocked by serotonin antagonists. There is a case report of inhibition of a stress-induced increase in serum prolactin by cyproheptadine - a serotonin antagonist. The control is mediated by a prolactin membrane receptor and by the role of monoamines both in the hypothalamus and pituitary, as well as by a prolactin inhibiting factor which has not yet been isolated - though it might be dopamine itself. Circulating prolactin shows a circadian rhythm with a peak between 1 and 5 A.M., which is not synchronized with TSH or ACTH.

Schizophrenia

Meltzer and Fang (1976) studied serum prolactin levels in 27 newly admitted schizophrenic patients before and after phenothiazine administration. In 72 hours, all 27 patients showed a persistently elevated serum prolactin. There was a lag between this rise in prolactin and the clinical response. The levels tended to be higher on thioridazine than chlorpromazine or trifluoperazine. There was suggestive evidence that the magnitude of prolactin elevation correlated with the clinical response.

In a study by Johnstone and others (1977), Prolactin FSH, LH, and TSH were measured in repeated samples of serum from sixteen unmedicated male patients with chronic schizophrenia. Changes in mental status were found to correlate with changes in certain hormone levels. For example, there was an inverse relationship between incoherence of speech and plasma prolactin with greater incoherence correlated with lower prolactin. Follicle stimulating hormone was inversely correlated with poverty of speech. On the other hand, a significant positive correlation occurred between FSH and delusions. In this study, it was felt that the relationship between symptom change and change in prolactin secretion was consistent with the dopaminergic hypothesis as applied to the tuberoinfundibular system. In a recent study by Crow and Johnstone (1977), two isomers of flupenthixol which differed in their ability to block the dopamine sensitive adenylate cyclase (Miller and others, 1974) (which is related to the dopamine receptor) were tested in acute schizophrenic patients for their therapeutic effect as well as their effect on serum prolactin. α-Flupenthixol caused a 376% and 470% rise in prolactin at the end of the first and fourth week respectively compared with pretreatment levels. Trans β-flupenthixol, on the other hand, caused a 172% and 151% increase only. In the group treated with α-flupenthixol, no precise relationship was observed between prolactin concentration and clinical improvement. The increase usually preceded improvement by two weeks.

In rats, α-flupenthixol is 245 times more active in elevating plasma prolactin than β-flupenthixol. This type of discrepancy is even more marked between (+) butaclamol and (-) butaclamol, where (+) butaclamol is the effective antipsychotic agent (Meltzer and others, 1977).

However plasma prolactin increases to single doses of chlorpromazine and decreases to single doses of L-dopa have been found to be no different in normals and subjects suffering from schizophrenia (Gruen and others, 1978). Neuroleptic drugs of all chemical classes which are active against schizophrenic symptoms stimulate prolactin release while chemically related drugs and other psychotropic agents which are ineffective in schizophrenia do not. It is also interesting to note that tolerance does not develop since tolerance does not develop to antipsychotic effects and the response is present in all patients. The dose response curve for the prolactin response reaches an upper limit of sensitivity at doses which are below the therapeutic range. However, the prolactin-stimulating potency in humans of chlorpromazine, thioridazine, trifluoperazine, butaperazine, and haloperidol does correlate well with their relative clinical potencies. The prolactin response therefore offers no support to the dopamine hypothesis of schizophrenia, though it may be a useful addition to screening devices for potentially antischizophrenic drugs. This may result in part from the fact that a significant degree of the control of prolactin secretion by dopamine is directly on the pituitary itself. It remains possible that some other dopamine system other than the nigro-striatal or tubero-infundibular is the one affected, for example, a cortical dopamine system.

In a recent study, sixteen severely ill patients with schizophrenia were treated with a new and chemically different neuroleptic drug called sulpiride. It is a member of a class called othopramides. Its chemical name is N[(1-ethyl-2-pyrrolindinyl)-methyl]-2-methoxy-5-sulfamoylbenzamide. It was found to have a positive antipsychotic potential as well as a low incidence of extrapyramidal side effects. Most of the subjects showed an increase in prolactin levels but two patients who did not show an increase in prolactin did have a good therapeutic effect, suggesting that central dopaminergic blockade in the hypothalamic area is not a prerequisite for antipsychotic activity. In this study, while low doses rapidly raised serum prolactin, higher doses produced no further increase. Growth hormone levels, on the contrary, were depressed by sulpiride over time (Mielke and others, 1977).

It is possible that CSF prolactin levels may provide a more sensitive correlation with clinical state than blood levels. In a study by Wode-Helgodt and others (1977), prolactin was measured in CSF and plasma before and two and four weeks following treatment with chlorpromazine at different doses. Before treatment low levels were found in the CSF of most patients with a concentration about 20% of that in the plasma. It was higher in women than men. Following treatment with chlorpromazine, prolactin levels rose in both CSF and plasma after two and four weeks. In this study, there was a positive relationship between prolactin and dose of chlorpromazine. Moreover, there was no change in total protein, follicle stimulating hormone, luteinizing hormone, thyroid stimulating hormone or oestradiol in either CSF or plasma. There have also been several reports indicating a positive therapeutic effect in schizophrenia with high doses of propanolol, a β-adrenergic blocking agent (up to 6000 mgm/day). In view of these therapeutic effects, it is interesting to note that high doses of propanolol causes an increase in plasma prolactin in rats, whereas low doses do not (Nasrallah and others, 1977). One report indicated that serum prolactin does increase transiently shortly after propanolol administration to patients with schizophrenia, but another reported a fall in prolactin after doses of 120-1280 mgm/day (Hanssen and others, 1978). It may be that the doses used in this latter study were too low to see either the therapeutic or the prolactin effect. It may be added here that plasma prolactin does not appear to be altered at all during chronic lithium administration (Nielsen and others, 1977).

Another use of the prolactin index of central dopaminergic activity has been to test the hypothesis that tardive dyskinesia is due to dopamine receptor supersensitivity. Tamminga and others, (1977) looked for an increased response of growth hormone and prolactin to dopamine agonists in chronic schizophrenic patients with tardive dyskinesia. They were not able to find any difference between patients with tardive dyskinesia and those without. Instead, there was a significantly decreased response to dopaminergic stimulation in the total chronic schizophrenic group. This, of course, would be expected if there is indeed chronic excess dopaminergic activity in such patients.

These findings are confirmatory of those of Ettigi and others (1976), who also found raised baseline levels of growth hormone in six out of seventeen of the schizophrenic patients but none of their controls.

Depression

In view of the facts that the somatic signs of depression suggest hypothalamic dysfunction and that several of the brain neurotransmitters, particulary the catecholamines, but also serotonin which have been suggested as playing a role in depression, regulate neuroendocrine function, it is of interest to study neuroendocrine function in affective illness.

Sachar and others (1976) have demonstrated a marked increase in the secretion of cortisol unrelated to stress or sleep disturbance. There is also a distortion of the normal 24-hour cycle with elevations in late afternoon, evening and early morning when cortisol is usually low.

The growth hormone responses to hypoglycaemia but not to L-dopa are significantly reduced. It had been previously reported that bipolar depressive patients had a significantly larger peak growth hormone response to L-dopa than healthy controls and unipolar depressive patients. These patients were on a controlled monoamine diet which might have accounted for the difference from Sachar (Gold and others, 1976). However, Mendlewicz and others (1977) who also used a controlled monoamine diet agreed with Sachar in not finding a significant difference in growth hormone peak between bipolar and unipolar depressives. They did find, however, a difference in the response between premenopausal and postmenopausal women and emphasize the importance of taking this factor into account. These workers also reported a paradoxical rise in prolactin secretion 30-90 min after L-dopa, followed by a suppression in bipolar patients. This peak in prolactin was not found in unipolar patients. It is clear that in evaluating such findings it is most important to take into account stress factors and estrogen levels. Postmenopausal depressed women secrete less LH than normal postmenopausal women. Sachar points out that since all these abnormalities can be reproduced by depletion of brain norepinephrine, these findings offer some support for the hypothesis of reduced nordrenergic activity in certain types of depression.

Plasma prolactin levels are doubled in depressive patients treated with monoamine-oxidase inhibitors, clorgyline and pargyline. This occurs without significant changes in plasma cortisol and is not due therefore to non specific stress (Slater and others, 1977).

In a medical OP clinic population, no difference was found in the prolactin levels between depressed and non depressed patients matched for age and sex (Arana and others, 1977).

Meltzer and others (1977) found no changes in plasma prolactin with either acute or chronic treatment with imipramine or amitryptyline in depressed patients and concluded that blockade of serotonin uptake does not affect basal prolactin levels.

While recent reports have been negative regarding the effect of TRH in depression, a recent report found that the TSH response to TRH was significantly lower in unipolar depressed patients and this was associated with a negative correlation with 5 hydroxyindoleacetic acid in the cerebrospinal fluid (Gold and others, 1977). This neuroendocrine response may therefore constitute a marker of specific monoamine dysfunction in certain subgroups of patients with affective illness.

Stress

There is some evidence from animal experiments that prolactin may play a role in the organism's response to stress. For example, rats bred selectively for behavioral differences in susceptibility to mild stress showed differences in serum prolactin and hypothalamic dopamine. The more reactive rats had a higher serum prolactin and higher levels of hypothalamic dopamine. They also showed a greater increase in serum prolactin one hour after blockade of catecholamine synthesis with L-AMPT (Blizard and others, 1977).

Surges of prolactin are known to occur in several physiological as well as stressful states. These include sleep, nipple stimulation, general anesthesia and insulin-induced hypoglycaemia. These surges may be mediated by a prolactin-releasing factor or by inhibition of a prolactin-inhibiting factor. A technique for comparing the effect of stress operating via the hypothalamus or via the pituitary is to give thyrotrophin releasing hormone which causes prolactin release directly from the pituitary and is not blocked by drugs such as cyproheptadine.

Aono and others (1976) reported on serum gonadotropin levels following surgical stress and general anesthesia. In male patients but not in females, LH was increased at 30 min and 1 hour post anesthesia. LH dropped slightly thereafter returning to baseline on the seventh postoperative day. No changes in FSH were found. In males, there were significant intra and post operative changes in testosterone levels.

The hormonal pattern of anterior pituitary response to stress in males engendered by treadmill exercise, diagnostic gastroscopy, and elective surgery with general anesthesia has been reported by Somers and others (1977). Serum TSH is depressed following all three stressful procedures, while serum prolactin, growth hormone and cortisol are all elevated. In addition, LH is elevated following gastroscopy and surgery. There were no significant changes in FSH. The depression in TSH may result from the suppressive effect of high serum levels of cortisol at the hypothalamic pituitary level.

Electroconvulsive therapy produces a rapid stimulation of acth-cortisol production in all subjects but no consistent changes in FSH, LH, TSH, HGH, or cyclic AMP (Ylikorkala and others, 1976). Another study found a 10-50 fold increase in serum prolactin 15 minutes after ECT in eight out of nine patients. In four patient controls undergoing the same anesthesia for minor gynaecological operations, there was no significant change in prolactin (Ohman and others, 1976).

HYPOTHALAMIC-PITUITARY-GONADAL FUNCTION

Schizophrenia

The literature is conflicting with regard to alterations in androgen metabolism in schizophrenia. Early reports suggested no consistent abnormality in the excretion of 17 ketosteroids. Brooksbank and Pryse-Phillips (1964) found that the average androsterol urinary excretion was significantly lower for male patients with schizophrenia. Tourney and Hatfield (1972) found that schizophrenic groups (acute, chronic institutionalized, and chronic noninstitutionalized) showed no difference from controls for plasma levels of testosterone and androstenedione. However, the chronic groups had a significantly lower level of dehydroandrosterone. Since this compound is derived predominantly from the adrenal, it suggests reduced adrenal cortical functioning in chronic schizophrenia.

Brambella and others (1975) reported the effects of 30 days of haloperidol therapy on sixty-two male chronic schizophrenic patients whose duration of illness varied between two and twenty-nine years. Pretreatment levels revealed decreased secretion of total gonadotropins, FSH, LH, ACTH and testosterone and increased insulin secretion. Haloperidol stimulated secretion of FSH, LH, total gonadotropins, ACTH and testosterone up to normal or low normal levels. More recent studies by Brambella and others (1977) have also continued to find evidence for reduced pituitary-gonadal function in chronic schizophrenics. They find a reduced secretion of FSH, LH and testosterone in male chronic schizophrenics. This data agrees with that of Suwa and others (1966), Ohawa (1966) and Persky and others (1968). Brambella and others (1976) also found increased responsed to GnRH of both FSH and LH. Using the clomiphene citrate test, also in male chronic schizophrenics, they found pretest levels of FSH, LH and testosterone was significantly lower than the controls and that while FSH showed a normal increase to clomiphene, the LH and testosterone responses were blunted. Phenothiazines or haloperidol apparently had no effect on the test. This result suggests a partial hypothalamic gonadotropin deficiency. (Clomiphene is an analogue of the non-steroidal estrogen chlortrianisene. It acts at a hypothalamic level to block estrogen and androgen sensitive receptors and blocks their inhibition of gonadotropin release).

Depression

There is a demonstrated relationship between testosterone and aggressive and sexual behavior in animals, while in depression there is a marked loss of libido and positive assertiveness. It therefore is worthwhile to study testosterone in depression. Sachar and others (1973) found, however, that in fifteen depressed men age 46-78, there were no meaningful changes in either urinary or plasma testosterone when illness and recovery values were compared. There was also no relationship between changes in testosterone and changes in severity of illness, nor was there any relationship between testosterone and cortisol production rate. It may be, however, that this group of males are too old to show testosterone changes. In a study by Doering and others (1975), the association between mood and plasma testosterone was investigated in twenty normal young men over a period of two months. They found a positive intersubject correlation between depression and testosterone.

Premenstrual Tension Syndrome

There is a reported association with low progesterone (14%) during luteal phase and increased prolactin levels. Serum oestradiol levels may be slightly increased in late luteal phase. Treatment with dihydrogesterone has produced some positive therapeutic effects in patients with low progesterone.

In a study of fifteen women with premenstrual tension, a significant correlation between oestrogen levels and symptoms of anxiety, irritability, anxiety plus irritability and depression. No significant correlation was found between progesterone and symptoms (Backstrom and Mattson, 1975). So it is evident that more research is necessary in this condition to resolve some of the discrepancies.

Aggression

In the study by Doering and others just quoted, no correlation was found between testosterone and angry effect. Indeed, in humans the interrelationship between testosterone and aggression is very controversial.

Persky and others (1971) found a significant relationship between testosterone production rate and self-administered hostility and aggression indicators in young men. Kreuz and Rose (1972) found that testosterone levels did not correlate with aggressive behavior in a young criminal population in prison, but did correlate with a prior history of fighting behavior in early adolescence.

Ehrenkranz and others (1976) determined plasma testosterone in three groups of male prisoners. One group showed chronic assaultive behavior in and out of prison, one group was socially dominant and tough in the prison hierarchy, and one group was neither physically aggressive or socially dominant. There was a significantly higher level of testosterone in the aggressive group as compared with the nonaggressive group or the other two groups combined. The socially dominant group also had a significantly higher testosterone than the non-aggressive group.

In a double blind study of lithium in impulsive aggressive delinquent males, we found a significant reduction of violent assaultive episodes. This reduction was associated with an increase in the level of serum LH without a change in serum testosterone. It is also of interest to note that in this study we found no correlation between self-administered ratings of hostility or aggression and actual aggressive behavior. This suggests that future studies attempting to correlate testosterone and aggression need to include a measurement of overt aggressive behavior.

Endorphins

Endorphin is the generic name for endogenous morphinomimetic peptides. Enkephalins are penta peptides, a subgroup of endorphins. Both are components of beta-lipotropin. The C terminal fragment of which containing 31 amino acids is the most powerful morphine-like peptide yet isolated and is called beta-endorphin. Many of the actions of these agents are reversible with morphine antagonists such as naloxone. Since morphine-like substances have profound effects on mood, it was of interest to investigate the action of narcotic antagonists in mood disorders. It was also of interest in schizophrenia in view of finding that these substances could produce catatonic-like states when injected into animal brain.

Terenius and others (1976) have reported increased levels of endorphins in the CSF in chronic psychosis as well as in depression (1977). Treatment with naloxone showed no positive effect on mood, but in two cases a rapid worsening of mood on discontinuing the naloxone. In the C.S.F. Endorphin Fraction I decreased, while Fraction II showed no distinct trend. An interesting finding was that 5-hydroxyindole acetic acid increased in the C.S.F. suggesting an effect on serotonin metabolism or release.

References

Aono, T., K. Kurachi, M. Miyata, A. Nakasima, and K. Koshiyama (1976). Influence of surgical stress under general anesthesia on serum gonadotropin levels in male and female patients. J. Clin. Endocrinol. Metab., 42, 144-148.

Backstrom, T. and B. Mattson (1975). Correlation of symptoms in premenstrual tension to oestrogen and progesterone concentrations in blood plasma. Neuropsychobiol., 1, 80-86.

Blizard, D.A., J. Slater, B. Liang, and L. Shenkman (1977). Serum prolactin and hypothalamic dopamine in rat strains selectively bred for behavioral differences in susceptibility to stress. Neuroendocrin., 23 297-305.

Brambella, F., A. Guerrini, A. Guastalla, C. Rovere, and F. Riggi (1975). Neuroendocrine effects of haloperidol therapy in chronic schizophrenia. Psychopharmacologia, 44, 17-22.

Brooksbank, B. and W. Pryse-Phillips (1964). Urinary 16 - Androsten-3-ol, 17-oxosteroids and mental illness. Brit. Med. J., 112, 1602-1609.

Carlsson, A. and M. Lundquist (1963). Effect of chlorpromazine and haloperidol on formation of 3-methoxytryptamine and normetanephrine in mouse brain. Acta. Pharmac. Tox., 20, 140-144.

Corenblum, B. and M. Whitaker, (1977). Inhibition of stress-induced hyperprolactinaemia. Brit. Med. J., 2, 1328.

Cotes, P.M., T.J. Crow, and E.C. Johnstone (1977). Serum prolactin as an index of dopamine receptor blockade in acute schizophrenia. Proc. B. P. S., 651.

Doering, C.H., H.K. Brodie, H.C. Kraemer, R.H. Moos, H.B. Becker, and D.A. Hamburg (1975). Negative affect and plasma testosterone: A longitudinal human study. Psychosom. Med., 37, 484-491.

Ehrenkranz, J., E. Bliss, and M.H. Sheard (1974). Plasma testosterone: Correlation with aggressive behavior and social dominance in man. Psychosom. Med., 36, 469-475.

Ettigi, P., N.P.V. Nair, S. Lal, P. Cervantes, and H. Guyda (1976). Effect of apomorphine on growth hormone and prolactin secretion in schizophrenic patients, with or without oral dyskinesia withdrawn from chronic neuroleptic therapy. J. Neurol. Neurosurg. Psychiat., 39, 870-876.

Fuxe, K., T. Hökfelt, and O. Nilsson (1969). Factors involved in the control of the activity of the tubero infundibular dopamine neurons during pregnancy and lactation. Neuroendocrinology, 5, 257-270.

Gruen, P.H., E.J. Sachar, G. Langer, N. Altman, M. Leifer, A. Frantz, and F.S. Halpern (1978). Prolactin responses to neuroleptics in normals and schizophrenic subjects. Arch. Gen. Psychiat., 35, 108-116.

Hanssen, T., T. Heyden, I. Sundberg, L. Wetterberg, and P. Eneroth (1978). Decrease in serum prolactin after propanolol in schizophrenia. Lancet, 1, 101-102.

Johnstone, E.C., J.J. Crow, and K. Mashiter (1977). Anterior pituitary hormone secretion in chronic schizophrenia: An approach to neurohumoral mechanisms. Psychol. Med., 7, 223-228.

Kreuz, L.E. and R.M. Rose (1972). Assessment of aggressive behavior and plasma testosterone in a young criminal population. Psychosom. Med., 34, 331-339.

Meltzer, H.Y. and V.S. Fang (1976). The effect of neuroleptics on serum prolactin in schizophrenic patients. Arch. Gen. Psychiat., 33, 279-286.

Meltzer, H.Y., S.M. Paul, and V.S. Fang (1977). Effect of flupenthixol and butaclamol isomers on prolactin secretion in rats. Psychopharmacol., 51, 181-183.

Mendlewicz, J., P. Linkowski, and H. Brauman (1977). Growth hormone and prolactin response to levodopa in affective illness. Lancet, 1, 652-653.

Mielke, D.H., D.M. Gallant, and C. Kessler (1977). An evaluation of a unique new antipsychotic agent, sulpiride: Effects on serum prolactin and growth hormone levels. Am. J. Psychiatry, 134, 1371-1375.

Miller, R.J., A.S. Horn, and L.L. Iverson (1974). The action of neuroleptic drugs on dopamine stimulated adenosine cyclic 3'5' monophosphate production in rat neostriatum and limbic forebrain. Mol. Pharmac., 10, 759-766.

Nasrallah, H.A., W.J. Freed, A. Rogol, and R.J. Wyatt (1977). Propanolol and prolactin. Lancet, 2, 1175-1176.

Ohman, R., J. Walinder, J. Balldin, and L. Wallin (1976). Prolactin response to electro convulsive therapy. Lancet, 2, 936-937.

Persky, H., K.D. Smith, and G.K. Basu (1971). Relation of psychologic measures of aggression and hostility to testosterone production in man. Psychosom. Med., 33, 265-269.

Sachar, E.J., F. Halpern, R.S. Rosenfeld, T.F. Gallagher, and L. Hellman (1973). Plasma and urinary testosterone levels in the depressed man. Arch. Gen. Psychiat., 28, 15-18.

Sachar, E.J., H.P. Roffwarg, P.H. Gruen, N. Altman, and J. Sassin. Neuroendocrine studies of depressive illness. Pharmakopsychiatr. Neuropsychopharmakol., 9, 11-17.

Sheard, M.H., J.L. Marini, C.I. Bridges, and E. Wagner (1976). The effect of lithium on impulsive aggressive behavior in man. Am. J. Psychiat., 133, 1409-1413.

Sheard, M.H., J.L. Marini, and S. Giddings (1977). The effect of lithium on testosterone and luteinizing hormone. J. Nerv. Dis., 38, 765-769.

Terenius, L., A. Wahlström, and H. Agren (1977). Naloxone (Narcam) treatment in depression: Clinical observations and effects on C.S.F. endorphins and monoamine metabolites. Psychopharmacol., 54, 31-33.

Tourney, G. and L.M. Hatfield (1973). Androgen metabolism in schizophrenics, homosexuals and normal controls. Biol. Psychiat., 6, 23-35.

Ylikurkala, O., A. Kauppila, J. Haapalahti, and H. Karppanen (1976). The effect of electroconvulsive therapy on the circulating concentrations of pituitary hormones, cortisol and cyclic adenosine monophosphate. Clin. Endocrin., 5, 571-574.

Concluding Remarks

H. LOO

Service Hospitalo-Universitaire de Santé Mentale et de Thérapeutique
(Pr. P. Deniker) Hôpital Ste-Anne, 1, rue Cabanis, 75014 Paris, France

Before concluding this symposium I would like to thank the different speakers and the participants from the floor who took part in the discussion.

After the general survey of the correlations between psychiatric disorders and biological modifications presented by Doctor E.Zarifian,Doctor D.J.Boullin gave us a very stimulating picture of the only reliable peripheral model i.e blood platelets. After this presentation it seems that platelets are not only a good model for MAO and serotonin modifications but can also be used for studying psychotropic drugs.

Doctor S.Z.Langer made a very brilliant but prudent inventory of the role of the pre and post-synaptic noradrenergic receptors in the CNS. Nevertheless we have now pharmacological arguments to think that extrapolation from the periphery to the brain is not unreasonable when we consider noradrenergic transmission.

Doctor H.Beckmann gave us a very complete and critical landscape of the measurements of neurotransmitter metabolites in human fluids. In fact, too many factors can modify the relevance of these mesures and now we understand better why the results are so questionable or contradictory.

Doctor M.H.Sheard opened up perspectives on the future with his review of endocrinological changes and endogenous peptides. The relationship between monoamines and brain hormons seem the most interesting. But, in my opinion, it is doubtfull that the so-called endorphins are going to play a major role from a practical point of view.

In fact all these biological factors are only elements of a big puzzle. It is not a reason to be discouraged and we must go on further in searching for new correlations between psychiatric disorders and biological changes. Nevertheless we have to be modest and very prudent in our interpretations.

Thank you again to all our brilliant speakers and thank you to the audience for your participation and attention.

Diagnostic and Pharmacotherapeutic Aspects of Child Psychiatry

Neuropsychopharmacology of Hyperkinetic Children

RACHEL GITTELMAN-KLEIN

New York State Psychiatric Institute, New York, New York 10032, U.S.A.

ABSTRACT

Psychostimulants have been found to improve markedly the symptoms of hyperkinesis, overactivity, impulsivity, inattention, and social adjustment. In addition, performance on a range of cognitive tests is also improved by the drugs.

Neuroleptics exert symptomatic relief on hyperactivity, overexcitability, and unmanageability, but are not as effective as the stimulants. Though a non-pharmacological treatment, behavior modification, induces clinical change, the impact of this intervention is inferior to that of stimulant treatment. Several studies seem to support the contention that the hyperkinetic disorder of childhood is linked to adult alcoholism, sociopathy, and hysteria, though not conclusively in view of lack of appropriate research design.

Theories of the disorder are discussed. Efforts to identify predictors of pharmacological effect have yielded weak results.

Keywords: hyperkinesis stimulants phenothiazines children

DIAGNOSIS OF HYPERKINETIC DISORDER

There is general consensus among clinicians that children diagnosed as hyperactive display, for their age, excessive motor activity, impulsivity, short attention span, low tolerance for frustration, in the absence of schizophrenic or other psychotic symptoms. Secondary clinical complications are not uncommon, typically consisting of poor peer relationships, aggression, and school failure. The above symptoms are of long duration and by the time the child is seen for treatment, typically difficulties have been of long-standing. The critical diagnostic issues in hyperkinesis do not revolve around the nature of the key symptoms, but rather when these traits can be considered pathological, how many of these characteristics are necessary for the diagnosis, under what circumstances do the symptoms have to be manifest before a child may be diagnosed as hyperkinetic (Gittelman-Klein and Klein, 1975).

There are no clear-cut objective criteria for the diagnosis. Nor are there rules indicating which, and how many of the symptoms justify considering them as representing the full syndrome. A complicating factor in the diagnostic process is that the behavior of children who share some or all of the traits may be extremely variable, so that difficulties may vary both in intensity, and across situations. However, behavioral inconsistency does not preclude the diagnosis. A useful rule of thumb is to consider the disorder as present when the symptoms interfere with the child's functioning in at least one important setting, such as school.

Group situations, and demands for self-application aggravate the symptoms of hyperkinetic children. Therefore, difficulties are most prominent in the classroom. One should be very cautious in diagnosing hyperactivity in children who are dysfunctional at home, and not in school. The diagnosis of hyperactivity is probably inappropriate for such youngsters and a critical evaluation of familial interactions and discipline is in order.

Central to the diagnosis is a report by teachers of the child's inability to stick to his work, difficulty in completing work. Parents rarely report hyperactivity *per se*; rather, they complain of lack of cooperation, of difficulty in following through on instructions, poor work habits. In addition, a history of such difficulties is extremely common. It is not unusual for the symptoms to be absent during office visits. The failure to observe directly the signs of the disorder does not preclude its presence.

It has been repeatedly demonstrated that the disorder is much more prevalent in boys than girls.

PHARMACOLOGICAL TREATMENT

In spite of diagnostic ambiguity very marked drug effects have been demonstrated among children diagnosed as hyperkinetic, thereby indicating that this state of diagnostic uncertainty does not preclude discerning clear patterns of outcome.

A number of compounds have been carefully investigated, stimulants, phenothiazines, other neuroleptics, and a tricyclic.

Stimulants

The psychostimulants are the treatment of choice for hyperkinetic children. When a good effect is obtained, the child is not only "better", but his behavior is indistinguishable from that of normal children (Gittelman-Klein, and co-workers, 1979). In addition, a very large proportion of hyperkinetic children respond to stimulants. Therefore, the drugs have a broad as well as potent therapeutic impact.

Of all pediatric psychopharmacological interventions, the therapeutic effect of stimulants on the syndrome of hyperkinesis in children is the best substantiated. Their short-term usefulness has been demonstrated in several controlled studies and a critical perusal of the literature clearly points to the conclusion that the therapeutic value of stimulants has been overwhelmingly established for the amelioration of gross motor hyperactivity and short attention span.

Among the stimulants, methylphenidate (Ritalin), dextroamphetamine (Dexedrine), magnesium pemoline (Cylert), and deanol (Deaner), have been shown to have positive therapeutic effect.

In 1973, caffeine was reported to be effective as well, with the advantage of being inexpensive and readily available (Schnackenberg, 1973). Unfortunately, placebo controlled studies of caffeine have failed to demonstrate significant therapeutic advantage for caffeine over placebo and we must conclude that caffeine does not offer a clinical alternative in the management of hyperkinetic children (Conners, 1975a; Garfinkel, Webster and Sloman, 1975; Huestis, Arnold and Smeltzer, 1975).

There are no clinical differences between methylphenidate and dextroamphetamine. Both are short acting in their effect and last from two to six hours. Interestingly, there are instances when a child will obtain less than an optimal effect from one of these, and respond very well to the other. Dosage requirements vary widely. For the most part, dextroamphetamine dosage ranges between 5 to 40 mg/day, methylphenidate dosage between 10 to 80 mg/day. Side effects are very similar for the two compounds, consisting typically of loss or reduction of appetite and delay in onset of sleep which occur in about 30% of children treated with moderately high doses. More rarely, mood changes consisting of interpersonal sensitivity or "touchiness" and a sad demeanor may occur. The latter side effects are most marked at the initiation of treatment and often diminish over time. In a child who responds well, the presence of the untoward effects should not lead to a premature termination of treatment. Rather, the child should be followed over several weeks, if there is no adaptation to the medication, dosage should be reduced, and subsequently increased very gradually if clinically indicated. Our clinical observation is that side effects are less likely to occur if dosage is built up in small increments.

There is suggestive data that stimulants, especially dextroamphetamine, may have an inhibiting effect on growth (Safer and Allen, 1975). Consequently, methylphenidate might be the drug of choice since with regard to this consideration it may be less noxious; however, this side effect is not established yet. A recent investigation failed to find a reduction in growth among early adolescents treated with stimulants in childhood (Gross, 1976).

From the data published on growth inhibition, there is very wide variation in this effect. The variability indicates that it is only a subgroup of the total treated sample who are vulnerable to this side effect. Further, larger children seem more at risk than others. These results are reassuring to the extent that the growth of most of the children will probably not be affected deleteriously. Nevertheless, a growth chart should be kept on all children treated with stimulants so that the clinician might be alerted to the possible presence of growth inhibition. In such cases, dosage reduction as well as drug holidays should be considered.

For children on moderate to high doses, medication should not be terminated abruptly since doing so may lead to a marked worsening, even to the appearance of unusual behaviors during the withdrawal period.

Because of the stimulant properties of magnesium pemoline in adults, its efficacy in the treatment of hyperactive children was investigated in several well designed studies (Conners and co-workers, 1972; Page and co-workers, 1974). The major differences in the activity of the drug compared to other stimulants is a one to two week delay in inducing significant clinical effects and its long-acting property.

In contrast to the other stimulants, the use of magnesium pemoline necessitates blood tests for liver function at regular intervals since there may be an elevation SOGT values reported. The abnormality may not be sustained and its significance is unclear; nevertheless, discontinuation is called for if the pathological findings are consistent over time.

Phenothiazines and Other Neuroleptics

Total refractoriness to stimulant treatment is extremely rare (about 10% or less) but may occur. In some instances, there may be intolerance to the stimulants. In such cases, other therapeutic options exist. The child may be treated with phenothiazines or tricyclics.

The effects of phenothiazines are not as well documented as those of the stimulants. One study (Cytryn, Gilbert, and Eisenberg, 1960) failed to observe improvements differences between prochlorperazine and placebo in hyperactive children. In contrast, significant therapeutic effects have been found for chlorpromazine, thioridazine and haloperidol (Gittelman-Klein, and Klein, 1976; Greenberg, Deem, and McMahon, 1972; Weiss and co-workers, 1968; Werry, Weiss, and Douglass, 1966; Werry and Aman, 1975). Phenothiazines are as effective as stimulants in reducing the level of motor activity among hyperactive children. However, improvement with stimulants is broader than with phenothiazines. Though phenothiazines reduce motor activity, they do not affect other behaviors as markedly as the stimulants.

Dosages up to 200 mg equivalent of thioridazine or chlorpromazine are necessary. Beyond this level, no clinical advantage is accrued and side effects increase considerably. The side effects associated with phenothiazine treatment in children are very different from those associated with stimulants. Drowsiness and weight gain are typical. With thioridazine, enuresis (usually nocturnal, very occasionally diurnal as well) may occur.

Tricyclics

Imipramine has been demonstrated to improve the behavior of hyperkinetic children (Greenberg and co-workers, 1975; Rapoport and co-workers, 1974) and offers certain practical advantages in that it is long-acting, eliminating or reducing the need for multiple dosages through the day. Further, clinical side-effects are reported to be negligible. However, as with the phenothiazines, the effect of imipramine is not as complete as with stimulants and many children fail to sustain their initially good response (Gittelman-Klein, 1974). There have been recent reports of cardiotoxic EKG effects with imipramine treatment in children thereby limiting the potential usefulness of high dosage of this drug (for a review see Saraf and co-workers, 1978).

Length of Therapy

The question arises as to how long stimulants can be used in hyperkinetic children. It used to be thought that the disorder reflected a maturational lag, and did not linger beyond puberty. Hence, treatment was limited to middle childhood. Though the symptom of hyperactivity diminishes markedly with age, attentional and social handicaps frequently remain through adolescence (Minde, Weiss and co-workers, 1972; Weiss and co-workers, 1971).

In adulthood, impulsivity appears to be a continuing problem for a significant number of formerly hyperactive youngsters (Weiss, Hechtman, and Perlman (in press). Our own clinical experience, treating children into adolescence is that stimulants continue to exert a positive effect, without concurrent euphoria, in grown-up hyperkinetic children with residual symptomatology. The risk for amphetamine abuse has been invoked to argue against the use of stimulants at any age level. However, all data available so far have failed to reveal an increased prevalence of drug abuse in youngsters treated with stimulants (Laufer, 1971; Weiss and co-workers, in press).

Further, even this remote danger is markedly reduced, perhaps even eliminated with magnesium pemoline which does not have euphoriant effects at therapeutic dose levels and therefore would not trigger a possible vicious cycle of positive mood effect, tolerance, increased intake, and so on, eventuating in an addictive pattern. Interestingly, adults believed to have been hyperactive in childhood have been reported to respond to stimulant treatment (Wood, Reimherr, and Wender, 1976).

Many studies have used heterogeneous groups of children with a variety of behavior problems and learning problems. That in spite of the sample heterogeneity hyperactivity is regularly reduced by pharmacological treatment attests to the marked value of medications in this disorder. At the same time, it is also conceivable that the stimulants have a broader spectrum of action and could play a useful role in the treatment of other childhood behavior disorders. So far, this issue has not been studied systematically, and the only valid conclusion which may be drawn from the empirical findings available is the unequivocal value of stimulants in the treatment of the hyperkinetic syndrome.

Non-Treatment Factors Influencing Drug Response

Empirical findings are ambiguous regarding the contention that medications have a selective effect on brain damaged hyperactive children (Laufer and Denhoff, 1957; Satterfield, Cantwell, and Saul, 1973; Steinberg, Troshinsky, and Steinberg, 1971) have reported greater improvement in MBD children with both EEG and neurological abnormality as compared to MBD children without either EEG or neurological abnormality. However, the proportion of children improved in each group did not differ statistically. Further, it is conceivable that children with both EEG and neurological abnormality were more behaviorally disturbed, so that the difference in degree of improvement might reflect differences in symptomatology. Since the children were not selected for hyperactivity it is not known how many were hyperactive and therefore the generalizability of the findings is problematical.

In addition to the role of brain dysfunction in mediating drug response, the relationship of clinical improvement to other physiological characteristics, autonomic nervous system measures, such as skin resistance and CNS evoked potentials, has been examined (Buchsbaum and Wender, 1973; Halliday and co-workers, 1976; Prichep, Sutton, and Hakerem, 1976; Satterfield and co-workers, 1972).

On the whole, the research data support the notion that stimulant drugs activate the nervous system. As a result, it has been argued that hyperactive children who are "underaroused" are more likely to respond. The evidence bearing upon this point is contradictory. Though this work has considerable theoretical importance, it offers no guidance to the clinician as of yet.

Aspects of psychopathology not related to diagnosis such as severity or stability of symptoms do not discriminate between responders and non-responders. Environmental factors, such as quality of home and mother-child relationship, have failed also to relate to drug therapy outcome (Weiss and co-workers, 1968; Werry, Weiss, and Douglass, 1966).

Age is positively related to outcome. Young, preschool hyperactive children show a more variable response to the stimulants. The lack of drug effect in a large proportion of very young children as compared to older ones may reflect greater diagnostic ambiguity and therefore diagnostic inaccuracy among the younger group (Conners, 1975b; Schleifer, Weiss, and Cohen, 1975). At the same time, there is age-related physiological variability in drug metabolism which affects drug response.

In summary, it appears that brain dysfunction and level of physiological reactivity may be relevant dimensions in the prediction of drug effects among hyperactive children but these factors are not powerful predictors. One of the major difficulties in predicting hyperkinetic children's response to stimulants is the lack of variance in outcome. The vast majority of the treated children have a remarkably good short-term response. Therefore, in prediction research, one is faced with the task of identifying a rare event (non-response)-- a very difficult task.

STIMULANT VERSUS NON-PHARMACOLOGICAL TREATMENTS

Much controversy surrounds the use of medications for the management of behavior disorders in children. Behavior therapy has been suggested as an effective alternative to pharmacotherapy. Indeed, some investigators have demonstrated the clinical efficacy of behavioral techniques in hyperactive children. We have conducted a study comparing behavior modification techniques to methylphenidate in a large sample of hyperactive children. Children received either methylphenidate, behavior therapy with placebo, or behavior therapy with methylphenidate. Though all treatments produced clinical improvement, the combination of methylphenidate with behavior therapy was regularly the best, but not significantly superior to methylphenidate alone.

Children receiving medication were significantly more improved than the children who received behavior therapy and placebo. Therefore, though the behavioral techniques are useful interventions, they are not as effective as methylphenidate in hyperkinetic children (Gittelman-Klein and co-workers, 1979).

THEORIES OF PSYCHOSTIMULANT EFFECT AND HYPERKINESIS

Three major theories related to the action of stimulants of hyperkinesis have been advanced.

The first, a biological hypothesis, argues that a defect of central monamine synthesis leading to a dopamine deficiency accounts for the hyperkinetic syndrome (Wender, 1971, 1975). The clinical efficacy of dextroamphetamine can therefore be understood by its dopaminergic action. By normalizing dopamine levels, the drug reverses the basic pathophysiology. The argument that a single central biological defect is rectified by stimulants is spurred by the dramatic therapeutic impact of the drugs giving the impression that a specific crucial biochemical dysregulation has been reversed.

There has been no critical test of the dopamine theory of childhood hyperkinesis, though there is some data from animal and human research supporting the notion that dopamine levels and motor activity level are correlated (Shaywitz, Yager, and Klopper, 1976). Low levels of cerebrospinal HVA, the principal dopamine metabolite, have been found in a small group of hyperkinetic children (though the authors failed to account for the effect of probenecid on the level of HVA)(Shaywitz, Cohen, and Bowers, 1977). The finding is consonant with the dopamine theory of hyperkinesis.

However, problems also abound. It is not clear that all psychostimulants are good dopamine agonists. For instance, levoamphetamine has been reported relatively inactive in this respect, and yet seems no different from dextroamphetamine in overall clinical efficacy in the treatment of hyperkinesis. Even more problematic for the dopamine theory is the effectiveness of neuroleptics, since these are dopamine blockers. It is true that the impact of the neuroleptics is not as broad and dramatic as that of stimulants, yet, if low dopamine levels were the key to the behavior disorder, neuroleptics should aggravate the disorder not improve it. Moreover, if the dopamine theory were correct, a phenothiazine should interfere with the therapeutic impact of stimulants. Yet, we have found just the opposite: adding thioridazine to methylphenidate enhances the behavioral improvement obtained with the latter drug alone. Therefore, the pattern of drug effect in this disorder does not fit with the catecholamine hypothesis.

The other two theories of hyperkinesis are related and may be seen as consistent with the dopamine theory. They are a physiological and psychological theory which propose that the central basic dysfunction in hyperkinesis is a defect in attention regulating mechanisms, the physiological view is that the children are underaroused. The children are viewed as being unable primarily to sustain focused attention. Some of the children with this attentional difficulty go on to develop secondary symptoms such as hyperactivity, impulsivity, academic difficulties, etc. This view is being integrated in the nomenclature by the American Psychiatric Association Diagnostic and Statistical Manual (DSM III), since the hyperkinetic disorder has been renamed Attention Deficit Disorder with Hyperactivity.

In order to quantify attention dysregulation in hyperkinetic children, a number of psychophysiological indices, and stimulant effects on these measures have been studied. Central measures of arousal i.e., EEG variables, pupil diameter, as well as peripheral ones (such as heart rate, blood flow volume, skin conductance, and respiration rate) have been examined. The data obtained are far from conclusive with contradictory findings abounding. The evidence gives weak support to the notion that the attention deficit in hyperkinetic children consists of a lower level of arousal. In turn, the stimulants have been found, on some occasions, to normalize the arousal level (i.e., they stimulate CNS activity). It is therefore argued that the children are underactivated, that the stimulants bring them to a level of normal arousal. The theory further holds that improvement in ability to focus and sustain attention leads to a diminution of excessive motor activity, to less impulsive behavior, to general behavioral change.

There is no uniform finding that hyperkinetic children are physiologically under-aroused, and there is no unanimity concerning the expected negative relationship between level of arousal and positive drug effect (the expectation that the children with lower arousal should be better drug responders). As a matter of fact, one study using skin conductance level as a measure of arousal obtained results indicating that hyperkinetic children with relatively high level of arousal were the best responders (Zahn, Abate, and Little, 1975). Further, as of now, we are lacking the evidence that the various measures used to tap CNS activation are intercorrelated and cannot assume that they tap the same cerebral function.

Another problem for the attention theory of hyperkinesis is created by the failure to find that behavioral improvement is strongly correlated with improvement on cognitive measures used to estimate changes in attention (Gittelman-Klein and Klein, 1975). It is possible to improve measures of attention and CNS arousal with caffeine without affecting behavior significantly (1975b). The notion that the behavior of hyperkinetic children improves because their attentional processes have been ameliorated is unsupported. Furthermore, the postulation of a defect in attention is not essential to an explanation or theory of stimulant activity in hyperkinesis. It has been found that stimulants improve attention and reduce motor activity in children without clear attention deficits such as children with pure reading disabilities (Gittelman-Klein and Klein, 1976), and normal children (Rapoport, and co-workers, 1978). Consequently, evocation of defective dopamine levels or pathological arousal mechanisms are superfluous to an interpretation of the effect of psychostimulants on hyperkinetic children. What seems established conclusively is that there is no "paradoxical" stimulant effect on hyperactive youngsters -- their response is qualitatively similar to that of other children.

GENETICS OF HYPERKINESIS

All clinicians working with hyperkinetic children have been struck by the frequent report of similar behavior among the parents, especially the fathers, of such youngsters.

The notion that this disorder is associated with a specific familiar pattern of psychopathology has been advanced.

Several studies have investigated the diagnostic characteristics of parents of hyperactive children compared to normals. Morrison and Stewart (1971) reported a nonsignificant elevated prevalence for alcoholism and sociopathy in the fathers of hyperactive youngsters. Hysteria was more frequent in the mothers of the probands than among controls, also nonsignificant. The above clinical differences become significant when combined, and the overall level of psychiatric illness significantly differentiated the two groups of parents. Affective disorders were not found to be more frequent among the parents of the hyperactive children than among the controls.

In a further study, Stewart and Morrison (1973) compared the above two groups to the adoptive parents of 35 hyperactive children and failed to find a difference in prevalence of affective disorder among the three groups.

Cantwell (1975) evaluated the biological and adoptive parents of hyperactive children being treated in private and public facilities and parents of normal controls whose children were receiving routine pediatric care.

The natural fathers of the hyperactive children were found to have a higher rate of alcoholism than the nonbiological comparisons and the controls. The difference between the natural and adoptive fathers was significant; controls not being significantly different from them. In addition, these natural fathers were also rated as having significantly greater frequency of sociopathy than the adoptive or control parents.

The natural mothers of the hyperactive children were found to have a significantly higher rate of alcoholism and hysteria than the other two mother groups.

Combining all psychiatric findings, the natural mothers and fathers of hyperactive children had significantly more psychiatric disturbance than the adoptive parents of similar children, than parents of normal children.

The three groups were no different with regard to frequency of diagnosable affective disorders, either unipolar or bipolar.

The consistency in findings obtained in these two studies is striking and remarkable. A shortcoming is that the evaluations were not done blindly. These findings require corroboration.

A retrospective study of adopted male alcoholics also linked this adult disorder to the hyperactivity syndrome (Goodwin and co-workers, 1975). More reports of behavior difficulties in childhood, including hyperactivity, were obtained retrospectively in the histories of the alcoholic males than those of an adopted control group.

References

Buchsbaum, M., and P. Wender (1973). Average evoked responses in normal and minimally brain dysfunctioned children treated with amphetamine. Arch. Gen. Psychiat., 29, 764-770.

Cantwell, D. P. (1975). Genetic studies of hyperactive children: Psychiatric illness in biologic and adopting parents. In J. R. Morrison and M. A. Stewart (Eds.), Genetic Research in Psychiatry. University Press, New York. pp. 273-280.

Conners, C. K., E. Taylor, G. Meo, M. A. Kurtz, and M. Fournier (1972). Magnesium pemoline and dextroamphetamine: A controlled study in children with minimal brain dysfunction. Psychopharmacologia, 26, 321-336.

Conners, C. K. (1975a). Controlled trial of methylphenidate in preschool children with minimal brain dysfunction; in R. Gittelman-Klein (Ed.), Recent Advances in Psychopharmacology. Human Sciences Press, New York. pp. 64-78.

Conners, C. K. (1975b). A placebo-crossover study of caffeine treatment of hyperkinetic children; in R. Gittelman-Klein (Ed.), Recent Advances in Child Psychopharmacology. Human Sciences Press, New York. pp. 136-148.

Cytryn, L., L. Gilbert, and L. Eisenberg (1960). The effectiveness of tranquilizing drugs plus supportive psychotherapy in treating behavior disorders of children: A double blind study of eighty outpatients. Amer. J. Orthopsychiat., 30, 113-129.

Garfinkel, B., C. Webster, and J. Sloman (1975). Methylphenidate and caffeine in the treatment of children with minimal brain dysfunction. Amer. J. Psychiat., 132, 723-728.

Gittelman-Klein, R. (1974). Pilot clinical trial of imipramine in hyperkinetic children. In C. K. Conners (Ed.), Clinical Use of Stimulant Drug in Children. Excerpta Medica, The Hague. pp. 192-201.

Gittelman-Klein, R., and D. F. Klein (1975). Are behavioral and psychometric changes related in methylphenidate-treated hyperactive children? in R. Gittelman-Klein (Ed.), Recent Advances in Child Psychopharmacology. Human Sciences Press, New York. pp. 185-201.

Gittelman-Klein, R. and D. F. Klein (1976). Methylphenidate effects in learning disabilities. I. Psychometric changes. Arch. Gen. Psychiat., 33, 655-664.

Gittelman-Klein, R., H. Abikoff, E. Pollack, and D. F. Klein (1979). A controlled trial of behavior modification and methylphenidate in hyperactive children. In C. Whalen and B. Henker (Eds.). Hyperactive Children: The Social Ecology of Identification and Treatment. Academic Press, New York.

Gittelman-Klein, R., D. F. Klein, S. Katz, K. Saraf, and E. Pollack (1976). Comparative effects of methylphenidate and thioridazine in hyperkinetic children. Arch. Gen. Psychiat., 33, 1217-1231.

Goodwin, D. W., F. Schelsinger, L. Hermansen, S. B. Guze and G. Winokur (1975). Alcoholism and the hyperactive child syndrome. J. Nerv. Ment. Dis., 160, 349-353.

Greenberg, L. M., M. A. Deem, and S. McMahon (1972). Effects of dextroamphetamine, chlorpromazine and hydroxyzine on behavior and performance in hyperactive children. Amer. J. Psychiat., 129, 532-539.

Greenberg, L. M., A. M. Yellin, C. Spring, and M. Metcalf (1975). Clinical effects of imipramine and methylphenidate in hyperactive children. In R. Gittelman-Klein (Ed.), Recent Advances in Child Psychopharmacology. Human Sciences Press, New York.

Gross, M. D. (1976) Growth of hyperkinetic children taking methylphenidate, dextroamphetamine, or imipramine/desipramine. Pediatrics, 58, 424-431.

Halliday, R., J. H. Rosenthal, H. Naylor, and E. Callaway (1976). Averaged evoked potential predictors of clinical improvement in hyperactive children treated with methylphenidate: An initial study and replication. Psychophysiology, 13, 429-439.

Huestis, R. D., I. E. Arnold, and D. J. Smeltzer (1975). Caffeine versus methylphenidate and d-amphetamine in minimal brain dysfunction: A double-blind comparison. Am. J. Psychiat., 132, 868-870.

Laufer, M. (1971). Long-term management of some follow-up findings on the use of drugs with minimal brain dysfunction. Pediatrics, 39, 55-58.

Laufer, M. S., and E. Denhoff (1957). Hyperkinetic behavior syndrome in children. J. Pediat., 50, 463-474.

Minde, K., G. Weiss, and W. Mendelson (1972). A five year follow-up study of 91 hyperactive school children. J. Amer. Acad. Child Psychiat., 11, 595-610.

Page, J., J. Bernstein, R. Janicki, and F. Michelli (1974). A multiclinic trial of pemoline in childhood hyperkinesis. In: C. K. Conners (Ed.), Clinical Use of Stimulant Drugs in Children. Excerpta Medica, Amsterdam. pp. 98-123.

Prichep, L. S., S. Sutton, and C. Hakarem (1976). Evoked potentials in hyperkinetic and normal children under certainty and uncertainty: A placebo and methylphenidate study. Psychophysiology, 13, 419-428.

Rapoport, J. L., M. Buchsbaum, T. Zahn, H. Weingartner, C. Ludlow, and E. Mikkelsen (1978). Dextroamphetamine: Cognitive and behavioral effects in normal prepubertal boys. Science, 199, 511-514.

Rapoport, J. L., P. Quinn, G. Bradbard, D. Riddle, and E. Brookes. Imipramine and methylphenidate treatments of hyperactive boys: A double blind comparison. Arch. Gen. Psychiat., 30, 789-793.

Safer, D. J., and R. P. Allen (1975). Side effects from long-term use of stimulants in children. In R. Gittelman-Klein (Ed.), Recent Advances in Child Psychopharmacology. Human Sciences Press, New York. pp. 109-122.

Saraf, K. R., D. F. Klein, R. Gittelman-Klein, N. Gootman, and P. Greenhill (1977). EKG effects of imipramine treatment in children. J. Acad. Child Psychiat., 17, 60-69.

Satterfield, J. H., D. Cantwell, L. Lesser, and R. Podosin (1972). Physiological studies of the hyperkinetic child: I. Amer. J. Psychiat., 128, 1418-1424.

Satterfield, J. H., D. P. Cantwell, and R. E. Saul (1973). Response to stimulant drug treatment in hyperactive children: Prediction from EEG and neurological finding. J. Autism Child Schiz., 3, 36-48.

Schleifer, M., G. Weiss, and N. Cohen (1975). Hyperactivity in preschoolers and the effect of methylphenidate. Am. J. Orthopsychiat., 45, 38-50.

Schnackenburg, R. C. (1973). Caffeine as a substitute for Schedule II stimulants in hyperkinetic children. Amer. J. Psychiat., 130, 796-798.

Shaywitz, B. A., D. J. Cohen, and M. B. Bowers (1977). CSF monoamine metabolites in children with minimal brain dysfunction: Evidence for alteration of brain dopamine. J. Pediat., 90, 67-71.

Shaywitz, B. A., R. D. Yager, and H. J. Klopper (1976). An experimental model of minimal brain dysfunction (MBD) in developing rats. Science, 191, 305-307.

Steinberg, G. S., C. Troshinsky, and H. C. Steinberg (1971). Dextroamphetamine-responsive behavior disorder in school children. Amer. J. Psychiat., 128, 174-179.

Stewart, M. A., and J. R. Morrison (1973). Affective disorder among the relatives of hyperactive children. J. Child Psychol. Psychiat., 14, 209-212.

Weiss, G., L. Hechtman, and T. Perlman (in press). Hyperactive children as young adults: A controlled prospective 10 year follow-up of the psychiatric status of 75 hyperactive children. Arch. Gen. Psychiat.

Weiss, G., K. Minde, J. Werry, V. Douglas, and E. Nemeth (1971). Studies on the hyperactive child. Arch. Gen. Psychiat., 24, 409-414

Weiss, G., J. Werry, K. Minde, V. Douglas, and D. Sykes (1968). Studies on the hyperactive child. V. The effects of dextroamphetamine and chlorpromazine on behavior and intellectual functioning. J. Child Psychol. Psychiat., 9, 145-156.

Wender, P. H. (1971). Minimal Brain Dysfunction. Wiley and Sons, New York.

Wender, P. H. (1975). Speculations conceiving a possible biochemical basis of minimal brain dysfunction. in R. Gittelman-Klein (Ed.), Recent Advances in Child Psychopharmacology. Human Sciences Press, New York. pp. 14-30

Werry, J. S., and M. G. Aman (1975). Methylphenidate and haloperidol in children. Arch. Gen. Psychiat., 32, 790-795.

Werry, J. S., G. Weiss, and V. I. Douglas (1966). Studies on the hyperactive child. III. The effect of chlorpromazine upon behavior and learning ability. J. Am. Acad. Child Psychiat., 5, 292-312.

Wood, D. R., F. W. Reimherr, and P. H. Wender (1976). Diagnosis and treatment of minimal brain dysfunction in adults. Arch. Gen. Psychiat., 33, 1453-1460.

Zahn, T. P., F. Abate, and B. C. Little (1975). Minimal brain dysfunction, stimulant drugs, and autonomic nervous system activity. Arch. Gen. Psychiat., 32, 381-387.

Neuropsychopharmacology of Childhood Psychoses

M. CAMPBELL

Department of Psychiatry, New York University Medical Center,
550 First Avenue, New York, N.Y. 10016, U.S.A.

ABSTRACT

The interaction of clinical and basic research in the expansion of knowledge of central nervous system (CNS) biochemistry, childhood psychoses and treatment is presented. An overview of the literature on pre- and perinatal assaults of the CNS, physical, biochemical, and neuroendocrine findings in this population is given. The need for defining subgroups within the etiologically heterogeneous group of childhood psychotics by a variety of parameters is emphasized. The results of selected drug studies with both therapeutic and untoward effects are summarized. Methodologically sound studies, using objective rating scales and designed to answer crucial questions, are required in order to place the psychoactive drugs currently available for psychoses of childhood in the right perspective.

Keywords: Autism, Childhood schizophrenia, Subgroups, Clinical research, Basic research, Psychopharmacological treatment

The status of childhood psychoses remains unresolved: classification and diagnosis are subjects of emotional discussions among researchers. The clinician is often in a dilemma when assessing the young, severely disturbed child and planning treatment and disposition.

Eisenberg (1966) classified childhood psychoses into 2 major categories: those associated with impairment of brain tissue dysfunction (e.g. degenerative disorders, convulsive disorders, etc.) and those without known impairment of brain tissue function. The latter are subdivided into 5 groups, which include autistic psychoses, the schizophrenias, psychoses associated with maturation failure (e.g. childhood schizophrenia of Bender), folie à deux, and manic-depressive psychosis. The classification of the group for the Advancement of Psychiatry (GAP, 1966) is along similar lines. Kolvin (1971) divides psychoses into early onset (infantile) and late onset (childhood schizophrenia). The ICD-9 (International Classification of Diseases, Ninth Edition, 1977), a tri-axial classification system, lists infantile psychoses, disintegrative psychoses, schizophrenia, and manic-depressive illness. DSM II (1968) has included only childhood schizophrenia; DSM III (1978), a multi-axial classification system, discards childhood schizophrenia, and, under pervasive developmental disorders, lists infantile autism and atypical childhood psychosis, as well as residual state, for both. The ICD-9 category of disintegrative psychosis is being diagnosed as dementia, and manic-depressive illness is not listed. Fish (1975) and Bender (1967) maintain that infantile autism is the earliest expression of childhood schizophrenia; Rutter (1972) and Eisenberg (1972) consider these separate entities.

Several authors developed diagnostic criteria for infantile autism or childhood psychosis (Creak, 1964; Kanner, 1943; Rimland, 1964; Rutter, 1966, 1978); the diagnostic criteria of DSM III are based on the above. Infantile autism has an onset prior to 30 months of age, with symptoms of "autism," gross deficits in language, peculiar speech patterns, if speech exists, and bizarre responses to environment (resistance to change, peculiar attachments, etc.). The essential features of atypical childhood psychosis are a deep disturbance of relationship with people (lack of appropriate affective interaction, inappropriate clinging, lack of empathy, social ineptitude, etc.) and various bizarre behaviors (anxiety, unusual affective reactions, resistance to change, repetitive and ritualistic behavior, speech abnormalities, self-mutilation, etc.) developing between the ages of 30 months and 12 years.

Clearly, the diagnostic criteria are purely descriptive and thus not satisfactory for treatment plans. Since most childhood psychotics remain severely deviant throughout life, further basic and clinical research into neurophysiology, biochemistry, and neuroendocrinology is required as well as assessment of the impact of psychoactive medication in order to develop more rational therapies which take etiology into account.

Cohen and Young (1977), Fish and Ritvo (1978), and Ornitz and Ritvo (1976) have recently reviewed the research considering biological basis of infantile autism and the technical and methodological difficulties involved; these issues will not be discussed here.

Since the late nineteen fifties several investigators found serotonin abnormalities in whole blood and in efflux from blood platelets though not all concurred on the latter (for review, see Campbell and co-workers, 1975; Ritvo and co-workers, 1978). Since a significant elevation of blood serotonin levels was found in autistic children as compared to controls, Ritvo and co-workers (1971) wished to determine whether, by administration of L-dopa, a lowering of blood serotonin levels can be produced, and, if so, whether this will be accompanied by behavioral improvement. L-dopa was given to 4 autistics, ages 3 to 13 years, orally, over 6 months, in doses of 2,000 to 4,000 mgs per day, in a double-blind, controlled fashion. In the 3 younger children, ages 3 to 9 years, a significant decrease in blood serotonin was observed ($p = < .05$); however, no decrease in symptoms was noted. In a double-blind crossover study, Campbell and co-workers (1976b) administered L-dopa to 12 psychotic children, ages 3 to 6 9/12 years in daily doses of 900 to 2,250 mgs. Five of the 12 children showed clinical improvements though the changes did not reach statistical significance. The most marked effects were in decrease of negativism, and an increase in play, energy, and motor initiation in the 6 hypoactive children. Four of the children showed increase in language production, vocabulary, and affective responsiveness, and decrease in irritability. There was no relationship between behavioral and blood serotonin response to L-dopa; there was a 23% to 82% decrease of serotonin levels in 4 patients, none of whom showed global improvement; there was essentially no change in 3, and in 5 there was a 23% to 76% increase of serotonin levels. Luteinizing (LH) and follicle stimulating hormone (FSH) were elevated on baseline in plasma; no significant changes were seen during L-dopa administration, while prolactin decreased. Of the 12 children, 7 had retarded bone age; at termination, there was no change except for maturation. On the basis of these 2 studies no conclusions can be drawn, since both involved a small sample of patients and had methodological flaws.

If elevation of serotonin is a pathogenic factor in some autistic children, the increase of serotonin by imipramine administration could be related to the worsening of psychosis in half of a sample of 10 children (Campbell and co-workers, 1971b).

On the other hand, Cohen and Young (1977) suggest that an overactivity of dopaminergic system exists in autistic children, which is associated with stereotypies, and other abnormal motor movements. This is based on cerebrospinal fluid (CSF) studies and clinical observations. Administration of dopamine blocking psychoactive drugs, such as the neuroleptics, results in decrease of autistic symptoms, whereas the dopamine releasing stimulant drugs (e.g. amphetamines) usually yield worsening of preexisting symptoms in autistic children. The latter has been confirmed by clinical studies (Campbell and co-workers, 1972a, 1972b, 1976b; Fish, 1971). Regarding the suggestion that overactivity of dopaminergic systems may be one of the aspects of autism (Cohen and Young, 1977), it is noteworthy that in a crossover study (Campbell and co-workers, 1976b), an increase of preexisting stereotypies or stereotypies de novo were observed on daily doses of 300 to 2,250 mgs of L-dopa in 8 of the 12 subjects during dose regulation or on optimal doses. The same was recorded among other behavioral side effects in 9 of the 11 children, on 3.5 to 24.5 mgs of L-amphetamine.

However, clinical observations have indicated that even on very low doses of the sedative type of neuroleptics, such as chlorpromazine, the young autistic child may get excessively sedated, or disorganized. He responds more favorably to a "stimulating" type of neuroleptic, such as thiothixene, haloperidol, or trifluoperazine (Fish, 1970; for review, see Campbell, 1975, 1978a; Campbell and co-workers, 1978b; Engelhardt and co-workers, 1973; Faretra, Dooher and Dowling, 1970).

In a controlled study involving 40 autistic children, ages 2.6 to 7.2 years, haloperidol was statistically significantly superior to placebo or behavior therapy in decreasing symptoms of stereotypies and withdrawal in the children who were 4.5 years of age or older (Campbell and co-workers, 1978a). The combination of haloperidol and behavior therapy was significantly more effective in facilitating imitative speech than each given alone, or their respective placebo controls.

Research involving platelet monoamine oxidase (MAO) activity in autistic children (Campbell and co-workers, 1976a; Cohen, Young and Roth, 1977) did not reveal any abnormalities, as compared to the MAO activity of siblings, parents, and other children used as controls. MAO is thought of by some as a genetic marker in schizophrenia of adults (for review, see Campbell and co-workers, 1976a; Cohen and Young, 1977; Cohen, Young and Roth, 1977).

Studies of serum dopamine-β-hydroxylase (DBH) levels in autistic children showed a great variability (Coleman and others, 1974; Young, Ross and Cohen, 1977).

Clearly, more methodologically sound biochemical research is indicated in this area.

Systematic neuroendocrine studies are almost completely absent in this population. In a few studies involving small patient samples, evaluation of LH and/or FSH levels was reported (Campbell and co-workers, 1976b, 1978e). Because of a suggestion that some autistic children may have somewhat elevated levels of thyroxine iodine (T_4) (Campbell and co-workers, 1973), that retardation of bone age is frequent (Campbell and co-workers, 1976b, 1978e, 1978f; Dutton, 1964; Simon and Gillies, 1964), and that a hypothalamic dysfunction may exist in some of these children (Campbell and Hollander, in preparation), investigation of the thyroid system was initiated in a somewhat more systematic fashion.

Thyrotropin-releasing hormone (TRH) was given intravenously in a small pilot study involving 10 children, ages 2 6/12 to 7 7/12 years (Campbell and co-workers, 1978e). Timed venous samples were obtained for determination of the plasma triiodothyronine (T_3), thyroid stimulating hormone (TSH), and, in some patients, of prolactin. In most of the children the responses to TRH were compatible with, but not diagnostic of, hypothalamic disease. Blunted or delayed T_3 response, followed by slow and prolonged rise, and delayed, exaggerated, or subnormal TSH response were the most uniform and prominent features. One of the children was biochemically hyperthyroid, and another was so 8 months prior to TRH administration; neither showed clinical evidence of hyperthyroidism. It was suggested that a genetic vulnerability and/or associated pre- or perinatal insult to the brain may result in a variety of abnormalities, which include behavioral and neuroendocrine parameters.

In a study (Campbell and co-workers, 1978f) of 30 autistic children, ages 2 3/12 to 7 2/12 years, all of whom were euthyroid clinically, 13 had somewhat elevated T_3 levels on baseline (172 ng/100 ml; normal values for children 3 to 4 years, 138 $\pm$ 2.6 ng/100 ml; 5 to 7 years, 142 $\pm$ 4.7 ng/100 ml, Av Ruskin and others, 1973). Maintenance administration of T_3 to these 30 children under double blind conditions resulted in significant decrease of stereotypies at the hospital, and had a beneficial overall effect on autistic symptoms at home, as compared to placebo. Overall improvement appeared to correlate with changes in thyroxine (T_4) blood levels. Interestingly, in 3 children the bone age was retarded by more than 2SD on baseline; it became normal at the end of treatment. Elevated baseline T_3 level (299 ng/100 ml) returned to normal (188 ng/100 ml) in one child after a maintenance of L-dopa (Campbell and co-workers, 1976b).

Changes of behavioral and endocrine parameters with various biological treatments were investigated in schizophrenic adolescents and retarded children suggesting that simultaneous treatment of both parameters may yield better and more lasting behavioral results (Brambilla and Penati, 1971; Reiss, 1958). Reiss (1971), administering human chorionic gonadotropin (HCG) on long-term basis to socially deprived children with stunted linear and mental growth and retarded gonadal development, produced an increase in the rate of 17-ketosteroid excretion and in the rate of growth. This was associated with behavioral and academic improvement and rise in IQ. Increase in growth hormone (GH) content of blood was noted on the first day of therapy. Prior to HCG administration, these children failed to improve in an enriched therapeutic environment.

It is noteworthy that autistic children are shorter and have a retarded bone age when compared to children in the general population (Campbell, 1978b; Dutton, 1964; Simon and Gillies, 1964), and to their own siblings (Campbell, 1978b). Currently, we are analyzing growth hormone (GH) responses to oral L-dopa administration in a sample of preschool autistics (collaborative study with Dr. Edward J. Sachar).

Reports indicate that pre- and perinatal complications are more often found in autistics than in controls (for review, see Campbell, 1977; Folstein and Rutter, 1977; Ornitz and Ritvo, 1976), suggesting that there is an association between the two, though premature birth is not significantly associated with autism (Campbell and colleagues, 1978d; for review, see Ornitz and Ritvo, 1976). The high degree of central nervous system (CNS) involvement in some autistics could explain Fish's (1970) clinical observation that small doses of the "sedative" type of neuroleptic, such as chlorpromazine, lead to sedation in the autistic child, while a therapeutic response may be elicited by the more stimulating agents, such as trifluperidol (Fish and co-workers, 1969), haloperidol (Campbell and co-workers, 1978a), thiothixene (Campbell and co-workers, 1970; Simeon and co-workers, 1973), and molindone (Campbell and co-workers, 1971a; for review, see Campbell, 1973, 1978a; Simeon, 1976). In a trial of L-dopa (Campbell and co-workers, 1976b), children who responded to the drug had a variety of pre- and perinatal complications, while those who failed to respond had none. However, in another study, involving T_3 administration, there was no association between complications of pregnancy and clinical response to drug (Campbell and co-workers, 1978f).

Minor physical or congenital anomalies stemming from embryonic and early fetal maldevelopment have a high incidence in various developmental disorders, including autism (Campbell and co-workers, 1978c; Links and co-workers, 1978). It was suggested (Steg and Rapoport, 1975; Waldrop and Halverson, 1971) that the high incidence of these anomalies may be associated with a genetically determined behavioral disorder, or it could be a result of a CNS insult during embryonic or early fetal development. In a study (Campbell and co-workers, 1978c) involving 52 autistic children, ages 2 6/12 to 5 11/12 years (mean, 3.8 years), the total number of anomalies and the weighted anomaly scores were significantly higher than for either their siblings or the normal controls. The correlation between scores of patients and their siblings was not significant (0.203, $p > .05$). Of the 52 patients, 17 had a history of complications during the first trimester of pregnancy; the anomaly scores were higher in this group than in the rest of the patients though the difference did not reach statistical significance.

We plan to investigate the relationship between complications of pregnancy, minor physical anomalies, IQs, symptoms and clinical response to psychoactive agents. Complications of pregnancy are rated on a questionnaire developed by us (Campbell, 1977) which represents a template to the CPDI and CSH of the ECDEU Pediatric Packet of NIMH (Psychopharmacology Bulletin, 1973). In 2 studies (Campbell and co-workers, 1978f; Fish and co-workers, 1966) the drug responders were those children with lower IQs. There is still a controversy concerning the effect of neuroleptics on learning; systematic research is needed in this area. Werry and Aman (1975) have shown that in non-psychotic children the adverse effect of haloperidol on learning was an effect of dose. We found no such effect of this drug at optimal doses (mean, 1.65 mg/day) in young autistic children (Campbell and co-workers, 1978a). However, at doses above optimal, sedation and motor retardation were the most common side effects, and clearly a function of dose. In addition to behavioral symptoms, we plan to investigate the effects of haloperidol on discrimination learning and selective attention, with the aid of an automated data collection system, and to correlate these dependent variables with bioavailability of drug. We will be using both subjective (Children's Psychiatric Rating Scale, CPRS, Psychopharmacology Bulletin, 1973; Children's Behavior Inventory, CBI, Burdock and Hardesty, 1967) and objective (Cohen, Anderson and Campbell, 1978) rating scales. Assessing the frequency of behavior by objective scales seems to be particularly useful in retarded (Sprague and Baxley, 1978) and autistic children (Cohen, Anderson and Campbell, 1978).

A few reports indicate that after withdrawal of neuroleptics some children may develop symptoms resembling tardive dyskinesia of adults (Engelhardt and Polizos, 1978; McAndrew, Case and Treffert, 1972). We will investigate the occurrence of this syndrome in our long-term prospective study of haloperidol.

In summary, there is a great need for defining subgroups within the etiologically heterogeneous childhood psychotics by a variety of parameters (Conners and Applebee, 1978). Methodologically sound studies designed to answer crucial questions, using objective rating scales, are required in order to place the role of currently available psychoactive drugs in the right perspective: are they helpful in the management or in the treatment of autistic children?

ACKNOWLEDGMENT

This work was supported by United States Public Health Service Grant MH 04665 from the National Institute of Mental Health.

REFERENCES

AvRuskin, T. W., S. C. Tang, L. Shenkman, T. Mitsuma, and C. S. Hollander (1973). Serum triiodothyronine concentrations in infancy, childhood, adolescence and pediatric thyroid disorders. J. Clin. Endocrinol. Metab., 37 (No. 2), 235-237.

Bender, L. (1967). Theory and treatment of childhood schizophrenia. Acta Paedopsychiat., 34, 298-307.

Brambilla, F. and G. Penati (1971). Hormones and behavior in schizophrenia. In D. H. Ford (Ed.), Influence of Hormones on the Nervous System. Karger, Basel. pp. 482-494.

Burdock, E. I. and A. S. Hardesty (1967). Contrasting behavior patterns of mentally retarded and emotionally disturbed children. In J. Zubin and G. A. Jervis (Eds.), Psychopathology of Mental Development. Grune & Stratton, New York. pp. 370-386.

Campbell, M. (1973). Biological interventions in psychoses of childhood. J. Autism Child. Schizo., 3, 347-373.

Campbell, M. (1975). Pharmacotherapy in early infantile autism. Biol. Psychiat. 10, 399-423.

Campbell, M. (1977). Demographic parameters of disturbed children: A template to the CPDI and CSH, its rationale and significance. Psychopharm. Bull., 13, 30-33.

Campbell, M. (1978a). The use of drug treatment in infantile autism and childhood schizophrenia. A review. In M. A. Lipton, A. DiMascio, and K. F. Killam (Eds.), Psychopharmacology: A Generation of Progress. Raven Press, New York. pp. 1451-1461.

Campbell, M. (1978b). Early detection, diagnosis, treatment and outcome: Seventeen years of work with autistic children. Annual Meeting and Conference of the National Society for Autistic Children, Dallas, Texas, June 29-July 1, 1978.

Campbell, M., B. Fish, T. Shapiro, and A. Floyd, Jr. (1970). Thiothixene in young disturbed children: A pilot study. Arch. Gen. Psychiat., 23, 70-72.

Campbell, M., B. Fish, T. Shapiro, and A. Floyd, Jr. (1971a). Study of molindone in disturbed preschool children. Curr. Therap. Res., 13, 28-33.

Campbell, M., B. Fish, T. Shapiro, and A. Floyd, Jr. (1971b). Imipramine in preschool autistic and schizophrenic children. J. Autism Child. Schizo., 1, 267-282.

Campbell, M., B. Fish, R. David, T. Shapiro, P. J. Collins, and C. Koh (1972a). Response to triiodothyronine and dextroamphetamine: A study of preschool schizophrenic children. J. Autism Child. Schizo., 2, 343-358.

Campbell, M., B. Fish, T. Shapiro, and A. Floyd, Jr. (1972b). Acute responses of schizophrenic children to a sedative and a "stimulating" neuroleptic: A pharmacologic yardstick. Curr. Therap. Res., 14, 759-766.

Campbell, M., B. Fish, R. David, T. Shapiro, P. J. Collins, and C. Koh (1973). Liothyronine treatment in psychotic and nonpsychotic children under six years. Arch. Gen. Psychiat., 29, 602-608.

Campbell, M., E. Friedman, W. H. Green, P. J. Collins, A. M. Small, and H. Breuer (1975). Blood serotonin in schizophrenic children. A preliminary study. Int. Pharmacopsychiat., 10, 213-221.

Campbell, M., E. Friedman, W. H. Green, A. M. Small, and E. I. Burdock (1976a). Blood platelet monoamine oxidase activity in schizophrenic children and their families: A preliminary study. Neuropsychobiology, 2, 239-246.

Campbell, M., A. M. Small, P. J. Collins, E. Friedman, R. David, and N. B. Genieser (1976b). Levodopa and levoamphetamine: A crossover study in schizophrenic children. Curr. Therap. Res., 18, 70-86.

Campbell, M., L. T. Anderson, M. Meier, I. L. Cohen, A. M. Small, C. Samit, and E. J. Sachar (1978a, in press). A comparison of haloperidol and behavior therapy and their interaction in autistic children. J. Amer. Acad. Child Psychiat.

Campbell, M., B. Geller, I. L. Cohen (1978b, in press). Current status of drug research and treatment with autistic children. J. Ped. Psychol.

Campbell, M., B. Geller, A. M. Small, T. Petti, and S. Ferris (1978c). Minor physical anomalies in young psychotic children. Amer. J. Psychiat., 135, 573-575.

Campbell, M., A. S. Hardesty, E. I. Burdock, P. A. Cleary, N. Polevoy, and B. Geller (1978d). Demographic and paranatal profile of 105 autistic children. A preliminary report. Psychopharm. Bull., 14, 36-39.

Campbell, M., C. S. Hollander, S. Ferris, and L. W. Greene (1978e, in press). Response to thyrotropin-releasing hormone stimulation in young psychotic children. A pilot study. Psychoneuroendocrinology.

Campbell, M., A. M. Small, C. S. Hollander, J. Korein, I. L. Cohen, M. Kalmijn, and S. Ferris (1978f, in press). A controlled crossover study of triiodothyronine in autistic children. J. Autism Child. Schizo.

Cohen, D. J., and J. G. Young (1977). Neurochemistry and child psychiatry. J. Amer. Acad. Child Psychiat., 16, 353-411.

Cohen, D. J., J. G. Young, and J. A. Roth (1977). Platelet monoamine oxidase in early childhood autism. Arch. Gen. Psychiat., 34, 534-537.

Cohen, I. L., L. T. Anderson, and M. Campbell (1978, in press). Measurement of drug effects in autistic children. Psychopharm. Bull.

Coleman, M., M. Campbell, L. S. Freedman, M. Roffman, R. P. Ebstein, and M. Goldstein (1974). Serum dopamine-B-hydroxylase levels in Down's syndrome. Clin. Genetics, 5, 312-315.

Conners, C. K., and A. Applebee (1978, in press). Methods for delineating subtypes of minimal brain dysfunction. J. Abnormal Child Psychol.

Creak, M. (1964). Schizophrenic syndrome in childhood. Further progress report of a working party (April 1964). Develop. Med. Child Neurol., 6, 530-535.

Diagnostic and Statistical Manual of Mental Disorders (DSM II) (1968). 2nd ed. American Psychiatric Association, Washington, D.C.

Diagnostic and Statistical Manual of Mental Disorders (DSM III) (1978). 3rd ed. American Psychiatric Association, Washington, D.C.

Dutton, G. (1964). The growth pattern of psychotic boys. Brit. J. Psychiat., 110, 101-103.

Eisenberg, L. (1966). The classification of the psychotic disorders in childhood. In L. D. Eron (Ed.), The Classification of Behavior Disorders. Aldine Publishing Company, Chicago. pp. 87-114.

Eisenberg, L. (1972). The classification of childhood psychosis reconsidered. J. Autism Child. Schizo., 2, 338-342.

Engelhardt, D. M., P. Polizos, J. Waizer, and S. P. Hoffman (1973). A double-blind comparison of fluphenazine and haloperidol. J. Autism Child. Schizo., 3, 128-137.

Engelhardt, D. M., and P. Polizos (1978). Adverse effects of pharmacotherapy in childhood psychosis. In M. A. Lipton, A. DiMascio, and K. F. Killam (Eds.), Psychopharmacology: A Generation of Progress. Raven Press, New York. pp. 1463-1469.

Faretra, G., L. Dooher, and J. Dowling (1970). Comparison of haloperidol and fluphenazine in disturbed children. Amer. J. Psychiat., 126, 1670-1673.

Fish, B. (1970). Psychopharmacologic response of chronic schizophrenic adults as predictors of responses in young schizophrenic children. Psychopharm. Bull., 6, 12-15.

Fish, B. (1971). The "one child, one drug" myth of stimulants in hyperkinesis. Importance of diagnostic categories in evaluating treatment. Arch. Gen. Psychiat., 25, 193-203.

Fish, B. (1975). Biological antecedents of psychosis in children. In D. X. Freedman (Ed.), The Biology of the Major Psychoses: A Comparative Analysis. Raven Press, New York. pp. 59-83.

Fish, B., T. Shapiro, and M. Campbell (1966). Long term prognosis and the response of schizophrenic children to drug therapy: a controlled study of trifluoperazine. Amer. J. Psychiat., 123, 32-39.

Fish, B., M. Campbell, T. Shapiro, and A. Floyd, Jr. (1969). Comparison of trifluperidol, trifluoperazine and chlorpromazine in pre-school schizophrenic children: The value of less sedative antipsychotic agents. Curr. Therap. Res., 11, 589-595.

Fish, B., and E. R. Ritvo (1978, in press). Psychosis of childhood. In J. D. Noshpitz (Ed.), Basic Handbook of Child Psychiatry. Basic Books, New York.

Folstein, S., and M. Rutter (1977). Genetic influences and infantile autism. Nature, 265, 726-728.

Group for the Advancement of Psychiatry (GAP) (1966). Psychopathological disorders in childhood: Theoretical considerations and a proposed classification. Vol. VI, Report No. 62.

ICD-9, International Classification of Diseases (1977). Manual of the International Statistical Classification of Diseases, Injuries and Causes of Death. Vol. I, World Health Organization, Geneva.

Kanner, L. (1943). Autistic disturbances of affective contact. Nervous Child, 2, 217-250.

Kolvin, I. (1971). Psychoses in childhood - A comparative study. In M. Rutter (Ed.), Infantile Autism: Concepts, Characteristics and Treatment. Churchill Livingstone, Edinburgh. pp. 7-26.

Links, P. S., M. Mastronardi, F. Abichandani, and J. Simeon (1978). Minor physical anomalies in autism: their relationship to pre- and perinatal complications. Paper presented at the Canadian Psychiatric Association Annual Meeting.

McAndrew, J. B., Q. Case, and D. A. Treffert (1972). Effects of prolonged phenothiazine intake on psychotic and other hospitalized children. J. Autism Child. Schizo., 2, 75-91.

Ornitz, E. M., and E. R. Ritvo (1976). The syndrome of autism: A critical review. Amer. J. Psychiat., 133, 609-621.

Psychopharmacology Bulletin, Special Issue (1973). Pharmacotherapy of Children.

Reiss, M. (1958) (Ed.), Psychoendocrinology. Grune & Stratton, New York.

Reiss, M. (1971). Clinical and basic neuroendocrine investigations in some states of mental retardation. In D. H. Ford (Ed.), Influence of Hormones on the Nervous System. Karger, Basel.

Rimland, B. (1964). Infantile Autism. Appleton-Century-Crofts, New York.

Ritvo, E. R., A. Yuwiler, E. Geller, A. Kales, S. Rashkis, A. Schicor, S. Plotkin, R. Axelrod, and C. Howard (1971). Effects of L-dopa in autism. J. Autism Child. Schizo., 1, 190-205.

Ritvo, E. R., K. Rabin, A. Yuwiler, B. J. Freeman, and E. Geller (1978). Biochemical and hematologic studies: A critical review. In M. Rutter and E. Schopler (Eds.), Autism. A Reappraisal of Concepts and Treatment. Plenum Press, New York. pp. 163-183.

Rutter, M. (1966). Behavioural and cognitive characteristics of a series of psychotic children. In J. K. Wing (Ed.), Early Childhood Autism, Clinical, Educational and Social Aspects. Pergamon Press, Oxford. pp. 51-81.

Rutter, M. (1972). Childhood schizophrenia reconsidered. J. Autism Child. Schizo., 2, 315-337.

Rutter, M. (1978). Diagnosis and definition. In M. Rutter and E. Schopler (Eds.), Autism. A Reappraisal of Concepts and Treatment. Plenum Press, New York. pp. 1-25.

Simeon, J. (1976). Pediatric psychopharmacology - A review of our findings and experience. In D. V. Sankar (Ed.), Psychopharmacology of Childhood. P.J.D. Publications Ltd., Westbury, New York. pp. 140-178.

Simeon, J., B. Saletu, M. Saletu, T. M. Itil, and J. DaSilva (1973). Thiothixene in childhood psychoses. Presented at the Third International Symposium on Phenothiazines, Rockville, Maryland.

Simon, G. B. and S. M. Gillies (1964). Some physical characteristics of a group of psychotic children. Brit. J. Psychiat., 110, 104-107.

Sprague, R. L. and G. B. Baxley (1978). Drugs used for the management of behavior in mental retardation. In J. Wortis (Ed.), Mental Retardation, Vol. 10. Grune & Stratton, New York. pp. 92-107.

Steg, J. P. and J. L. Rapoport (1975). Minor physical anomalies in normal, neurotic, learning disabled, and severely disturbed children. J. Autism Child. Schizo., 5, 299-307.

Waldrop, M., and C. E. Halverson (1971). Minor physical anomalies and hyperactive behavior in young children. In J. Hellmuth (Ed.), Exceptional Infant. Studies of Abnormalities, Vol. II. Brunner/Mazel, New York. pp. 343-380.

Werry, J.S. and M. G. Aman (1975). Methylphenidate and haloperidol in children. Arch. Gen. Psychiat., 32, 790-795.

Young, G., N. Ross, and D. J. Cohen (1977). Serum dopamine-beta-hydroxylase activity: clinical applications in child psychiatry. Presented at the Twenty-Fourth Annual Meeting of the American Academy of Child Psychiatry, Houston, Texas, October 19-23, 1977.

Neurophysiology and Child Psychiatry

JOVAN SIMEON* and BERND SALETU**

*Professor of Psychiatry, Department of Psychiatry, School of Medicine, University of Ottawa, Ottawa, Ontario
**Dozent, Section of Pharmacopsychiatry, Psychiatrisvhe Universitätsklinik Wien, Austria

ABSTRACT

The usefulness of the conventional EEG in psychiatry has been very limited, as the complex EEG variables cannot be analysed. In child psychiatry EEG abnormalities usually confirm the presence of organic pathology, and are neither diagnostic, nor useful as a guide to therapy. Computerized EEG analyses and other special techniques (evoked potential, sleep, CNV) have greatly facilitated neurophysiological research in children, resulting in significant findings in behavioural and sleep disorders, psychosis, mental retardation, etc. Advances have been made in the study of normal and abnormal development, and of differences between various diagnostic groups; the identification of high-risk children; the classification of specific EEG patterns of psychotropic drugs; the use of drugs to explore behavioural-neurophysiological associations and differences between drug-responders and non-responders, and in the identification of predictors of therapeutic outcome. Neurophysiological investigations of brain mechanisms and their association with clinical, biological and psychological phenomena may provide a more scientific basis for a classification of psychiatric disorders and the selection of therapy in children. The clinical significance of the various neurophysiological findings in relation to psychiatric diagnosis, therapy, and prognosis remains to be clarified.

I INTRODUCTION

Neurophysiological research has contributed very little to the diagnosis and therapy of the vast majority of children with psychiatric disorders. New strategies in the study of the behavioral significance of neurophysiological findings indicate that we are only beginning to understand the complex dynamic integration of the whole brain in relation to conscious experience, cognitive processes, memory and psychopathology. The mechanisms of arousal, habituation, language, attention and hemispheric specialization are of special relevance to child psychiatry disorders such as developmental delays, infantile autism, dyslexia, hyperkinesis and sleep disorders.

The conventional visual analysis of the EEG applications in psychiatry suffers from severe limitations, since the complexity of variables, minute pattern alterations, activity in the very fast frequencies, and variability of frequency and amplitude over relatively long periods of time cannot be adequately measured, and therefore are usually reduced to various so-called EEG abnormalities or normal variations. Recently, various computerised quantification techniques have been applied in the recording and analysis of human brain functions. The electronic processing of conventional EEG data and their further automated evaluation has been applied in pediatrics in the study of maturational processes, metabolic disorders, mental retardation, and sleep and neurological impairment (Dumermuth, 1971).

In this paper neurophysiological findings in child psychiatry disorders, pediatric psychopharmacology and sleep studies in children will be briefly reviewed.

II Child Psychiatry Disorders

A. Behaviour disorders:

In general, children with psychiatric disorders have a high incidence of EEG abnormalities which are consistently greater than in normal children (Harris,1977). These abnormalities depend more upon co-existing neurological defects, even slight, than upon a particular psychiatric condition, and are rarely a guide to the management or drug treatment of a patient. The main indication for EEG in child psychiatry remains the confirmation of a presence of organic disorders. There is frequent parallelism between the clinical and the EEG improvement, indicating the functional rather than the structural implications of EEG abnormalities in many children. EEG abnormalities tend to diminish or disappear during later childhood, adolescence and early adulthood (Harris,1977).

The inclusion of children with organic brain disorders confuses the relevance of the EEG abnormality to the various psychiatric disorders. In children with affective disorders only, EEG abnormalities are around 20% (Lairy and Harrison,1968). If children with epilepsy, neurological defects and an I.Q. below 70 to 75 are excluded, the percentage of EEG abnormalities in behavior disorders is about 40% to 50% (Aird and Yamamoto,1966; Bayrakal,1965; Spilimbergo and Nissen,1971). About 40% of children with minimal brain dysfunction have EEG abnormalities (Capute et al.,1968; Paine et al.,1968). A high correlation was found between an abnormal EEG, and poor impulse control and motor incoordination (Bayrakal, 1965). In 53% of hyperkinetic children with epilepsy or some neurological defects an EEG abnormality is found, while 30% of those with no neurological problems or epilepsy have abnormal EEGs (Klinkerfuss et al.,1965). The most common abnormality was an excess of slow wave activity, with focal findings predominant in children with neurological impairment. Children with school behaviour problems but no neurological disease have greater slow EEG activity than normal controls, indicating brain dysfunction (Wikler et al.,1970). The EEG abnormalities found by various authors include a variety of phenomena such as 6-7 and 14/ sec. positive spikes, slow waves, sharp waves, excessive theta and persistent after-effects in response to hyperventilation. The most prominent finding is an excess of slow waves. The significance of these abnormalities is complicated by the presence of spikes, sharp waves and large amplitude slow waves in focal or diffuse bursts in 15% of normal children (Eeg-Olofsson,1970), while only 68% of normal children have a "normal" EEG free from any paroxysmal or slow wave activity. Further, the 14 and 6/sec. positive spikes were found in 58% of normal 13-15 year old boys (Lombroso, et al.,1966). Some investigators have attempted to correlate particular abnormalities with specific symptoms (Stevens et al.,1968; Lucas et al.,1965), but in general, although focal changes may predominate in neurologically handicapped children, there are no positive correlations between the type and location of EEG abnormality and the different kinds of behavioural disorders. In 6 to 14 year old patients with psychomotor and language problems but no evidence of epilepsy or encephalopathy, with an IQ above 75 and spike foci, motor problems occurred most often with rolandic unilateral spikes; visual or oculomotor problems with occipital foci; and perceptual motor problems with left occipital foci; multiple symptoms were found in children with multiple spikes (Lairy et al.,1969). Clinical improvement was paralleled by EEG improvement, but half of the patients with persistent focal abnormalities continued to have clinical - mainly affective - problems. None of those with spike foci developed epilepsy, and anticonvulsant drugs were never given. The presence of spikes was seen as a sign of cerebral dysfunction in the immature brain. The view that children with behaviour disorders with spike discharges do not benefit from anticonvulsants is reinforced by other similar findings (Egli et al.,1975).

Neurophysiological studies may clarify the possible relationship between hyperkinetic, and antisocial and delinquent behaviour. In delinquents 13 to 18 years of age, free from organicity or mental retardation, no significant EEG difference from normal boys of the same age were reported in one study (Wiener et al.,1966). Diffuse EEG abnormalities in children with antisocial and aggressive behaviour (Stevens, et al., 1968) and excessive EEG slow wave activity in hyperkinetic children (Capute et al.,1968; Hughes,1971; Klinkerfuss et al.,1965) and sociopaths (Hare,1970; Klinkerfuss et al.,1965) have been reported in a number of studies. Violent patients often have diffuse slow wave EEG activity. About half sociopathic patients have an EEG abnormality (Hill and Watterson, 1942), which is not specific and is not limited to the temporal lobe. Abnormal EEGs have also been found in unmotivated and psychotic murderers, and recurrently violent individuals (Bender, 1959; Sayed, et al., 1969). While focal (predominantly temporal lobe) EEG abnormalities have been found in 67% of children with behaviour disorders (Aird and Yamamoto, 1966), others have reported negative correlations between focal EEG abnormalities and antisocial and aggressive children (Stevens, et al., 1968; Stevens, 1970). In hyperkinetic and aggressive children a statistically significant correlation between the computer analysed EEG measurements, and conduct and anti-social factors derived from teachers' ratings (Conners,1979) was found. Children with greater aggression scores had more amplitude variability in their EEGs, and smaller amounts of fast frequencies (Simeon,1975).

Event-related potentials (ERP) have been a most active area of human neurophysiology research as they reflect specific mental functions (John et al.,1977). Children with learning disabilities and hyperkinesis have been most often investigated. Differences in ERP amplitude responses between dyslexics and good readers have been reported (Conners,1971). Language underachievers have shown left hemispheric departure from normal ERP patterns, while arithmetic underachievers showed a markedly different pattern (H.Ahn, unpublished doctoral dissertation). In groups of children with learning disabilities, left parietal components of the visual evoked potentials (VEP) were attenuated, latencies in the occipital region increased (Conners,1971), while others reported smaller amplitudes and longer latencies (Satterfield et al.,1973,1974). In dull children VEPs were different from those in bright children, and poor readers had unusual wave forms. In specific reading difficulties the percentage of EEG abnormality is similar to a clinically mixed group of children with behaviour disorders (Ayers and Torres,1967).

Using computerised analysis of the EEG, hyperactives were found to have less power (power density spectra) in the 10 cps band and significantly higher within hemisphere coherence (up to 8 cps) than controls (Montagu,1975). In dyslexics there was more energy in the 3-7 cps and 16-32 cps bands compared to normals, and the most discriminating feature was the pattern of coherence between various scalp leads: normals had greater coherences between symmetrical positions in both hemispheres (Sklar, et al.,1972,1973). In a group of learning disabled (LD) children compared to normals, factor analysed EEG variables could discriminate better between LD and normal children than psychometric measures. Stepwise discriminant function analyses were able to identify 5 subgroups of LD children. The auditory evoked responses (AERs) in 3 different evoked potential (EP) conditions showed distinctive features for each sub-group (John et al.,1977). In behaviourally disturbed children, significant correlations were found between the quantitative and qualitative EEG changes and the behavioural changes (Itil et al.,1967).

The measurement of the contingent negative variation (CNV) is another new avenue in the study of the development of the neurophysiological correlates of attention and learning (Tecce,1971; Tecce and Scheff,1969). Therefore, it could be a useful approach in the study of hyperkinesis and other attention deficit disorders. In 3-year-olds the CNV response is much larger and persistent than in adults. The response highly correlated with general interest, attention and motivation (Gullickson,1971). In 2-year-olds both attention and CNV are diminished. CNV was absent in dyslexic children.

B. Childhood Psychoses

A variety of electroencephalographic (EEG) investigations have been undertaken to clarify the nature of childhood psychosis and determine its neurophysiological correlates. While the EEG findings indicate significant neurobiological differences between psychotic children and normal controls, the problems of etiology, classification, and differential diagnosis remain confused (Simeon and Itil,1975). High incidences of abnormal EEGs have been reported in many studies of psychotic, schizophrenic, and autistic children (Jasper et al.,1938; Kennard,1947,1948,1953; Cattell and Pacella,1950; Ingvar and Koersner,1952; Schain and Yannet,1960; Bray,1962; Goldman and Rosenberg, 1962; Chao,1963; White et al.,1964; Hutt et al.,1964, 1965; Fish and Shapiro,1965; Ward and Hoddinott,1965; Creak and Pampiglione,1969; Kolvin et al.,1971) ranging from about one-third (Kolvin et al.,1971) to 83% (Creak and Pampiglione, 1969) of the cases studied. Significant changes of the EEGs of psychotic children have been reported following convulsive therapy (Kennard,1948) and pharmacotherapy (Goldman and Rosenberg,1962). EEG abnormalities have been correlated with the presence of psychosis or severe neurosis in the family (Kennard,1947), lower age (Kennard,1948), stereotypies (Hutt et al.,1964), severity of illness (Goldman and Rosenberg,1962), and seizure activity (Schain and Yannet,1960; Bray,1962; Chao,1963; White et al.,1964; Kolvin et al.,1971), the range of the latter varying in different series from 13% to 42%. These EEG abnormalities were most often characterized by irregular paroxysmal spike and wave complexes (White et al.,1964), or low voltage irregular activity without a dominant rhythm ("flat" records) (Hutt, et al.,1964; Kolvin et al.,1971). More recent studies of the electrical brain activity of psychotic children generated during sleep and dreaming (Ornitz et al., 1968; Ornitz et al.,1969), and evoked by external sensory stimuli (Hermelin and O'Connor,1968; Small,1970; Walter et al.,1970) indicate differences in patterns from those of normal controls.

It is difficult to interpret these EEG findings and to relate them to diagnostic categories of unknown etiology, since the EEG is only an expression of brain function. Not all psychotic children manifest EEG abnormalities and normal variations, and when present, these are neither pathognomonic nor diagnostic. Further, criteria for EEG normality vary, as only 68% of children selected as normal according to strict criteria have a totally normal EEG (Eeg-Olofsson,1971). In such normal children, nonrhythmic low frequency at rest, paroxysmal effects, and 14 and 6 cps spike activity were manifested in 14%, 15%, and 16%, respectively. Further longitudinal studies will be required to obtain normative EEG data, and to determine whether some EEG characteristics in normal children are a variation of normal maturation or an unknown minor brain injury (Eeg-Olofsson,1971).

In our studies of a heterogenous group of psychotic children, we have used averaged evoked potential responses and computerised EEG (CEEG) analysis, including period analysis, amplitude variability and analog frequency analysis. We investigated psychotic children before and after pharmacotherapy (Simeon et al.,1974), and compared them to normal controls and high risk for schizophrenia children (Itil et al.,1976; Simeon and Itil,1975; Saletu et al.,1975b). The evoked potentials (visual, auditory and somatosensory) showed significant differences between the psychotic children and the normal controls (Saletu et al.,1975a). The EP latencies of psychotic children were shorter and the amplitudes smaller than in the normals. There were also significant hemispheric differences, as well as differences in the variabilities of the latency and amplitude, and in habituation. The "high risk" children also had shorter EP latencies than a control group. The decrease of the EP latencies found in the psychotic and "high risk" children (Saletu et al.,1975b) have also been reported in adult schizophrenics (Saletu et al.,1973). In the CEEG analyses the psychotic children had a significantly greater percentage of slow activity and of fast activity, and higher frequency and frequency deviation. High risk children also had more slow, more fast, and less alpha activity, as well as a decrease of the average absolute amplitude, as compared to matched normal controls. Findings in these two groups of children are similar to those in adult schizophrenics (Itil et al.,1972; Itil et al.,1974). Based on step-wise discriminant function analysis of the EP and CEEG findings, the psychotic children could clearly be separated from normal controls (Simeon and Itil,1975).

It is essential to determine if the CEEG differences are indeed a manifestation of mechanisms responsible for the psychosis, or of secondary phenomena such as attention, anxiety, and intelligence. The interhemispheric differences in the EP of our psychotic children, the differences in drug-induced alterations, and the possible associations with diagnosis or intelligence ought to be further explored. Our findings lent further support to theories of cerebral "dysfunction" in childhood psychosis. In our patients the different degrees of improvement in some symptoms were associated with partial "normalization" of certain aspects of the CEEG and EP, indicating a lesser efficacy for antipsychotic drugs in these children than in adult schizophrenics.

III Pediatric Psychopharmacology

A growing number of children with various psychiatric disorders are treated with a wide variety of psychotropic drugs (Simeon et al.,1975). The selection of a particular drug, and the evaluation of its efficacy is largely based on the clinical judgement and experience of the therapist. There are, as yet, no reliable medical procedures that can help the therapist determine whether to prescribe a drug, which specific drug, what dosage and for how long. Recent neurophysiological studies have used averaged evoked potential responses, computerized programs and the CNV to investigate drug-induced changes. The effects of psychotropic drugs on the CNV, mediated probably by attention, distraction and arousal, can be accurately and objectively measured by this event-related brain potential (Tecce et al.,1978). D-amphetamine and methylphenidate increased the CNV in hyperkinetic children (Andreasen,1976).

In children with behaviour disorders treated with stimulant medication, a decrease in abnormal EEG patterns and an increase in alpha activity have been reported (Lindsley and Henry,1941; MacKay et al.,1973; Shetty,1971). The results of stimulant medication effects on the EP reported in various studies have not been consistent (Saletu et al.,1975c; Satterfield et al.,1972; Buchsbaum and Wender,1973; Conners,1975; Halliday et al.,1976; Sroufe,1975; Weber and Sulzbacher,1975).

In our studies, d-amphetamine increased the latencies and amplitudes of the VEP (Saletu et al.,1975c). Thioridazine increased the latencies but decreased the amplitudes of the EP. Shorter pretreatment latencies and higher amplitudes were found in the more disturbed children. Predictors of good therapeutic outcome were short latencies and small amplitudes with thioridazine, and short latencies and high amplitudes with d-amphetamine. A greater clinical improvement was associated with a drug-induced increase of latencies. In another study, to assess the need for further treatment with a thioridazine/d-amphetamine combination, thioridazine was discontinued first and d-amphetamine later. There was a significant latency decrease in the VEP during each of the drug withdrawal periods (Simeon et al.,1973). The neurophysiological changes (EP and CEEG) preceeded the observable clinical relapses during d-amphetamine withdrawal. Changes in the CEEG with both thioridazine and d-amphetamine differed significantly from those with placebo (Itil and Simeon,1974; Saletu et al.,1975c). Compared to the pretreatment CEEG, the two drugs produced a significant increase in fast (20 - 26.6 cps) activity. The CEEG profiles of the two drugs were surprisingly similar, in contrast to findings in adults. No significant changes in the CEEG occurred after 8 weeks of placebo treatment. Withdrawal of thioridazine from the thioridazine/d-amphetamine combined therapy resulted in an increase of fast CEEG activity; d-amphetamine withdrawal resulted in an increase of slow CEEG activity and a decrease of fast activity (Simeon et al.,1973). Following retreatment with the drug combination, CEEG changes in the opposite direction occurred. The patients responding best to therapy exhibited a marked increase of average CEEG frequency, frequency deviation and fast activity, as well as a decrease of slow activity, amplitude and amplitude variability compared to the pre-drug placebo. The treatment resistant patients, however, showed no such changes.

Of the antipsychotic drugs, chlorpromazine therapy has been associated with a decrease of alpha EEG activity (Campbell et al.,1972; Korien et al.,1971), a decrease of focal abnormalities (Campbell et al.,1972) and increases of slow EEG activity (Campbell et al.,1972; Korien et al.,1971) and previous asymmetries (Korien et al.,1971). In our studies of thiothixene and fluphenazine therapy of psychotic children, both EP latencies and amplitudes increased (Saletu et al.,1975d; Simeon et al.,1974). The increase of EP amplitudes with both thiothixene and fluphenazine are unlike those found in adult patients. The increases of latencies and amplitudes represent a shift of brain functions towards normality, as the EP of psychotic children had shorter latencies and smaller amplitudes than the normal controls. With thiothixene, the CEEG showed an increase of fast theta and slow alpha activity, and a decrease of fast alpha and beta activity. Our neurophysiological findings related to psychotropic drugs are summarised in Figures 1 and 2.

In summary, psychotropic drugs in children produce significant quantitative EEG and EP changes, which are sometimes different from those in adults. The use of psychotropic drugs as tools in exploring behavioural -

neurophysiological associations may provide a more scientific basis for the understanding of brain mechanisms in the developing organism and in mental illness. The growing sophistication of neurophysiological methods and analysis will hopefully elucidate the mechanisms responsible for psychotropic drug action, and help determine the optimal type of therapy.

Drug	CEEG				Evoked Potential	
	Slow Waves	Alpha	Fast Waves	Amplitude	Latency	Amplitude
D-AMPHETAMINE			↑		↑	↑ (trend)
THIORIDAZINE			↑		↑	↓ (trend)
THIORIDAZINE & D-AMPHETAMINE - IMPROVED PATIENTS	↓		↑	↓	↓	↑
THIORIDAZINE & D-AMPHETAMINE - RESISTANT PATIENTS	↑		↓	↑		↑
THIORIDAZINE WITHDRAWAL & D-AMPHETAMINE			↑	↑ (trend)	↓	↑
D-AMPHETAMINE WITHDRAWAL	↓	↑	↓	↑ (trend)	↓	

INCREASE ↑ DECREASE ↓ TREND ↑↓ (trend)

Fig.1. Drug Effects in Hyperkinetic Children

Drug	CEEG				Evoked Potential	
	Slow Waves	Alpha	Fast Waves	Amplitude	Latency	Amplitude
TRIHEXYPHENIDYL					↓	↓↑
THIOTHIXENE	↑	↑↓	↓	↑ (trend)	↑	↑
FLUPHENAZINE			↓		↑	↑

INCREASE ↑ DECREASE ↓ OR TREND ↑↓ (trend)

Fig.2. Drug Effects in Psychotic Children

IV Sleep EEG Studies

A great deal of research in children has been undertaken in this area. Significant progress has been made in the understanding of sleep mechanisms of various sleep disorders, such as nightmares, sleep-walking, sleep-talking, nocturnal enuresis and bruxism; the development of sleep patterns in the newborn, and during childhood, as well as in medical disorders such as the premature infant, brain damage, mental retardation and epilepsy; and the patterns of hormonal activity related to the circadian rhythm. Sleep studies in pediatric psychopharmacology have been a most neglected area, compared to the extensive research in adults. Very few sleep EEG findings have been reported in childhood psychosis, and practically none in unmedicated children with hyperkinetic, aggressive or learning disorders. In a relatively short period, sleep EEG investigations have facilitated the diagnosis and treatment of many childhood disorders.

V Discussion

Neurophysiological studies are complex, expensive, time- consuming, and require a well co-ordinated multidisciplinary effort. As most psychiatric disorders in adults have their origins in childhood, such studies may clarify not only the biological substrates of clinical conditions in children, but also help understand the development of adult disorders. In correlating sets of complex behavioural and neurophysiological variables, it is essential to determine whether the significant CEEG differences are indeed a manifestation of specific mechanisms responsible for a particular syndrome or of unspecific factors such as attention, anxiety, intelligence, organic damage and other secondary phenomena. Only then can neurophysiological findings contribute in the formulation of a scientific diagnostic classification, and the CEEG profile of individual patients help determine a more precise prognosis and more rational therapy. Similar brain mechanisms do not necessarily imply a similar etiology and therefore the CEEG characteristics of a patient may be unrelated to the etiology of his illness. To develop a meaningful diagnostic classification and a rational approach to the selection of therapy, quantitative neurophysiological correlations of heterogeneous groups of children using precise and comprehensive descriptions of their behavior (such as the ECDEU Assessment Battery for Pediatric Psychopharmacology, 1973) are essential. The separation of many disorders into "distinct" categories based on descriptive criteria, such as childhood psychosis, is still premature. Longitudinal research and careful single case studies can result in significant further progress.

The significant associations between behavioural and CEEG changes induced rapidly with psychotropic drugs can provide useful models in testing biochemical and neurophysiological theories of child psychiatry disorders.

REFERENCES

Aird, R.B., and T.Yamamoto (1966). Behaviour disorders of childhood. Electroencephalogr. Clin. Neurophysiol., 21, 148-156.

Andreasen, N.J.C., J.F.Peters and J.R.Knott (1976). CNVs in hyperactive children: Effects of chemotherapy. In W.C.McCallum and J.R.Knott (Eds.), The Responsive Brain, John Wright and Sons, Bristol, England.

Ayers, F.W., and F.Torres (1967). The incidence of EEG abnormalities in a dyslexic and a control group. J.Clin.Psychol., 23, 334-336.

Bayrakal, S. (1965). The significance of electroencephalographic abnormality in behaviour-problem children. Can.Psychiatr.Assoc.J., 10, 387-392.

Bender, L. (1959). The concept of pseudopsychopathic schizophrenia in adolescence. Amer.J.Orthopsychiat.,29, 471.

Bray, P.F. (1962). Temporal lobe syndrome in children. Modern Medicine, 30, 117.

Buchsbaum, M., and P.Wender (1973). Average evoked responses in normal and minimally brain dysfunctioned children treated with amphetamine. Arch.Gen.Psychiatry, 29, 764-770.

Campbell, M., B.Fish, J.Korein, T.Shapiro, P.Collins and C.Koh (1972). Lithium and chlorpromazine: A controlled crossover study of hyperactive severely disturbed young children. J.Autism Child Schizophr., 2, 234-263.

Capute, A.J., E.F.Neidermeyer, and F.Richardson (1968). The electroencephalogram in children with minimal cerebral dysfunction. Pediatrics, 41, 1104-1114.

Cattell, J.P., and B.L.Pacella (1950). An electroencephalographic and clinical study of children with primary behavior disorders. Am.J. Psychiatry, 107, 25-33.

Chao, D. (1963). The autistic child. Med.Records and Ann., 56, 247-248.

Conners, C.K. (1969). A teacher rating scale for use in drug studies with children. Am.J.Psychiatry, 126, 152-156.

Conners, C.K. (1971). Cortical visual evoked response in children with learning disorders. Psychophysiology, 7, 3, 418-428.

Conners, C. (1975). Minimal brain dysfunction and psychopathology in children. In A. Davids (Ed.), Child Personality and Psychopathology: Current Topics, Vol. 2, John Wiley and Sons, New York.

Creak, M., and G. Pampiglione (1969). Clinical and EEG studies on a group of 35 psychotic children. Dev.Med.Child Neurol., 11, 218.

Dumermuth, G. (1971). Electronic data processing in pediatric EEG research. Neuropaediatrie, 2, 4, 349-374.

Eeg-Olofsson, O. (1971). The development of the electroencephalogram in normal children and adolescents from the age of 1 through 21 years. Acta Paediatr.Scand., (Suppl.) 208, 7-46.

Egli, M., and I.Graf (1975). The use of anticonvulsant treatment of behaviorally disturbed children with bio-electric epilepsy. A follow-up study of 76 cases. Acta Paedopsychiatr., (Basel) 41, 54-69.

Fish, B., and D.A. Shapiro (1965). A typology of children's psychiatric disorders: Its application to a controlled evaluation of treatment. J.Am.Acad.Child Psychiatry, 4, 35-52.

Goldman, D., and B.Rosenberg (1962). Electroencephalographic observations in psychotic children. Compr.Psychiatry, 3, 93-112.

Gullickson, G.R. (1971). Contingent negative variation and attention in two and three year old children. Psychophysiology, 8, 249.

Halliday, R., J.Rosenthal, H.Naylor and E.Callaway (1976). Average evoked potential predictors of clinical improvement in hyperactive children treated with methylphenidate: An initial study and replication. Psychophysiology, 13, 429-440.

Hare, R.D. (1970). Psychopathy: Theory and Research, John Wiley & Sons, New York.

Harris, R. (1977). The EEG. In M.Rutter and L.Hersov (Eds.), Child Psychiatry. Modern Approaches, Blackwell Scientific Publications, Oxford.

Hermelin, B., and N.O'Connor (1968). Measures of the occipital alpha rhythm in normal, subnormal, and autistic children. Br.J. Psychiatry, 114, 603-610.

Hill, D., and D.Watterson (1942). Electroencephalographic studies of psychopathic personalities. J.Neurol.Psychol., 5, 47.

Hughes,J.R. (1971). Electroencephalography and learning disabilities. In H.Myklebust (Ed.) Progress in Learning Disabilities, Vol.2, Grune & Stratton, New York. pp. 113-146.

Hutt, C., S.J.Hutt, D.Lee and C.Ounsted (1964). Arousal and childhood autism. Nature, 204, 908-909.

Hutt, S.J., C.Hutt, D.Lee and C. Ounsted (1965). A behavioral and electroencephalographic study of autistic children. J.Psychiatr.Res.,3, 118-197.

Ingvar, N., and P.Koersner (1952). Electroencephalography and cerebral lesions: A clinical investigation on children. J.Clin.Exp. Psychopathology, 13, 164-174.

Itil, T.M., W.Hsu, B.Saletu and S.Mednick (1974). Computer EEG and auditory evoked potential investigations in children at high risk for schizophrenia. Am.J.Psychiatry, 131, 8, 892-900.

Itil, T.M., A.E.Rizzo and D.M.Shapiro (1967). Study of behavior and EEG correlation during treatment of disturbed children. Dis.Nerv.Syst., 28, 731-736.

Itil, T.M., B.Saletu, and S.Davis (1972). EEG findings in chronic schizophrenics based on digital computer period analysis and analog power spectra. Biol.Psychiatry, 5, 1-13.

Itil, T.M. and J.Simeon (1974). Computerized EEG in the prediction of outcome of drug therapy in hyperactive childhood behavior disorders. Psychopharmacology Bulletin, 10, 4, 36 (abridged).

Itil, T.M., J.Simeon and C.Coffin (1976). Qualitative and quantitative EEG in psychotic children. Dis.Nerv.Syst., 37, 247-252.

Jasper, H.H., P.Solomon and C.E.Bradley (1938). An analysis of behavior problem children. Am.J.Psychiatry, 95, 641-658.

John, E.R., B.Z.Karmel, W.C.Corning, P.Easton, D.Brown, H.Ahn, M.John, T.Harmony, L.Prichep, A.Toro, I.Gerson, F.Bartlett, R.Thatcher, H.Kaye, P.Valdes, and E.Schwartz (1977). Neurometrics. Numerical taxonomy identifies different profiles of brain functions within groups of behaviorally similar people. Science, 196, 1393-1410.

Kennard, M.A. (1947). Inheritance of electroencephalogram patterns in the families of children with behavior disorders. Trans.Am.Neurol.Assoc., 72, 177-179.

Kennard, M.A. (1948). Factors affecting the electroencephalogram in children and adolescents. J.Nerv.Ment.Dis., 108, 442-444.

Kennard, M.A. (1953). The electroencephalogram in psychological disorders: A review. Psychosom.Med., 15, 95-115.

Klinkerfuss, G.H., P.H.Lange, W.A.Weinberg and J.L.O'Leary (1965). Electroencephalographic abnormalities of children with hyperkinetic behaviour. Neurology, (Minneap.) 15, 889.

Kolvin, C., C.Ounsted and M.Roth (1971). Cerebral dysfunction and childhood psychoses. Br.J.Psychiatry, 118, 407-414.

Korein, J., B.Fish, T.Shapiro, E.Gevner and L.Levidow (1971). EEG and behavioral effects of drug therapy in children. Arch.Gen.Psychiatry, 24, 552-563.

Lairy, G.C. and A.Harrison (1968). Functional aspects of EEG foci in children. In P.Kellaway and O.Petersen (Eds.), Clinical Electroencephalography in Children, Grune & Stratton, New York.

Lairy, G.C., A.Remond, H.Rieger and N.Lesevre (1969). The alpha average: III. Clinical application in children. Electroencephalogr.Clin.Neurophysiol., 26, 453-467.

Lindsley, D., and C.Henry (1941). The effect of drugs on behavior and the electroencephalograms of children with behavior disorder. Psychosom.Med., 4, 140-149.

Lombroso, C.T., I.H.Schwartz, D.M.Clark, H.Muench and J.Barry (1966). Ctenoids in healthy youths. Neurology, 16, 1152-1158.

Lucas, A.R., and E.A.Rodin (1973). Electroencephalogram in Gilles de la Tourette's disease. Dis.Nerv.Syst., 34, 85-89.

Lucas, A.R., E.A.Rodin and C.B. Simson (1965). Neurological assessment of children with early school problems. Dev.Med.Child Neurol., 7, 145-156.

MacKay,M., L.Beck and R.Taylor (1973). Methylphenidate for adolescents with minimal brain dysfunction. N.Y.State J.Med., 73, 550-554.

Montagu, J.D. (1975). The hyperkinetic child: a behavioural, electrodermal and EEG investigation. Dev.Med.Child Neurol., 17, 299-305.

Ornitz, E.M., E.R.Ritvo, M.B.Brown, S.LaFranchi, T.Parmelee and R.D.Walter (1969). The EEG and rapid eye movements during REM sleep in normal and autistic children. Electroencephalogr.Clin. Neurophysiol., 26, 167-175.

Ornitz, E.M., E.R.Ritvo, L.H.Panman, V.H.Lee, E.M.Carr and R.D.Walter (1968). The auditory evoked response in normal and autistic children during sleep. Electroencephalogr.Clin.Neurophysiol.,25, 221-230.

Paine, R.S., J.S.Werry and H.C.Quay (1968). A study of 'minimal cerebral dysfunction'. Dev.Med.Child Neurol., 10, 505-520.

Saletu, B., M.Saletu and T.M.Itil (1973). The relationship between psychopathology and evoked responses before, during and after psychotropic drug treatment. Biol.Psychiatry, 6, 45-74.

Saletu, B., M.Saletu, T.M.Itil and J.Simeon (1975a). Brain function analysis in childhood psychosis: Evoked responses. Clin.Electroencephalogr., 6, 2, 44-53.

Saletu, B., M.Saletu, J.Marasa, S.Mednick and F.Schulsinger (1975b). Acoustic evoked potentials in offspring of schizophrenic mothers ('high risk' children for schizophrenia). Clin.Electroencephalogr., 6, 253-257.

Saletu, B., M.Saletu, J.Simeon and J.Marasa (1975d). Fluphenazine treatment in the psychotic child: Clinical evoked potential correlations. Compr.Psychiatry, 6, 3, 265-277.

Saletu, B., M.Saletu, J.Simeon, G.Viamontes and T.M.Itil (1975c). Comparative symptomatological and evoked potential studies with d-amphetamine, thioridazine and placebo in hyperkinetic children. Biol.Psychiatry, 10, 3, 253-275.

Satterfield, J., D.Cantwell, L.Lesser and R.Podosin (1972). Physiological studies of the hyperkinetic child. I. Am.J.Psychiatry, 123, 1418-1424.

Satterfield, J.H., D.P.Cantwell and B.T.Satterfield (1974). Pathophysiology of the hyperactive child syndrome.Arch.Gen.Psychiatry, 31, 839-844.

Satterfield, J.H., L.I.Lesser, R.E.Saul and D.P.Cantwell (1973). EEG aspects in the diagnosis and treatment of minimal brain dysfunction. Ann.N.Y.Acad.of Sci., 205, 274-282.

Sayed, Z.A., S.A.Lewis and R.P.Britain (1969). An electroencephalographic and psychiatric study of 32 insane murderers. Electroencephalogr.Clin. Neurophysiol., 27, 335.

Schain, R.J., and H.Yannet (1960). Infantile autism: An analysis of 50 cases and a consideration of certain relevant neurophysiological concepts. J.Pediatr., 57, 560-567.

Shetty, J. (1971). Alpha rhythms in the hyperkinetic child. Nature, 234, 476.

Simeon, J. (1975). The study and treatment of aggression in childhood behavior disorders. Presented at G.W.A.N. Meeting, Louisville, Kentucky.

Simeon, J., and T.M.Itil (1975). Computerized electroencephalogram: A model of understanding the brain function in childhood psychosis and its treatment. J.Autism Child.Schizophr., 3, 247-265.

Simeon, J., B.Saletu, M.Saletu, T.M.Itil and J.DaSilva (1974). Thiothixene in childhood psychosis. In I.S.Forrest, C.J.Carr and E.Usdin (Eds.), The Phenothiazines and Structurally Related Drugs, Vol.9, Raven Press, New York. pp. 519-534.

Simeon, J., B.Saletu, G.Viamontes, M.,Saletu and T.M. Itil (1973). Clinical and neurophysiological investigations of combined thioridazine - d-amphetamine maintenance therapy and withdrawal in childhood behavior disorders. Proceedings of the VIII Congress of the Collegium Internationale Neuropsychopharmacologium (CINP), Avecenum - Czechoslovak Medical Press, Prague, 270-292.

Simeon, J., C.Utech and S. Simeon (1975). Twenty-three psychotropic drugs used in children abroad which were not recommended in the United States. Psychopharmacol.Bull.,11,2,31-38.

Sklar, B., J.Hanley and W.W.Simmons (1972). An EEG experiment aimed toward identifying dyslexic children. Nature, 240, 414-416.

Sklar, B., J.Hanley and W.W.Simmons (1973). A computer analysis of EEG spectral signatures from normal and dyslexic children. IEEE Transactions on Biomedical Engineering, 1, 20-26.

Small, J.G. (1970). Sensory evoked responses of autistic children. In D.W.Churchill, G.D.Alpern and M.DeMyer (Eds.), Infantile Autism: Proceedings of the Indiana University Colloquium, Springfield, Illinois.

Spilimbergo, A. and G.Nissen (1971). Verhaltensstorungen und EEG - veranderungen bei Kindern. Acta Paedopsychiatr., (Basel) 38, 59-65.

Sroufe, L. (1975). Drug treatment of children with behavior problems. In F.Horowitz (Ed.), Review of Child Development Research, Vol. 4, University of Chicago Press, Chicago.

Stevens, J.R. (1970). EEG in psychiatric disorders. Am.J.Dis.Child., 120, 182-192.

Stevens, J.R., K.Sachdev and V.Milstein (1968). Behavior disorders of childhood and the electroencephalogram. Arch.Neurol., 18, 160-177.

Tecce, J.J. (1971). Contingent negative variation and individual differences. A new approach in brain research. Arch.Gen.Psychiatry, 24, 1-16.

Tecce, J.J., J.Savignano-Bowman and J.O.Cole (1978). Drug effects on contingent negative variation and eyeblinks: The distraction-arousal hypothesis. In M.A.Lipton, A.DiMascio and K.F.Killam (Eds.), Psychopharmacology: A Generation of Progress, Raven Press, New York.

Tecce, J.J. and N.M. Scheff (1969). Attention reduction and suppressed direct-current potentials in the human brain. Science, 164, 331-333.

Walter, S.G., V.J.Aldridge, R.Cooper, G.O'Gorman, C.McCallum and A.L.Winter (1970). Report on: Neurophysiological correlates of apparent defects of sensori-motor integration in autistic children. In D.W.Churchill, G.D.Alpern and M.DeMyer (Eds.), Infantile Autism: Proceedings of the Indiana University Colloquium, Springfield, Illinois.

Ward, T.F., and B.A.Hoddinott (1965). A study of childhood schizophrenia and early infantile autism. Part I - Description of the sample. Can.Psychiatr.Assoc.J., 10, 377-382.

Weber, B., and S.Sulzbacher (1975). Use of CNS stimulant medication in average electroencephalic audiometry with children with MBD. J.Learning Disabilities, 8, 300-303.

White, P.T., W.DeMyer and M.DeMyer (1964). EEG abnormalities in early childhood schizophrenia: A double-blind study of psychiatrically disturbed and normal children during promazine sedation. Am.J.Psychiatry, 120, 950-958.

Wiener, J.M., J.G.Delano and D.W.Klass (1966). An EEG study of delinquent and non-delinquent adolescents. Arch.Gen.Psychiatry, 15, 144-150.

Wikler, A., J.F.Dixon and J.B.Parker Jr., (1970). Brain function in problem children and controls - psychometric neurological and electroencephalographic comparisons. Am.J.Psychiatry, 127, 644-645.

The Relevance of Quantitative EEG and Sleep Investigations

EEG Effects of Clozapine: Assocation or Dissocation of EEG and Behavior?

MAX FINK

Department of Psychiatry and Behavioral Science, School of Medicine, SUNY at Stony Brook, Stony Brook, New York

In the past two decades, both a theory of the association of EEG and behavior and a methodology designed to predict the useful role of new psychoactive drugs has been developed. The theory states that psychoactive drugs systematically affect brain functions such that distinctive EEG patterns are elicited which are directly related to the behavioral effects in man. Drugs with similar EEG patterns have similar behavioral effects; and drugs which fail to elicit EEG effects fail to have systematic behavioral effects.

The theory was first challenged by pharmacologic studies with anticholinergic drugs in which surface EEG electrodes showed slow frequency high voltage patterns characteristic of sleep while the animal was restless, exhibited running movements, and vocalized. These studies were justifiably criticized for limiting the observations to measures of motor activity and of vigilance, and for using gross estimates of brain function (Bradley and Fink, 1968). In contrast to animal studies, those in man allow a wide repertoire of behavioral measures, better control of the parameters of the experiments, and minimum interference from adventitious movement and changes in vigilance. In human studies also, more sophisticated and more reliable computer based measures of brain function have been used.

Theory of Association

From the human studies of the effects of drugs on EEG and behavior, we are able to define relations between changes in EEG pattern, amplitude, and variability with specific behaviors. For example, drugs which alter thought processes, reduce delusions and hallucinations, and inhibit psychomotor activity are associated with a slowing of EEG frequencies, a decrease of fast frequencies, an increase in amplitudes, and a regularity of the background rhythms. This is usually seen with antipsychotic drugs such as phenothiazines (e.g., chlorpromazine and fluphenazine) and butyrophenones (haloperidol).

An increase in EEG slow waves and in fast frequencies, a decrease in alpha amplitudes, an increase in variability of frequencies, and a decrease in rhythmicity is associated with heightened mood, increased psychomotor activity, and decreased vigilance and alertness. These effects are seen with the tricyclic and tetracyclic thymoleptic antidepressant drugs, (*e.g.*, imipramine, amitriptyline, and mianserin).

An increase in EEG fast frequencies and in rhythmicity is associated with increased sedation, relaxation, decreased anxiety, and at higher doses, sleep and anesthesia. These associations are seen with anxiolytic and sedative drugs such as benzodiazepines (diazepam, chlordiazepoxide) and barbiturates.

Compounds may also decrease amplitudes, the amounts of slow and alpha EEG activities, as well as the regularity and rhythmicity of the records. These changes are associated with increased mental activity, irritability, anxiety, hallucinations, illusions, and imagery and are seen with psychotomimetic drugs (*e.g.*. LSD, mescaline). The same desynchronization of EEG frequencies but with an increase in delta activity is associated with obtunding of consciousness and delirium, and is seen after anticholinergic drugs (*e.g.*, scopolamine, atropine) and in alcoholic deliruim.

Prediction of Drug Activity

These observations have had a special application in predicting the clinical effects of new drugs. Thus, doxepin and mianserin have been identified as antidepressants and mesterolone as an anxiolytic agent using this methodology. But some problems in this methodology remain, and these are the basis of this discussion. There are two types of problems: the assertion of clinical activity for compounds for which no EEG profile has been demonstrated; and clinically useful compounds with an EEG profile that does not fit the anticipated clinical activity. Examination of noötropic compounds, diphenylhydantoin, and some stimulant drugs are examples of the first problem. The single clear example of the second problem is the EEG and behavioral relations of clozapine.

Noötropic Compounds

Based on the effects observed in pharmacologic and *in vitro* studies, clinical activity has been predicted for piracetam, Gerdaxyl, EMD 21,657, pyrroxan, and ACTH 4-10. These compounds affect vigilance or alter oxygen metabolism, and have been given the class name of "noötropic". But EEG studies of the compounds have failed to demonstrate systematic changes in EEG patterns or in behavior under laboratory conditions. If the theory of association of EEG and behavior is correct, these compounds should have no consistent effects in clinical trials. And this is indeed the present situation for each compound. While some clinical reports are available, they are either uncontrolled open studies or the samples are too small to be convincing. Yet, some of the compounds are advocated for clinical use. Only further study will determine if the EEG trials were unsatisfactory; and the compounds do elicit an EEG profile, whether the clinical trials reflect a placebo (non-cerebral) effect; or, if the compounds are examples of the dissociation of EEG and behavior after drugs.

Some observers have been unable to define an EEG profile for some compounds with defined CNS effects. An example is the failure to define EEG effects for diphenylhydantoin (DPH) in the background alert EEG at dosage levels that are deemed non-toxic. We recently examined the EEG effects of DPH in normal volunteers and did not find a systematic effect for single doses of 700 mg. When we examined the plasma levels, we found that the levels were below 7.1 ng/ml --- levels generally considered ineffective in clinical studies. Higher doses, 500 mg and 500 mg given at a two hour interval, elicited plasma levels between 8.0 and 12.8 ng/ml, and at these levels the EEG demonstrated increases in fast (18-29 Hz) frequencies and in average frequency, and a decrease in theta (4-7 Hz) activity. An understanding of the metabolism and pharmacokinetics of DPH is essential to establish its EEG profile. Perhaps, the failure to observe EEG patterns for other compounds cited as psychoactive may be due to a failure to achieve effective blood levels in the time and at the dosages administered ?

EEG Study of Clozapine

The study of clozapine exemplifies the second type of problem. This novel sedative compound lacks the characteristic effects of antipsychotic drugs on the dopaminergic system (*e.g.*, it does not stimulate a plasma elevation of prolactin), and exhibits considerable anticholinergic activity. In clinical trials it is highly sedating, lowers blood pressure, and reduces psychotic ideation (Gross and Langer, 1966; DeMaio, 1968; Angst, *et al.*, 1971a, b; Singer and Lam, 1973; Ionescu, *et al.*, 1973; Simpson and Varga, 1974; Matz, *et al.*, 1974). Some authors have described clinical antidepressant activity for clozapine (Kogan and Nikolenko, 1974; Nahunek *et al.*, 1975, Klik *et al.*, 1976). Parkinsonsim is not elicited. From its clinical activity, clozapine may be classified as a unique antipsychotic agent without antiparkinson features.

We examined the EEG effects of clozapine in normal volunteers and in psychiatric patients. In volunteers, we first determined the effects of 5 and 10 mg oral clozapine on EEG, heart rate, blood pressure, critical flicker fusion frequency (CFF), and behavioral measures. Both the physiologic and behavioral measures were altered within 2 hours of ingestion at each dose level. In a double-blind crossover study of 5 mg and 10 mg clozapine and of placebo in four subjects, EEG spectral analysis showed an increase in theta (4-7 Hz) and in high beta (21-35 Hz) activity with a decrease in the alpha (8-13 Hz) frequencies. Delta activity increased in two subjects with 5 mg and in all four subjects with 10 mg clozapine. The dose-response relationship was well defined. In the behavioral measures, there was a decrease in alertness in the self-ratings, but no effect in heart rate, blood pressure, or CFF. Self reports showed sedation, blurred vision, and decreased ability to concentrate. These findings were interpreted as consistent with a pattern seen with thymoleptic antidepressants (Fink, 1969).

In clinical trials with clozapine in chronic schizophrenic patients, we obtained EEG records in four patients, including records during the drug free period. Examinations were done at 3 and 5 hours after the first 5 mg dose, and again after four weeks of daily clozapine administration. In comparison with the drug free record, delta (1-3.5 Hz), low theta (3.5-5.5 Hz), and high beta (23-29 Hz) EEG activities increased, low alpha activity (7.5-9.5 Hz) decreased, and amplitudes and high theta activity (5.5-7.5 Hz) were variable. These effects also were interpreted as similar to those seen with thymoleptic antidepressants (Fink, Irwin, and Weinhold, in preparation).

We carried out both power spectral density and period analyses. While there are some differences in the frequency bands affected, the overall patterns were not distinguishable between the two methods.

These observations can be compared to prior analyses reported by Roubicek and Major (1977). These authors also found an increase in theta and high beta activities, a decrease in alpha activity, and no change in delta and low beta bands (Table 1). They used both power spectral density and iterative analyses, again with a greater similarity than differences among the findings by the two methods. They concluded that the EEG profile of clozapine resembled that of a thymoleptic antidepressant drug more than that of an antipsychotic drug.

Table 1

EEG PROFILE OF CLOZAPINE

		ANALYSIS TYPE	FREQUENCY (Hz) 0-3.5	3.5-7.5	7.5-13	13-16	16-20	+20	AMPLITUDE
BASLE	CLOZAPINE	Pwr	++	++	--	(+)	(-)	+	(+)
		I.I.	0	++	--	0	++	++	
NEW YORK	CLOZAPINE	Pwr	++	++	-	(±)	(±)	+	-
		Per	+	++	--	0	++	++	
	CHLORPROMAZINE	Pwr	+	++	±	0	0	-	+
	MIANSERIN	Pwr	+	++	-	(+)	(+)	+	-

Pwr: Power Spectral Density Analysis (relative power)
I.I.: Iterative Interval Analysis
Per: Baseline Cross Period Analysis
( ): Not different from Placebo

Discussion

These analyses find the EEG activity of clozapine to fit that of an antidepressant drug more closely than any other drug class, and we would anticipate that clinically clozapine should be an active thymoleptic antidepressant. While some clinical trials have found clozapine to be antidepressant, others have reported it to act as an antipsychotic drug. Controlled clinical trials are few. For the most part, the patients selected have been the most chronic of the psychotic populations, and many have had tardive dyskinesia. One recent report, that of van Praag, Korf and Dols (1976) is of special interest, as they find clozapine to be sedative without specific antipsychotic activity in the prototypic symptoms of hallucinations and delusions.

How is one to integrate this apparent discrepancy into the present theory of association of EEG and behavior after psychoactive drugs ? Clozapine is a difficult drug to classify by modern pharmacologic means, for in its effects on dopaminergic and cholinergic systems, on motor systems, and on psychosis it differs from other antipsychotic drugs. Is it possible that the expectation of antipsychotic activity which was suggested by the first pharmacologic studies and the initial drug trials dominated the clinical assessments ? The premature cessation of the clinical trials precludes the operation of the clinical marketplace to better define the activity of the new compounds as it has done with doxepin (first anxiolytic, later antidepressant) and convulsive therapy (first anxiolytic, later antidepressant).

Unfortunately, clozapine has evinced toxic hematopoetic activity so that clinical trials have been suspended, and a resolution of the discrepancy between the EEG and the clinical findings is no longer possible.

Conclusion

With the observation that psychoactive drugs elicit distinctive patterns in the alert EEG, a theory of the association of EEG and behavior was developed. Inconsistencies in studies of anticholinergic drugs in animals was seen as resulting from the limited measures of behavior used, e.g. motor activity and gross estimates of sleep-wakefulness. More recent challenges are observations that active drugs like diphenylhydantoin (DPH) provide no measurable EEG effect; that noötropic compounds with irregular behavioral effects elicit no EEG effects; and the EEG classification of clozapine.

The EEG profile of DPH was recently determined by attention to its pharmacodynamic properties. An EEG profile was readily defined when clinically active plasma levels were achieved.

Analysis of the noötropic drugs is as yet incomplete, since the EEG and clinical studies are inadequate and only further study will determine whether these substances are active CNS agents without EEG effects.

Clozapine elicited EEG profiles of a thymoleptic drug in two studies. In clinical trials, both antipsychotic and antidepressant activity were defined. Termination of the clinical studies because of toxicity preclude resolution of this discrepancy.

The EEG profile analysis of clozapine represents the single most difficult challenge to the EEG and behavior association hypothesis.

Acknowledgements: The studies reported here were done in association with Peter Irwin, Yannis Papakostas, Walter Sannita, and Paul Weinhold.

Aided, in part, by grant MH 28471 of the National Institute of Mental Health and Sandoz Pharmacenticals.

Presented at the XI CINP Congress, Vienna, July 12, 1978.

References

Angst, J. Bente, D, Berner, P., Helmann, H., Helmchen, H., Hippius, H. Das Klinische Wirkungsbild von Clozapin (Untersuchung mit dem AMP-System). Pharmakopsychiat. 4: 201-211, 1971.

Angst, J., Jaenicke, U., Padrutt, A. Scharfetter, C. Ergebnisse eines Doppelblind Versuches von HF 1854 (8-chlor-11-14-methy 1-1-piperazinyll 5-H-dibenzo [b,e,] [4,4] diazepin) in Vergleich zu Levomepromazin. Pharmakopsychiat. 4: 192 (1971).

Bradley, P. and Fink, M. (Eds.): Anticholinergic Drugs and Brain Functions in Animals and Man. Amsterdam, Elsevier Publishing, 194 pp., 1968.

deMaio, D. Preliminary clinical evaluation of a new neuroleptic agent: HF-1854. In: The present status of psychotropic drugs. Pharmacological and clinical aspects - Proceedings of the VIth International Congress of Collogium Internationale Neuro-Psycho- Pharmacologicum; Tarragona, April, 1968. Cerletti. A., Bové, J. (Eds.): 485-488, 1969. Amsterdam, Excerpta Medica Foundation 1969 (International Congress Series 180).

Fink, M. EEG and human psychopharmacology. Ann. Rev. Pharmacol. 9: 241-258, 1969.

Fink, M., Irwin, P. and Weinhold, P. EEG effects of clozapine in psychotic patients. In preparation.

Gross, H., Langer, E. Das Wirkungsprofil eines Chemisch-neuartigen Breitband-neuroleptikums der Dibenzodiazepine-gruppe. Wien. Med. Wochenschr. 116: 814-816, 1966.

Klik, J., Krausova, J., Krizova, A., Maresvova, H., Vencovsky, E. Experience with clozapine in psychiatric home practice. Cesk. Psychiatr. 72: 197-201, 1976.

Kogan, W., Nikolaenko, N. New drugs in the treatment of nervous and mental diseases. Leningrad Bechterev Psychoneurological Research Institute Report, 40-41, 1974.

Matz, R., Rick, W., Oh, D., Thompson, H. Gershon, S. Clozapine - a potential antipsychotic agent without extrapyramidal manifestations. Current Ther. Res. 16: 687-695, 1974.

Nahunek, K., Svestka, J., Misurec, J., Rodova, A. Experiences with clozapine. Cesk. Psychiat. 71: 11-15, 1975.

Van Praag, H.M., Korf, J., Dols, L.C.W. Clozapine versus perphenazine: the value of the biochemical mode of aciton of neuroleptics in predicting their therapeutic activity. Br. J. Psychiat. 129: 547-555, 1976.

Roubicek, J., Major, I. EEG profile and behavioral changes after a single dose of clozapine in normals and schizophrenics. Biological Psychiatry 12: 613-633, 1977.

Simpson, G.M., Varga, E. Clozapine - a new antipsychotic agent. Current Therapeutic Res. 16: 679-686, 1974.

Singer, K., Lam, C.M. Evaluation of Leponex (clozapine) in schizophrenia with acute symptomatology. J. Int. Med. Res. 1: 627, 1973.

Acute Efficacy of 20 Psychotropic Drugs on Human EEG Power Spectrum Variables Shown by Multivariate and Univariate Statistics

W. M. HERRMANN*, K. FICHTE, T. M. ITIL*** and St. KUBICKI******

*Departments of Clinical Neuropsychopharmacology
Biometrics and Statistics
**SCHERING AG, Berlin/Bergkamen, West Germany
***Division of Biological Psychiatry, New York Medical College, New York, U.S.A.
****Department of Clinical Neurophysiology, Freie Universität, Berlin, West Germany

ABSTRACT

The acute efficacy of single oral dosages of 20 psychotropic drugs, 5 neuroleptics, 5 anxiolytics, 5 antidepressants and 5 psychostimulants plus 5 placebos has been tested in 5 basic studies simultaneously designed and performed and involving 75 healthy male volunteers. Each study was done in a Latin square double-blind design with 15 subjects, each receiving one placebo and one compound of each of the four clinical therapeutic psychotropic drug classes. Three 5-minute EEG recordings (pre, 1 hr. and 3 hr. post drug intake) are taken to represent the drug effects. The differences in drug efficacy were tested by multivariate analysis of variance using 3 x 7 power spectrum estimates selected from these 3 EEG recordings. 14 of the 20 substances could be distinguished from placebo at a 5%, 16 at a 10% level.

In order to demonstrate the results visually, examples of the mean relative power estimates as well as the standard q-score profiles of the 7 variables at three times are given. All 7 variables selected contribute to the differences between the drugs. However, some variables seem to be more specific for a defined drug class than others: $\vartheta^F = 5.5 - 8.5$ Hz for the neuroleptics, $\beta_1{}^F = 12.0 - 18.0$ Hz for the anxiolytics, $\alpha_1{}^F = 8.5 - 10.5$ Hz for the psychostimulants and a combination of $\delta^F = 1.5 - 3.5$ Hz, ϑ^F and $\alpha_1{}^F$ for the antidepressants.

KEYWORDS

EEG-effects, normal awake volunteers, psychotropic drugs, power spectrum analysis, multivariate statistics.

INTRODUCTION

The main aim of the five so-called basic studies including 20 psychotropic drugs and 5 placebos was to develop an objective rule for the classification of new testsubstances to one of the four hypothetical psychotropic drug classes using EEG power spectrum variables of human volunteers.
For this purpose the 5 studies were treated as parts of a commonly designed multicentre study. The results have been described by Herrmann, Fichte and others (1979).

At the same time each individual study is an example of a standard design for quantitative pharmaco electroencephalography in human volunteers after single oral administration to test the null hypothesis on treatment effects of psychotropic substances.

The aim of this article therefore is to describe the efficacy of these substances using EEG power spectrum estimates.

Psychotropic drugs have systematic effects on the human EEG and substances belonging to one of the four clinical therapeutic drug classes have class specific effects, as has been described in quantitative EEG work done in the past few decades.

Neuroleptics show an increase in δ- and ϑ-, and a decrease in β-wave activity (Borenstein a. oth., 1970; Itil, 1969a; Itil and others, 1969), anxiolytics show an increase in the slow β-activity, mainly in the range of 13.0 to 21.0 Hz (Fink and others, 1976; Itil, 1974), tricyclic antidepressants an increase in δ- and ϑ-, a decrease in α- and an increase in β-activity, mainly above 21.0 Hz (Fink, 1969; Itil 1975), while psychostimulants show either an increase in α-activity and a decrease in δ- and ϑ- and β-actitivity, mainly above 21.0 Hz as with dextroamphetamine (Fink and others, 1971; Itil, 1975), or a total shift into low voltage fast β-activity, as with LSD_{25} (Akpinar and others, 1972).

In another pilot trial Herrmann und McDonald (1978) demonstrated in a single experiment that the typical representatives of all four clinical therapeutic drug classes, diazepam 10 mg, dextroamphetamine-sulfate 18 mg, chlorpromazine 75 mg and amitriptyline 75 mg, could be discriminated from placebo and showed EEG effects which allowed them to be distinguished from each other by visual comparison of the results of the power spectrum standard t-score profiles.

Selecting for each of the 5 studies one typical neuroleptic, antidepressant, anxiolytic and psychostimulant on the basis of their clinical therapeutic properties, we hypothesized that, if trials are performed in populations with comparable inclusion/exclusion criteria and identical study design, then substances belonging to one of the four clinical therapeutic drug classes will show similar EEG changes. This hypothesis will be tested in the present experiment.

Since 5 substances were involved in one trial and since 3 x 7 variables were selected for the parametrisation of the EEG the test problem was both a multiple and a multivariate one. The adequate test method was multivariate analysis. However, to allow interpretation of the results, graphs were plotted from univariate statistics.

Based on our experience, the working hypothesis is therefore:
Using multivariate statistics we can test, and using univariate tests we can demonstrate visually the acute efficacy of psychotropic drugs in human volunteers and determine among the 7 variables selected those which are relevant for differentiation in pairwise drug comparisons.

MATERIAL AND METHODS

Drugs and Dosages

The drugs and dosages used in the studies are shown in Table 1. The drugs were selected from a clinical point of view. The neuroleptics had to have proven therapeutical efficacy in schizophrenia, the antidepressants in psychotic depression, the anxiolytics in anxiety neurosis. The psychostimulants selected had to have proven CNS-stimulatory properties in humans as measurable by quantitative EEG-changes, mood elevation and improvement in motor and/or mental performance. Monoamine oxidase inhibitors, though used therapeutically in certain forms of depression, were assigned to the clinical therapeutic class of psychostimulants because of their general CNS-stimulatory properties.

TABLE 1

Basic Studies: Drugs and Dosages

Study Number	**NEUROLEPTICS**	**ANXIOLYTICS**	**ANTI-DEPRESSANTS**	**PSYCHO-STIMULANTS**
HUM 110	CHL 75 mg Chlorpromazine	CDO 30 mg Chlor-diazepoxide	IMI 75 mg Imipramine	MET 30 mg Methyl-phenidate
HUM 111	HAL 3 mg Haloperidol	DIA 10 mg Diazepam	AMI 75 mg Amitriptyline	DEX 20 mg Dextroamphet-amine Sulfate
HUM 114	CLO 50 mg Clozapine	CLA 15 mg Dipotassium Chlorazepate	MIA 30 mg Mianserin	CAF 200 mg Caffeine
HUM 115	TIO 30 mg Tiotixene	MEP 600 mg Meprobamate	NOR 75 mg Nortriptyline-HCL	TRA 20 mg Tranylcypro-mine Sulfate
HUM 116	MOL 30 mg Molindone	LOR 3 mg Lorazepam	DES 75 mg Desipramine	PHE 30 mg Phenelzine Sulfate

The selection of the dosages was based on clinical therapeutic daily dosages and/or on our own experience with the substances in EEG trials.

Subjects

For each of the five studies 17 male subjects (2 as replacements) were selected. The age range was 21 to 45 years, body-weight: Germans 60 to 80 kg, Americans 70 to 90 kg and Turkish volunteers 50 to 70 kg. Each subject underwent a physical examination, a psychiatric screening interview and a battery of laboratory tests, including ECG and a clinical EEG. All the subjects selected were physically healthy, had no history of mental disorder and were receiving neither psychotropic medication nor any other type of medical treatment.

The subjects had to be within the ± 1σ-range of the mean of the German norm-values (Eggert, 1974) in the EPI (Eysenck Personality Inventory, Eysenck, 1957). Additional inclusion criteria were a score less than 20 in the VELA (vegetative lability, Fahrenberg, 1965) questionnaire and an occipital α-rhythm. Those who had predominantly frequencies below 8.0 Hz or an α-amplitude below 10 μV, ECG or muscle artefacts or relevant abnormalities in the EEG were excluded.

All subjects gave their informed consent, and were paid for their participation.

Study Design

We decided to perform the five studies simultaneously using three different laboratories – two studies (study numbers HUM 110 and HUM111) in the laboratory of the Department of Clinical Neuropsychopharmacology of Schering AG, Berlin/Bergkamen, two studies (study numbers HUM 114 and HUM 116) in the laboratories of the HZI Neuropsychiatric Foundation in Istanbul, Turkey, and one study (study number HUM 115) in the EEG-laboratories of the Division of Biological Psychiatry, Department of Psychiatry, New York Medical College, New York. The design of one basic study (study number HUM 110) can be seen from Table 2. After an adaptation session with a single-blind placebo, the four psychotropic drugs, one neuroleptic, one psychostimulant, one antidepressant, one anxiolytic and a placebo were administered in a Latin square design under double-blind conditions. Then, in each study, either two hormones or one hormone and a placebo were given.

TABLE 2

Design of One Basic Study (HUM 110)

sequence	subject code	study day 1	2	3	4	5	6	7	8
			latin square						
I	038 102 110	PLA	CHL	MET	IMI	CDO	PLA	L-NGL	D-NGL
II	039 101 112	PLA	IMI	CDO	PLA	CHL	MET	D-NGL	L-NGL
III	040 100 114	PLA	MET	IMI	CDO	PLA	CHL	L-NGL	D-NGL
IV	045 096 109 113	PLA	CDO	PLA	CHL	MET	IMI	D-NGL	L-NGL
V	078 079 103 111	PLA	PLA	CHL	MET	IMI	CDO	D-NGL L-NGL D-NGL L-NGL	L-NGL D-NGL L-NGL D-NGL

To achieve comparability of the data from three different EEG-laboratories several precautions were taken; all studies were done at about the same time, as described in the previous section; subjects/inclusion/exclusion criteria were uniform in all three laboratories. The electronic device in all three laboratories was controlled by one engineer, the same type of filters were used, the calibration of the EEG-machines was done with highly stable battery-operated sine wave generators of 100 μV peak-to-peak amplitude and a frequency of 30.0 Hz through the electrode-boxes. The generators were all of the same type.

The EEG data were FM-recorded on AMPEX tape recorders. Detection of artefacts, refiltering, digitalisation and parametrisation of the data were carried out by the department of research data processing of Schering AG, Berlin.

The subjects were tested at weekly intervals, either at 8.00 or 9.00 o'clock in the morning. A prerecording was made, the drug administered and the subjects were retested one hour and three hours after drug intake. All subjects had a light breakfast. They were requested not to drink alcohol the night before and to refrain from drinking any stimulatory beverage such as coffee, tea or Coca-Cola that morning; these beverages were also withheld for the rest of the day.

The testing sequence was as follows:
1. Physiological measurement EEG recording, 5 minutes resting recording (RR) and 5 minutes auditory evoked potential recording (AEP).
2. Subjective verbal reporting by self-rating reporting check lists, duration 10—15 minutes.
3. Performance test battery consisting of vigilance tests, psychomotor tests, sensual motor coordination and higher mental performance, duration about 30 minutes.

The results of the self-reporting check lists, the performance test battery and the auditory evoked potential recordings will be reported elsewhere. This paper describes only the results of the resting recording EEG. Resting recording means that the subjects sat in a comfortable chair, in a sound-proof shielded and air conditioned room with dim light, with their eyes closed and their hands resting comfortably on arm rests. They were required to press a thumb-operated button. If the button was released, a 70 dB 1000 Hz sine wave tone was given.
Vigilance during the 5 minutes was free floating. The subjects were generally fully awake and in the A_1 to A_4 stages of Bente's (1964) categories which is broadly equivalent to the A_0 to A_2 stages of the Kugler et al. (1978) classification. If the subjects reached a B-stage a sound signal was given. During the 5-minute recording subjects were therefore predominantly in the A-stages, only very seldom in the B-stages, and never in a C-stage.

EEG-Methodology

For a detailed description of the method see Herrmann & McDonald (1978) and Herrmann/Fichte and others (1979).
For the recording the time constant was 0.3 s. and notch filters were used, 50 Hz for West-Berlin and Istanbul, and 60 Hz for New York. A low pass filter was not used during the recording procedure. Atechnician observed the plotted analogue signals and identified and marked the artefacts.
At the beginning of each recording calibration was carried out with the sine wave generator described above.
During computer playback of the data an independent EEG-technician rechecked the recordings for artefacts: ECG, muscle, movement, opening eyes etc. This he did blind without knowledge of the drug key. EEG-epochs (10 s.) with artefacts were excluded from the analysis. Only the O_2A_2 lead was analyzed.

Parametrisation of EEG Time Series

The treatment-unit of each subject and study day in the Latin square is called a subject-treatment-unit. The total number of subject-treatment-units is 375.

Due to missing data, a total of 364 subject-treatment-units were available. Each unit is represented by three (pre, 1 hr. and 3 hr. post) 5 min. EEG-recordings under RR conditions. In the following symbolic vector ($\underline{x}$) representing a subject-treatment-unit

$$\underline{x} = \begin{matrix} \text{EEG} - \text{pre} \\ \text{EEG} - 1 \text{ hr. post} \\ \text{EEG} - 3 \text{ hr. post} \end{matrix}$$

each component is a vector itself, the five-minute EEG-recording being represented by 7 parameters. Therefore each subject-treatment-unit is represented by a 3 x 7 component vector. While epochs with artefacts were excluded, 30 epochs of 10 sec. were included. Each epoch is represented by 1000 values, which give the time-serie in $\Delta = \frac{1}{100}$ sec. intervals. The spectrum is estimated by Fourier-transformation of the modified autocovariance function using hamming-window with lags of up to 1 sec. (= 1/10 of the epoch).
For each power spectrum the following variables were calculated:
relative power in

δF = 1.5 – 5.5 Hz	$\alpha_1 F$ = 8.5 – 10.5 Hz	$\beta_1 F$ = 12.0 – 18.0 Hz
ϑF = 5.5 – 8.5 Hz	$\alpha_2 F$ = 10.5 – 12.0 Hz	$\beta_3 F$ = 21.0 – 30.0 Hz

and the total power (1.5 – 30.0 Hz).

Selection of variables was based on factor analysis by Herrmann/Fichte/Kubicki (1978).

Statistical Models

From the study plan models can be derived which involve as systematic effects
sequences of treatments (S)
treatments (T)
probands (P) hierarchical in the sequences (random effect),
interaction between sequences and treatments:

$$\underline{y}_{ijk} = \underline{\mu} + \underline{\alpha}_i^S + \underline{\alpha}_j^T + \underline{a}_{ik}^P + \underline{\alpha}_{ij}^{ST} + \underline{e}_{ijk}$$

$i = 1, 2, \ldots, 5$
$j = 1, 2, 3, \ldots, 5$
$k = 1, 2, 3$ (see study design)

This is a multivariate model, because variables from the same subject are taken to be correlated.

It should be mentioned that in developing the above model or any other that would fit the study plan, we encounter – among others (e.g. missing values) – two difficulties, if we are willing to perform tests giving α-risks. The first we call the „multivariate problem"; the second arises from the fact that more than two treatments are given in each study and is called the „multiple problem". Up to now, there has been no practicable way for us to solve both problems simultaneously (e.g. a multivariate Scheffé or Tukey test).

This is why two kinds of test statistics were used on the same data:
a) Multivariate statistics with two groups
b) Univariate statistics with five groups and adequate multiple testing (Tukey).

In a) attention is paid to correlation of the variables, neglecting the fact that 10 tests have to be performed, if one is interested in all pairwise comparisons.

In b) attention is paid to the fact that we are handling 5 groups and the multivariate problem is ignored. Each subject treatment unit is represented by a vector of 21 components:

$$(\underbrace{\delta^F, \vartheta^F, \alpha_1{}^F, \alpha_2{}^F, \beta_1{}^F, \beta_3{}^F, P}_{\text{pre}}; \underbrace{\delta^F, \ldots, P}_{\text{1 hour post}}, \underbrace{\delta^F, \ldots, P}_{\text{3 hours post}})$$

The formal results of multivariate statistics, shown in Table 3, are based on vectors with three components, e.g.

$(\delta^F,$	$\delta^F,$	$\delta^F)$
pre	1 h	3 h

Examples of the Tukey test are given in Figs. 2 and 3.

RESULTS

Multivariate Statistics

The multivariate pairwise comparisons have been done using Wilk's U-statistics for each of the 7 variables at three time periods (pre, 1 hr. post and 3 hr. post). The results for each of the five basic studies are shown in Table 3. There are 10 multivariate comparisons for each study and for each variable set, making a total of 70 tests for each study. Assuming the variables are independent, we could expect 7 tests at a 10% level and 4 tests at a 5% level to be false positive by chance. However, the average number of significances for the five studies is 18 at the 10% level and 11 at the 5% level, indicating that the differences revealed by the multivariate statistics are not attributable solely to chance.

Assuming that a tested drug has an effect on the EEG, if there is a difference in at least one variable at the 5% level in the multivariate pairwise comparisons, then out of the 20 substances 14 show differences versus placebo (at the 10% level: 16 of the 20 substances). Those which show no differences at the 10% level are methylphenidate, meprobamate, tranylcypromine-sulfate and phenelzine-sulfate. The lack of

TABLE 3

The effects of the psychotropic drugs on the 7 selected EEG power spectrum estimates are tested by multivariate (3 time periods, pre, 1 hr. and 3 hr. post) analyses of variance with the factors treatment and subject. The 5 treatments per study (HUM 110, 111, 114, 115, 116) have been compared pairwise. No α-adjustment was made. For the variables listed in the table, the null hypothesis of no difference is rejected. 14 of the 20 substances could be distinguished from placebo on a 5% and 16 on a 10% level.

Effects of Psychotropic Drugs on EEG Power Spectrum Variables
Results of the Multivariate Analysis of Variance (MANOVA)

	CHL	CDO	PLA	IMI	MET	HUM 110 RR, n=13
Haloperidol HAL		ϑ^F (β_1^F)	δ^F ϑ^F (α_1^F)	(ϑ^F) (P)	δ^F ϑ^F	CHL Chlorpromazine
Diazepam DIA	ϑ^F (β_1^F)		(α_1^F) β_1^F (P)	δ^F α_1^F	ϑ^F (β_1^F)	CDO Chlordiazepoxide
Placebo PLA	(ϑ^F) α_2^F (β_1^F)	(α_2^F)		δ^F (α_1^F) ϑ^F (β_3^F)		PLA Placebo
Amitriptyline AMI	(α_1^F) (β_1^F)	ϑ^F α_1^F (β_1^F)	(ϑ^F)		δ^F (α_1^F) (ϑ^F) (β_3^F)	IMI Imipramine
Dextroamphetamine Sulfate DEX	(α_1^F) (ϑ^F) P	(δ^F) α_1^F β_1^F P	δ^F (α_1^F) P	δ^F ϑ^F P		MET Methylphenidate
HUM 111 RR, n=16	HAL	DIA	PLA	AMI	DEX	

	CLO	CLA	PLA	MIA	CAF	HUM 114 RR, n=16
Tiotixene TIO			δ^F	(δ^F)	δ^F (ϑ^F) α_2^F	CLO Clozapine
Meprobamate MEP	ϑ^F		ϑ^F	δ^F α_1^F ϑ^F α_2^F	β_3^F	CLA Dipotassium Chlorazepate
Placebo PLA	β_1^F			δ^F α_1^F ϑ^F	P	PLA Placebo
Nortriptyline-HCl NOR			(P)		δ α_1 ϑ α_2	MIA Mianserin
Tranylcypromine Sulfate TRA	(α_1^F) (P)			(β_1^F) ϑ^F β_3^F		CAF Caffeine
HUM 115 RR, n=14	TIO	MEP	PLA	NOR	TRA	

	MOL	LOR	PLA	DES	PHE	HUM 116 RR, n=16
		α_1^F (β_3^F) β_1^F	(β_3^F) (ϑ^F) P	ϑ^F	(α_2^F) β_1^F	MOL Molindone
			β_3^F β_1^F	β_3^F	α_1^F (β_1^F)	LOR Lorazepam
				ϑ^F		PLA Placebo
						DES Desipramine
						PHE Phenelzine Sulfate

P = total power 1.5-30.0 Hz
δ^F = 1.5- 5.5 Hz
ϑ^F = 5.5- 8.5 Hz
α_1^F = 8.5-10.5 Hz
α_2^F = 10.5-12.0 Hz
β_1^F = 12.0-18.0 Hz
β_3^F = 21.0-30.0 Hz
$\delta^F \triangleq p < .05$, $(\delta^F) \triangleq p < .10$ taking the frequency band δ^F
MANOVA for each variable at 3 times (pre, 1 h post, 3 h post)
RR = Resting Recording

Figure 1

Time dependent drug effects are shown by the mean values of the EEG power spectrum estimates (6 frequency bands and total power) and their standard deviation.
An example for one representative of each psychotropic drug class is given. A change in the relative power can only be interpreted with reference to the absolute power.

Figure 2

Standard EEG q-score profiles of the substances shown in Figure 1 are plotted against placebo. The q-scores are obtained by Tukey tests. These profiles are examples of the visual demonstration of test results by multiple univariate comparisons.

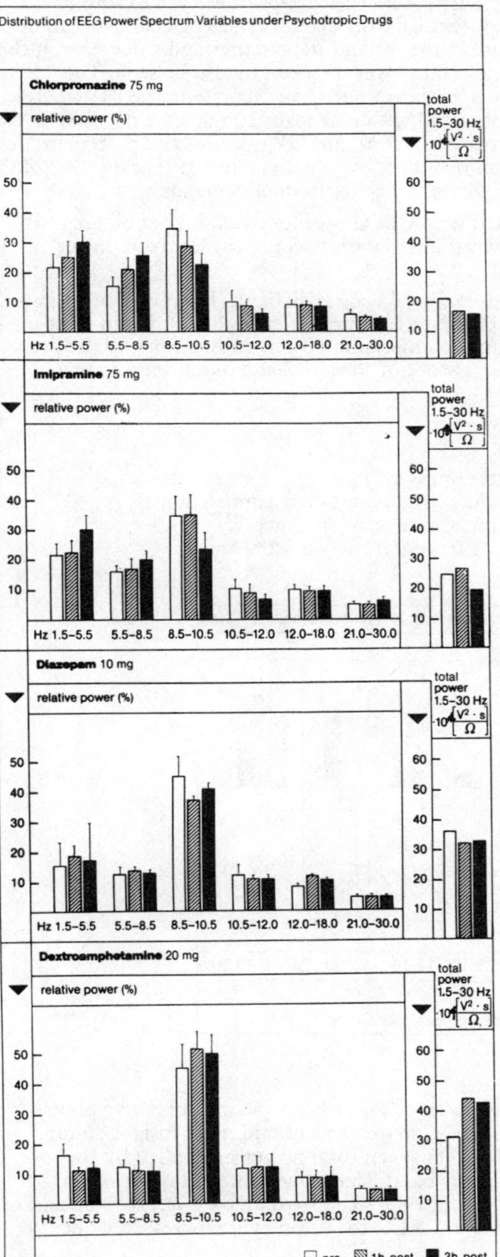

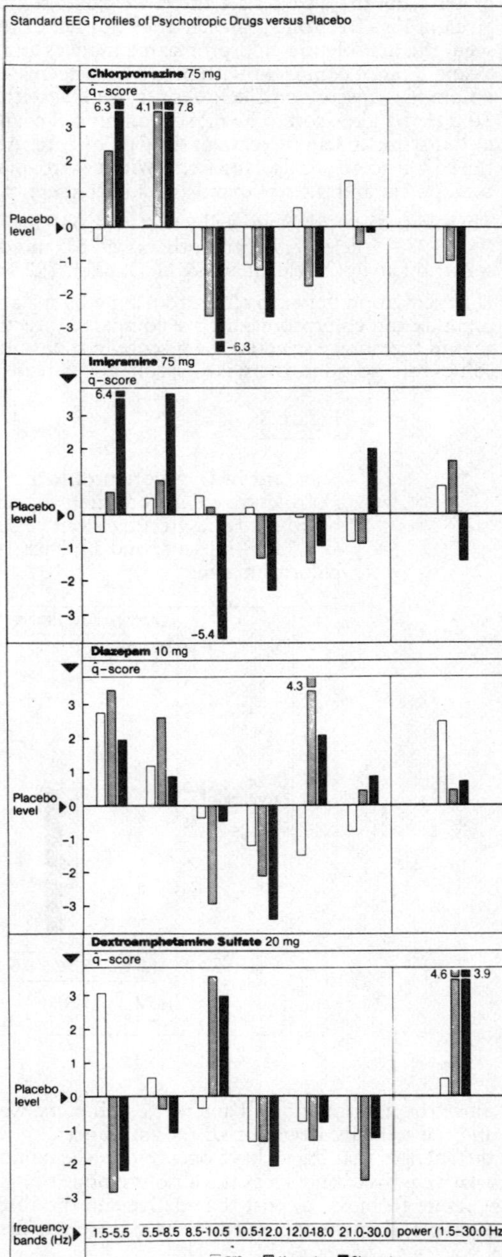

efficacy of these compounds may be due to the selection of the subjects (α-subjects) and/or the applied methodology (power spectrum analysis without high frequency β-activity) and/or may be due to the dosages selected.

Univariate Statistics

The results of the test statistics obtained by multivariate statistics are relatively abstract. We therefore used multiple Tukey tests which demonstrate changes in a more concrete manner. 21 Tukey tests are needed for each study (one for each variable at three time periods) which leads to 210 decisions about treatment effects. The results of these are not interpreted as statistical tests giving α-levels and the profiles drawn from the q-values are therefore called standard EEG-profiles (q-score-profiles). An example is given in Fig. 2 for one representative of each of the hypothetical drug classes versus placebo. As can be seen, the neuroleptic chlorpromazine induces an increase in the δ^F and ϑ^F q-scores and a decrease in the α- and β-range compared with placebo. A decrease in the total power q-score can also be seen. The imipramine q-score-profile looks very similar with one exception: there is an increase in the $\beta_3{}^F = 21.0 - 30.0$ Hz band q-score. The most pronounced changes obtained with diazepam 10 mg are a decrease in the $\alpha_2{}^F$ q-score and an increase in the $\beta_1{}^F$ q-score. An increase in the δ^F and ϑ^F q-scores and a decrease in the $\alpha_1{}^F$ q-score are also apparent. With dextroamphetamine sulfate there is an increase in the q-scores of the total power and the $\alpha_1{}^F$-band and a decrease in the q-score of all other frequency bands.

These results correspond well with those obtained by Itil with CEEG profiles based on period-analysis (Itil, 1974; Itil 1977; Itil and others, 1975), and our own findings with t-score profiles from power spectrum analysis (Herrmann & McDonald, 1978).

Differentiation between chlorpromazine 75 mg and imipramine 75 mg is difficult. However, when imipramine and chlorpromazine are compared directly with the q-score profile, as in Fig. 3, it can be seen that in the dosage selected the q-score in the ϑ^F-band under imipramine is lower. Also, taking the pre-values into account, there is a reasonable increase in the q-score of the $\beta_3{}^F$-band under imipramine.

Figure 3

Standard EEG q-score profile of the antidepressant imipramine versus the neuroleptic chlorpromazine as example of a drug versus drug comparison based on Tukey tests. As can be seen, imipramine causes a lower $\vartheta^F = 5.5 - 8.5$ Hz – q-score and a higher $\beta_3{}^F = 21.0 - 30.0$ Hz – q-score than chlorpromazine.

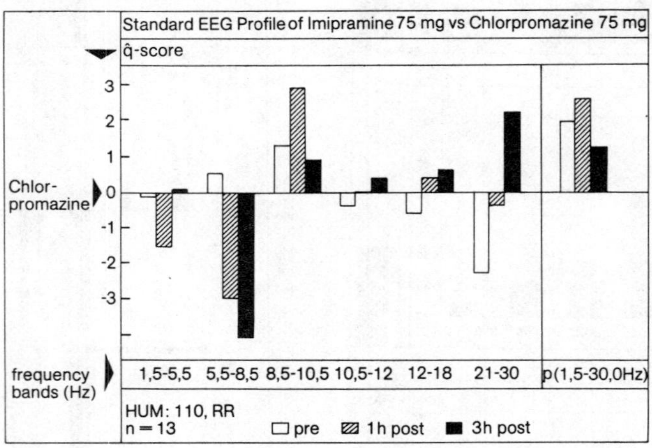

Since the q-scores are still abstract parameters, we have drawn in Fig. 1 both the mean relative power and the standard deviation of the substances, shown in Fig. 2, in order to obtain more insight about the changes that might have occurred in the clinical EEG. The given total power multiplied by the relative power value gives the absolute power in a frequency band. Hence, we can readily ascertain whether from pre to post the relative and the absolute power values change under a given substance. For example, it might appear from the q-score profiles that in the EEG the α-waves are increased while the

β-waves are decreased. Looking at the relative power distribution, this impression might be confirmed. However, the total power shows a 30% increase of the $\beta_3{}^F = 21.0 - 30.0$ Hz. The clinical picture of dextroamphetamine (Herrmann & McDonald, 1978) might well be interpreted as showing an increase in the α-waves and a decrease in the percentage of β-waves. However, the β-waves are obviously still existent, their total power is increased and they may only be hidden from view in the high amplitude α-waves.

DISCUSSION

Recalling our working hypothesis the following can be stated: The question as to whether the substances belonging to a particular substance class show similar EEG changes can be answered by looking at the variables which show significant differences in pairwise comparisons (see Table 3). In order to separate relevant from non relevant results it was decided to list in Table 4 only those variables which showed differences in corresponding pairwise comparisons in at least two out of the five studies. The arrow in Table 4 also shows the direction of the change. As can be seen, all 7 variables selected are involved in obtaining the differences between two substances. However, for the differences between the substances of one drug class and those of another drug class certain variables seem to be more relevant than others.

TABLE 4

As a summary of the results of the multivariate pairwise comparisons shown in Table 3, the relevant variables for differentiation among representatives of 5 defined drug classes are listed. A variable is deemed relevant if in at least two of the five studies the null hypothesis can be rejected. The *number* of arrows indicates the number of studies in which significant results in corresponding pairwise comparisons have been obtained. The *direction* of an arrow indicates the direction of the change at 1 hr. and 3 hr. post. Access to the Table is horizontal, from left to right. Example: In row 1, the neuroleptics are listed. If one goes to column 3 (PLA), then the arrows indicate that neuroleptics increase δ^F, ϑ^F and decrease $\beta_1{}^F$ in comparison to placebo.

Relevant Variables for the Differentiation Among Representatives of the 5 Defined Drug Classes

Summary of the Results of the Multivariate Pairwise Comparisons

Drug Class	**NEU**	**ANX**	**PLA**	**ANT**	**PSY**
NEUroleptics		ϑ^F ↑↑↑ $\beta_1{}^F$ ↓⇣⇣	δ^F ↑↑ ϑ^F ↑⇡⇡ $\beta_1{}^F$ ↓↓	ϑ^F ↑⇡	δ^F ↑↑ ϑ^F ↑⇡⇡ $\alpha_2{}^F$ ↓⇣ $\alpha_1{}^F$ ⇣⇣ p↓⇣
ANXiolytics	ϑ^F ↓↓↓ $\beta_1{}^F$ ↑⇡⇡		$\beta_1{}^F$ ↑↑	δ^F ↓↑ ϑ^F ↓↑ $\alpha_1{}^F$ ↑↑↓	$\alpha_1{}^F$ ↓↓ $\beta_1{}^F$ ↑⇡⇡
PLAcebos	δ^F ↓↓ ϑ^F ↓⇣⇣ $\beta_1{}^F$ ↑↑	$\beta_1{}^F$ ↓↓		δ^F ↓↓ ϑ^F ↓↓↓⇣ $\alpha_1{}^F$ ↑↑	p↓↓
ANTidepressants	ϑ^F ↓⇣	δ^F ↑↓ ϑ^F ↑↓ $\alpha_1{}^F$ ↓↓↑	δ^F ↑↑ ϑ^F ↑↑↑⇡ $\alpha_1{}^F$ ↓↓		δ^F ↑↑↑ ϑ^F ↑↑↑⇡ $\alpha_1{}^F$ ↓↓ $\beta_3{}^F$ ⇡⇡
PSYchostimulants	δ^F ↓↓ ϑ^F ↓↓⇣ $\alpha_2{}^F$ ↑⇡ $\alpha_1{}^F$ ⇡⇡ p↑⇡	$\alpha_1{}^F$ ↑↑ $\beta_1{}^F$ ↓⇣⇣	p↑↑	δ^F ↓↓↓ ϑ^F ↓↓↓⇣ $\alpha_1{}^F$ ↑↑ $\beta_3{}^F$ ⇣⇣	

↑ (↓) ≙ $p<.05$ } increase (decrease) in the EEG variable
⇡ (⇣) ≙ $p<.10$ }

It can be seen that in the pairwise comparisons of the neuroleptics with all other substances $\vartheta^F = 5.5 - 8.5$ Hz is involved. As we know from Itil (Itil, 1969a), the neuroleptics produced δ- and ϑ-waves. When we look at the comparison of neuroleptics with placebo we find this also true of the δ^F- and ϑ^F-band. The fact that, if neuroleptics are tested versus anxiolytics and antidepressants, ϑ^F seems to be more relevant than δ^F can be interpreted in two ways: Either δ^F is not a relevant variable for differentiation because the other substance classes also cause increase in δ^F-activity, or the slow waves induced by neuroleptics are more in the ϑ^F- than the δ^F-frequency band range.
For the anxiolytics, $\beta_1{}^F = 12.0 - 18.0$ Hz seems to be an important variable. This is in accordance with the findings of Itil (Itil, 1974) and Fink (Fink and others, 1976), and our own findings (Herrmann & McDonald, 1978). The benzodiazepine anxiolytics induce a shift from the fast α- into the slow β-wave range, and therefore made the $\beta_1{}^F$ variable a discriminatory one. Only in comparison with the antide-

pressants which themselves cause an increase in the relative β-power does the $\beta_1{}^F$ fail to contribute to the differentiation.

For the antidepressants, the differences compared with other substance classes – with the exception of neuroleptics – are obtained by the δ^F-, ϑ^F- and $\alpha_1{}^F$- (8.5 – 10.5 Hz) frequency bands. In comparison to placebo there is an increase in δ^F- and ϑ^F-, and a decrease in $\alpha_1{}^F$-activity. This is in accordance with interpretations of Itil (Itil, 1974; Itil, 1975), Fink (Fink, 1961), and our own earlier findings (Herrmann & McDonald, 1978). However, it must be taken into account that comparability of the results is limited due to differences in methodology (EEG parametrisation and statistics).

When testing the psychostimulants versus substances of the other drug classes – with the exception of placebo – $\alpha_1{}^F$ is involved. There is an increase in slow α-activity when stages of reduced vigilance with α-dissolution are permitted during recordings. In the case of the psychostimulants an increase in the α-amplitude, and α-percent can be obtained (Itil, 1976; Fink and others, 1971).

This is also in accordance with the power spectrum estimates as can be seen from Fig. 1 and also with the standard q-score profile (Fig. 2).

The differences between neuroleptics and antidepressants, which are fairly small when using discriminant function analysis (Herrmann/Fichte et al., 1979), and also visually when comparing amitriptyline 75 mg with chlorpromazine 75 mg (Herrmann & McDonald, 1978), have been described in more detail by Itil (Itil, 1974) using the standard CEEG profiles and interval analysis mainly in the interval classes of higher frequencies (30 – 90 Hz). While antidepressants cause an increase in the fast β-wave activity, neuroleptics cause a decrease. In the basic studies using power spectrum variables up to 30.0 Hz, only imipramine showed a marked increase in the $\beta_3{}^F$-range in comparison to placebo.

Visual demonstration of drug efficacy using the relative power values for the 6 frequency bands and the total power in combination with the q-score standard profiles seems to be an adequate method. The power distribution gives information about the quality and quantity of the power estimates obtained, and is a good link between the clinical EEG picture and the abstract results obtained in the q-score standard profiles. The q-score profiles, on the other hand, are a necessary link between the variables used for statistics and the test results obtained by multivariate statistics, which could hardly be interpreted without them.

REFERENCES

Akpinar, S., T.M. Itil, J. Marasa, A. Marazzi (1972). Blocking Effect of Chlorpromazine on LSD_{25} Induced Clinical and Digital Computer Analyzed EEG Changes. Clin. Electroenceph., 3, 4, 224 – 232.

Bente, D. (1964). Die Insuffizienz des Vigilitätstonus. Habilitationsschrift. Universität Erlangen-Nürnberg.

Borenstein, P., M. Dongier, M. Fink, V. Florio, T.M. Itil, V.G. Longo, F. Mellerio, R. Naquet, G. Pampiglione, J. Titeca, G. Verdeaux (1970). Clinical and experimental electroencephalography. In: Modern Problems of Pharmacopsychiatry, 5. Karger, Basel, pp. 109 – 125

Eggert, D. (1974). Eysenck-Persönlichkeits-Inventar E-P-I (Manual). Verlag für Psychologie, Dr. C.J. Hogrefe, Göttingen.

Eysenck, H.J. (1957). Drugs and Personality. I. Theory and Methodology. J. Ment. Sci., 103,119 131.

Fahrenberg, J. (1965). Ein itemanalysierter Fragebogen funktionell-körperlicher Beschwerden (VELA). Diagnostica, 11, 141–153.

Fink, M. (1961). Quantitative Electroencephalography and Human Psychopharmacology. I: Frequency Spectra and Drug Action. Med. Exp., 5, 364 – 369.

Fink, M. (1969). Drugs, EEG and Behavior. In: Black: Drugs and the Brain. Hopkins, Baltimore. pp. 149–160.

Fink, M., P. Irwin, R.E. Weinfeld, M.A. Schwartz, A.H. Conney (1976). Blood levels and electroencephalographic effects of diazepam and bromazepam. Clin. Pharmacol. Ther., 20, 2, 184–191.

Fink, M., D.M. Shapiro, T.M. Itil (1971). EEG profiles of fenfluramine, amobarbital and dextroamphetamine in normal volunteers. Psychopharmacologia (Berl.), 22, 369–383.

Herrmann, W.M., K. Fichte, T.M. Itil, St. Kubicki (1979). Development of a classification rule for four clinical therapeutic psychotropic drug classes with EEG power-spectrum variables of human volunteers. Pharmakopsych., in press

Herrmann, W.M., K. Fichte, St. Kubicki (1978). Mathematische Rationale für die klinischen EEG-Frequenzbänder. 1. Faktorenanalyse mit Powerspektralschätzungen zur Definition von Frequenzbändern. EEG – EMG, 9, 146 – 154.

Herrmann, W.M., R.J. McDonald (1978). A multidimensional test approach for the description of the CNS acitivity of drugs in human pharmacology. Pharmakopsych., 11, pp. 247 – 265.

Itil, T.M. (1969). Definition and Classification of Neuroleptics from the EEG Point of View. In D.P. Bobon (ed.), Reprints of the Interdisciplinary Week on Neuroleptics. University of Liege. pp. 167 – 169.

Itil, T.M., D.M. Shapiro, M. Fink, N. Kiremitci, C. Hickmann (1969). Quantitative EEG Studies of Chlordiazepoxide, Chlorpromazine and Imipramine in Volunteers and Schizophrenic Subjects. In W.O. Evans and N.S. Kline (eds.), The Psychopharmacology of the Normal Human. C.C. Thomas, Springfield, Ill. pp. 219 – 237.

Itil, T.M. (1974). Quantitative Pharmaco-Electroencephalography. The Use of Computerized Cerebral Biopotentials in Psychotropic Drug Research. In T.M. Itil (ed.): Modern Problems of Pharmacopsychiatry, 8. Karger, Basel. pp. 43 – 75.

Itil, T.M. (1975). Computer EEG-Profiles of Antidepressants. In S. Fielding and H. Lal (eds.), Industrial Pharmacology, Vol. II. Futura Publishing Company, Mt. Kisco, New York. pp. 319 – 351.

Itil, T.M. (1976). The Neurophysiological Models in the Development of Psychotropic Hormones. In T.M. Itil, G. Laudahn and W.M. Herrmann (eds.): Psychotropic Action of Hormones. Spectrum Publications, New York. pp. 53 – 77.

Kugler, J., K.-J. Johannes, M. Laub, K. Tuluweit (1978). Elektroenzephalografische Vigilanzbestimmung nach Amitriptylin-N-oxid. Arzneim.-Forsch. 28, 3, 475 – 479.

Strategy of Statistical Spectral Analysis in Drug Studies. A Methodological Synopsis

P. ETEVENON, B. PIDOUX* and P. RIOUX**

Section d'E.E.G. Quantitative du S.H.U. de Santé Mentale et de Thérapeutique du Centre Hospitalier Sainte-Anne
*Service d'Exploration Fonctionnelle du Système Nerveux du Centre Hospitalier Sainte-Anne, 1 rue Cabanis, F. 75674 Paris, Cédex 14
**Groupe U 88 de l'INSERM, F. 75013 Paris

ABSTRACT

A theoretical and experimental comparison between 4 classical methods of EEG analysis has been conducted : amplitude histograms, spectral analysis, integrative method of Drohocki and zero-crossing. Specific advantages and disadvantages, proper data reduction, comparisons were made between mean values and coefficients of variation. Spectral Fourier analysis can sum up and add more than the three other methods.

After considering the basic strategy of Fourier analysis, for periodic, random or transient data, we present the strategy of statistical spectral analysis : on-line interactive A/D conversion with double rejection of artifacts, followed by Fourier analysis and data reduction allowing first statistical and graphical results. The last step is an increasing digital data base and further multivariate analysis.

Finally, we present two examples of multivariate cluster analysis between quantified EEGs. The first is a dichotomic classification of 240 recordings obtained in 10 normal volunteers, providing a high spectral intensity alpha sub-group vs. a low alpha intensity and high bêta intensity sub-group. The second is a classified 5 clusters graph, between 103 quantified EEG recordings, from normal and psychotic patients, where one cluster contained mostly paranoïd EEGs with low spectral alpha intensity and one another contained mostly hebephrenic EEGs with high alpha frequency and alpha spectral intensity.
KEYWORDS: spectral analysis, quantitative EEG, schizophrenia, methodology, statistics

INTRODUCTION

Progresses in EEG data analysis have been successively related in collective books devoted almost every year since 1973 to quantitative electroencephalography by specialists in the field (2, 4, 9, 10, 11, 12, 14, 16), besides monographies written on this topic from different points of view (3, 5, 15).

Before presenting the statistical spectral analysis that we are now applying to drug-studies, we will have to compare the classical methods of E.E.G. analysis and then consider the strategy of Fourier analysis. Later, after a discussion of the basic statistics that we have applied to the spectral parameters chosen as good descriptors of a quantified E.E.G. recording, we will briefly underline the last step of E.E.G. analysis, which is also the most sophisticated one and implies the use of statistical multivariate techniques.

COMPARISON BETWEEN METHODS OF EEG ANALYSIS

In different quantitative EEG laboratories, different analyses are used providing after data reduction different parameters. In 1977, we have made in our dissertation (5) a theoretical as well as experimental comparison of the most classical methods of EEG analysis. We will now present briefly our conclusions.

Four Methods have been compared :

I. The probability density distributions obtained by the computation of amplitude histograms.
2. The power spectrum or spectral analysis providing electrical power values in ordinates vs. frequency in abscissae, based on Fourier analysis.
3. The integrative method of Drohocki based on surface computation between the rectified EEG and its base-line.
4. The zero-crossing method or period analysis providing mean frequency computation.

Specific Advantages and Disadvantages of each of these Methods

I. The first one is very easy to handle. However the amplitude histograms are gaussian or non-gaussian depending on the chosen sampling frequency. Therefore, a parametrisation of this method is biased by this dependency, which in fact depends on the second order statistical properties of the EEG signal which are considered in spectral analysis. This method neglects the frequency and the phase variables.
2. The spectral analysis is still more costly to apply than the other techniques. It needs a second step of data reduction with a proper choice of spectral parameters as we will see later. Theoretically, the analysed EEG signal should be independent of the origin of time. This is called the stationarity property. Practically, there are recordings where it is not the case and this is a practical difficulty which can be solved by analysing the time changes of the set of spectral parameters. Measurements of power spectra neglects the phase variable but Fourier transform analysis allows phase analysis under specific conditions.
3. The integrative method neglects the frequency and the phase variables. However, it is the cheapest of all the methods of EEG analysis.
4. The zero-crossing analysis neglects the amplitude and the phase variables. Computation of errors have not yet been properly established. This method was applied by using specially built analogic electronic circuits which were biased by the fact that the signal/noise ratio was sensitive to high frequency components present in the EEG. Therefore, mean frequencies computed for the first or the second time derivative of the EEG signal, were biased measurements. Moreover, computation of errors are very difficult to be applied. However, new techniques such as iterative interval analysis of Hjorth parameters of mobility (mean frequency) and complexity, can be considered as derived from the classical zero-crossing method and provide better data reduction parameters.

DATA REDUCTION

The next step of data reduction or choice of proper parameters is crucial for the statistical quantification of the EEG.

I. From the amplitude histograms, standard deviations around the means are good descriptors of the EEG distributions. The deviations form normality can be computed, but it depends on the chosen statistics : chi-square, test of Shapiro and Wilk or skewness and kurtosis measurements. These last two parameters have been computed for instance by Dumermuth (in 4).

2. From the power spectrum or the power spectrum density curve, a number of very descriptive and highly relevant 16 parameters can be computed for each quantified EEG channel :
   - 8 spectral parameters related to Zetterberg (17) analysis and characterizing the delta peak and the alpha peak of the power spectrum : the peak spectral intensity with its standard deviation and the peak dominant frequency with its standard deviation.
   - 4 broad frequency bands : integrated spectral intensities which are usually expressed in % of the surface of the spectrum and related to delta, theta, α and bêta 1 frequency ranges familiar to electroencephalographers.
   - Statistical spectral parameters such as the mean power value, the integral of the power spectrum, the variance of the EEG signal computed together with its root-mean-square, which is the RMS amplitude value expressed in microvolts.
   - Then, the mean frequency N (or mobility coefficient of Hjorth) computed from spectral formulas.
   - The resonance coefficient k, that we finally compute is depending only on the shape of the spectrum and is scale free. This coefficient characterizing the variability of a spectrum, is equal to 1 for a pure sine-wave and to 0.1 for a pure white noise.
3. With the integrative method, an EEG recording of 5 min., analysed for every successive 10 s. epoch, provides 30 measurements. From these values, a mean value I with a standard deviation s around the mean can be easily computed. The ratio I/s provides also a coefficient of variation which characterizes the variability of the analysed recording.
4. From the zero-crossing method, the main parameters are the mean frequency N (or its inverse called the major period) of the EEG signal and the mean frequency N 1 of the first derivative (or its inverse called the intermediate period). Hjorth has also proposed a "complexity" coefficient which depends on N and N 1. It is equal to zero for a sine-wave and has increasing values when the analysed signal approaches a white noise with equal intensities of frequency components.

Comparisons between the Methods

If we want to sum up our findings, we have to consider separately the mean values obtained in each method from their dispersion measurements.

We have shown a linear proportionality between the standard deviation of the amplitude histogram, the RMS value computed from the power spectrum and the mean value given by the integrative method. These parameters are proportional to the standard deviation of the EEG time-signal and that is why they are basic descriptors of the EEG signal.

Perhaps more interesting is the proportionality between coefficients of variation of the spectral analysis (proportional to the resonance coefficient k easily computed by : $k^2 = (\Sigma G^2) / (\Sigma G)^2$ where G is the power spectrum) and of the integrative method.

Each coefficient of variation is proportional to the inverse of the square-root of T the period of analysis. This means that when the time window of analysis decreases, the coefficients of variation are increasing. As a direct consequence, it is very important, when comparing different results in different laboratories which are obtained with these methods, to check if the periods of analysis have the same value.

Finally, the zero-crossing method can be applied not only on the rough EEG but on broad-band filtered EEGs, providing results which are not far from frequency or spectral analysis measurements, in terms of EEG frequency bands or broad-band integrated spectral values. This has been empirically demonstrated by Irwin and Fink (8). Now, the computations of N 1 is difficult to be accurate, because of the derivation of the EEG signal which enhances the fast frequencies and then decreases the signal/noise ratio. The same bias occurs in the computation of the complexity coefficient of Hjorth, which is less accurate than the coefficient of resonance k that we prefer to compute from the spectral values.

We consider presently that statistical spectral analysis provides all the basic parameters of the three other methods of EEG analysis that we have considered.

Before presenting the procedure involved in statistical spectral analysis applied to the quantification of EEG data, it is important to review the basic strategy of Fourier analysis which depends on the nature of the analysed signal.

BASIC STRATEGY OF FOURIER ANALYSIS

In 1807, Fourier presented a general solution for the problem of vibrating strings. A periodic function of time was decomposed as a sum of sinusoïdal and cosinusoïdal terms, which was called later a Fourier serie. It was only in 1930 and 1933 that Wiener extended the Fourier analysis to random signals by applying Fourier transforms. However these integral relationships, relating time properties of the signal to the frequency domain, were difficult to manage until the discovery in 1965 by Cooley and Tukey of the Fast Fourier Transform (FFT) algorithm. Presently the FFT computation time, microprogrammed in recent minicomputers, takes 125 ms or less for a data block of 1024 channels, representing for instance 10 s of EEG. However, transient signals decaying rapidly with time, were not usually analysed by Fourier analysis until the introduction of distribution theory and extensive use of Dirac functions by Schwartz (1, 5).

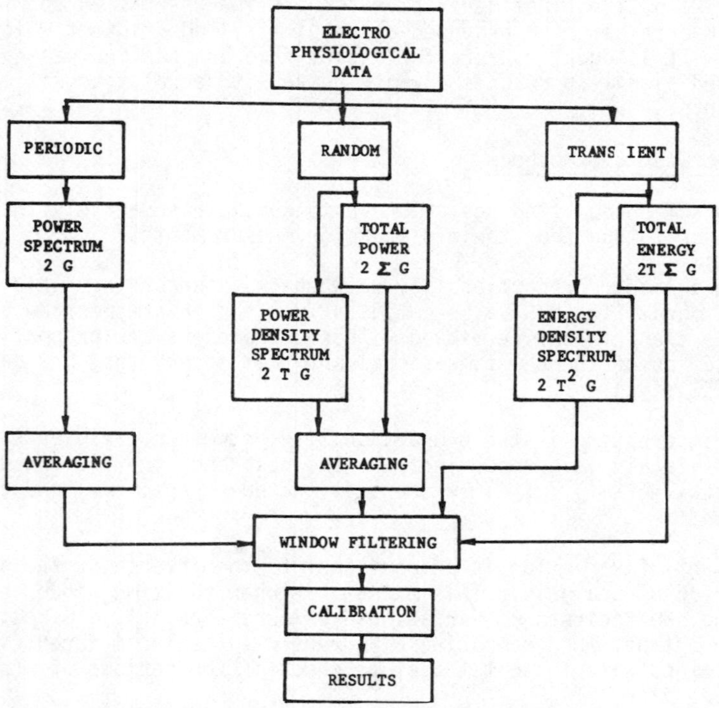

Fig.1. Strategy of Fourier analysis.

Depending on the nature of incoming signal, electrophysiological data can be considered as periodic (EKG, breath), random (EEG, EMG) or transient (isolated spikes, evoked potentials). Therefore, they will be submitted to different computations, based on Fourier series or Fourier transforms properties, providing power spectrum, power spectrum density or energy density spectrum.

STRATEGY OF STATISTICAL SPECTRAL ANALYSIS

Our interest being centered on EEG analysis, we shall consider now in Fig. 2, the general flow-chart which is usually followed in quantitative EEG laboratories.

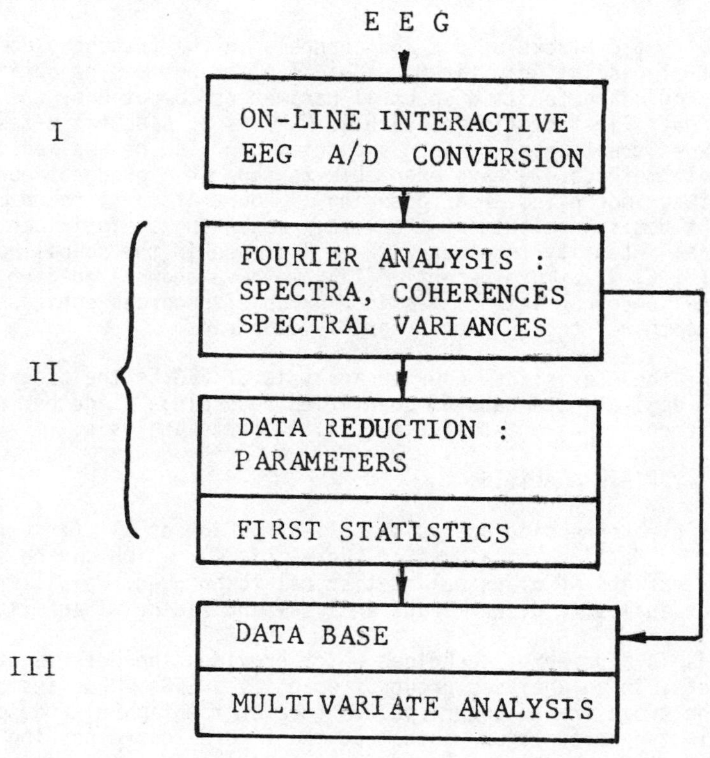

Fig. 2. Strategy of statistical Fourier analysis of EEG.

In the first step, occurs a real time analog to digital conversion of EEG recording. This implies analog pre-processing of the EEG such as fast frequency filtering, on-line A/D conversion at proper sampling rate (200 Hz for 2.5 s. of 4 EEG channels in our case), on-line digital pre-processing (such as direct courant component removal) together with proper calibration of the digitalized EEG and rejection of artifacts. We have already described elsewhere (5, 6, 7), the existing interactive double rejection of artifacts (one automatic rejection based on a predetermined amplitude threshold and one manual delayed rejection). This real time programme called "SANTE" is working on a Fourier Analyzer (5451 B Hewlett-Packard) with 32 K memory (2100 S microprogrammable minicomputer) equipped with mass memory (disc and digital magnetic tape). On the disc, 6 successive EEG sequences of 5 mn. of 4 simultaneously recorded channels, can be digitalized almost in real time (not considering the 10 s. delay needed for the delayed manual rejection of artifacts). For each sequence, 30 epochs of 10 s.

each are stored on disc. The program (written in assembly language) can be stopped at any time and started again. It ends automatically after the 30th converted sample.

The second step is the proper Fourier analysis which can be run in real time for the computation and digital storage of successive evolutive spectra (of successive 10 s. epochs of EEGs), according to Bickford's method of Compressed Spectral Array. It can also be run in 12 min. for the computation and digital storage of averaged spectral results : 4 auto power spectra with their 4 spectral variances, 6 cross-spectra (computed in double precision) and 6 coherences between the 4 analysed EEG channels.

From these results (26 blocks of 2 x 256 channels in the frequency domain, with 0.4 Hz of spectral resolution), first graphical plottings can be obtained and first listings of characteristic spectral parameters computed by the next program of data reduction. First statistics such as MANOVAs or spectral t-tests between sequences, between treatments, between subjects, can also be applied immediately. With these simple methods, we have been able to show in a group of normal subjects differences between occipital areas occuring 14 hours after nitrazepam administration : The right hemisphere but not the left, presenting a significant decrease in alpha spectral intensity together with an increase in the so-called benzodiazepine spindles (5, 6, 7). More recently (13), we have shown a greater symmetry (α%) between occipital spectral intensities in a group of recorded schizophrenic patients, when compared to a group of normal volunteers.

The last step of the statistical Fourier analysis of EEG is the progressive increase of the digital data base of quantified recordings, together with applications of different kinds of statistical multivariate analysis.

MULTIVARIATE ANALYSIS

Apart from multiple regression analysis applied by Fink et al. (in reference 4), MANOVAs applied by Matejcek et al. (12), Künkel (in 4), which can be seen as multivariate extensions of classical statistical techniques, we will now briefly consider cluster analysis, discriminant analysis and factorial analysis.

Cluster analysis is a powerful technique which provides the determination of sub-sets, of clusters, in an analysed group of quantified EEGs. For instance, figure 3 represents the two averaged power spectra (top of the figure) and power density spectra (in relative percentages, bottom of the figure) corresponding to each of the first two clusters which were found in 10 normal subjects having provided 240 quantified EEG sequences (Etevenon et al. in reference 14).

These clusters were respectively a high alpha sub-group and a low alpha sub-group. Moreover, each sub-group reacted differently to a same dosage of anxiolytic compound. The high alpha group decreased in alpha intensity towards the theta range whereas the low alpha group increased in alpha intensity following the oral administration of 10 mg of chlordiazepoxide.

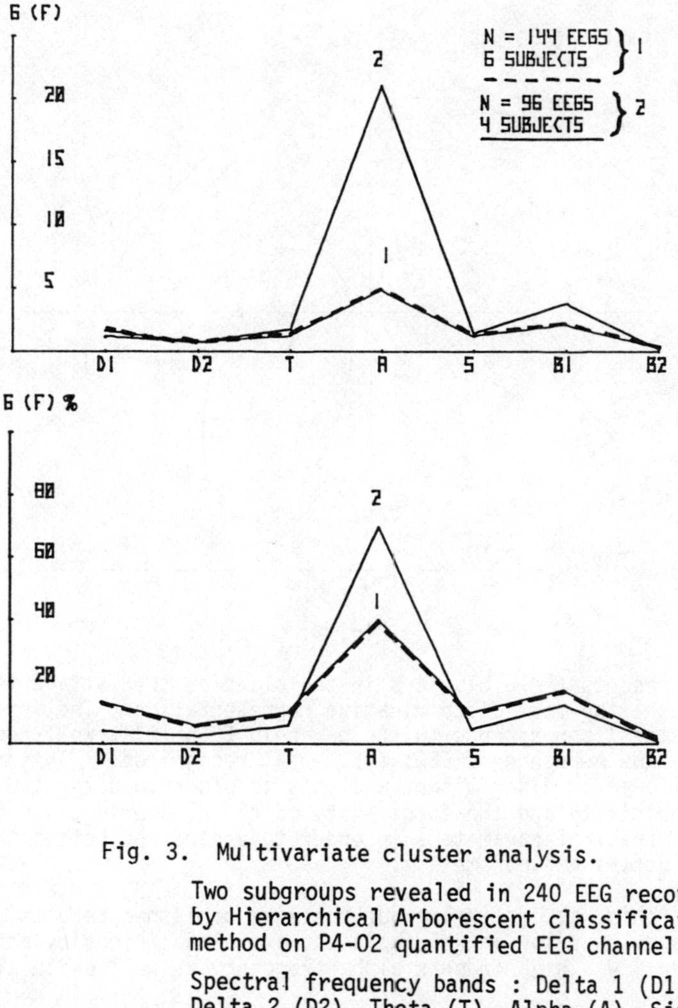

Fig. 3. Multivariate cluster analysis.

Two subgroups revealed in 240 EEG recordings by Hierarchical Arborescent classification method on P4-O2 quantified EEG channel.

Spectral frequency bands : Delta 1 (D1), Delta 2 (D2), Theta (T), Alpha (A), Sigma (S), Beta 1 (B1), Beta 2 (B2), from 0 to 50 Hz.

We will give a second example of multivariate cluster analysis from our recent findings, which will soon be published in details. Thirty subjects were recorded an average of 3 times, under the same conditions : eyes closed, 4 posterior EEG channels, providing 103 EEG recorded sequences which were submitted to statistical spectral analysis and data reduction. For each EEG channel 6 parameters were only computed : spectral intensity of the alpha peak and its standard deviation, spectral frequency of the alpha peak together with its standard deviation. Five clusters were determined from 103 quantified EEG recordings. These quantified EEGs were recorded from a group of human volunteers (28 EEGs from 14 subjects), of psychotic but non-schizophrenic patients (23 EEGs from 7 patients), and of schizophrenic patients (36 EEGs from 6 hebephrenic patients and 16 from 5 paranoid patients).

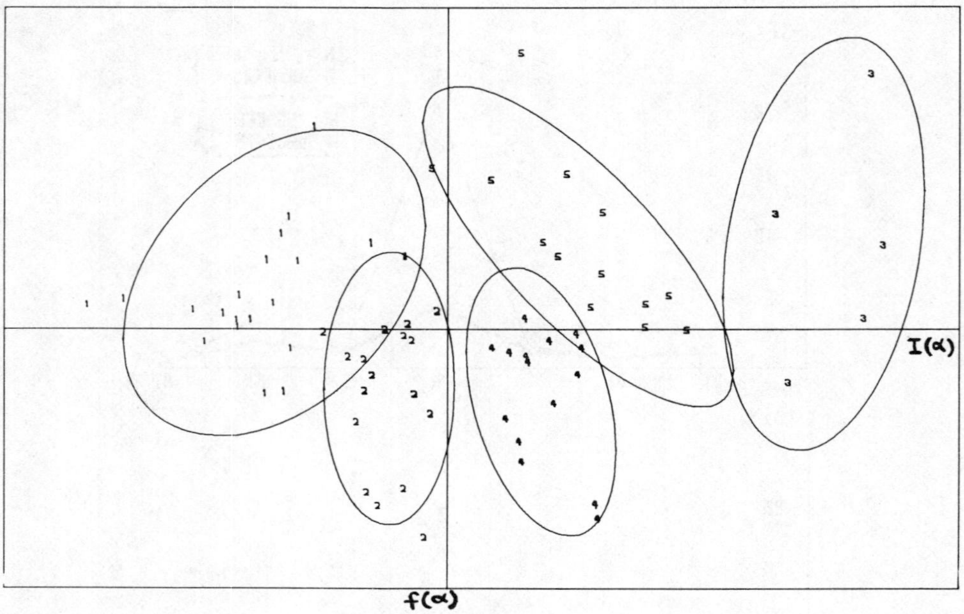

Fig. 4.

The figure 4 represents the 5 clusters in the plane of the 1st and the 3rd axis, which appears to be the most discriminative representation. The interesting fact is that the cluster 1 corresponds to the paranoid EEGs (81 % well recognized) and the cluster 4 to the hebephrenic EEGs (65 % well recognized). This multivariate analysis was followed by discriminant analysis in order to determine with a better accuracy the sensitivity and the specificity of the clustering, and by factorial analysis between spectral parameters in order to understand better the relationships between clusters and parameters.

In our case, and this was confirming our previous published results (6), the paranoid sub-group 1 was low in RMS amplitude and alpha intensity and the hebephrenic sub-group 4 was high in peak alpha frequency as well as in alpha intensity.

ACKNOWLEDGEMENTS.

We are grateful to Dr PERON-MAGNAN, Chargé de Recherches INSERM, for clinical global diagnosis and follow up of the schizophrenic patients.
We wish also to thank Mr LETEL for his skillful EEG recordings.

This work was supported by French INSERM Grants ATP 39-76-71, 65-78-97 and UER Cochin-Port-Royal.

REFERENCES

1. Bendat, J.S. and A.G. Piersol (1971). Random data : analysis and measurement procedures. Wiley-Intersciences, New York.
2. Burch, N. and H.L. Altshuler (Eds.) (1975). Behavior and brain electrical activity, Plenum Press, New York.
3. Callaway, E. (1975). Brain electrical potentials and individual psychological differences, Grune and Stratton, New York.
4. Dolce, G. and H. Kunkel (Eds.) (1975). CEAN computerized EEG analysis, Gustav Fischer Verlag, Stuttgart.
5. Etevenon, P. (1977). Etude méthodologique de l'électroencéphalographie quantitative. Application à quelques exemples. Thèse D. Sc., Paris, Faculté des Sciences, Université de Paris VI.
6. Etevenon, P. and B. Pidoux (1977). From biparametric to multidimensional analysis of EEG. In A. Remond (Ed.), EEG Informatics. A didactic review of methods and applications of EEG data processing, Elsevier/North Holland, Amsterdam, pp. 193-214.
7. Etevenon, P., B. Pidoux, P. Peron-Magnan, P. Rioux, G. Verdeaux, J.R. Boissier and P. Deniker (1978, in press). Electroencephalography statistical spectral analysis of quantitative electroencephalography. In P. Deniker (Ed.), Proc. Xth Intl. Congress C.I.N.P., Pergamon Press, Oxford, pp. 1141-1150.
8. Irwin, P.M. and M. Fink (1975). An empirical comparison of three EEG digital conversion techniques : baseline cross analysis, power spectral density analysis and Hjorth analysis. In M. Matejcek and G.K. Schenk (Eds.), Quantitative analysis of the EEG, AEG Telefunken, Konstanz, pp. 379-393.
9. Itil, T.M. (Ed.), (1974). Psychotropic drugs and the human EEG. Mod. Probl. Pharmacopsychiatry, Vol. 8, Karger, Bâle.
10. Kellaway, P. (Ed.), (1976). Quantitative analytic studies in epilepsy, Raven Press, New York.
11. Kellaway, P. and I. Petersen (Eds.), (1973). Automation of clinical electroencephalography, Raven Press, New York.
12. Matejcek, M. and G.K. Schenk (1975). Quantitative analysis of the EEG. Proc. of 2nd symp. study group for EEG-methodology, AEG-Telefunken, Konstanz.
13. Pidoux, B., P. Etevenon, G. Verdeaux and P. Deniker (1978, in press). L'activité alpha dans un groupe de schizophrènes : Analyse spectrale et comparaison avec un groupe témoin. Rev. EEG Neurophysiol. clin.
14. Remond, A. (Ed.), (1977). EEG informatics. A didactic review of methods and applications of EEG data processing, Elsevier, Amsterdam.
15. Saletu, B. (1976). Psychopharmaka, Gehirntätigkeit und Bibliotheca Psychiatrika, No. 155, Karger, Bâle.
16. Schenk, G.K. (1973). Die quantifizierung des elektroencephalogramms, AEG-Telefunken, Konstanz.
17. Zetterberg, L.H. (1969). Estimation of parameters for a linear difference equation with application to EEG analysis. Math. Biosci., 5, 227-275.

Drawing Inferences about the Therapeutic Efficacy of Drugs in Patients from their CNS Effect in Normals: Comparative Quantitative Pharmaco-EEG and Clinical Investigations

B. SALETU*, M. SALETU, J. GRÜNBERGER* and R. MADER****

*Section of Pharmacopsychiatry, Psychiatric University Clinic, Vienna, Austria
**Anton Proksch Institute, Vienna, Austria

ABSTRACT

In two subsequent studies the question was explored to which extent short-term drug effects in the EEG of normal subjects are predictive of clinical and EEG effects in patients. Early Phase I EEG trials in volunteers suggested that D-12524 (lopirazepam - a new pyridodiazepine) is a CNS-effective substance which differs significantly from placebo and produces a pharmaco-EEG profile typical for the "anxiolytic" drugs. Indeed, a subsequent clinical study in alcoholic patients with an anxiety syndrome confirmed this prediction. During a three-week treatment period with this drug a marked and significant improvement was noted in clinical symptomatology as evaluated by means of the global score, Hamilton, Zung and Erlanger anxiety score, of somatic symptoms and side effect rating scale and by psychometric test methods. Comparing the central effects of a certain dosage of the drug (at the same time after oral administration) in the two different populations, it was found that lopirazepam produced the same "anxiolytic" type of EEG changes, although some quantitative differences - especially in the slow waves (sedative effect) - were obvious. But then there were also significant baseline differences between the brain activity of alcoholics and normals. Single dose EEG effects in patients were highly correlated to EEG alterations after three weeks of chronic administration of the drug. Moreover, the drug-induced EEG changes during therapy were significantly linked to clinical improvement or deterioration. Finally, the relationships between single-dose effects in brain activity and therapeutic outcome was investigated.

KEYWORDS

EEG analysis, anxiolytics, lopirazepam, classification, pharmacodynamics, alcoholics, anxiety syndrome, therapeutic efficacy, psychopathology, side effects, psychometrics, clinical-neurophysiological correlation, predication of outcome.

INTRODUCTION

Recently Wittenborn (1977) stated in his guidelines for clinical trials of psychotropic drugs: "Since adequate animal models of human psychiatric illnesses are nonexistent, the initiation of Phase I studies could be based on considerations other than specific pharmacological activity in animals, e.g., on possible effects on brain biochemistry or electro-physiological parameters". Indeed, the quantitatively analyzed EEG in combination with certain statistical procedures seems to be such a method giving valuable information about a drug's encephalotropic, psychotropic and pharmaco-dynamic properties in man at an early stage in drug development (Fink, 1969; Itil, 1974; Saletu, 1976). Although on the first view the method seems alike to the retrospective animal pharmacology model (predicting psychoactive properties based on similarities of effects to actions observed in marketed and clinically effective drugs), it has the principal advantage that the CNS effects are observed in humans. Moreover, as the same techniques can be applied in normal volunteers and in patients, one may obtain valuable information concerning the relationship between CNS-effects (in normals) and therapeutic efficacy (in patients)! Indeed, there are already some (although mainly indirect) data available demonstrating such relationships (Itil, 1974, 1976; Itil and Saletu, 1973; Itil and co-workers, 1972, 1973; Matejcek and Devos, 1976; Roubicek and Majors, 1977; Saletu, 1976). Utilizing quantitative EEG and evoked potential methods, the effects of representatives of the major psychopharmaceutical classes were investigated in normals and in patients in a systematic manner. The analyses demonstrated that neuroleptics and anxiolytics induce similar CNS changes - or better - the same type of CNS alterations in both populations and furthermore that these neurophysiological changes were linked to changes in psychopathology (Itil, 1974; Itil and co-workers, 1972, 1973, 1975; Saletu and co-workers, 1971a, 1971b, 1971c, 1974, 1975; B. Saletu, M. Saletu and Itil, 1972 and 1973a). In the last three years we had the opportunity to investigate one and the same drug (D-12524 - lopirazepam[1]) initially in a normal population with the aim of classifying and determining its cerebral bioavailability by quantitative EEG methods and to subsequently carry out an open Phase I clinical trial in an alcoholic patient population with an anxiety syndrome. Thus, we could compare the effect of a certain dosage of a drug in a normal and psychiatric population and collect some data concerning the relationship between CNS effectiveness and therapeutic efficacy of a drug.

METHOD

In the initial double-blind placebo-controlled pharmaco-EEG study, 10 healthy normal volunteers in the age between 24 and 34 years (27 years) were included. They were not allowed to take any psychoactive substances 3 weeks prior to and during the time of the investigations. They received randomized in weekly intervals single oral doses or 3 mg, 5 mg, and 10 mg lopirazepam as well as 10 mg prazepam and placebo. Lopirazepam is chemically a 3-hydroxy-5(O-chlorphenyl-)7-chlor-1,2-dihydro-3H-pyrido[3,2-e]-1,4 diazepine-2-one (Homburg, 1976), whose pharmacology was described elsewhere (Saletu and co-workers, in press). Quantitative pharmaco-EEG, psychometric and clinical investigations were carried out before as well as 2, 4, 6 and 8 hours after drug. The former included 5-minute resting EEG records by means of an eight channel SLE-electroencephalograph polygraph with the subjects lying relaxed and with eyes closed in an electrically-shielded room. Electrodes were attached according to the international 10/20 system on the scalp. 4 leads (O2-Cz, O1-Cz, O3-Cz, O4-Cz) were recorded on a Hewlett-Packard 3960 tape recorder and were analyzed off-line by a digital computer system (PDP-12; Intertechnique Plurimat S) utilizing period analysis programs (Burch and co-workers, 1964). These programs permit analysis of 22 EEG measurements in 10/20 sec. epochs: the average frequency (AVG), frequency deviation (DEV) and the percentage distribution of the bioelectrical activity in eight different frequency bands of the "primary wave" (PW) and the "first derivative" (FD) as well as of the average absolute amplitude (AMPLIT)

[1]Lopirazepam was kindly supplied by Chemiewerk HOMBURG/GB. Pharma d. DEGUSSA, Frankfurt, Germany.

and amplitude variability (DRHOKI). At the end of each R-EEG period, means and sigmas of the 22 variables are calculated.

In the subsequent clinical (open Phase I) study 20 hospitalized male alcoholic patients with an anxiety syndrome in the age-range of 26-50 (mean 35) years were included. At the onset of the study there had to be a minimum of 10 days off any psychoactive medication and at least 24 hours off alcohol. They were treated for 3 weeks with lopirazepam and received no other psychoactive medication during that time; in the first week the lopirazepam dosage was titrated by the psychiatrist to a clinically optimal mean daily dosage of 33.6 mg (range: 11-58 mg), while the mean daily dosage in the following 2 weeks was 23.6 mg (range: 5-50 mg).

Clinical evaluations included the ECDEU Global Clinical Impression Rating Scale, the Hamilton Anxiety Rating Scale, the Zung Self-Rating Scale for Anxiety, a Somatic Symptom and Side-Effect Rating Scale, as well as measurements of pulse, systolic and diastolic blood pressure and was carried out on days 0, 7 and 21 of treatment and 3 days after discontinuation of the drug. At these times also the following psychometric parameters were tested: the AD-test (alphabetischer Durchstreichtest = alphabetical cross-out test) for quantification of attention and concentration (Grünberger, 1977), the psychomotor activity test for determination of changes in motor activity and drive (Grünberger, 1977), the von Zerssen Befindlichkeitsskala for quantification of mood (Zerssen, Koeller and Rey,1970). On days 0 and 21 the CFF, the after-effect according to the Archimedean Spiral, the reaction time as determined on the Wiener Reaktionsgerät, the affectivity (semantic differential polarity profile according to Osgood, Suci and Tannenbaum, 1974), time estimation of 1, 2 and 3 second tones and the Freiburger personality inventory (FPI) was evaluated. The Erlanger Anxiety Rating Scale (EAS) was completed daily by each patient. Blood was drawn on days 0, 7 and 21 for determination of SGOT, SGPT, γ-GT and LDH. EEG recordings were done before drug, 2 hours after one single dose of 10 mg lopirazepam as well as on day 21 of treatment (again 0 and 2 hours after an additional dose of 10 mg).

RESULTS

Predictive Pharmaco-EEG Trials in Normals

Digital computer period analysis of the R-EEG in normals after single doses of 3 mg, 5 mg and 10 mg lopirazepam, placebo and 10 mg prazepam demonstrated only some minor changes after administration of placebo. In contrast lopirazepam induced a pharmaco-EEG profile characterized by a dose-dependent increase of beta activity, average frequency and frequency deviation in both the primary wave and first derivative measurements, and a dose-dependent decrease in alpha activity and amplitude. The augmentation of beta activity was maximally pronounced in the 20-26 cps band. Slow activities indicating sleep-inducing properties were only significantly increased after the highest dosage (10 mg) lopirazepam, 10 mg prazepam induced the same type of changes and was most similar to 5 mg lopirazepam.

Statistical comparison of lopirazepam-induced changes at the hours 2, 4,6 and 8 after administration with alterations after placebo showed a significant augmentation of beta activity and average frequency already after the lowest dosage (3 mg) lasting up to the 4th hour post drug (Fig. 1). The 5 mg dosage produced the same type of changes up to the 6th hour, the 10 mg dosage up to the 8th hour after oral administration. 10 mg D-12524 produced also a significant augmentation of slow waves (delta and theta range) in the 4th and 6th hour post drug indicating hypnotic qualities of this dosage in normals at these times.

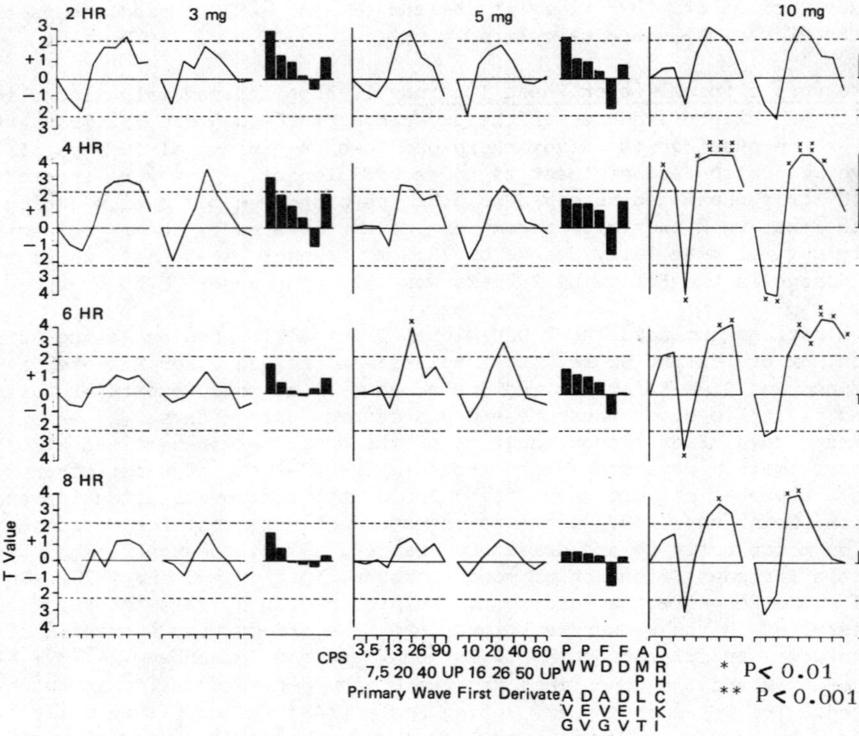

Fig. 1. Quantitative EEG changes at different times after different doses of lopirazepam (D-12524) as compared with placebo.

Twenty-two digital computer period analyzed EEG variables are represented in the abscissas, drug-induced changes as compared to placebo are shown in terms of t-values in the ordinates. The zero line = placebo. While 3 mg lopirazepam induces significant anxiolytic EEG alterations up to the 4th hour, 5 mg does so up to the 6th and 10 mg up to the 8th hour. Generally, the peak effect seems to be in the 4th hour post drug. The highest dosage (10 mg) produces an additional increase in slow activities, which indicates sleep-inducing properties.

Dose-efficacy and time-efficacy relationships were calculated by means of the non-parametric Friedman's rank analysis of variance (ANOVA) utilizing the placebo- corrected drug-induced changes in all 22 EEG variables (e.g., the placebo-induced or spontaneous alterations were subtracted from the drug-induced ones, thus calculating the "pure" drug effect; as positive and negative changes are regarded as equally important, the sign was neglected). A statistically significant dose-efficacy relationship was observed in as much as 5 mg lopirazepam were slightly more effective than 3 mg, while 10 mg were almost twice as effective than 5 mg. Concerning time-efficacy relationships the overall peak effect was seen in the 4th hour after drug administration. While 3 mg induced a sharp rise in CNS effect up to the 4th hour and thereafter a drop, 5 mg showed the same efficacy in the 2nd and 6th hour (besides the peak efficacy in the 4th hour post drug), while 10 mg produced longer lasting effects (up to the 8th hour).

In conclusion, quantitative pharmaco-EEG trials in normals demonstrated that 1) lopirazepam is CNS effective as compared with placebo; 2) it induces a pharmaco-

EEG profile seen after representative drugs of the "anxiolytic class"; 3) produces dose-dependent changes (minimal effecitve dosage was 3 mg as compared with placebo); 4) its CNS effect is already present in 2nd hour post drug, peaks in the 4th hour and lasts after 5 mg up to the 6th and after 10 mg up to the 8th hour post drug. Based on this data, we suggested that the drug should be tried in anxiety syndrome patients.

Clinical Findings in Anxiety Patients

Evaluation of the Clinical Global Impression Score demonstrated that the overall clinical symptomatology of alcoholic patients with an anxiety syndrome improved significantly (P 0.01, Wilcoxon test), from a pretreatment value of 5.0 to 3.6 and 2.8 at the end of the 1st and 3rd week of lopirazepam therapy. After discontinuation of the drug there was a slight rebound to 3.2 (P 0.05).

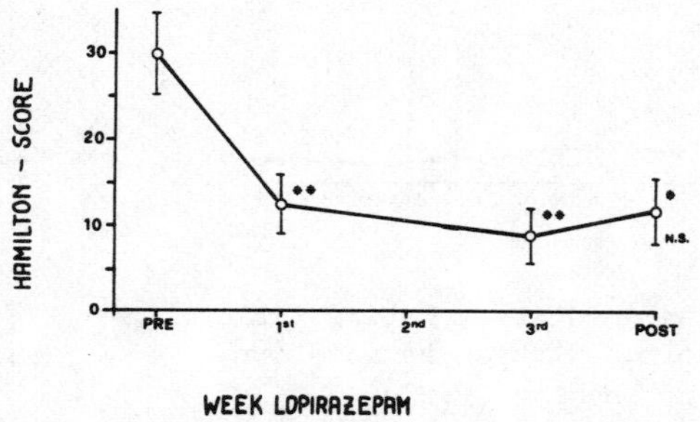

Fig. 2. Improvement in the Hamilton-Score (HAMA) of alcoholics with an anxiety syndrome during lopirazepam therapy (N:20).

• $P \leq 0,05$ (WILCOXON)
•• $P \leq 0,01$
▲ $P < 0,05$ (3rd W-POST)
▲▲ $P < 0,01$

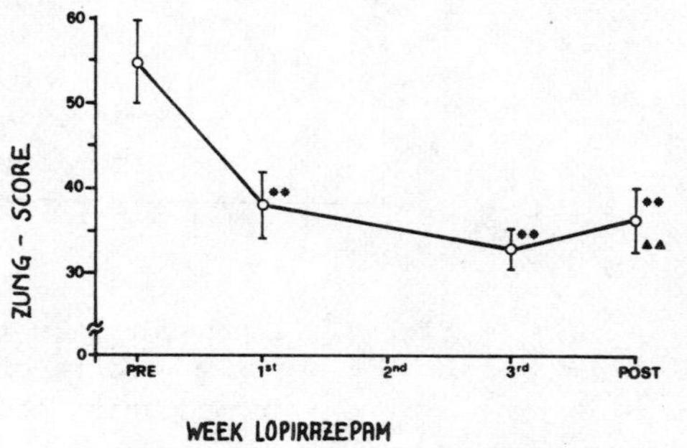

Fig. 3. Improvement in the Zung-Score (SAS) of alcoholics with an anxiety syndrome during lopirazepam therapy (N:20).

Evaluation of the patients psychopathology on the Hamilton Anxiety Scale (HAMA) showed a significant ($P < 0.01$, Wilcoxon) improvement from a pretreatment score of 29.1 to 12.4 and 8.8 at the end of the 1st and 3rd weeks of lopirazepam therapy (Fig. 2). After discontinuation there was a non-significant slight increase to 11.8.

The patients rated themselves significantly ($P < 0.01$, Wilcoxon) improved based on the Zung Self-Rating Anxiety Scale (SAS). The Zung score dropped from a pretreatment value of 54.6 to 38.0 and 32.7 at the end of the 1st and 3rd weeks, while after discontinuation of therapy the score increased again to 36.3 (Fig. 3).

Evaluation of the daily completed Erlanger Anxiety Self-Rating Scale (EAS) showed also a significant ($P < 0.01$, Wilcoxon) improvement from a pretreatment score of 23.5 down to 6.8, 3.8 and 3.4 at the end of week 1, 2 and 3. Based on this rating scale there was no deterioration after discontinuation of the drug (EAS score: 3.7). Figure 4 demonstrates the day by day change of the EAS score. As can be seen, the most improvement occurs already during the 1st week of treatment, which indicates a true drug effect as the withdrawal symptomatology of alcoholic patients grows worse during the 1st week of abstinence.

Pulse rate decreased from a pretreatment value of 87 to 82, 77 ($P < 0.05$, t-test) and 69 ($P < 0.01$) at week 1, 3 and after discontinuation of the drug, respectively. Systolic blood pressure decreased from a pretreatment value of 132 mm/Hg to 117

($P < 0.05$), 112 and 113 ($P < 0.01$) at week 1, 3 and after discontinuation of lopirazepam. Similarily, the diastolic blood pressure decreased from 85 to 76, 75 and 73 ($P < 0.01$) in the respective treatment periods. There were no cardio-vascular complaints by the patients. On the contrary, hypotonic dysregulations were noted in 8 patients during the pretreatment period and improved in all subjects.

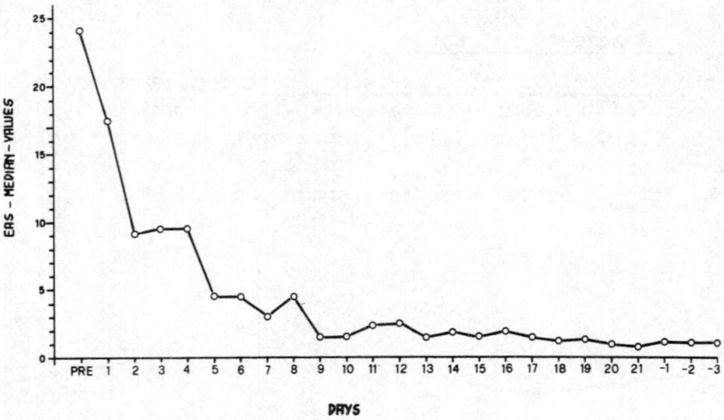

Fig. 4. Improvement in the Erlanger Anxiety Rating Scale (EAS) - Score of alcoholics with an anxiety syndrome during lopirazepam therapy (N:20).

The enzyme SGOT, which was elevated in 14 patients (above 18 U/L), improved in all but 2 patients in whom the SGOT remained borderline (19). In one patient SGOT increased from 18 to 22 U/L. The mean values and standard deviations of the total population decreased from a pretreatment value of 31 (standard deviation 13) to 24 (10) and 20 (6) on days 7 and 21 ($P < 0.01$, t-test). SGPT was elevated in 13 patients (above 22 U/L), who all showed improvement during therapy. In one patient SGPT increased from 15 to 23 U/L. The means and standard deviations for days 0, 7 and 21 were 34 (15), 26 (10) and 23 (6) U/L, respectively, with the improvement reaching the level of statistical significance ($P < 0.05$, 0.01, respectively). γ-GT was elevated in 14 patients (above 28 U/L), who improved all during the 3 weeks treatment. The mean values and standard deviations decreased from a pretreatment value of 73 (62) to 46 (29) and 29 (14) U/L on days 7 ($P < 0.05$) and 21 ($P < 0.01$). LDH was elevated in 6 patients (above 240 U/L), but improved in all patients. The means and standard deviations dropped from a pretreatment value of 209 (40) to 197 (50) and 181 (34) U/L on days 7 and 21, respectively.

Evaluation of somatic findings and side effects demonstrated an improvement in early, middle and late insomnia in all 20 patients. After discontinuation of the drug, a slight and temporary increase in early, middle and late insomnia was noted in 10, 5 and 8 patients, respectively, while 1 patient continued to improve. Diurnal drowsiness improved in 17 patients and became worse in 3. In the post treatment period 8 patients improved and 2 deteriorated as compared with the treatment period. Dreams decreased in half of the population during therapy and rebounded minimally only in 1 patient thereafter. Appetite was increased in 16 patients during lopirazepam administration and continued to increase in 2 patients after discontinuation, while in 5 patients appetite decreased again. Thirst decreased in all but 1 patient during therapy, while in the post treatment period only 1 patient showed again an increase. Dryness of mouth improved in all patients during therapy and deteriorated in only 2 thereafter. Nausea and vomiting improved in all patients. Twelve patients showing diarrhea before start of the study improved all, while in 4 patients an increase in constipation was noted (the latter disappeared again in 2 of these 4 patients during post treatment). All patients complained in the pretreatment period about feeling hot and then again chilly, furthermore about flushing and sweating, but these symptoms improved in the total population on the drug. Thereafter sweating deteriorated again in 9 patients. Headaches and cardiac sensations were observed in 17 patients, and improved in all of them (1 patient relapsed after discontinuation of the drug). Fourteen patients complained about dizziness, 15 about paresthesias before treatment, but improved all during treatment (dizziness reappeared in 2 patients in the post treatment period). Regarding polyuria 14 patients demonstrated improvement and 1 deterioration during treatment. Libido increased in 12 patients and decreased in 3 patients, while after discontinuation an improvement was noted in 3 and a deterioration in 2 patients.

Psychometric Findings in Anxiety Patients

Assessment of attention based on the total score in the AD-test of Grünberger (1977) demonstrated no changes on day 7 (score 440.4) as compared with day 0 (442.1), but a significant improvement (P< 0.05, t-test) was noted on day 21 (503.7) (Fig. 5). There was a slight drop after discontinuation of the drug down to 477.7.

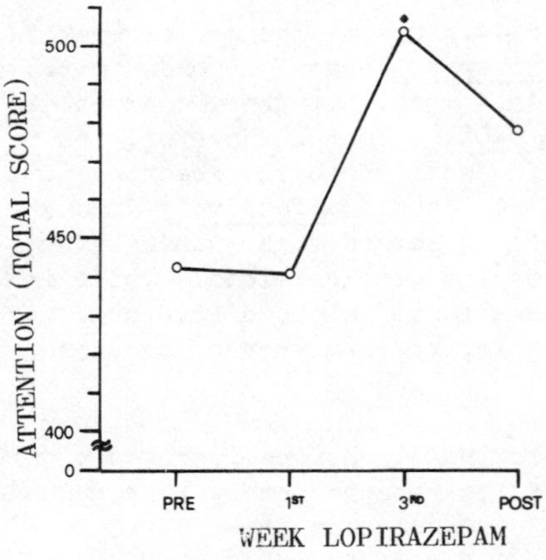

Fig. 5. Improvement in attention (total score, AD-test) of alcoholics during lopirazepam therapy (N:20; *P<0.05, t-test).

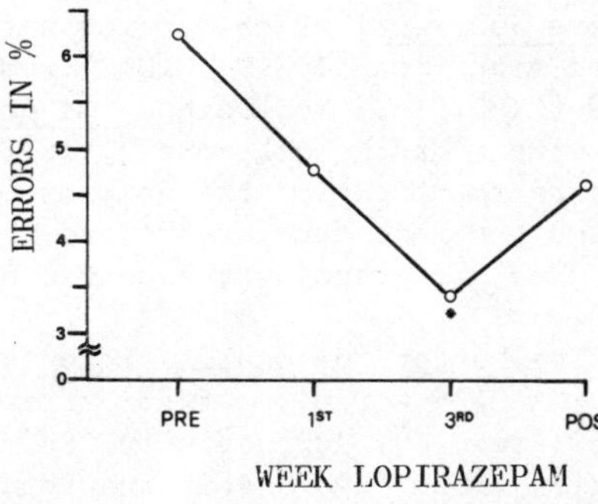

Fig. 6. Improvement in concentration (errors in % of total score) of alcoholics during lopirazepam therapy (N:20; *P<0.05, t-test).

Concentration as evaluated by the errors in the AD-test (in percent of the total score) improved from 6.2 errors to 4.8 and 3.4 at the end of week 1 and 3 (P< 0.05), and showed a rebound to 4.6 after the end of therapy (Fig. 6).

Psychomotor activity improved significantly (P< 0.05 - 0.01) throughout lopirazepam administration and increased from a pretreatment score (both hands) of 58.2 to 65.6, 68.1 and 69.3 in the respective assessment periods (Fig. 7).

Mood as evaluated based on the von Zerssen Befindlichkeitsskala showed significant (P< 0.01) improvement from a pretreatment score of 21.6 to 11.0, 7.7 and 10.1 at the end of week and 3 and in the post treatment period, respectively (Fig. 8).

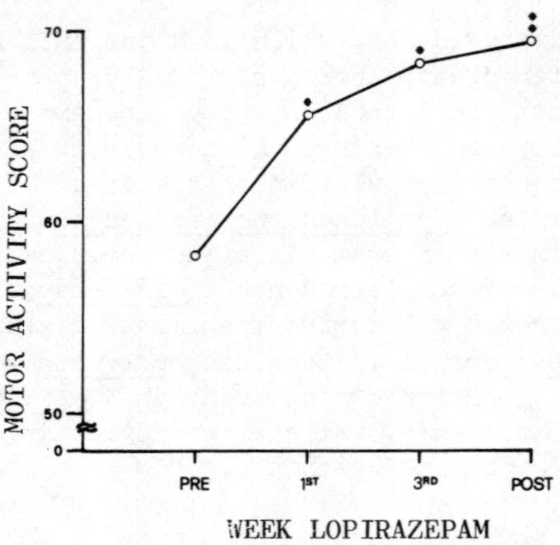

Fig. 7. Improvement in psychomotor activity of alcoholics with an anxiety syndrome during lopirazepam therapy (N:20; *P < 0.05; **P < 0.01, t-test).

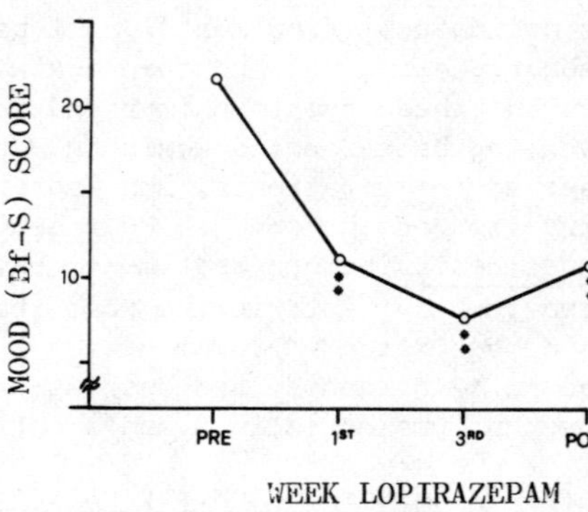

Fig. 8. Improvement in mood of alcoholics with an anxiety syndrome during lopirazepam therapy (N:20; **P < 0.01, t-test).

CFF (upper frequency) decreased from 45.4 cps to 44.8 cps at the end of week 3, as did the after effect according to the Archimedean spiral from 7 seconds to 6.5 seconds and the reaction time from 46.9 msec. to 46.4 msec. but these changes did not reach the level of statistical significance ($P < 0.05$, t-test). However, the reaction time quotient, which considers the errors in addition to the reaction time, improved significantly ($P < 0.05$) from 23.1 to 21.4, as did affectivity from 38.2 to 25.8 ($P < 0.01$). Regarding time estimation of a 2 second tone (randomly presented with 1 and 3 sec. tones) the following results were obtained: while in the pretreatment period the patients estimated the tone prolonged (2.8 sec.), they evaluated the same tone at the end of the 3 week lopirazepam therapy shortened (1.7 sec.). The difference was significant ($P < 0.05$).

In the Freiburger personality inventory the following dimensions improved significantly ($P < 0.05 - 0.01$, t-test) after 3 weeks of lopirazepam therapy: nervousness (from 6.1 to 4.6), aggressivity (from 5.1 to 4.3), depression (from 6.1 to 4.6), inhibition (from 5.2 to 4.2) and frankness (from 5.5 to 4.5).

Quantitative EEG Findings in Anxiety Patients

Oral administered single doses of 10 mg lopirazepam induced in alcoholic patients with an anxiety syndrome 2 hours post drug the same type of EEG changes as observed after the administration of the same dosage at the same time in normals (Fig. 9). Slow beta activity between 13-40 cps, and especially the 20-26 cps activity increased significantly, as did the average frequency, while alpha activity decreased. The amplitude showed a trend towards attenuation.

Chronic administration of the drug throughout 3 weeks resulted in the same type of EEG changes (Table I) and by means of a Spearman rank correlation analysis we could demonstrate that acute and chronic changes are highly correlated with each other (Table I).

However, while the normal and anxiety population generally showed the same type of EEG alterations after the administration of the same dosage of the same drug analyzed at the same time, nevertheless some quantitative and significant ($P < 0.05$,

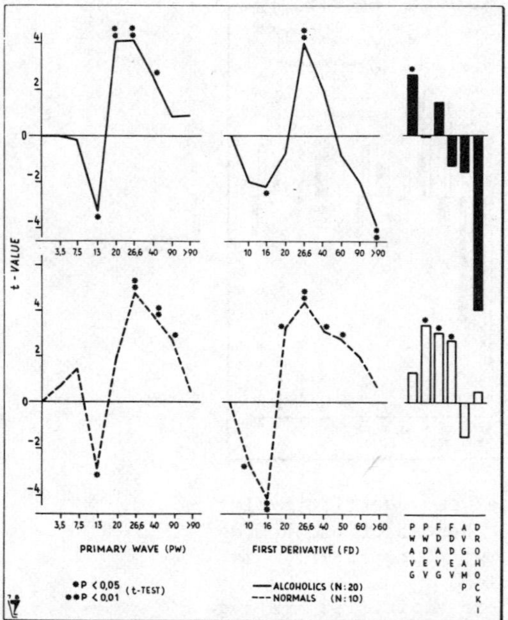

Fig. 9. Effect of 10 mg lopirazepam on the EEG of alcoholics and normals (period analysis; 5 min. R-EEG; O2-Cz). Twenty-two period analysis measurements are shown in the abscissa, drug-induced changes are indicated as t-values in the ordinate. Note the similarity of changes in the two different populations (alcoholics in the upper part; normals in the lower part of the figure).

TABLE I Relationships between EEG changes after a single dose of lopirazepam and EEG changes after 3 weeks therapy with lopirazepam in alcoholics (N:17)

EEG-VARIABLES	CHANGE ACUTE	CHANGE CHRONIC	CORRELATION
PW 1,3 - 3,5 cps	0	+ 0,01	+ 0,51
3,5 - 7,5	- 0,1	- 0,5	+ 0,61*
7,5 - 13	- 8,8	+ 2,7	+ 0,57*
13 - 20	+ 3,2	+ 3,01	+ 0,24
20 - 26	+ 2,5	+ 0,1	+ 0,51*
26 - 40	+ 2,2	- 1,99	+ 0,67*
40 - 90	+ 0,7	- 2,7	+ 0,61*
90	+ 0,2	- 0,72	+ 0,65*
FD 1,3 - 10 cps	- 2,4	+ 0,04	+ 0,85*
10 - 16	- 3,9	+ 3,08	+ 0,70*
16 - 20	- 0,8	+ 0,21	+ 0,04
20 - 26	+ 3,2	+ 2,02	+ 0,21
26 - 40	+ 2,8	- 3,44	+ 0,64*
40 - 60	- 0,1	- 3,02	+ 0,28
60	- 1,0	- 1,46	+ 0,58*
PW AVG FRQ	+ 1,0	- 0,86	+ 0,66*
FRQ DEV	- 0,2	- 5,52	+ 0,81*
FD AVG FRQ	+ 1,1	- 2,3	+ 0,64*
FRQ DEV	- 1,2	- 3,08	+ 0,52*
AMPLITUDE	- 2,9	- 0,14	+ 0,60*
DROHOCKI	-27,4	- 1,7	- 0,07

* P 0,05 (Spearman Rank Correlation)

Man-Whitney-test) differences could be observed (Fig. 10). Ten mg lopirazepam induced delta and theta waves in normals which was not seen in patients. Furthermore, normals showed an increase in the 16-20 cps band and frequency deviation, while oppositional alterations were observed in patients. The findings indicate that higher doses of an anxiolytic drug produce in normals more likely sedation than in anxiety patients, who exhibit, of course, a state of higher arousal in the CNS. The latter effect could be substantiated by comparing the pretreatment EEG with the baseline EEG of the normal population (Fig. 11). Alcoholic patients with an anxiety syndrome demonstrated significantly more fast beta activities, a higher average frequency and frequency deviation, as well as less slow waves and alpha waves in both the primary wave and first derivative measurements than normals (Fig. 11).

Clinical/Neurophysiological Correlations during Drug Treatment

Utilizing polynomial regression and Spearman rank correlation analyses we could demonstrate that there was a significant relationship between lopirazepam-induced changes in brain activity and clinical alterations at the end of the treatment period: the more increase in the middle fast 20-26 cps beta activity (which is the most characteristic EEG change for the class of anxiolytics), the better the

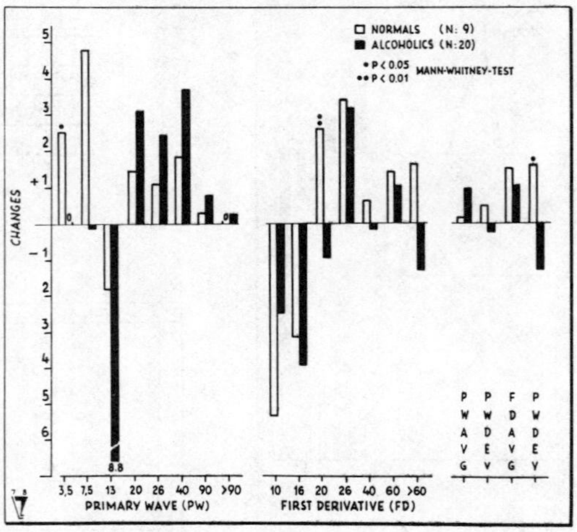

Fig. 10. Comparison between quantitatively analyzed EEG changes of alcoholics and normals two hours after 10 mg lopirazepam.
Delta and theta activities are augmented only in normals. Further significant intergroup differences can be observed in the 16-20 cps band and in the frequency deviation of the first derivative.

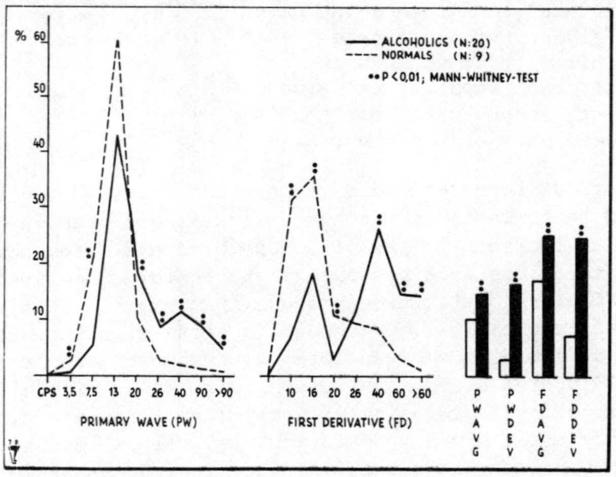

Fig. 11. Quantitatively analyzed EEG of alcoholic patients and normals (based on digital computer period analysis; 5 min. resting EEGs; O2-Cz).

clinical improvement in the Hamilton anxiety score (Fig. 12). The Spearman rank correlation coefficient was - 0.41. Moreover, the more decrease in fast beta activity (40-60 cps, FD) during lopirazepam therapy, the better the improvement as rated by the patients themselves on the EAS-scale (Fig. 13). The respective correlation coefficient was +0.51. Similarily, the more decrease in very fast beta activity (over 60 cps, FD), the better the improvement as rated by the patients on the Zung SAS scale (r_s = +0.42). The more decrease in frequency deviation of the first derivatives, the more decrease in the Hamilton score (r_s = +0.49) and Zung score (r_s = +0.46).

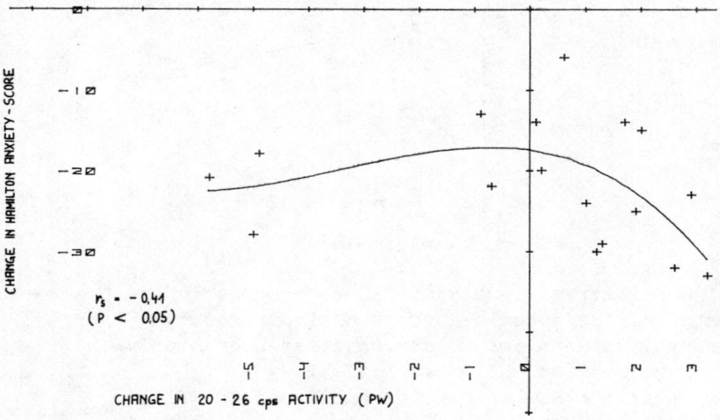

Fig. 12. The relationship between changes in EEG and Hamilton Anxiety score of alcoholics after 3 weeks of lopirazepam therapy (based on first degree polynomial regression analysis, N:17). EEG changes are shown in the abscissa, psychopathological alterations (HAMA) are represented in the ordinate.

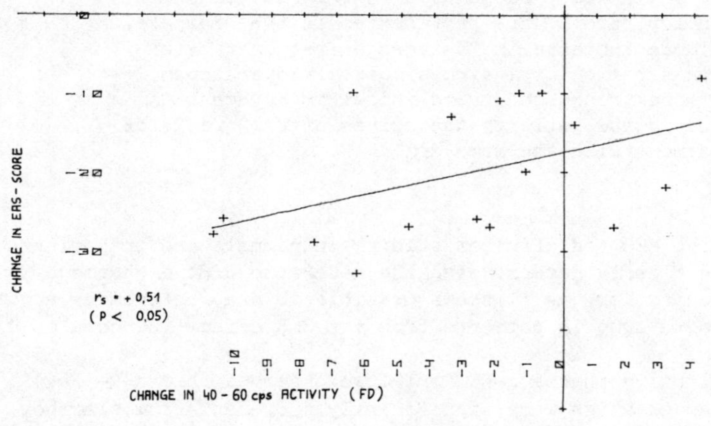

Fig. 13. Relationships between changes in EEG and the Erlanger Anxiety score (EAS) of alcoholics after 3 weeks of lopirazepam therapy (based on first degree polynomial regression analysis N:17).

Single Dose-EEG Effect as Prognostic Indicator

Since the utilization of quantitative neurophysiological techniques for prediction of therapeutic outcome would be of great clinical significance, we tried to correlate EEG changes after single oral doses of lopirazepam in alcoholic patients with the therapeutic outcome after 3 weeks of therapy with the same drug. The following significant relationship was observed: the greater the increase in average frequency (FD) 2 hours after administration of one single oral dosis of 10 mg lopirazepam, the more pronounced the clinical improvement (Zung score) in the alcoholic patients after 3 weeks of drug administration (r_s = -0.51((Fig. 14).

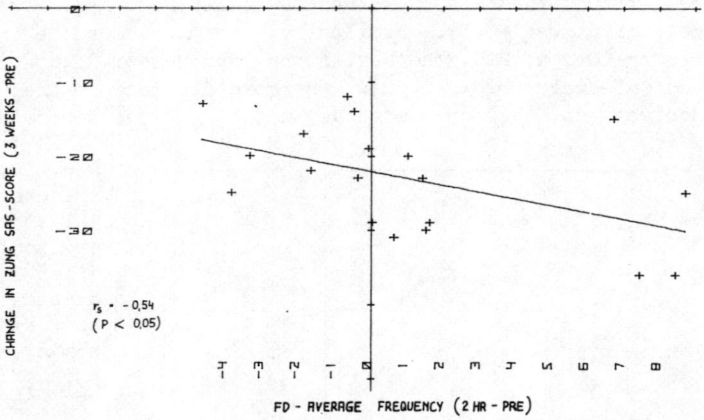

Fig. 14. The quantitatively analyzed EEG as prognostic indicator of therapeutic success of lopirazepam-therapy in alcoholics (based on first degree polynomial regression analysis, N:17).
Changes in the EEG average frequency of the first derivatives 2 hours after the administration of 1 single dose are shown in the abscissa; changes in the Zung Anxiety Score after 3 weeks of treatment with lopirazepam are represented in the ordinate. The more increase in FD-average frequency after administration of 1 single dose of lopirazepam, the more pronounced the clinical improvement as rated by the patients themselves after 3 weeks of treatment with the same drug.

DISCUSSION

Our comparative quantitative EEG and clinical studies in normals and in patients with a new pyridodiazepine clearly demonstrated the relevance of the pharmaco-EEG method for human psychopharmacology as it seems possible to draw inferences about the therapeutic efficacy of a drug in patients from its CNS effect in normals.

In an early Stage I quantitative pharmaco-EEG trial we observed that a D-12524 (lopirazepam) produced changes which were significantly different from placebo and were characterized by an increase in beta activity (especially in the 20-26 cps band), average frequency and frequency deviations as well as by a decrease of alpha activity and amplitude (Saletu and co-workers, in press). Slow activities were augmented after the highest given dosage indicating sedative properties of the drug in this dosage.

Such alterations were previously described as typical for the class of anxiolytics (Fink, 1969; Itil, 1974; Saletu, 1976) and as the most sensitive indicators of the benzodiazepine effect based on blood level-EEG correlations (Fink, 1975; Saletu and Grünberger, 1978). Moreover, they were found to be dose-dependent: while the smallest given dosage of 3 mg exerted a significant effect on the CNS lasting up to the 4th hour after oral administration, 5 mg did so up to the 6th and 10 mg up to the 8th hour. The peak effect was in the 4th hour. It was concluded that D-12524 is psychoactive and should be tried clinically in anxiety patients.

Indeed, clinical investigations in alcoholic patients with an anxiety syndrome demonstrated that D-12524 has anxiolytic qualities as substantiated by means of the global score, Hamilton score, Zung score and Erlanger anxiety score. Despite the fact that this was an open study, the data is conclusive as one would expect in such a patient population a marked deterioration of symptomatology within the 1st week of alcohol withdrawal. However, in the 1st week of the study psychopathology improved most, which was especially well demonstrated by means of the daily completed Erlanger Anxiety Self-Rating Scale. After discontinuation of the drug, a slight worsening was noted in the Zung score but not so in the Hamilton and EAS score. Somatic complaints and blood chemistry (SGOT, SGPT, γ-GT, LDH) improved also during the 3 weeks treatment period. Pulse rate and blood pressure decreased and as there were no cardiovascular complications (on the contrary, orthostatic dysregulations and cardiac sensations disappeared), these changes seemed to be due to a decrease of somatic anxiety. Psychometric variables such as attention, concentration, psychomotor activity, mood, affectivity and the reaction time quotient showed marked and significant improvement as did the FPI dimensions nervousness, aggressivity, depression, inhibition and frankness.

Most interesting were the results of the quantitative EEG analysis as we could compare the CNS effect of a certain dosage (10 mg) of the same drug measured at the same time (2 hrs post oral administration) in 2 different populations. As was seen, lopirazepam induced both in normals and anxiety patients the same type of EEG changes (pharmaco-EEG profile of the anxiolytic class), although some quantitative differences were observed: while slow waves were augmented in normals, this was not the case in patients. This data suggests that normals feel already much sooner sedative properties of a drug than anxiety patients, which in the present study might be due to the fact that alcoholics show a higher state of arousal in the CNS than normals. The latter was demonstrated by neurophysiological baseline differences between the two populations, as alcoholics showed less slow waves and alpha activity as well as more fast beta activity, a higher average frequency and frequency deviation than normals. Three weeks after the start of lopirazepam therapy the alcoholic patients showed still the same type of EEG changes which was demonstrated also by a correlation analysis investigating the relationship between acute and chronic drug effects. Thus our present paper confirms previous results indicating that the type of EEG changes after anxiolytics remains essentially the same whether a drug is administered in single doses or chronically (Itil and Saletu, 1973). Our present study confirms also previous observations regarding the similarity of pharmaco-EEG profiles of another benzodiazepine - U-31,889 (alprazolam) in normals and anxiety patients (Itil and co-workers, 1972, 1973).

The question arises whether or not certain typical EEG changes after benzodiazepine administration are related to anxiolytic effects of the drug noted by the clinician or patient himself. Thus, we correlated the most typical EEG change of benzodiazepines - the 20-26 cps beta activity - with symptomatological alterations as rated by means of the Hamilton score. Indeed, a statistically significant correlation was noted: the greater the increase in 20-26 cps activity, the better the clinical improvement of the patients. Of further interest was the positive correlation between fast beta activity and psychopathology: the more decrease in fast beta activity during lopirazepam therapy, the more reduction in anxiety was rated by the patients themselves on the EAS and Zung scale. This is of interest as we observed already previously similar correlations in schizophrenic populations, where we found a neuroleptic-induced decrease in fast beta activity to be correlated with clinical improvement (Saletu and co-workers, 1973b; Itil and co-workers, 1975). The data suggests that irregular low voltage fast beta activity reflects symptoms such as anxiety, agitation, restlessness, muscular tension, etc., which are reduced by both neuroleptic and anxiolytic drugs.

While the correlations between drug-induced changes in brain activity and clinical symptomatology are impressive, the utilization of quantitative neurophysiological techniques for prediction of therapeutic outcome is of still greater clinical significance. Thus, we tried to correlate EEG changes after single oral doses of lopirazepam in alcoholic patients with the therapeutic outcome after 3 weeks of therapy with the same drug. The following significant relationship was observed: the greater the increase in average frequency (FD) 2 hours after administration of 1 single oral dosis of 10 mg lopirazepam, the more pronounced the clinical improvement (Zung score) in the alcoholic patients after 3 weeks of drug administration. As the increase in average frequency is one of the typical EEG effects of anxiolytics, the correlation suggests that patients showing marked changes in brain activity after application of 1 single dose of a certain drug might be more therapy responsive to a subsequent long-term treatment with the same drug than patients exhibiting no or only minimal CNS changes. However, while these results indicate that single dose trials in connection with quantitative EEG analyses might be eventually an interesting prognostic tool, future studies have to show us exactly as to which extent a certain neurophysiological change predicts improvement of psychopathology on a certain scale in a certain patient.

REFERENCES

Burch, N. R., W. H. Nettleton, J. Sweeney, and R. J. Edwards (1964). Period analysis of electroencephalogram on a general purpose digital computer. Ann. N. Y. Acad. Sci., 115, 827-943.

Fink, M. (1969). EEG and human psychopharmacology. A. Rev. Pharmac., 9, 241-258.

Fink, M. (1975). Cerebral electrometry-quantitative EEG applied to human psychopharmacology. In G. Dolce and H. Künkel (Eds.), Computerized EEG Analysis, Fischer, Stuttgart, pp. 271-288.

Grünberger, J. (1977). Psychodiagnostik des Alkoholkranken. Methodischer Beitrag zur Bestimmung der Organizität in der Psychiatrie. Maudrich, Wien.

Homburg-Chemiewerk (1976). Homburg D-12524 (Lopirazepam)- vorläufiger wissenshaftlicher Prospekt.

Itil, T. M. (1974). Quantitative pharmaco-electroencephalography. In T. M. Itil (Ed.), Psychotropic drugs and the human EEG. Mod. Probl. Pharmacopsycho., Vol. 8, Nasel, Karger. pp. 43-75.

Itil, T.M. (1976). Neurophysiological effects of hormones in humans: computer EEG profiles of sex and hypothalamic hormones. In E. J. Sachar (Ed.) Hormones, Behavior, and Psychopathology, Raven Press, New York. pp. 31-40.

Itil, T. M. and B. Saletu (1973). Neurophysiologische Untersuchungsmethoden in der Psychopharmakologie. Nervenarzt, 44, 65-74.

Itil, T. M., B. Saletu, J. Marasa and A. N. Mucciardi (1972). Digital computer analyzed awake and sleep EEG (sleep prints) in predicting the effects of a triazolobenzodiazepine (U-31,889). Pharmakopsychiat., 5, 225-240.

Itil, T. M., N. Polvan, S. Egilmez, B. Saletu and J. Marasa (1973). Anxiolytic effects of a new triazolobenzodiazepine, U-31,889. Curr. Ther. Res., 15, 603-615.

Itil, T. M., J. Marasa, B. Saletu and S. Davis (1975). Computerized EEG: Predictor of outcome in schizophrenia. J. Nerv. Ment. Dis., 160, 188-203.

Matejcek, M. and J. E. Devos (1976). Selected methods of quantitative EEG analysis and their application in psychotropic drug research. In P. Kellaway and I. Peterson (Eds.), Quantitative analytic studies in epilepsy, Raven Press, New York. pp. 183-205.

Osgood, C. E., G. J. Suci, and P. H. Tannenbaum (1975). The Measurement of Meaning. Univ. Press, Urbana.

Roubicek, J. and I. Major (1977). EEG profile and behavioral changes after a single dose of clozapine in normals and schizophrenics. Biol. Psychiat., 12, 613-633.

Saletu, B. (1976). Psychopharmaka, Gehirntätigkeit und Schlaf. Bibliotheca Psychiatrica, No. 155. Karger, Basel.

Saletu, B., M. Saletu, T. M. Itil and J. Jones (1971a). Somatosensory evoked potential changes during thiothixene treatment in schizophrenic patients. Psychopharmacologia, 20, 242-252.

Saletu, B., M. Saletu, T. M. Itil, and W. Hsu (1971b). Changes in somatosensory evoked potentials during fluphenazine treatment. Pharmakopsychiat., 4, 158-168.

Saletu, B., M. Saletu and T. M. Itil (1972). Effect of minor tranquilizers on somatosensory evoked potentials. Psychopharmacologia, 24, 347-358.

Saletu, B., M. Saletu, T. M. Itil and J. Marasa (1971c). Somatosensory evoked potential changes during haloperidol treatment of chronic schizophrenics. Biol. Psychiat., 3, 299-308.

Saletu, B., M. Saletu, and T. M. Itil (1973a). The relationships between psychopathology and evoked responses before, during and after psychotropic drug treatment. Biol. Psychiat., 6, 45-74.

Saletu, B., T. M. Itil, M. Arat, and S. Akpinar (1973b). Long-term clinical and quantitative EEG effects of clopenthixol in schizophrenics: Clinical-neurophysiological correlations. Int. Pharmacopsychiat., 8, 193-207.

Saletu, B., J. Simeon, M. Saletu, T. M. Itil, and J. Dasilva (1974). Behavioral and neurophysiological effects of trihexyphenidyl and thiothixene in psychotic boys. Biol. Psychiat., 8, 177-189.

Saletu, B., M. Saletu, J. Simeon, and J. Marasa (1975). Fluphenazine treatment in the psychotic child: clinical-evoked potential correlations. Comp. Psychiat., 16, 265-278.

Saletu, B. and J. Grünberger (1978). Evaluation of pharmacodynamic properties of psychotropic drugs: quantitative EEG, psychometric and blood level investigations in normals and patients. Pharmacopsychiat. 11.

Saletu, B., J. Grünberger, L. Linzmayer, and R. Stadler (in press). Classification and assessment of cerebral bioavailability of lopirazepam (D-12524) by quantitative EEG and psychometric analysis. Arzneim. - Forsch.

Wittenborn, J. R. (1977). Guidelines for clinical trials of psychotropic drugs. Pharmacopsychiat., 10, 205-231.

Zerssen, V.D., von, D. M. Koeller, and E. R. Rey (1970). Die Befindlichkeitsskala (BF-S) - ein einfaches Instrument zur Objektivierung von Befindlichkeitsstörungen, insbesondere im Rahmen von Längsschnittuntersuchungen. Arzneim. Forsch., 20, 915-918.

Chronospectrogram Analysis in the Assessment of Spontaneous and Drug-induced Changes in Vigilance

M. MATEJCEK

Biological and Medical Research Division, SANDOZ Ltd., Basle, Switzerland

ABSTRACT

A quantitative EEG method (Chronospectrogram Analysis) for assessing spontaneous and drug-induced changes in vigilance, considering the dynamic properties of the EEG record is presented and its various applications are shown. The available evidence proved this method to be of remarkable sensitivity for studying effects of drugs on the central nervous system.

Keywords: Quantitative EEG, Chronospectrogram Analysis, Spectral Analysis, Drug Effects, Central Nervous System, Vigilance.

INTRODUCTION

Information extracted from the EEG might form a basis for a more objective evaluation of the characteristics of the mechanisms regulating *vigilance* and their changes in the course of time (Bente, 1964). Thus, the loss of alpha rhythm, especially in the occipital regions, when the EEG is recorded under resting conditions (i.e. the appearance of subvigilant phases), has been shown in numerous studies to be associated with impaired precision of the adaptive reactions orientated toward the environment. The scale of decreasing vigilance which the subject passes through, for example in the process of falling asleep, and its electroencephalographic correlates have been studied thoroughly. Thus, while falling asleep an individual requires a certain time in order to pass consecutively through the various EEG stages. The length of this period, the duration and sequence of each single EEG phase, etc., depend upon the state of the individual at the time, and one of the various ways in which it may be altered is by psychoactive drugs.

DESCRIPTION OF METHOD AND SOME APPLICATIONS

With a view to deriving the required information from the EEG in a form which can take sufficient account of rapid fluctuations in vigilance, power spectra from EEG leads are calculated for short, freely-selectable intervals, the shortest being one second. The pertinent variables are then extracted (such as absolute and relative power content of the EEG frequency bands: delta, theta, alpha, beta, various quotients etc.).

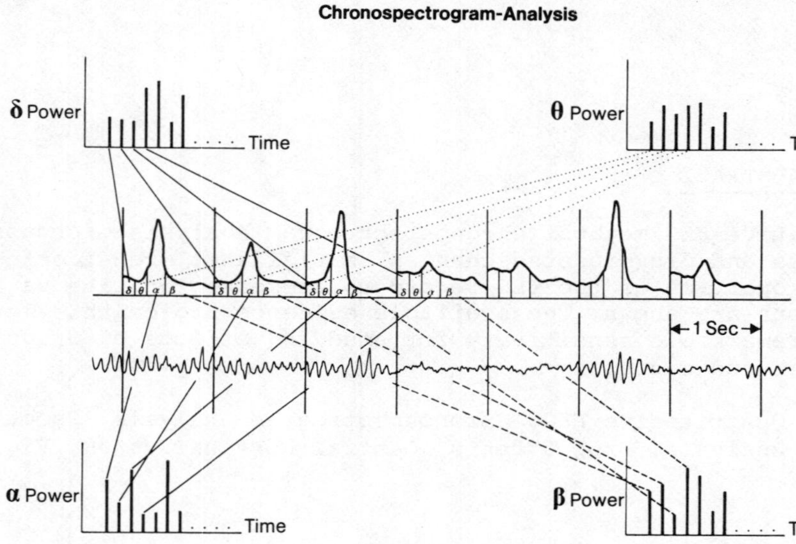

Fig. 1. Basic concept of the Chronospectrogram Analysis.

The evolution in time of the variables (see Fig. 2) constitutes a *chronospectrogram* which can be represented graphically and stored numerically in a data bank for statistical processing (Matejcek, 1975; Matejcek and Devos, 1977).

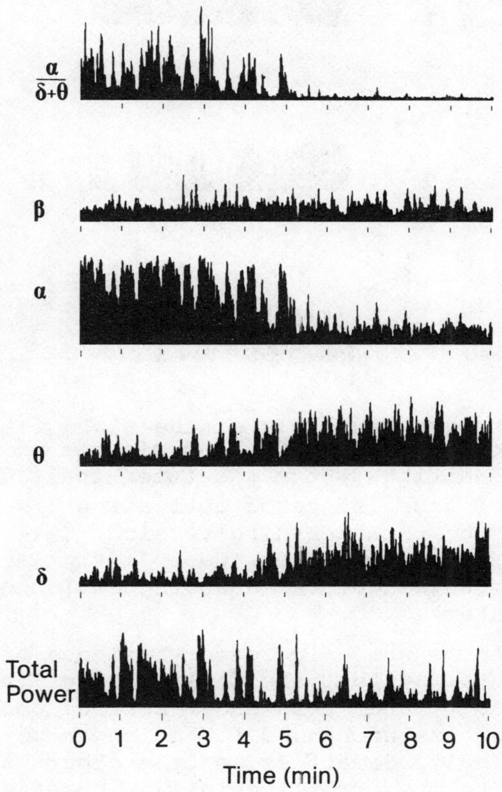

Fig. 2. Chronospectrogram analysis: various chronospectrograms of the total power and of the relative values of the delta, theta, alpha and beta activities and of the ratio $\alpha/(\delta+\theta)$ are shown (EEG dynamics). Lead O_2-C_z, ten minutes resting EEG, chronospectrogram resolution 1 second.

It is now possible to analyse two EEG channels simultaneously, thus permitting an appraisal of inter-hemispheric and intra-hemispheric relations, symmetry, scalp topography etc., as such parameters are essential in vigilance studies.

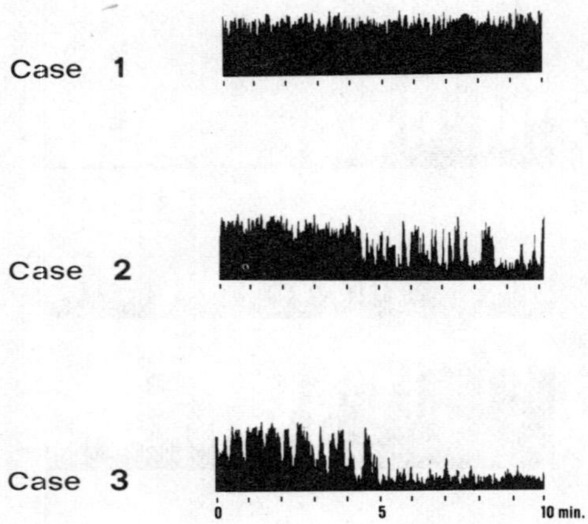

Fig. 3. Chronospectrogram analysis of the alpha frequency band in three subjects (lead O_2-C_z, ten minutes of resting EEG, standardized conditions). Note the inter-individual differences. Case 1: Vigilance (state of activation) is maintained unchanged during the recording session. Case 2: vigilance decrease after 4-5 minutes. Case 3: vigilance decrease after 4-5 minutes, slowed down regulation of vigilance (innert system).

For example, substances which increase vigilance affect the regulating process in such a way that the first subvigilant phases appear in the EEG appreciably later than under control conditions. The initial EEG pattern remains unchanged for a longer period, or changes appreciably more slowly. Sedatives, on the other hand, decrease the period elapsing up to the first subvigilant phase and this effect is dose-related.

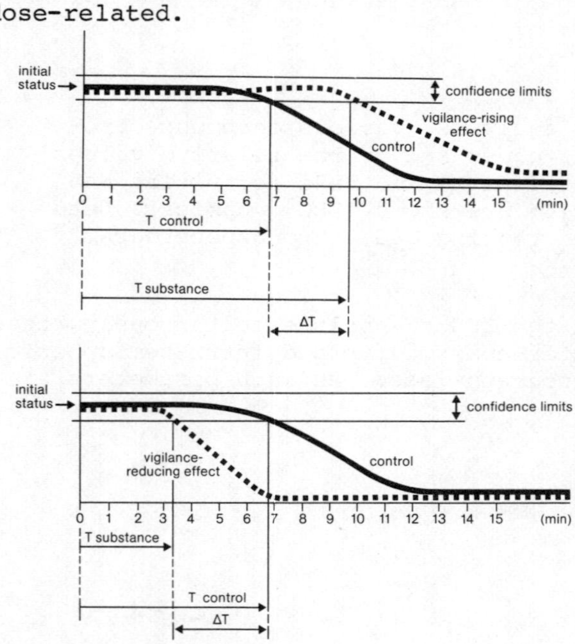

Fig. 4.

Schematic presentation of an application of chronospectrogram analysis for studying changes in vigilance. For statistical purposes, after calculation of mean chronospectrograms, confidence limits based on initial individual values can be defined. T = average time until the appearance of the first subvigilant phase under a defined condition; ΔT = difference between two average times (for example T control - T substance).

As shown in Fig. 4, the difference between the time required before subvigilant phases appear under the influence of drugs and that required under control conditions may, therefore, be employed not only to ascertain the intensity and dose-dependency of the effect of a drug, but also to study the nature of the drug's influence on vigilance.

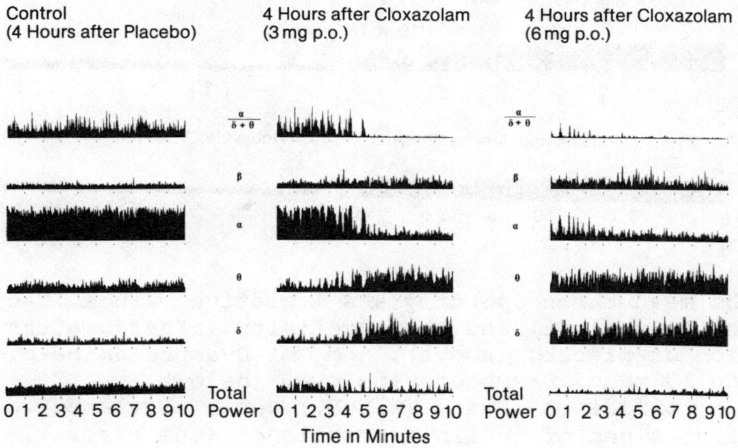

Fig. 5. Chronospectrogram analysis of ten minutes resting EEG, (normal subject, lead O_2-C_z, relative values, chronospectrogram resolution 1 second).
4 hours after placebo (left), 4 hours after 3 mg p.o. of cloxazolam (center) and 4 hours after 6 mg p.o. of cloxazolam (right).
Note the dose-dependent increase of slow activities (delta and theta), decrease of alpha activity and increase of beta activity, changes commonly observed after benzodiazepines. Dose-dependent changes can also be seen in total power and in the ratio $\alpha/(\delta+\theta)$.

ASSESSMENT OF THE VIGILANCE-STIMULATING EFFECT OF SINGLE DOSES OF D-AMPHETAMINE

In order to objectify the *vigilance-stimulating effect* of relatively low single doses of D-amphetamine, a study was carried out in six healthy volunteers. This took the form of an intra-individual, double-blind test in which preparations of 5 and 10 mg of D-amphetamine and placebo were randomly allocated. EEGs were recorded before and 2, 4, 6 and 8 hours after administration of the preparations. Each EEG was recorded under resting conditions for 20 minutes.

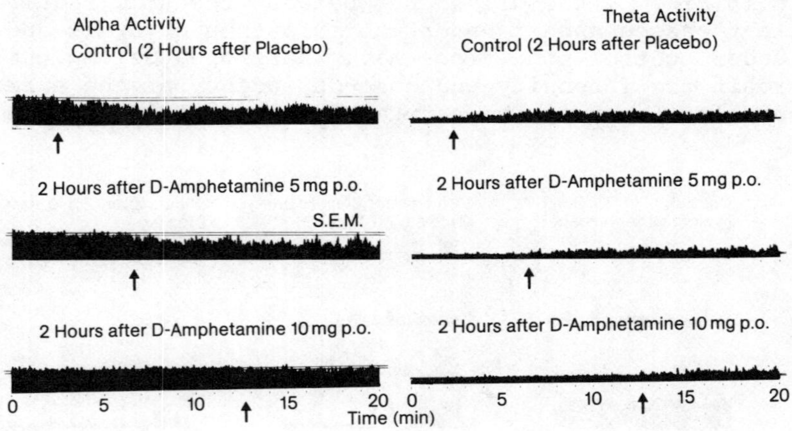

Fig. 6. The mean chronospectrograms (relative values, N=6) of alpha activity (left) and theta activity (right), after administration of placebo (above), 5 mg of D-amphetamine p.o. (center) and 10 mg of D-amphetamine p.o. (below).
2 σ confidence limits (S.E.M.) were calculated to detect first signs of declining vigilance (see arrows). Twenty minutes of resting EEG, lead O_2-C_z were analysed. Chronospectrogram resolution 1 second.

Figure 6 shows representative mean chronospectrograms 2 hours after administration. For clarity, only the alpha and theta activities are shown. These chronospectrograms indicate that after placebo the first signs of declining vigilance occurred, on average, 2 to 3 minutes (arrow) after the start of the EEG recording. After 5 mg of D-amphetamine, the decrease in vigilance was not obvious until 6 to 7 minutes after the start of the recording, while after 10 mg of D-amphetamine no notable decline in "mean vigilance" below the initial level was discernible in the subjects for at least 13 minutes.

ASSESSMENT OF VIGILANCE REDUCTION BY SINGLE DOSES OF CLOXAZOLAM

Chronospectrogram analysis was applied to EEG data from a study with the benzodiazepine derivative cloxazolam to elucidate the possible *vigilance-decreasing effect* of higher dosages. This was a double-blind intra-individual study with randomized allocation of the preparation sequences, carried out in 8 healthy volunteers. The resting EEG was recorded for 10 minutes.

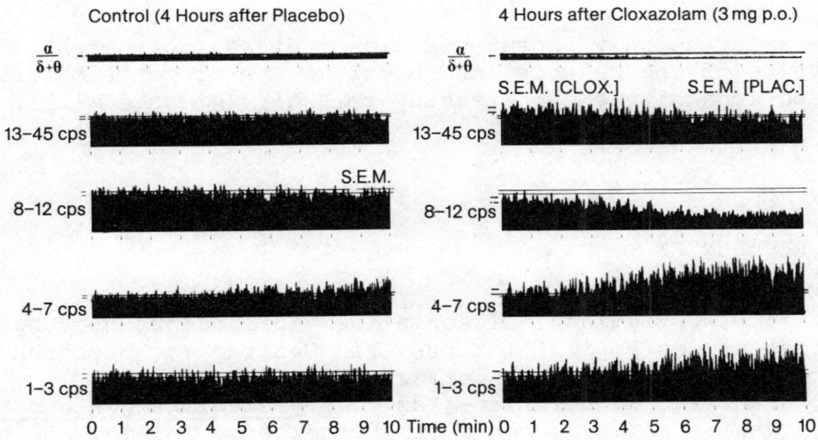

Fig. 7. Mean chronospectrograms (relative values, N=8) of the delta, theta, alpha, beta activities and the ratio $\alpha/(\delta+\theta)$ in the 4th hour after administration of placebo (left) and after 3 mg p.o. of cloxazolam (right). Increase of slow (delta and theta), decrease of alpha and increase of beta activities indicate vigilance-reducing properties of the dosage used. Ten minutes of resting-EEG, lead O_2-C_z were analyzed. Chronospectrogram resolution 1 second.

In Fig. 7 the situation 4 hours after administration of placebo and cloxazolam is shown. After placebo, the first changes were discernible only after 3 to 4 minutes, whereas after a 3 mg oral dosage of cloxazolam vigilance was decreased already from the onset, as is distinctly visible in the alpha frequency range. The decline in vigilance, as detectable from the time-course of alpha activity or from the rapidly increasing slow waves, was appreciably more pronounced after cloxazolam than after placebo. Also beta activity was markedly increased compared with placebo.

CONCLUDING REMARKS

The approach presented may be employed in a variety of situations. For example: It may be used to characterize the initial state of activation of subjects entering a study and to demonstrate the effects of compounds in either single or repeated dose experiments. The method could be applied to detect a possible improvement in vigilance after long-term treatment, especially important in the testing of geriatric compounds, but also with other preparations. This would not only provide proof of a general effect on the EEG, which Kewitz (1976), Coper and Kanowski (1976) stipulate as a requirement for all geriatric drugs, but would also furnish objective evidence on the quality of their influence (Matejcek, 1978).
It might even be possible with repeated measurements to determine the diurnal fluctuations in vigilance, which are otherwise difficult to detect.
It could be used for interaction studies and to charactize new drug combinations.

These few spontaneously chosen examples indicate the potentiality and the value of the methods for objective measurements of drug effects and emphasize the increasing role of vigilance within such studies.

REFERENCES

Bente, D. (1964). Vigilanz, dissoziative Vigilanzverschiebung und Insuffizienz des Vigilitätstonus. Ein Beitrag zur psychophysiologischen Fundierung der experimentellen Psychiatrie. In: H. Kranz and K. Heinrich (Eds.), Begleitwirkungen und Misserfolge der psychiatrischen Pharmakotherapie, Thieme, Stuttgart.

Coper, H. and S. Kanowski (1976). Geriatrika: Theoretische Grundlagen, Erwartungen, Prüfung, Kritik. Hippokrates, 47, 303-319.

Kewitz, H. (1975). Die sogenannten Geriatrika im Kreuzverhör. Internist. Prax., 16, 889-909.

Matejcek, M. and J.E. Devos (1977). Assessment of spontaneous and drug-induced changes in vigilance by means of a new modification of the short time spectral analysis of the EEG. Electroenceph. clin. Neurophysiol., 43, 4, 476.

Matejcek, M. (1978). Methodological considerations in Pharmaco-Encephalography. In: P. Deniker, C. Radouco-Thomas, A. Villeneuve (Eds.), Neuro-Psychopharmacology, Vol. V/2, Pergamon Press, Oxford, 1151-1164.

Matejcek, M. (1978). Elektroenzephalogramm am alternden Menschen. Medita, 10, 61-63.

Quantitative EEG in Relation to Plasma Concentration During Treatment with Antiepileptic Drugs

G. ROSADINI and W. G. SANNITA

Institute of Neurophysiopathology, University of Genoa, Centre for Cerebral Neurophysiology, National Council of Research, Genoa, Italy

ABSTRACT

The suitability of quantitative EEG methodologies in the estimation of cerebral bioavailability and central action of antiepileptic compounds has been tested in 44 patients during single-drug therapy with ethosuximide, diphenylhydantoin, valproic acid, or phenobarbital. Clinical conditions were monitored, and EEG and plasma samples were collected periodically during long-term treatment. The background EEG activity was quantified by spectral power analysis on signal epochs free from specific epileptic phenomena. Drug plasma concentrations were determined by gas liquid chromatographic methods. Consistent EEG modifications were observed during treatment with ethosuximide, valproic acid and phenobarbital, and found to be related to plasma concentration only in the case of phenobarbital. No changes were detected during therapy with diphenylhydantoin.

KEY WORDS

Quantitative EEG, power spectral analysis, plasma concentration, antiepileptic drugs, ethosuximide, diphenylhydantoin, valproic acid, phenobarbital, epilepsy.

INTRODUCTION

Theoretical and applicative motivation and rationale for quantitative EEG studies do not differ to any relevant extent whether antiepileptic drugs or compounds used in the treatment of psychiatric conditions are considered. Common intent is to seek information about the dynamics of drug action at the Central Nervous System level-action that can only be inferred from pharmacokinetic measures and the assessment of which has therefore to rely mostly on the monitoring of therapeutic efficacy.

Unlike psychoactive compounds (Fink, 1969, 1975, 1978; Itil, 1974; Saletu, 1976), data available on the effects of antiepileptic drugs on background EEG activity are based upon non-quantitative or semiquantitative studies (Little, 1949; Courjon and others, 1962; Gaenshirt, 1967; Riehl and McIntyre, 1968; Miribel and Marinier, 1968; Ketz, 1974; Bente, 1975) and scarsely conclusive.

Interest has been focused thus far mostly on critical and intercritical epileptic EEG alterations, regarded as more specific. Epilepsy is nevertheless characterized by clinical and EEG symptoms which are by definition recurrent, but lack predictable frequency of occurrence. The frequency of clinical seizures can be remarkably low and EEG recordings can show little intercritical alterations, or be borderline or normal. These eveniences are quite common, especially during therapy, and make the assessment of treatment modes a dilatory procedure, when based on clinical results.

Serial determinations of drug plasma concentration have been proposed to bypass these limitations, and are routinary applied for monitoring purposes (Woodbury and others,1972; Kutt and Penry,1974; Lund,1974; Schneider and others,1975; Gardner-Thorpe and others,1977; Pippenger and others,1978), relying on the existing correlation between plasma concentrations within the so-called therapeutic range and control of seizures. The approach concurred in improving the pharamcological management of the epilepsies. However, the "therapeutic range" has obvious statistical connotations, which limit the possibilities for a one-patient oriented monitoring of therapy.

Our intent has been therefore to verify - in a pilot study on patients - the suitability of quantitative analysis in defining patterns of EEG changes occurring during antiepileptic therapy, and to consider its possibilities of providing additional criteria for the individual monitoring and tailoring of the treatment modes.

METHOD

Four groups of outpatients, homogeneous for age and clinical conditions, have been selected among those referred to single-drug treatment with ethosuximide (ESM), diphenylhydantoin (DPH), valproic acid (VPA), or phenobarbital (PB). Subjects assigned to therapy with ESM (n=6), DPH (n=5), and VPA (n=4) were children with, respectively: generalized non-convulsive epilepsy; partial epilepsy with complex symptomatology; generalized non-convulsive epilepsy with photosensitivity. Patients on therapy with PB (n=29) were adults with generalized convulsive epilepsy. With the exception of those receiving PB, the patients had never been treated before and the evaluation of baseline conditions prior to therapy was possible.

Plasma samples were collected periodically during treatment and drug plasma concentrations were determined by gas liquid chromatography. EEG samples were concomitantly recorded (dermal electrodes; 10-20 International System) on magnetic tape, in standard conditions of vigilance, and processed off-line by power spectral analysis at 128 samples/s, in 8-s epochs, for the frequencies between 0.5 and 45 Hz and with a 0.5 Hz resolution (Rosadini,1975). Six bipolar leads (Fp1-C3; C3-O1; T1-C3; Fp2-C4; C4-O2; T2-C4) were processed. Epochs containing artifacts or specific epileptic alterations - such as spikes, spike and wave discharges and so on - were excluded from further analysis. For any sample, data were combined into preselected bandwidths (0.5-4; 4.5-8; 8.5-12; 12.5-16; 16.5-20, and above 20 Hz), for which mean power and standard error were computed; the measure of average frequency was included in the outprint.

A modified protocol was followed to study the EEG changes occurring during treatment with VPA. Five EEG and plasma samples were collected in the three hours following the administration of the first daily dose (20 mg/kg), in order to acquire information about the first dose effects; in addition, six samples were concentrated within the first weeks of therapy.

RESULTS

Ethosuximide

ESM doses ranging 18.5 to 47.6 mg/kg/day yielded drug plasma concentrations within the range usually referred to as therapeutic, and resulted in the complete control of seizures and the disappearance of spike and wave discharges at the conventional EEG recording, in all patients but one, whose daily dose was to be increased.

The modifications occurring in the background EEG signal are reported in Fig. 1.

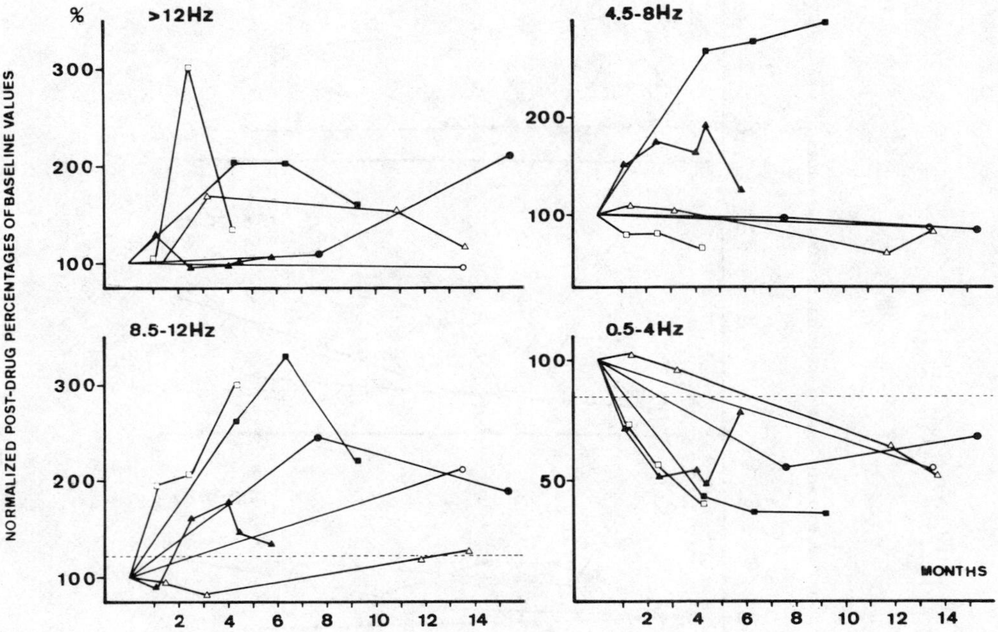

Fig. 1. Variations in the relative power, expressed as percentages of normalized pre-drug values, during treatment with ethosuximide. The dotted line represents the ≤ 0.01 level of significance (t-test).

A reduction in the relative power of the frequency components in the 0.5-4 Hz range and a concomitant increment in the power of the 8.5-12 Hz band was detected. An increment in the power of the 16.5-20 Hz segment occurred as well (Fig. 2). The EEG modifications were significant when compared to baseline ($p \leq 0.01$) and consistent over subjects, except the one (Δ in Fig. 1 and 2) whose initial ESM dose was inadequate. For this patient, the EEG variations in the 0.5-4 and 8.5-12 Hz spectral segments were delayed and dependent upon increment of ESM dose, while only incostant changes occurred in the 16.5-20 Hz frequency bandwidth. No other EEG modifications were observed. Both nature and time course of the EEG changes were analogous in all leads.

The variations in the relative power were not related, in either linear or exponential fashion, to the measures of ESM plasma concentration. No linear relation was found between EEG changes and period of sampling from the beginning of treatment; the correlation between these two variables was however approximated by an exponential function, which applied to the three frequency bandwidths 0.5-4; 8.5-12; 16.5-20 Hz, but attained statistical significance (coefficient of correlation: 0.52; $P \leq 0.05$) for the 0.5-4 Hz band only (Fig. 3).

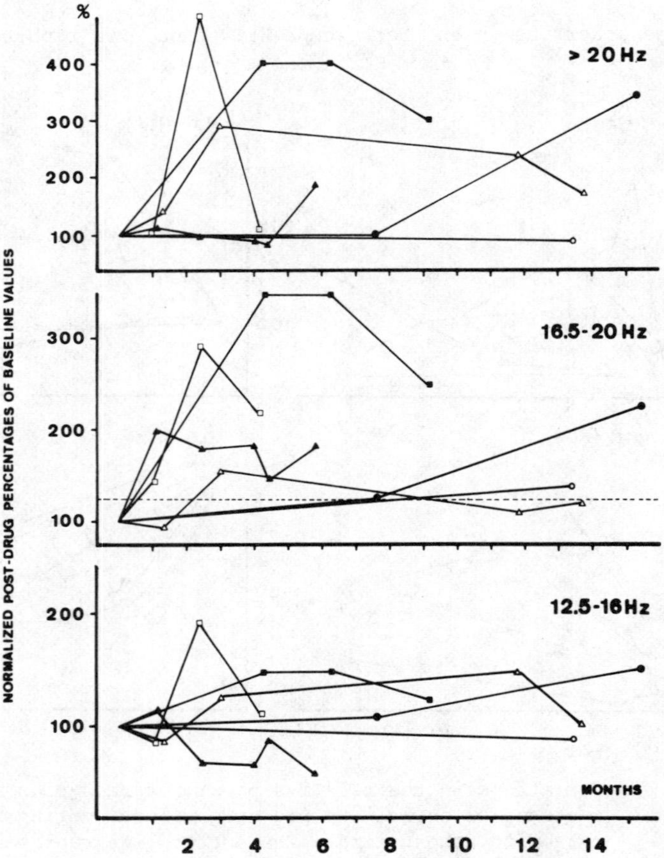

Fig. 2. Variations in the relative power of the fast frequency components, during treatment with ethosuximide

Diphenylhydantoin

Adequate drug plasma concentrations and control of seizures were obtained in all patients with DPH doses ranging 4.7 to 9.5 mg/kg/day. No EEG changes related to treatment have been however observed. The EEG variations (Fig. 4) were statistically significant when compared (t-test) to baseline values, but were neither consistent over subjects nor related to DPH plasma concentration, time of treatment or clinical effects.

Valproic Acid

Three subjects completed the study; one dropped at the fourth week for personal reasons. Control of seizures and reduction of photoconvulsive response to photic stimulation were achieved in all patients during the first three weeks of therapy.

Consistent EEG changes were observed only in the frequency components above 12.5 Hz, as reported in Fig. 5. The variations in the relative power which occurred in

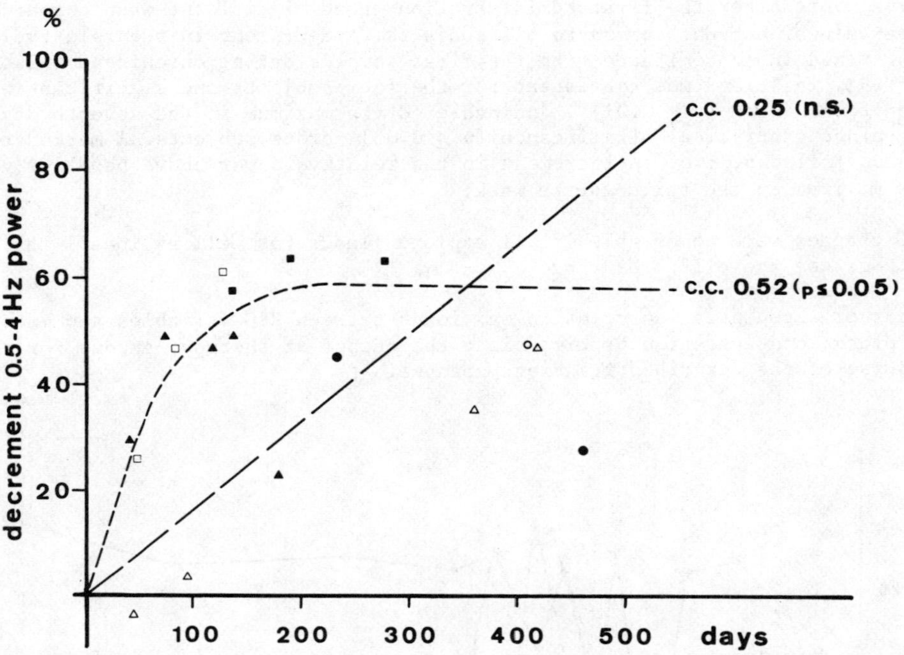

Fig. 3. Correlation (linear and exponential regression analysis) between decrement in 0.5-4 Hz relative power and time from the beginning of treatment with ethosuximide.

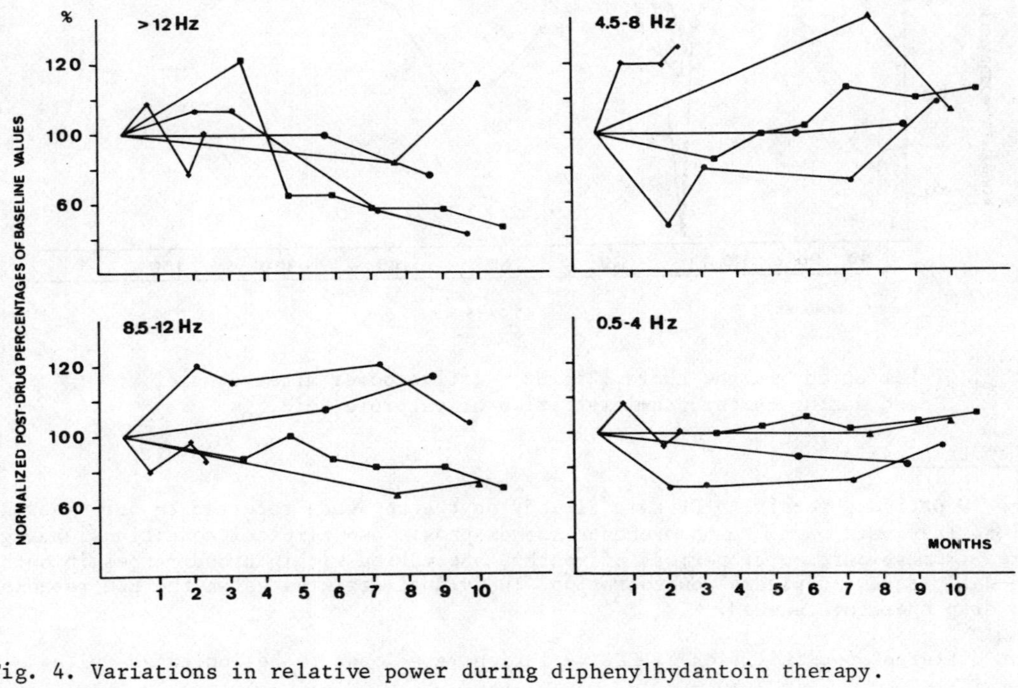

Fig. 4. Variations in relative power during diphenylhydantoin therapy.

the three hours after the first administration where significant when compared to baseline values, but not common to all subjects. A decrement in the relative power supervened in concomitance with the first samples during chronic administration of VPA. The trend was consistent for the four subjects and significant when compared to baseline ($p \leq 0.01$) , and achieved its maximum in the seventh day, when attained statistical significance ($p \leq 0.05$) across subjects. A marked rebound phenomenon followed, i.e. an increment in the relative power above baseline values, with its maximum in the third-fourth week.

The EEG changes were comparable in all explored leads, as well as in all the subsegments of the above 12.5 Hz range.

No linear or exponential correlation was found between EEG variables and measures of VPA plasma concentration or time since the outset of therapy, except for the time course of the described transient changes.

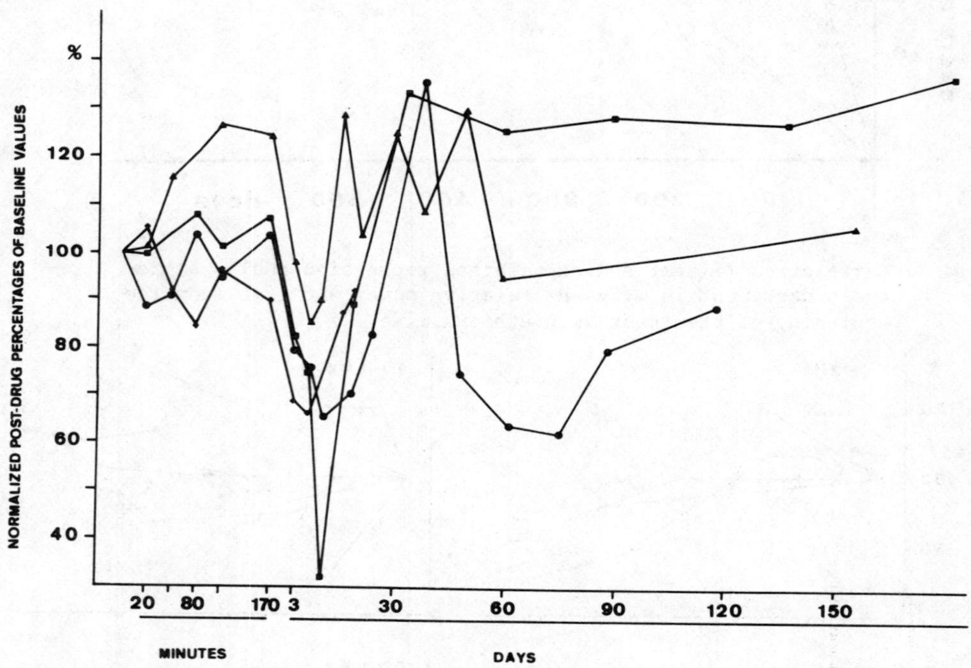

Fig. 5. Variations in the above 12.5 Hz relative power after single, and during chronic administration of valproic acid.

Phenobarbital

The 29 patients receiving PB were already on therapy when referred to our observation. They were therefore homogeneous for diagnosis and clinical conditions, being free from seizures over periods of months, but varied within broad ranges in both PB daily dose and plasma concentration. Individual differences in the EEG response to drug therefore ensued.

The different possibilities of EEG variation were found to be indicated with sufficient approximation by the measure of average frequency of the spectrum, as reported in Fig. 6. The average frequency was found to shift towards the fast frequency segment of the spectrum as drug plasma concentration increased; it conversely dropped at PB concentrations above 40-45 μg/ml. The statistical analysis was limited by the small number of samples with plasma concentration above this threshold. A significant linear correlation (coefficient of correlation: 0.34; $p \leq 0.1$) was nevertheless found for plasma concentration values below 40 μg/ml.

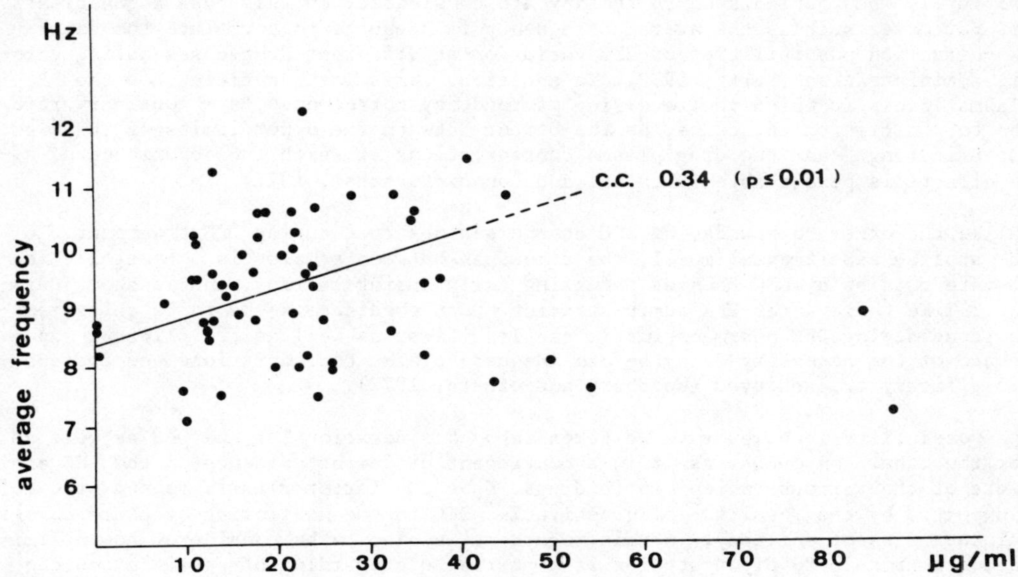

Fig. 6. Correlation (linear regression analysis) between EEG average frequency and phenobarbital plasma concentration.

DISCUSSION

The quantitative analysis of background activity has proved to be suitable in defining changes in the EEG pattern which occur during long-term treatment with antiepileptic drugs and are not confined to specific epileptic phenomena.

Relevant limitations nevertheless exist in relating these EEG variations to a direct and specific drug action. In fact, for what ESM and VPA are concerned, it has not been possible to determine any relation between drug plasma concentration and EEG changes, which appear to be rather dependent upon the time modes of treatment and parallel the clinical results. In the particular case of ESM, the EEG variations in background activity are, to this regard, in accordance with the reported ESM effects on the frequency of occurrence of spike and wave discharges (Penry and others, 1972).

The EEG changes during ESM therapy concern the whole EEG pattern and are consistent over the period of treatment; a qualitative analogy also exists with those modifications that the EEG undergoes during maturation processes (Petersen and others, 1976). The possibility of such an interference should however be ruled out by both the relatively short latency from the beginning of treatment and the different patients' age, unless it is speculated that the normalization induced on brain functions by ethosuximide makes it possible the acceleration of maturation processes interfered with by the pathological conditions.

An indirect "therapeutic" action seems conceivably accountable for the EEG variations detected for both ESM and VPA, possibly relevant enough to obscure other EEG changes, more directly drug-related.

Quantitative EEG appears to be more reliable, as an index of drug action at the CNS level, when patients on PB therapy are considered. In this case a quantitative EEG parameter such as the average frequency is adequate to correlate the described two-direction possibilities of EEG variation at different drug doses during chronic administration (Kurtz, 1977). In addition, it is worth noticing how the PB plasma levels to which the reversing of tendency corresponds, are routinary referred to, in clinical practice, as the border between the upper limits of the "therapeutic range" and the drug plasma concentrations at which the occurrence of side effects is predictable (Buchthal and Lennox-Buchthal, 1972).

Unlike the other compounds, no EEG change was observed during DPH treatment. In the applied experimental model, the time span between samples is potentially inadequate to display EEG changes occurring early during therapy, and of short duration, like those after VPA administration. Such evenience seems to be quite remote, considering DPH pharmacokinetic peculiarities, as well as the clinical experience of the necessary delay before adequate plasma concentrations and therapeutic efficacy are achieved (Woodbury and others, 1972).

The possibility is however to be taken into consideration for the DPH as well as for the other compounds, as it is a contingent different evidence of the EEG effects of the various antiepileptic drugs. Upon the latter clearly depends the role - supported by the results - of quantitative EEG in the monitoring of pharmacological therapies of epilepsy. To this regard it is also to be considered how a limitation intrinsic to pilot studies is a partial disregarding of possible sources of variability, which need larger samples to achieve relevance. In this case, systematic studies on epileptic patients are warranted, in which individual differences in physiopathological variables - especially response to drug action - can be minimized, and the limits of the approach can be defined.

The authors wish to acknowledge the contribution from Mrs. L.Gervasio, M.D, in providing part of the patients population, and P.Zagnoni, M.D., in determining part of the drugs plasma concentrations.

REFERENCES

Bente,D. (1975). Antikonvulsiva und elektroencephalogram. In H.Helmchen (ed.), Antiepileptische Langzeitmedication, Biblthca Psychiat., no. 151, Karger, Basel. pp.182-189.

Buchthal, F. and Lennox-Buchthal, M.A. (1972). Phenobarbital relation of serum concentration to control of seizures. In D.M. Woodbury, J.K. Penry and R.P. Schmidt (Eds), Antiepileptic Drugs, Raven Press, New York. pp. 335-343.

Courjon, J., Miribel, J., et Ferreno, E. (1962). Peut-on à l'heure actuelle préciser les indications et le mode d'administration de l'alpha-ethyl-alphaméthyl-succinimide dans le traitement de l'épilepsie? Rev.Neurol, 106, 394-401.

Fink, M. (1969). EEG and human psychopharmacology. Ann.Rev.Pharmacol., 9, 241.
Fink, M. (1975). Cerebral electrometry. Quantitative EEG applied to human psychopharmacology. In G.Dolce and H.Kunkel (Eds), CEAN - Computerized EEG analysis, Fischer Verlag, Stuttgart. pp. 271-288.
Fink, M. (1978). Psychoactive drugs and the waking EEG, 1966-1976. In M.A.Lipton, A. Di MAscio, and K.F.Killam (Eds), Psychopharmacology: a generation of progress, Raven Press, New York. pp.691-698.
Gaenshirt, H. (1967). Die behandlung der epilepsie in der nervenartzlichen sprechstunde. Nervenarzt, 38, 429-433.
Gardner-Thorpe, C., Janz, D., and Meinardi, H. (Eds). (1977). Antiepileptic drug monitoring. Pitman Medical Publ.Co.Ltd.,London.
Itil,T.(1974).(Ed).Psychotrppic drugs and the human EEG.Modern Problems of pharmacopsychiatry, Karger, Basel.
Ketz, E. (1974). Wirkung von antikonvulsiva und psychotropen drogen aut das EEG. Z. EEG-EMG, 5, 99-106.
Kurtz, D. (1977). The EEG in acute and chronic drug intoxication. In G.H. Glaser (Ed), Metabolic,endocrine and toxic diseases. In A.Remond (Ed. in chief), Handbook of Electroencephalography and Clinical Neurophysiology, Vol. 15C. Elsevier, Amsterdam. pp. 88-102.
Kutt, H., and Penry, K. (1974). Usefulness of blood levels of antiepileptic drugs. Arch.Neurol., 31, 283-288.
Little, C.S. (1949). Changes in the EEG following administration of mesantoin (methyl-phenyl-ethyl hydantoin). Electroenceph.clin.Neurophysiol., 1, 325-332.
Lund, L. (1974). Anticonvulsant effects of diphenylhydantoin relative to plasma levels. Arch.Neurol., 31, 289-294.
Miribel, J., and Marinier, R. (1968). Modifications éléctroencephalographiques chez les enfants traités par le Dépakene. Rev.Neurol., 119, 313-320.
Penry, J.K., Porter, R.J., Dreifuss, F.E. (1972). Ethosuximide relation of plasma levels to clinical control. In D.M. Woodbury, J.K. Penry, and R.P. Schmidt (Eds), Antiepileptic drugs, Raven Press, New York. pp. 431-441.
Petersen, I., Sellden, U., and Eeg-Olofsson, O. (1976). The evolution of the EEG in normal children and adolescents. In G.C. Lairy (Ed), The normal EEG throughout life. In A.Remond (Ed. in chief), Handbook of Electroencephalography and Clinical Neurophysiology, vol. 6B, Elsevier,Amsterdam. pp. 31-59.
Pippenger, C.E., Penry, J.K., and Kutt, H. (Eds), (1978). Antiepileptic drugs: quantitative analysis and interpretation. Raven Press, New York.
Riehl, J.L., and McIntyre, H.R. (1968). A quantitative study of the acute effects of diphenylhydantoin on the EEG of epileptic patients. Neurology, 18, 1107-1112.
Rosadini, G. (1975). Computerized EEG analysis in clinical neurophysiology. In G. Dolce and H.Kunkel (Eds), CEAN - Computerized EEG analysis, Fischer Verlag, Stuttgart. pp. 309-323.
Saletu, B. (1976). Psychopharmaka, gehirntatigkeit und schlaf. Bibl. Psychiat., no. 55, Karger, Basel.
Schneider, H., Gardner, C., Meinardi, H., and Sherwin, A.L. (Eds), (1975). Clinical pharmacology of anti-epileptic drugs, Springer Verlag, Berlin.
Woodbury, D.M., Penry, J.K., and Schmidt, R.P. (Eds), (1972). Antiepileptic Drugs, Raven Press, New York.

Naltrexone in Normal Men

J. VOLAVKA*, A. MALLYA*, J. PEVNICK*, D. CHO*, D. REKER*, B. JAMES*, J. BAUMAN and R. DORNBUSH*****

*University of Missouri Columbia-School of Medicine, at Missouri Institute of Psychiatry, St. Louis, Mo., U.S.A.
**Reproductive Biology Research Foundation, St. Louis, Mo., U.S.A.
***New York Medical College, Valhalla, New York, U.S.A.

INTRODUCTION

Since the discovery of endogenous opiate-like substances (endorphins) (Terenius and Wahlstrom, 1974; Hughes and co-workers, 1975; Pasternak, Goodman and Snyder, 1975), many experimental approaches have been devised to study their functions (Costa and Trabucchi, 1978). A strategy which has been used very widely consists in the administration of an opiate antagonist. It is assumed that the antagonists displace endorphins from their receptors; once this happens, any function for which endorphins are needed should be altered. It has been hypothesized that endorphins play a role in pain perception (Buchsbaum, Davis and Bunney, 1977; El-Sobky, Dostrovsky and Wall, 1976; Grevert and Goldstein, 1978; Hosobuchi, Adams and Linchitz, 1977), modulation of mood (Jones, 1978), sexual functioning (Goldstein and Hansteen, 1977), mental health (Watson and co-workers, 1978; Verebey, Volavka and Clouet, 1978) and other areas. These hypotheses were tested by the administration of the opiate antagonist naloxone. Another opiate antagonist, naltrexone, has also been used for similar experiments: it was administered to rats in order to study the function of endorphins in prolactin release (Guidotti and Grandison, 1978); it was also used in therapeutic experiments in psychotic patients (Simpson, Branchey and Lee, 1977; Gunne and Terenius, 1978; Gitlin and Rosenblatt, 1978). Opiate-naive subjects were used in these studies. The principal advantage of naltrexone against naloxone in human experiments were seen in its longer duration of action after oral administration. Clinical trials in ex-addicts have shown that naltrexone antagonizes the effects of heroin for up to 72 hours and that it is non-toxic in doses up to 200 mg/day (Volavka and co-workers, 1976).

One of the assumptions underlying such experiments is that the antagonist which is being used has essentially no other effects than that of blocking the opiate receptor. Should the antagonist have opiate-like effects of its own, the results of these experiments would be difficult to interpret. Naltrexone has been classified as a relatively pure narcotic antagonist (Martin, Jasinski and Mansky, 1973), and this classification was appropriate in its original context, i.e. with regard to treatment of heroin addiction. The fact that it caused a non-significant decrease of respiratory rate and pupillary size, and significant decrease of temperature was not considered important in view of the very small size of these effects observed in five ex-addicts (Martin, Jasinski and Mansky, 1973). The administration of opiates probably alters interactions between the opiate receptor and endorphins (Goldstein, 1976; Ehrlich and co-workers, 1978). For this reason, these issues are best studied in organisms that have not been exposed to opiates. We have found only two studies of naltrexone in opiate-naive normal humans. Ratings of mood and behavior obtained in one of these studies (Irwin and co-workers, 1974) indicated that naltrexone may have some opiate-like properties. Sleepiness, dysphoria, sexual ideation, penile erection, and an increase of luteinizing hormone were reported after 50 mg of naltrexone (Mendelson and co-workers, in press).

METHODS

In our present study, the subjects were 10 healthy male volunteers (age range 19-31). It was determined that none of them had a history of opiate use by questioning the subjects, and also by taking a urine sample for opiates at the beginning of each session. (No opiates were ever detected.) Each subject had three sessions which were separated from each other by at least a week. Either placebo or naltrexone 50 mg or 100 mg was given in tablets by mouth in each session. These substances were given in a counterbalanced order. We studied respiration rate (which was recorded using a strain gauge placed around the subject's chest), heart rate, blood pressure, oral temperature, and pupil size (pupil photographs were taken after a 10-minute adaptation to the dark; a Polaroid camera with circular flash was used). Electroencephalogram (EEG) was evaluated by subjecting ten-minute EEG records from the right and left occipital areas to power spectral analyses. We also assessed an opiate withdrawal questionnaire which consisted of 13 items: stomach cramps or stomach pain; nausea; bowel movement; eyes teary; nose runny; yawning; sweating; goosepimples; chills; muscle, joint or back pain; dizziness; anxiety-nervousness; loss of appetite. Each item was rated on a four-point scale (absent, slight, moderate, a lot). We also studied the subject's sensitivity to pain. This was determined by having the subjects immerse the nonwriting hand for two minutes into chipped ice. They indicated the time of pain onset; this was used as a measure of pain threshold. Severity of pain and the attitude toward pain were rated every 30 seconds during the immersion. Immediately after each pain test, a blood sample was drawn for the radioimmunoassays of luteinizing hormone (LH), prolactin, testosterone, ACTH and cortisol. Subjects were asked by a male nurse whether they were sexually aroused and/or had an erection. All these variables were assessed before the drug administration, then at 1, 2, 4 and 8 hours after the drug. Short unstructured interviews were done at the same time periods; an additional interview occurred 24 hours after the drug administration. All sessions started between 8 and 9 a.m.

Multiple hierarchical regression analyses were used to test the significance of the drug effects while accounting for the variance of the baseline (pre-drug) values. These procedures were analogous to analyses of covariance for repeated measures (Kerlinger and Pedhazur, 1973). Double-blind procedures were followed both in data acquisition and analyses.

RESULTS

Breathing rate and temperature were significantly lower after naltrexone than after placebo (Table 1). The pain threshold showed a highly significant interaction between baseline values and drug effect (Table 1, Figure 1). This interaction means that the subjects showing higher threshold (i.e. less sensitivity to pain) before the drug administration are more likely to experience the analgesic effect of naltrexone than those with low initial threshold (i.e. those who are more pain-sensitive). Pain threshold as measured by our method may be a relatively permanent individual attribute. The three baseline values (i.e. pre-placebo, pre-naltrexone 50 mg, and pre-naltrexone 100 mg) for individual subjects were correlated with each other (the average r was 0.65). Pain severity ratings did not yield significant results.

TABLE 1
EFFECTS OF NALTREXONE AND PLACEBO IN 10 SUBJECTS

	PLACEBO		NALTREXONE 50 mg		NALTREXONE 100 mg		Drug Effect on Post-value	Inter-action
	pre	post	pre	post	pre	post	p	p
Respiration rate (breaths/min)	15.9	16.7	16.0	15.4	16.0	15.1	0.005	n.s.
Oral temperature (°C)	36.69	36.83	36.63	36.60	36.58	36.53	0.005	n.s.
Pain threshold (sec) (cold pressor test)	17.3	17.7	14.5	17.2	15.8	21.9	n.a.	0.005
Luteinizing hormone (mIU/ml)	6.8	7.7	5.0	10.2	7.1	11.4	0.005	n.s.
Cortisol (ng/dl)	9.6	9.1	10.7	11.5	10.4	12.2	0.005	n.s.

The "post" values were obtained by averaging observations made at 1, 2, 4 and 8 hours after the drug administration. Each of these averages was used as the dependent variable in a multiple stepwise regression analysis. The baseline (pre-drug) values were entered as covariates, and the coded drug treatments were entered as the independent variables. The last steps in each of the analyses were the interactions between the drug effect and the pre-drug value.

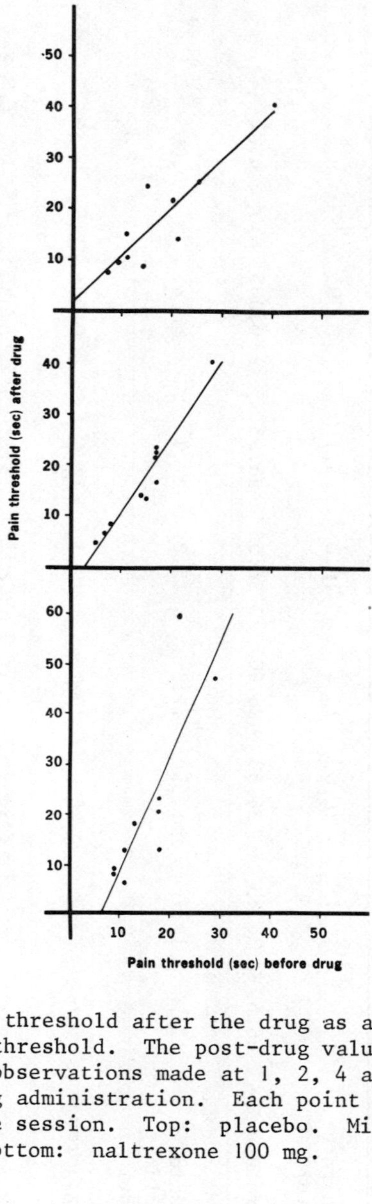

Fig. 1. Pain threshold after the drug as a function of the pre-drug threshold. The post-drug values were obtained by averaging observations made at 1, 2, 4 and 8 hours after the drug administration. Each point represents one subject in one session. Top: placebo. Middle: naltrexone 50 mg. Bottom: naltrexone 100 mg.

The global score on the opiate withdrawal questionnaire was significantly ($p < 0.05$) higher after naltrexone than after placebo. Naltrexone elicited a significant increase of LH and cortisol (Table 1). An increase of ACTH and prolactin was seen in the first hour after naltrexone; these and other hormonal data will be published elsewhere in greater detail. Pupillary diameter showed a slight non-significant decrease after naltrexone. The average frequency of the EEG alpha activity was significantly slower after naltrexone than after placebo; details are published elsewhere (Volavka and co-workers, in press). Nausea, abdominal cramps and/or decreased appetite occurred in six of the ten subjects after 100 mg, in one subject after 50 mg, and in two subjects after placebo. These complaints started at 8 or 24 hours after 100 mg of naltrexone. No difference between naltrexone and placebo was detected in reports of sexual arousal or erection.

DISCUSSION

These data indicated that naltrexone has opiate-like, as well as antagonist properties in opiate-naive humans. The reduction of breathing rate, temperature and EEG alpha frequency, as well as the effects on pain threshold suggest opiate-like activity. The presence of clinical symptoms usually associated with opiate withdrawal suggests that naltrexone also has antagonist activity. However, these symptoms are not specific for opiate withdrawal. Since morphine has a biphasic action on the secretion of ACTH (George, 1971) and LH (Zimmerman and Pang, 1976), the observed hormonal effects of naltrexone are difficult to interpret as either agonist or antagonist in nature. We confirm the increase of LH reported by Mendelson and co-workers (in press), but not their finding of sexual arousal.

Our observations of pain threshold effects differ from those published by Buchsbaum, Davis and Bunney (1977). They found that after naloxone, pain-insensitive subjects showed hyperalgesia whereas the pain-sensitive ones showed hypoalgesia. Since naltrexone apparently has much more agonist activity than naloxone, we have seen little or no hyperalgesia; however, the hypoalgesic effect of naltrexone was more pronounced in our pain-insensitive subjects. This discrepancy in observations may be due to the difference between naloxone and naltrexone, or to the differences in methodology. We agree in that the initial values strongly interact with the drug effect on pain perception. A slight analgesic effect of naltrexone was observed in the rat but not in the mouse (Blumberg and Dayton, 1972). We are not aware of any report of analgesic activity of naltrexone in humans.

The opiate-like effects we observed are too small to concern clinicians using naltrexone for the treatment of opiate addiction of overdose. However, they do have implications for endorphin research. Opiate antagonists do not generally exert large effects in opiate-naive humans (Buchsbaum, David and Bunney, 1977; El-Sobky, Dostrovsky and Wall, 1976; Grevert and Goldstin, 1978; Hosobuchi, Adams and Linchitz, 1977; Verebey, Volavka and Clouet, 1978). Therefore, even the relatively small effects detected in this study are important for experiments that use naltrexone to explore endorphin functions in opiate-naive organisms. In our opinion, the mixed effects of naltrexone make any results of those experiments difficult or impossible to interpret. Several such experiments are now in progress, and Watson and co-workers (1978) suggest that more naltrexone studies in psychiatric patients might be useful. We feel that our data do not encourage such hopes.

SUMMARY

Ten healthy males with no history of opiate dependence received a dose of placebo, 50 mg, and 100 mg of naltrexone. Naltrexone decreased breathing rate and oral temperature, and it increased pain threshold in certain subjects. It increased plasma levels of luteinizing hormone and cortisol. These findings have implications for endorphin research.

ACKNOWLEDGEMENT

This study was supported in part by a grant from the Missouri Institute of Psychiatry, University of Missouri-Columbia School of Medicine. We thank Dr. Karl Verebey and the Office of Drug Abuse Services, Brooklyn, New York, for the urine analyses. Naltrexone was a gift from Endo Laboratories.

REFERENCES

Blumberg, H. and Dayton, H.B. (1972). Narcotic antagonist studies with EN-1639A (N-Cyclopropylmethylnoroxymorphone hydrochloride). In *Fifth International Congress on Pharmacology, Volunteer Abstracts*. San Francisco, July, p. 23.

Buchsbaum, M.S., Davis, G.C. and Bunney, W.E. Jr. (1977). Naloxone alters pain perception and somatosensory evoked potentials in normal subjects. *Nature*, 270, 620-622.

Costa, E. and Trabucchi, M. (eds.) (1978). *The Endorphins. Advances in Biochemical Psychopharmacology*, Vol. 18, Raven Press, New York.

Ehrlich, Y.H., Bonnet, K.A., Davis, L.G., and Brunngraber, E.G. (1978). Decreased phosphorylation of specific proteins in neostriatal membranes from rats after long-term narcotic exposure. *Life Sciences*, 23, 137-146.

El-Sobky, A., Dostrovsky, J.O., and Wall, P.D. (1976). Lack of effect of naloxone on pain perception in humans. *Nature*, 263, 783-784.

George, R. (1971). Hypothalamus: Anterior pituitary gland. In D.H. Clouet (ed.), *Narcotic Drugs, Biochemical Pharmacology*, Plenum Press, New York.

Gitlin, M. and Rosenblatt, M. (1978). Possible withdrawal from endogenous opiates in schizophrenics. *Am. J. Psychiatry*, 135, 377-378.

Goldstein, A. (1976). Opioid peptides (endorphins) in pituitary and brain. *Science*, 193, 1081-1086.

Goldstein, A. and Hansteen, R.W. (1977). Evidence against involvement of endorphins in sexual arousal and orgasm in man. *Arch. Gen. Psychiat.*, 34, 1179-1180.

Grevert, P. and Goldstein, A. (1978). Endorphins: Naloxone fails to alter experimental pain or mood in humans. *Science*, 199, 1093-1095.

Guidotti, A. and Grandison, L. (1978). Participation of hypothalamic endorphins in the control of prolactin release. In E. Costa and M. Trabucchi (eds.), *The Endorphins. Advances in Biochemical Pharmacology*, Vol. 18, Raven Press, New York.

Gunne, L.M. and Terenius, L. (1978). Possible role of endorphins in schizophrenia and other psychiatric disorders. In E. Usdin, W.E. Bunney, Jr. and N.S. Kline (eds.) *Endorphins in Mental Health Research*, Macmillan Press, New York.

Hosobuchi, Y., Adams, J.E., and Linchitz, R. (1977). Pain relief by electrical stimulation of the central gray matter in humans and its reversal by naloxone. *Science*, 197, 183-186.

Hughes, J., Smith, T.W., Kosterlitz, H.W., Fothergill, L.A., Morgan, B.A. and Morris, H.R. (1975). Identification of two related pentapeptides from the brain with potent opiate agonist activity. *Nature*, 258, 577-579.

Irwin, S., Konohi, R.G., Coolet, P.M. and Bottomly, D.R. (1974). Acute time-dose-response effects of cyclazocine, naltrexone, and naloxone in man. *Proc. Committee on Problems of Drug Dependence*, Cambridge, Mass.

Jones, R. (1978). Naloxone-induced mood and physiologic changes in normal volunteers. In E. Usdin, W.E. Bunney Jr., and N.S. Kline (eds.) *Endorphins in Mental Health Research*, Macmillan Press, New York.

Kerlinger, F.N. and Pedhazur, E.J. (1973). *Multiple Regression in Behavioral Research*. Holt, Rinehart, Winston, New York.

Martin, W.R., Jasinski, D.R. and Mansky, P.A. (1973). Naltrexone, an antagonist for the treatment of heroin dependence. *Arch. Gen. Psychiat.*, 28, 784-791.

Mendelson, J.H., Ellingboe, J., Keuhnle, J.C. and Mello, N.K. Effects of naltrexone on mood and neuroendocrine function in normal adult males. *Psychoneuroendocrinology*, in press.

Pasternak, G.W., Goodman, R. and Snyder, S.H. (1975). Endogenous morphine-like factor in mammalian brain. *Life Sci.*, 16, 1765-1769.

Simpson, G.M., Branchey, M.H. and Lee, J.H. (1977). A trial of naltrexone in chronic schizophrenia. *Curr. Ther. Res.*, 22, 909-913.

Terenius, L. and Wahlstrom, A. (1974). Inhibitor(s) of narcotic receptor binding in brain extracts and cerebral spinal fluid. *Acta Pharmacol. Toxicol.*, 35 (Suppl. 1), 55.

Verebey, K., Volavka, J., and Clouet, D. (1978). Endorphins in psychiatry. *Arch. Gen. Psychiatry*, 35, 877-888.

Volavka, J., Resnick, R., Kestenbaum, R., and Freedman, A. (1976). Short-term effects of naltrexone in 155 heroin ex-addicts. *Biol. Psychiat.*, 11, 679-685.

Volavka, J., James, B., Reker, D., Mallya, A., Cho, D., and Pevnick, J. EEG and other effects of naltrexone and heroin in man. *Pharmakopsychiatrie Neuro-Psychopharmakologie*, in press.

Watson, S.J., Berger, P.A., Akil, H., Mills, M.J., and Barchas, J.D. (1978). Effects of naloxone on schizophrenia: reduction in hallucinations in a subpopulation of subjects. *Science*, 201, 73-76.

Zimmerman, E. and Pang, C.N. (1976). Acute effects of opiate administration on pituitary gonadotropin and prolactin release. In D.H. Ford and D.H. Clouet (eds.), *Tissue Responses to Addictive Drugs*, Spectrum, New York.

The Biological and Clinical Basis of the Therapeutic Effects of Benzodiazepines

Introduction

EVE C. JOHNSTONE

Division of Psychiatry, Clinical Research Centre, Watford Road, Harrow, Middlesex, HA1 3UJ, England

ABSTRACT

This summary of the 8 papers presented in the symposium under this heading indicates the various modes of action which recent basic studies have suggested may account for the anxiolytic action of benzodiazepine drugs. The many factors which may influence the pharmacokinetics of these various benzodiazepine derivatives and the psychophysiological and clinical aspects of their use are then discussed. The difficulties in identifying homogenous diagnostic categories and the problems of finding clinical predictors of benzodiazepine response are stressed.

Benzodiazepines; basic studies; clinical aspects

The first speaker in this symposium was Dr Sandra File who described her experiments in which the social behaviour of rats has been studied. The alterations in the behaviour of these animals produced by circumstances such as unfamiliarity are used as a model for anxiety. These changes in behaviour are reduced by benzodiazepines given on a chronic basis and are increased by the administration of ACTH. There is evidence to show that this effect is due to ACTH itself and not to secondarily produced steroids. Dr File hypothesised that the actions of the peptide ACTH upon the CNS involve 5HT pathways and produced evidence in support of this idea from experiments concerning the effects of ACTH upon suitably lesioned rats. Administration of chlordiazepoxide on a chronic basis reversed the behavioural changes produced in the rats by ACTH. Thus it was concluded that it is possible that one of the mechanisms of the anxiolytic action of the benzodiazepines is to counteract the action of ACTH on 5HT neurones. Dr Braestrup described in detail his experiments in which the presence of specific binding sites for pharmacologically active benzodiazepines has been demonstrated in the brains of humans and some animals. In evolutionary terms these binding sites develop rather late as they are not present in certain primitive animals. Presumably benzodiazepines are ineffective in these creatures and the endogenous ligand of the benzodiazepine receptors is not present in them. The existence and nature of the endogenous ligand is of course a most fascinating question. Dr Braestrup then went on to describe experiments which showed that the tolerance and abstinence syndromes which occur in relation to high dosage administration of benzodiazepines are not caused by changes in the benzodiazepine receptor.

Dr Haefely then gave a comprehensive summary of the effects of benzodiazepines upon the electrical activity of the CNS. He discussed the interaction of benzodiazepines with GABAergic transmission and the demonstration of the potentiation of GABAergic activity by benzodiazepine administration. He explained that the question of the contribution of the presynaptic and postsynaptic effects is as yet unsettled.

The remaining speakers discussed more clinical aspects of the use of benzodiazepines. Dr Shader described benzodiazepine pharmacokinetics in man discussing the considerable variation between individuals in the blood levels of the drugs which they achieve and the amounts and relative proportions of the metabolites which they produce. He pointed out the different rates of clinical effect of the different types of benzodiazepines and discussed the effects of food and of concurrent antacid administration upon the absorption of various benzodiazepine derivatives. He discussed the interaction of diazepam and alcohol and explained that this is a topic on which questions remain to be answered. Dr Hillestad then went on to discuss the effects of benzodiazepines in the physically ill. He pointed out the beneficial effects which benzodiazepines produce in coronary patients in terms of reduced need for analgesics and reduced incidence of malignant arrhythmias. He described the enhanced clinical effects of benzodiazepines in patients with hepatic and renal failure. These occur in the absence of significant change in the plasma half lives and he hypothesised that they are due to alterations in protein binding.

Dr Lader gave a clear description of the physical concomitants of anxiety, of the sensitive and reliable ways in which these physiological variables can be measured and of the ways in which these effects are modified by benzodiazepines and other drugs. He illustrated this by case material and concluded by producing a hypothetical psychophysiological model for anxiety.

Professor Rickels described his studies of very large numbers of neurotic patients. He explained the difficulties of identifying homogeneous diagnostic categories and pointed out that if depression is present in any severe degree it tends to over-ride anxiety. He gave results of discriminant function tests and these showed that the features particularly relevant for improvement in depressed patients differed from those relevant for improvement in anxious patients. In a similar way the symptom areas affected by antidepressants differed from those affected by diazepam.

The last paper concerned 240 neurotic patients who were not placed in any diagnostic category but who were assessed on various ratings of depression and anxiety during a four week placebo controlled study of diazepam and amitriptyline. The distinction between anxiety states and neurotic depression was unclear. Clinical factors were of low predictive value with regard to response to various drug regimes. Psychophysiological measures were of stronger predictive value but the relationships remained too weak to be useful in the individual case. These contributions ranged over a wide field and referred to very interesting results. Although they differed greatly they tended to share the common factor of answering one question only to raise another and it is clear that much more work remains to be done in this field.

ACTH as a Mediator in Anxiety

SANDRA E. FILE

Department of Pharmacology, The School of Pharmacy, University of London, 29/39 Brunswick Square, London WC1N 1AX, England

ABSTRACT

Using the social interaction test of anxiety we have shown that whereas in acute doses benzodiazepines have a sedative effect, with chronic (5 days) administration they have an anxiolytic (anxiety reducing) action. Corticotrophin ($ACTH_{1-24}$) has an anxiogenic action and when given in combination with benzodiazepines it can reverse their behavioural effects. The importance of 5-HT pathways is indicated by our findings: a) that chronic (5 days) administration of benzodiazepines reduces 5-HT turnover, whereas ACTH increases it; and b) that parachlorophenylalanine (an inhibitor of 5-HT synthesis) produces a behavioural profile similar to that seen with anxiolytic drugs. It is therefore suggested that ACTH exerts an anxiogenic action by acting on 5-HT pathways and that this effect can be counteracted by anxiolytic drugs. On the basis of our lesion studies we suggest that the 5-HT pathways ascending from the dorsal raphe nucleus might be of particular importance.

Animal Tests of Anxiety

For ethical and practical reasons investigations into the biochemistry of anxiety and the mechanisms of action of anxiolytic drugs cannot be conducted solely with human subjects. Animal models are needed to investigate the mode of action of existing drugs and to screen for potential new anxiolytics. The two most widely used animal tests of anxiety are the Geller-Seifter conflict test (Geller & Seifter, 1960) and the conditioned emotional response (Estes & Skinner, 1941). These tests use deprivation and electric shock and in the Geller-Seifter test, and usually in the conditioned emotional response test, the animal is required to make an operant response. The drawback of these tests is that it is not always possible to control adequately for drug-induced changes in sensory thresholds, in motivation, or in response performance.

We have recently devised a new animal test of anxiety (File & Hyde, 1978) that does not require lengthy pretraining of the animals or operant responding, and does not use deprivation or electric shock. The test exploits the social behaviour of rats, and the way in which this changes with manipulations of the test conditions. Pairs of male rats are tested in a wooden box in which neither rat has an established territory and thus in which the social interaction is not dominated by aggressive encounters. Most of the interaction is investigatory in nature, sniffing and following the partner, but sexual and aggressive behaviours do also occur, although relatively infrequently. The greatest amount of active interaction is seen when the rats are tested in a box with which they are familiar and which is lit with a low level of illumination. If the box is unfamiliar or if the light level is increased there is a decrease in the amount of active interaction.

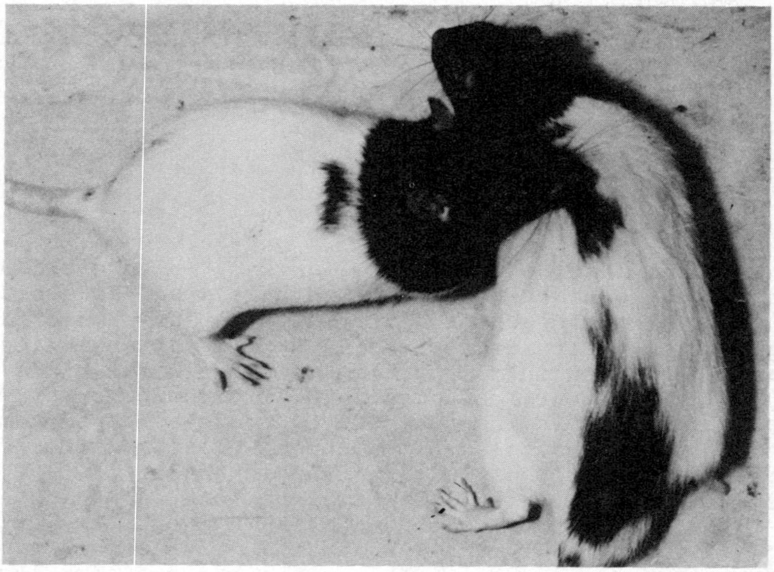

Fig. 1. This figure shows two rats in a brightly lit unfamiliar box. The one rat has been sniffing and grooming the back of the other rat, which is crawling away.

In manipulating unfamiliarity and light level we were hoping to change factors that would lead to an increase in anxiety. By putting the rats in an unfamiliar environment we were maximising uncertainty, a potent cause of anxiety: in an unfamiliar situation the nature, place or time of arrival of possible dangers are all unknown. The rat has an innate preference for low levels of illumination and thus by manipulating the light level we were hoping to increase anxiety.

There is no single behavioural, physiological or biochemical measure that can distinguish anxiety from other emotional states or even from states of physiological arousal after physical exercise. It is therefore difficult to validate any test of anxiety. Nevertheless, if the four test conditions are placed in the rank order shown on the abscissa of Fig. 2 then there is a significant decrease in the time spent in active interaction, and an increase in defecation, freezing and displacement behaviours, which are more traditional measures of emotional behaviour in the rat. It is impossible to prove that the decreased social interaction is caused by increasing anxiety, but two alternative explanations can be excluded. We have shown that the decrease in social interaction is not due to an increase in the time spent exploring the box when it is unfamiliar, and is not in response to changes in the olfactory cues emitted by the partner in the different test conditions (File & Hyde, 1978).

Anxiolytic Drugs

Another way of validating an animal test is to see whether the drugs that are used clinically to treat anxiety do indeed change the animal's test behaviour in the predicted manner. Since we have suggested the decrease in interaction is due to increased anxiety we would expect anxiolytic drugs to prevent, or significantly reduce, this decrease. This is just the result we found with the low doses of ethanol (File, Hyde & Pool, 1976) and with benzodiazepines, the drugs most widely used to treat anxiety. The pattern of results with the benzodiazepines was particularly interesting as it was the same as that found clinically. In acute doses, chlordiazepoxide (5 mg/kg) had a significantly sedative action, whereas given chronically (5 mg/kg for 5 days) it had a significant anxiolytic effect. This difference between acute and chronic administration is reflected in the effects on motor activity (see Table 1) and in the effects on active social interaction (see Fig. 2).

TABLE 1 The Effects of Acute and Chronic (5 days) Administration of Chlordiazepoxide (CDP 5 mg/kg) on Motor Activity (Mean ± S.E.M.)

	Controls		CDP	
Acute Treatment	266.2 ± 17.8	$p < .01$	200.3 ± 15.3	$p < .01$ (Acute CDP vs Chronic CDP)
Chronic Treatment	258.3 ± 38.7		270.5 ± 15.2	

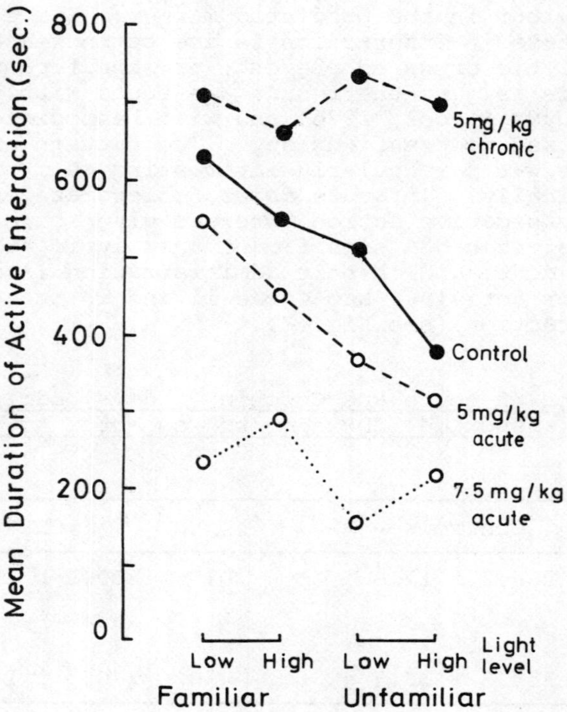

Fig. 2. The mean time spent in active social interaction by undrugged rats and by those given acute or chronic (5 days) chlordiazepoxide. Each data point is the mean score from an independent group of 6 pairs of rats.

Anxiogenic Agents

We have suggested that corticotrophin ($ACTH_{1-24}$ 5 μg/100 g) is anxiogenic (File & Vellucci, 1978). We found that ACTH significantly reduced active interaction in all the test conditions and that this behavioural effect could be counteracted by low doses of ethanol (see Fig. 3) or by chlordiazepoxide (5 mg/kg for 5 days).

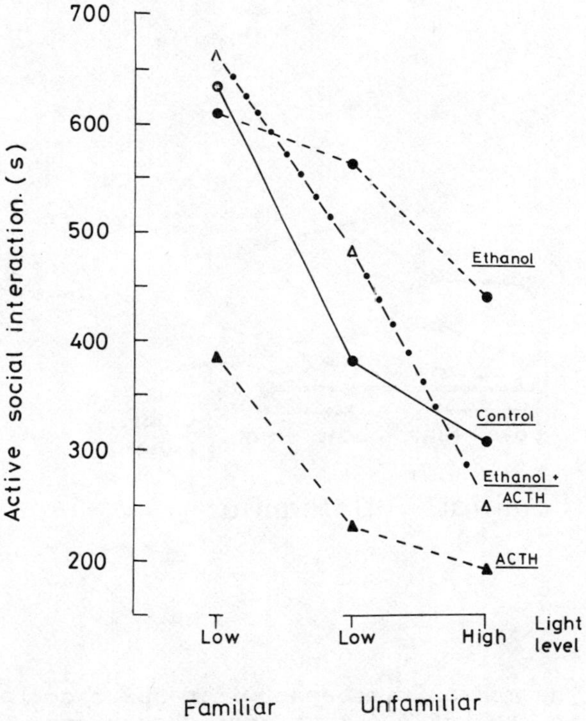

Fig. 3. The mean time spent in active interaction by rats injected with ethanol (0.4 g/kg), ACTH (5 μg/100 g), ethanol + ACTH, and by rats given control injections.

Since the effect of ACTH is to reduce active interaction, and this is also the effect seen with sedative drugs, it is necessary to distinguish between anxiogenic and sedative agents. There was no evidence from motor activity scores that ACTH was sedative. But there is also a measure from the social interaction test that reflects sedation. Passive contact is defined as the time that the rats spend sitting or lying with their bodies in contact, but without interacting with each other. This increases in a dose-related manner with administration of a sedative drug. Fig. 4 shows an example of this with acute administration of CDP. It can also be seen from Fig. 4 that there is little change in passive contact across the test conditions, i.e. with presumed changes in anxiety. There is no evidence from the passive contact scores that ACTH is sedative.

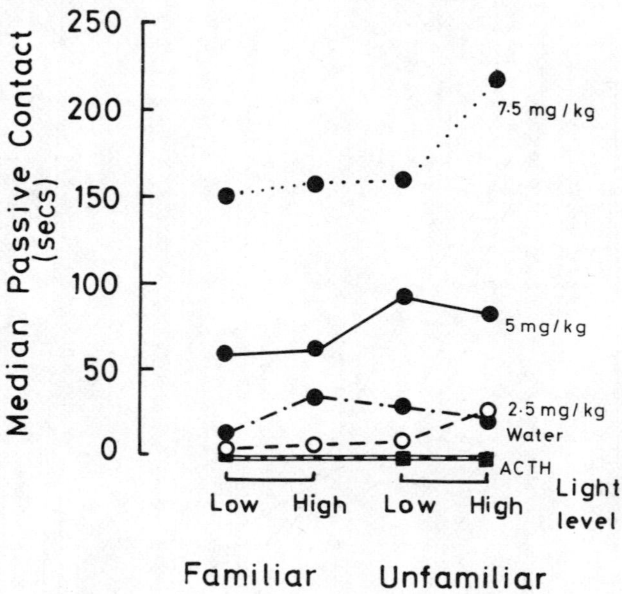

Fig. 4. The median time spent in passive contact in each of the four test conditions, for rats injected with ACTH (5 μg/100 g), CDP (2.5, 5 and 7.5 mg/kg, acute doses) and for water-injected controls.

5-HT and Anxiety

Stein, Wise and Berger (1973) proposed that a reduction in 5-HT turnover was important for anxiety reduction. In support of this we have found that parachlorophenylalanine, an inhibitor of 5-HT synthesis, produces an anxiolytic profile in the social interaction test (File & Hyde, 1977). Similar results have been reported from other animal tests (Robichaud & Sledge, 1969; Geller & Blum, 1970; Cook & Sepinwall, 1975). Our biochemical results also indicate the importance of a reduced 5-HT turnover in the mechanism of action of anxiolytic drugs (File & Vellucci, 1978). Chronic (5 days), but not acute, administration of chlordiazepoxide significantly increased 5-HT levels and reduced 5-HIAA levels (5-hydroxy-indoleacetic acid, the major metabolite of 5-HT). These changes are indicative of a reduced 5-HT turnover and were most marked in the hypothalamus, midbrain and cerebral cortex. Similar changes were found with acute administration of ethanol. In contrast, ACTH resulted in significant elevations of 5-HIAA, i.e. an indication of increased turnover, in the hypothalamus and midbrain (see Table 2).

TABLE 2 Ratio of 5-HIAA/5-HT in Various Brain Regions of Rats given Acute or Chronic (5 days) CDP (5 mg/kg), Ethanol (0.4 g/kg) and ACTH (5 μg/100 g).

	Hypothalamus	Midbrain	Hippocampus	Cortex
Acute CDP	-	-	-	-
Chronic CDP	* ↓	* ↓	-	** ↓
Acute Ethanol	-	* ↓	-	* ↓
ACTH	* ↑	** ↑	-	-

* $p < 0.05$, ** $p < 0.01$ compared with relevant control group; ↑ increase in ratio, ↓ decrease in ratio.

The biochemical results suggest that critical sites of action for anxiolytic drugs and for ACTH are 5-HT pathways in the midbrain and hypothalamus. This idea receives support from the results of a recent lesion study (File, Hyde, MacLeod, in preparation). Lesions of the median raphe nucleus, or of the dorsal raphe nucleus were made by microinjecting the neurotoxin 5,7-dihydroxytryptamine into each nucleus. Fig. 5 shows that rats with lesions of the median raphe nucleus were indistinguishable from the controls, whereas those with lesions of the dorsal raphe nucleus showed a behavioural profile similar to rats treated with PCPA and to those given anxiolytic drugs.

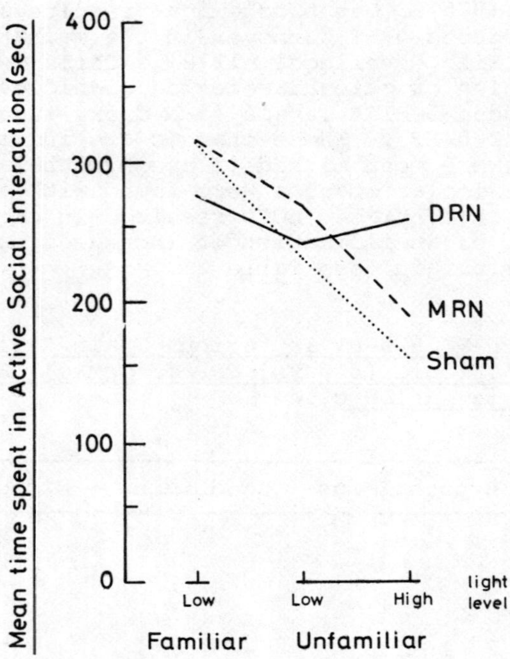

Fig. 5. The mean time spent in active interaction in the 4 test conditions, by rats with lesions of the median raphe nucleus (MRN), with lesions of the dorsal raphe nucleus (DRN) and by vehicle-injected controls (sham).

TABLE 3 Mean Time Spent in Active Social Interaction in the LF Test Condition after Injections of Saline or of $ACTH_{1-24}$ (5 μg/100 g).

Group	Saline	$ACTH_{1-24}$
Sham-operated control	314	189*
Median raphe lesion	315	208*
Dorsal raphe lesion	278	287

*Saline VS ACTH significantly different

We have suggested that ACTH exerts its anxiogenic effects by acting on 5-HT pathways in the midbrain and hypothalamus. The lesion experiment indicates that the pathways from the dorsal raphe nucleus are likely to be important. If critical sites for the action of ACTH are these particular 5-HT pathways, then ACTH should not produce any behavioural changes in rats with lesions of the dorsal raphe nucleus. Table 3 shows that this was, in fact, the case. Sham-operated controls and rats with lesions of the median raphe nucleus showed significantly less active interaction when injected with ACTH, compared with groups given saline injections. However, rats with dorsal raphe lesions showed no reduction after ACTH injections.

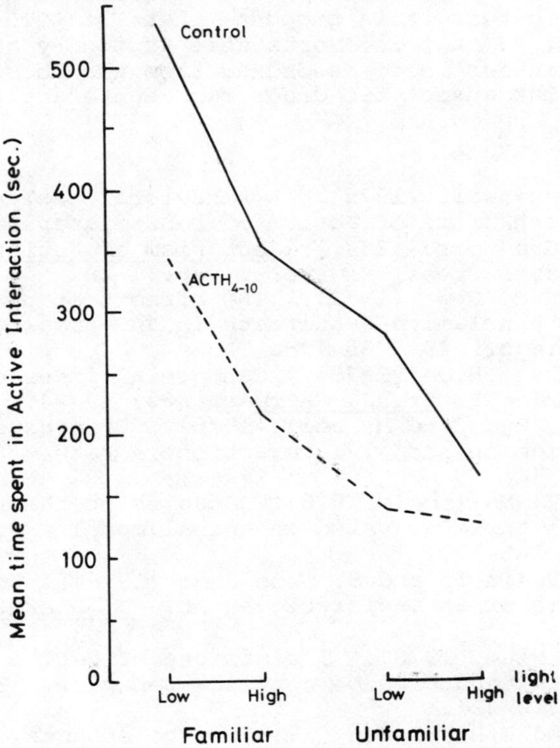

Fig. 6 The mean time spent in active interaction in the 4 test conditions by rats injected with $ACTH_{4-10}$ (4 μg/100 g) and by rats given control injections.

ACTH or Corticosterone?

There are several reasons for supposing that the behavioural changes seen with $ACTH_{1-24}$ are due to the action on CNS neurones of a fragment of ACTH itself, and are not due to the action of corticosteroids that are released by $ACTH_{1-24}$. The behavioural changes were greatest when the test (which lasts 10 mins) was started 3 mins after injection of ACTH, at which time the plasma glucocorticoid levels would not be significantly elevated. The effects of ACTH were no longer significant when a 30-min interval was allowed between injection and the start of testing, and by this time there would be considerable concentrations of glucocorticoids in the circulation. We have also shown that injected corticosterone, the principal corticosteroid in the rat, does not produce the same effects as injections of ACTH (File, Vellucci & Wendlandt, in press). And, finally, $ACTH_{4-10}$, which has no steroid-releasing properties, produces the same changes in social behaviour as $ACTH_{1-24}$ (See Fig. 6).

Summary

On the basis of the results from animal experiments using the social interaction anxiety test it is proposed that: 1) ACTH has an anxiogenic action; 2) that it exerts this action by acting on 5-HT pathways, in particular those ascending from the dorsal raphe nucleus; and 3) that anxiolytic drugs can counteract this action.

REFERENCES

Cook, L. and J. Sepinwall (1975). A behavioral analysis of the effects and mechanisms of action of benzodiazepines. In E. Costa and P. Greengard (Eds.), Mechanism of Action of Benzodiazepines, Raven Press, New York. pp. 1-28.

File, S.E. and J.R.G. Hyde (1977). The effects of p-chlorophenylalanine and ethanolamine-O-sulphate in an animal test of anxiety. J. Pharm. Pharmac., 29, 735-738.

File, S.E. and J.R.G. Hyde (1978). Can social interaction be used to measure anxiety? Br. J. Pharmac., 62, 19-24.

File, S.E., J.R.G. Hyde and M. Pool (1976). Effects of ethanol and chlordiazepoxide on social interaction in rats. Br. J. Pharmac., 58, 465P.

File, S.E. and S.V. Vellucci (1978). Studies on the role of ACTH and of 5-HT in anxiety, using an animal model. J. Pharm. Pharmac., 30, 105-110.

File, S.E., S.V. Vellucci and S. Wendlandt (1978). Corticosterone - an anxiogenic or an anxiolytic agent? J. Pharm. Pharmac., in press.

Geller, I. and K. Blum (1970). The effects of 5-HT on parachlorophenylalanine attenuation of conflict behavior. Eur. J. Pharmac., 9, 319-324.

Robichaud, R.C. and K.L. Sledge (1969). The effects of p-chlorophenylalanine on experimentally induced conflict in the rat. Life Sci., 8, 965-969.

Stein, L., C.D. Wise and B.D. Berger (1973). Antianxiety action of benzodiazepines: Decrease in activity of serotonin neurons in the punishment system. In S. Garattini (Ed.), The Benzodiazepines, Raven Press, New York. pp. 299-326.

Effects of Benzodiazepines on the Electrical Activity of the Central Nervous System: Correlation with Synaptic Pharmacology

W. HAEFELY, P. POLC, L. PIERI and R. SCHAFFNER

Pharma Research Department, F. Hoffmann-La Roche & Co. Ltd., Basle, Switzerland

ABSTRACT

The study of spontaneous and evoked bioelectrical phenomena in the central nervous system (CNS) has, until very recently, been the most successful approach in elucidating the mode of action of benzodiazepines. A vast body of evidence indicates that the preferential, and possibly exclusive, primary effect of these drugs in therapeutically relevant doses is an enhancement of GABA ergic synaptic transmission at all levels of the CNS. This generalized modulating effect on one distinct type of chemical inhibitory synapse accounts very well for the numerous changes of bioelectrical phenomena which benzodiazepines have been found to produce in most of the central nervous regions studied. To illustrate this correlation, some effects of benzodiazepines on spontaneous and evoked electrical activity in the spinal cord, the brainstem reticular formation and the limbic system are discussed against the background of a modulation of GABA ergic transmission.

KEYWORDS

benzodiazepines - GABA ergic transmission - presynaptic inhibition - postsynaptic inhibition - spinal cord - brainstem reticular formation - limbic system - cuneate nucleus - cerebellar cortex - substantia nigra

INTRODUCTION

The effect of psychotropic drugs on the CNS can be assessed by studying behavioural responses and by measuring bioelectrical phenomena and biochemical parameters. Although behavioural effects of drugs in animals are still the most direct indications for a potential therapeutic application in man, even the most sophisticated behavioural studies can by themselves hardly increase our understanding of the mechanisms of action in terms of cellular and molecular events. The bioelectrical and the biochemical approaches, which theoretically should be most efficient when used in combination, have, in fact, contributed to a very differing degree to our understanding of psychotropic drug action. For instance, biochemical psychopharmacology has contributed most to our present knowledge of the part played by the biogenic amines in the action of antipsychotics and antidepressants, while the effects of these drugs on the electrical activity of the CNS, in particular on single synapses is very incompletely known for various reasons. In contrast, biochemical neuropsychopharmacology has, until very recently, contributed little to our understanding of the mode of action of minor tranquillizers, except perhaps to show that the monoaminergic and cholinergic systems are unlikely to be their primary site of action. Two lines of research initiated very recently, namely the characterization of benzodiazepine receptors (Braestrup and Squires, 1978; Möhler and Okada, 1978) and the interactions of benzodiazepines with regulatory proteins determining the affinity of GABA for its receptor (Costa, Guidotti and Toffano, 1978), open a new era of biochemical studies of this type of compounds.

The use of electrophysiological methods was more successful in the analysis of the effects of antianxiety agents and, in particular of benzodiazepines, than the earlier biochemical studies, for reasons which we shall try to make clear. At the last C.I.N.P. meeting we presented data from our laboratory which strongly suggested that benzodiazepines interact very specifically with one type of chemical synapse, namely the GABA ergic synapse (Haefely and co-workers, 1978). In the past two years several investigators have added impressive evidence to support our view, with the result that the facilitatory effect of benzodiazepines on GABA ergic transmission is now being increasingly accepted. In the first part of this presentation a brief survey will be given on what is presently known of the interaction of benzodiazepines with GABA ergic transmission, and in the second part, we shall discuss against the background of this synaptic pharmacology a few of the effects on the electrical activity of the CNS which have been considered to be characteristic for benzodiazepines.

GABA ERGIC TRANSMISSION

We may start with a few words about GABA as a neurotransmitter - as opposed to monoamines. Whereas monoaminergic neurones make up an extremely small proportion of central neurones - which by the way does not tell us very much about their functional importance - neurones, which use GABA as neurotransmitter, probably overweight any other neurotransmitter system in the CNS, and it has been calculated that more than 1/3 of all synapses in the brain are GABA ergic. The effect of GABA at synapses is well known - again in contrast to that of monoamines: its role in synaptic transmission is exclusively inhibitory. This inhibition is brought about in two ways. GABA that is released at synapses on cell bodies or dendrites of a target cell (Fig. 1 e) increases selectively the conductance of the subsynaptic membrane for chloride. Usually, but not always, this conductance increase results in hyperpolarization (inhibitory postsynaptic potential, IPSP), but always counteracts the effect of excitatory transmitters which tend to decrease the membrane potential below the critical value from which a propagated action potential arises (excitatory postsynaptic potential, EPSP). This type of inhibition is called <u>post</u>synaptic inhibition. Another type of inhibition produced by GABA occurs at axo-axonal synapses; these are synapses formed between GABA ergic nerve terminals and axon terminals of primary afferent neurones in spinal and cranial nerves, which release their excitatory transmitter on motoneurones (Fig. 1 a), second order sensory neurones or interneurones. At these axo-axonal synapses GABA also increases chloride conductance; however, due to a particular distribution of chloride ions between the extracellular space and the interior of primary afferent endings, this conductance increase for chloride does not result in hyperpolarization, but in a partial depolarization (primary afferent depolarization). An action potential that arrives at the nerve terminal partially depolarized by GABA will have a smaller amplitude than in the absence of GABA. Since the amplitude of the action potential at the ending appears to determine the amount of transmitter which is liberated, primary afferent depolarization reduces the amount of excitatory transmitter released. This type of inhibition is called presynaptic inhibition. Most

GABA ergic neurones are interneurones, i.e. they have short axons, which do not leave the structure in which their cell body is located, and they exert their inhibitory effect in close vicinity of their cell body. Besides the interneurones, which are part of the presynaptic inhibitory pathways, GABA ergic interneurones

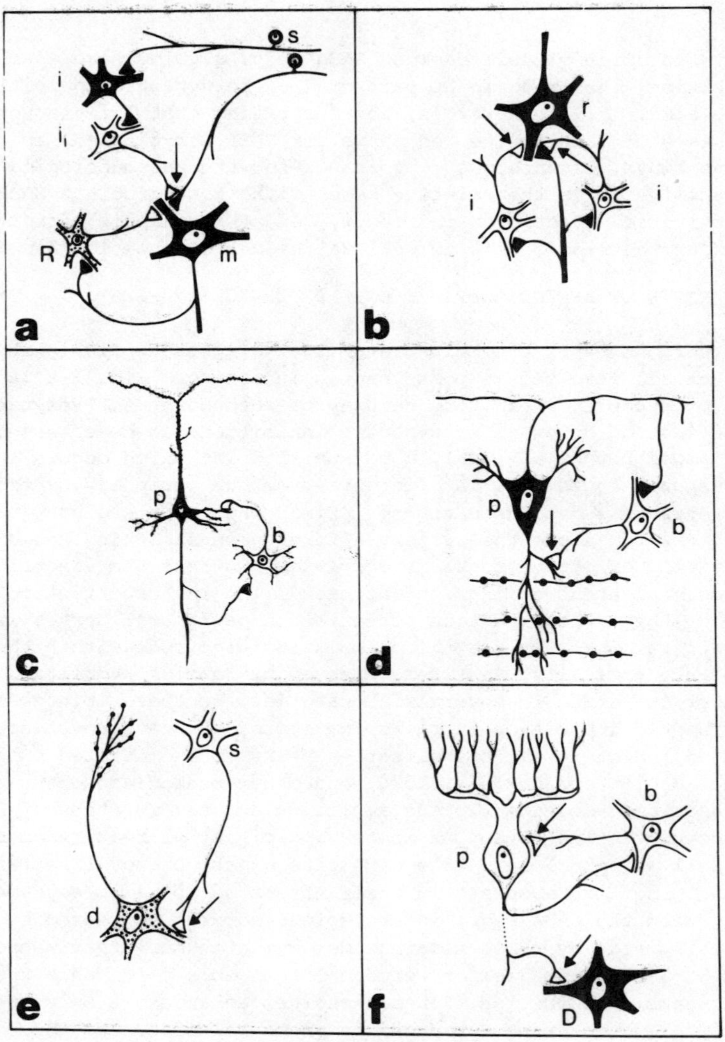

Fig. 1. Schematic synaptic arrangements of GABA ergic neurones (white) with excitatory (black) or other inhibitory neurones (stippled). a) Spinal cord (m motoneurone, s spinal ganglion cell, i excitatory interneurone, i_1 inhibitory GABA ergic interneurone, R Renshaw cell) b) cuneate nucleus (r cuneothalamic relay cell, i GABA ergic inhibitory interneurones) c) cerebral cortex (p pyramidal cell, b basket cell) d) hippocampus (p pyramidal cell, b basket cell) e) substantia nigra (d dopaminergic neurone, s GABA ergic striato-nigral neurone) f) cerebellar cortex and Deiters' nucleus (p Purkinje cell, b basket cell, D Deiters' neurone).

occur in pathways of recurrent (Fig. 1 c, d) and collateral (Fig. 1 b) inhibition. Probably all principal output neurones of the various central structures are protected from excessive and long-lasting overactivity by recurrent and collateral inhibition. In addition to interneurones, GABA ergic neurones also exist as projection neurones which produce postsynaptic inhibition at some distance from their site of origin (Fig. 1 e, f).

Although other neurotransmitters besides GABA (e.g. glycine) are also involved in synaptic inhibition, the predominant part of GABA in synaptic inhibition can hardly be overestimated. It is, therefore, not surprising that life is not possible when the synthesis of GABA or the receptors for GABA are blocked, in contrast again with monoamines. Of uppermost importance for the pharmacological study of GABA ergic transmission is the relative ease, with which distinct GABA ergic pathways can be activated directly or indirectly, and the synaptic effect on target cells measured at the single cell as well as the cell population level.

EFFECTS OF BENZODIAZEPINES ON GABA ERGIC SYNAPSES

In the spinal cord, GABA is the main transmitter of presynaptic inhibition, but is little or not at all involved in postsynaptic inhibition. Fig. 1 a is a simplified scheme of the presynaptic inhibitory pathway to motoneurones. Presynaptic inhibition and the effect of drugs on presynaptic inhibition can be assessed by recording the dorsal root potential (DRP), a potential shift which occurs in dorsal rootlets in response to stimuli in afferents from the periphery or from the medulla and which represents depolarization of primary afferent endings conducted electrotonically backwards along the primary afferent axons. During the DRP, the monosynaptic excitation of motoneurones is depressed, whereas the electrical excitability of primary afferent endings is increased. The latter effect is measured by the amplitude of the compound action potential in peripheral nerves initiated in primary afferent terminals by a small stimulating electrode within the gray matter and conducted antidromically. As first observed by Schmidt, Vogel and Zimmermann (1967) and later confirmed in several laboratories, benzodiazepines enhance all signs of presynaptic inhibition in the spinal cord, but have no effect on postsynaptic inhibition, which in the spinal cord appears to be mediated by glycine. Diazepam (Polc, Möhler and Haefely, 1974) and other benzodiazepines (unpublished results) increase dose-dependently the amplitude and the duration of DRP's and accentuate presynaptic inhibition of monosynaptic ventral root responses in decerebrate as well as spinal cats. The GABA antagonist, bicuculline, and benzodiazepines are reciprocal antagonists in their effect on spinal presynaptic inhibition. However, when the GABA level in the spinal cord is decreased by an inhibitor of GABA synthesis, e.g. by thiosemicarbazide, which in our experiments depleted GABA by about 60 %, benzodiazepines were no longer able to enhance the virtually abolished presynaptic inhibition. Benzodiazepines enhance not only presynaptic inhibition of spinal motoneurones produced by segmental afferents, but also that produced by stimulation of medullary centers.

In the cuneate nucleus, as indicated in Fig. 1 b, primary afferents running in the dorsal columns synapse with cuneothalamic relay cells and, in addition, with GABA ergic interneurones which, in contrast to the spinal cord, mediate both presynaptic inhibition and collateral postsynaptic inhibition. Our study of this structure was particularly important, because it showed that benzodiazepines enhance to almost the same degree presynaptic and postsynaptic inhibition, where the latter is mediated by GABA (Polc and Haefely, 1976).

In the cerebral cortex, Raabe and Gumnit (1977) observed that benzodiazepines enhanced postsynaptic GABA ergic inhibition of pyramidal tract cells. This inhibition is initiated by the excitation of GABA ergic interneurones via recurrent collaterals of pyramidal cells (Fig. 1 c). To show this, axons in the pyramidal tract were stimulated antidromically and the recovery time for antidromic invasion of pyramidal cells measured after a preceding volley. In the sensorimotor cortex of the rabbit, Kozhechkin and Ostrovskaya (1977) and Zakusov and co-workers (1977) showed that diazepam did not antagonize the inhibitory effect of a high amount of GABA iontophorized on pyramidal cells and clearly enhanced the effect of low doses of GABA.

In the hippocampus, a similar arrangement of GABA interneurones mediates recurrent inhibition of hippocampal pyramidal cells (Fig. 1 d). Wolf and Haas (1977) observed with two diazepines a potentiation of recurrent inhibition produced by stimulation of pyramidal cells, and Tsuchiya and Fukushima (1978) obtained similar results with fludiazepam.

Recurrent inhibition also occurs in the hypothalamus. In cultured hypothalami of the rat, Geller, Taylor and Hoffer (1978) observed a marked potentiation of recurrent inhibition by diazepam.

In the cerebellar cortex, the only output neurone, the Purkinje cell, is GABA ergic, and so are 3 out of the 4 types of interneurones (Fig. 1 f). The basket/stellate cell-mediated postsynaptic inhibition of Purkinje cells was enhanced by diazepam (Curtis and co-workers, 1976 ; Geller, Taylor and Hoffer, 1978). Diazepam also enhanced the inhibitory effect of GABA applied iontophoretically on Purkinje cells. These findings provide the direct proof for our suggestion that benzodiazepines enhance basket cell inhibition of Purkinje cells, based on a consistent depressant effect of various benzodiazepines on the spontaneous firing rate of cerebellar Purkinje cells (Pieri and Haefely, 1977).

Benzodiazepines enhance not only presynaptic and postsynaptic inhibition produced by GABA ergic interneurones, but also postsynaptic inhibition mediated by GABA ergic projection neurones. A GABA ergic pathway originates in the caudate nucleus and ends at dopamine cell bodies in the substantia nigra (Fig. 1 e). We found that single stimuli in the caudate nucleus evoked a potential in the substantia nigra, which was dose-dependently reduced by the GABA antagonists, bicuculline and picrotoxin, but not by the glycine antagonist, strychnine. Benzodiazepines had no consistent effect on this evoked potential, but were very potent in preventing or reversing the depressant effect of picrotoxin (Haefely and co-workers, 1978). In confirmation of these electrophysiological findings, studies of the dopamine turnover clearly indicated a facilitatory effect of benzodiazepines on GABA ergic inhibition of dopamine cells (Keller, Schaffner and Haefely, 1976).

The cerebellar Purkinje cell is another example of a GABA ergic projection neurone. One of the target structures of Purkinje cells is the lateral vestibular nucleus of Deiters' (Fig. 1 f). Stimulation of Purkinje cell axons in the cerebellar white matter produces a complex evoked potential in Deiters' nucleus. One component of this evoked potential is selectively abolished by picrotoxin and bicuculline. Benzodiazepines reverse this depressant effect of picrotoxin (Haefely and co-workers, 1978).

Two other structures in the brain, where GABA ergic terminals are present, although the detailed neuronal connections are not yet known, are the locus coeruleus, an important site of origin of noradrenergic neurones, and the raphe nuclei, where serotoninergic cell bodies are located. Circumstantial evidence obtained in studies of ponto-geniculo-occipital (PGO) waves suggested to us that benzodiazepines may enhance a GABA ergic input to noradrenergic locus coeruleus cells (Haefely, Jalfre and Ruch-Monachon, 1975). In the dorsal raphe nucleus, Gallagher (1978) recently found that benzodiazepines enhance the inhibitory effect of iontophoretically applied GABA. Benzodiazepines had a negligible effect on the spontaneous discharge rate of raphe neurones, however, they depressed the firing of these cells when an inhibitor of GABA metabolism, aminooxyacetic acid (AOAA) was given beforehand, suggesting that the tonic GABA ergic input was probably too small in this experimental situation to be enhanced by benzodiazepines, but high enough after AOAA to permit these drugs to produce their effect.

The findings presented so far conclusively show that benzodiazepines are very potent in facilitating ongoing GABA ergic activity at presynaptic and postsynaptic inhibitory synapses in various structures of the CNS. Dr. Braestrup (this Symposium) reviewed the findings which clearly show that the receptive sites, through which benzodiazepines produce their effects, are highly selective for this class of drugs. An important open question remains to be answered, namely whether the benzodiazepines act presynaptically at GABA ergic nerve terminals, e.g. by improving excitation-secretion coupling, or postsynaptically in the vicinity of GABA receptors and chloride channels. At a recent meeting, Costa, Guidotti and Toffano (1978) reported the very exciting data suggesting that benzodiazepines increase the affinity of GABA for its receptor sites, probably by interfering with an endogenous regulatory protein which normally reduces the affinity of GABA for its receptor.

CORRELATION BETWEEN SYNAPTIC PHARMACOLOGY AND THE EFFECTS ON THE ELECTRICAL ACTIVITY OF CERTAIN BRAIN STRUCTURES

In the second part of this presentation we shall examine whether the recently acquired knowledge of the synaptic pharmacology of benzodiazepines could explain changes of the electrical activity of the CNS which have been found to be characteristic for benzodiazepines. Only 3 structures will be considered, namely the spinal cord, the reticular formation of the brainstem, and the limbic system.

Spinal Cord

The potent muscle relaxant action of benzodiazepines point to the spinal cord as a possible site of their action. While there is no doubt that benzodiazepines can affect spinal cord activities by a primary action on supraspinal mechanisms, it is easy to demonstrate direct effects of benzodiazepines at the level of the spinal cord, e.g. in spinal cats. Using such preparations, we have found - as many other investigators - that benzodiazepines reduce in a dose-dependent manner the amplitude of both monosynaptic and polysynaptic segmental reflexes and depress the spontaneous and evoked γ-motoneurone activity (see Schallek, Schlosser and Randall, 1972; Schallek, Horst and Schlosser, 1978). Depression of spinal reflexes is observed with a great number of centrally active compounds. The term "interneurone blocking agents" was coined for these drugs, in particular for propanedioles and benzodiazepines, because it was thought that they preferentially depress excitatory interneurones. It seems that the concept of "interneurone block" has to be revised, since Curtis, Game and Lodge (1976) in a direct study did not observe a depression of dorsal horn interneurones by benzodiazepines. We asked ourselves whether the enhancement of GABA ergic presynaptic inhibition at primary afferent endings might fully account for the depression of monosynaptic and polysynaptic reflexes as well as of γ-motoneurone activity (Polc, Möhler and Haefely, 1974). In favour of this view is our finding that depression of reflexes and enhancement of presynaptic inhibition become visible and reach their maximum at identical doses. In addition, thiosemicarbazide, which inhibits the synthesis of GABA, almost completely blocks presynaptic inhibition and increases the amplitude of the monosynaptic reflex. After such a depletion of GABA, diazepam was no longer able to enhance presynaptic inhibition nor to depress the monosynaptic reflex. However, results with the GABA antagonist, bicuculline, and the inhibitor of GABA catabolism, aminooxyacetic acid, gave less convincing results. Therefore, it cannot be definitively stated that all effects of benzodiazepines on the spinal cord are accounted for by facilitation of presynaptic inhibition. We believe that the spinal cord is an excellent structure on which to study the question whether facilitation of GABA ergic transmission is the only mechanism of action of benzodiazepines or just one of the several ways by which these drugs affect neuronal activity in a given structure.

Brainstem Reticular Formation

Some investigators have focused their attention on the role of the brainstem reticular formation in the effects of benzodiazepines. The changes produced by these drugs in the spontaneous and evoked activity of the reticular neurones are difficult to interpret. For instance, Hernandez-Peón and co-workers (1964) observed a moderate depression of auditory evoked potentials in the mesencephalic reticular formation of freely moving cats, and Olds and Baldrighi (1968) found a mild depression of visual evoked potentials in this structure. The latter authors suggested that benzodiazepines had a stimulant effect on the activating reticular formation, because it is known that sensory input is depressed by stimulation of the activating system. However, in a later study in unrestrained rats, Olds and Olds (1969) found that diazepam depressed the spontaneous firing rate of mesencephalic reticular neurones. Similar findings were obtained by Przybyla and Wang (1968) and Guerrero-Figueroa and co-workers (1973). Multiunit activity in the mesencephalic reticular formation was reduced by benzodiazepines in all phases of the sleep-wakefulness cycle in studies of Tsuchiya and Fukushima (1977). Surprisingly, these investigators obtained increased wakefulness and a decrease of slow wave sleep by local injection of benzodiazepines into the mesencephalic reticular formation. Unfortunately, the identification of GABA ergic synapses in the reticular formation is only at its beginning and it remains to be shown, how exactly benzodiazepines affect the various parts of the brainstem reticular formation. At present, it seems safe to state that benzodiazepines do not depress the reticular formation in a general nonspecific manner, but rather affect its various functions quite selectively. The specific effect on GABA ergic synapses could well explain this discriminative action. On the whole, benzodiazepines appear to affect the neuronal activity of the brainstem less markedly than that of other central nervous structures. It does not seem unreasonable to relate this to the fact that the brainstem contains relatively low quantities of GABA and the smallest density of benzodiazepine binding sites of the cerebral gray matter (Möhler and Okada, 1978).

Limbic System

The limbic system has been postulated long ago to play a primordial part in the behavioural and anticonvulsant actions of benzodiazepines. One electrophysiological approach has been the study of evoked potentials in the hippocampus elicited by stimulation of other limbic areas or extralimbic structures. A most intensively studied connection is that between the basolateral nucleus of the amygdaloid complex and the ventral hippocampus. In an earlier study we found that benzodiazepines are most potent in depressing the amplitude of the amygdalo-hippocampal evoked potential and in increasing its latency (Jalfre, Monachon and Haefely,

1971). Tsuchiya (1977) obtained similar findings on the amygdalo-hippocampal potential and, in addition, a depressant effect on the hippocampal response to stimulation of the central gray matter.

Other techniques used in the study of limbic activity are the so-called after-discharges; repetitive stimulation of a structure above a certain intensity induces paroxysmal activity in the stimulated structure as well as in distant areas, which outlasts the period of stimulation. Benzodiazepines were found to be most potent in raising the threshold for the induction of after-discharges and in shortening the duration and reducing the amplitude of after-discharges (Schallek, Zabransky and Kuehn, 1964). The structures found to be most sensitive to the action of benzodiazepines are those in the limbic system and parts of the thalamus.

The spontaneous activity of single neurones in the hippocampus was found to be consistently depressed by benzodiazepines in studies of Olds and Olds (1969) in freely moving rats. In immobilized cats, Chou and Wang (1977) observed a strong depression of the spontaneous firing rate of neurones in the amygdala and the hippocampus by benzodiazepines. About half of the neurones tested were responsive to the drugs, but could not be characterized in relation to the non-responsive units. Most interestingly, morphine, which produces fear and rage reactions in the cat very similar to those obtained by electrical stimulation of either the amygdala or the hippocampus, increased the firing rate of amygdala and hippocampal neurones. The activating effect of morphine was potently antagonized by benzodiazepines.

Considering the prominent facilitatory effect of benzodiazepines on recurrent GABA ergic inhibition in the hippocampus, it appears reasonable to assume that a more effective recurrent inhibition of principal output cells in the hippocampus, and perhaps also in the amygdala and the septum, are the basis of the drug effects on the multiple electrical phenomena in limbic structures.

CONCLUSION

In conclusion, benzodiazepines have been shown, on the one hand, to affect the electrical activity of virtually all central sturctures. On the other hand, they have a specific effect on one type of chemical synapse. It might well be that those sites, in which the effect of these drugs are most prominent, were those in which the inhibitory influence of GABA ergic neurones is most critically required for an appropriate balance between excitatory and inhibitory synaptic mechanisms. These areas of the CNS, whose activity is very easily increased by all kinds of stimuli, are also the ones that are intimately connected with behavioural and vegetative functions in emotional reactions as well as with epileptoid phenomena. It is, therefore, not surprising that drugs, which enhance synaptic inhibitory mechanisms throughout the CNS, produce their therapeutic effects primarily by reducing such a pathologic hyperactivity in some highly vulnerable areas.

REFERENCES

Braestrup, C., and R.F. Squires (1978). Brain specific benzodiazepine receptors. Brit. J. Psychiat., 133, 249-260.

Chou, D.T., and S.C. Wang (1977). Unit activity of amygdala and hippocampal neurons: effects of morphine and benzodiazepines. Brain Research, 126, 427-440.

Costa, E., A. Guidotti, and G. Toffano (1978). Molecular mechanisms mediating the action of diazepam on GABA receptors. Brit. J. Psychiat., 133, 239-248.

Curtis, D.R., C.J.A. Game, and D. Lodge (1976). Benzodiazepines and central glycine receptors. Br. J. Pharmacol., 56, 307-311.

Curtis, D.R., D. Lodge, G.A.R. Johnston, and S.J. Brand (1976). Central actions of benzodiazepines. Brain Research, 118, 344-347.

Geller, H.M., D.A. Taylor, and B.J. Hoffer (1978). Benzodiazepines and central inhibitory mechanisms. Naunyn-Schmiedeberg's Arch. Pharmacol. In Press.

Guerrero-Figueroa, R., D.M. Gallant, C. Guerrero-Figueroa, and J. Gallant (1973). Electrophysiological analysis of the action of four benzodiazepine derivatives on the central nervous system. In S. Garattini, E. Mussini and L.O. Randall (Eds.), The benzodiazepines. Raven Press, New York. pp. 489-511.

Haefely, W. (1978). Central actions of benzodiazepines: general introduction. Brit. J. Psychiat., 133, 231-238.

Haefely, W., M. Jalfre, and M.-A. Ruch-Monachon (1975). A pathway and neurotransmitters involved in the control of noradrenergic locus coeruleus neurons. In O. Almgren, A. Carlsson and J. Engel (Eds.), Chemical Tools in Catecholamine Research. North-Holland, Amsterdam. pp. 135-142.

Haefely, W., P. Polc, R. Schaffner, H.H. Keller, L. Pieri, and H. Möhler (1979). Facilitation of GABAergic transmission by drugs. In H. Kofod and P. Krogsgaard-Larsen (Eds.), GABA-Neurotransmitters. Munksgaard, Copenhagen. In press.

Haefely, W., H.H. Keller, L. Pieri, P. Polc, R. Schaffner, and R. Zihlmann (1978). Interaction of minor tranquillizers with synaptic processes mediated by GABA. In P. Deniker, C. Radouco-Thomas and A. Villeneuve (Eds.), Neuro-Psychopharmacology. Pergamon Press, Oxford. pp. 907-916.

Hernandez-Peón, R., J.A. Rojas-Ramirez, J.J. O'Flaherty, and A.L. Mazzuchelli-O'Flaherty (1964). An experimental study of the anticonvulsive and relaxant actions of valium. Int. J. Neuropharmacol., 3, 405-412.

Jalfre, M., M.-A. Monachon, and W. Haefely (1971). Effects on the amygdalo-hippocampal evoked potential in the cat of four benzodiazepines and some other psychotropic drugs. Naunyn-Schmiedeberg's Arch. Pharmacol., 270, 180-191.

Keller, H.H., R. Schaffner, and W. Haefely (1976). Interaction of benzodiazepines with neuroleptics at central dopamine neurons. Naunyn-Schmiedeberg's Arch. Pharmacol., 294, 1-7.

Kozhechkin, S.N., and R.U. Ostrovskaya (1977). Are benzodiazepines GABA antagonists? Nature, 269, 72-73.

Möhler, H., and T. Okada (1978). The benzodiazepine receptor in normal and pathological human brain. Brit. J. Psychiat., 133, 261-268.

Olds, M.E., and G. Baldrighi (1968). Effects of meprobamate, chlordiazepoxide, diazepam, and sodium pentobarbital on visually evoked responses in the tectotegmental area of the rat. Int. J. Neuropharmacol., 7, 231-239.

Olds, M.E., and J. Olds (1969). Effects of anxiety-relieving drugs on unit discharges in hippocampus, reticular midbrain, and pre-optic area in the freely moving rat. Int. J. Neuropharmacol., 8, 87-103.

Pieri, L., and W. Haefely (1976). The effects of diphenylhydantoin, diazepam and clonazepam on the activity of Purkinje cells in the rat cerebellum. Naunyn-Schmiedeberg's Arch. Pharmacol., 296, 1-4.

Polc, P., and W. Haefely (1976). Effects of two benzodiazepines, phenobarbitone, and baclofen on synaptic transmission in the cat cuneate nucleus. Naunyn-Schmiedeberg's Arch. Pharmacol., 294, 121-131.

Polc, P., H. Möhler, and W. Haefely (1974). The effects of diazepam on spinal cord activities: possible sites and mechanisms of action. Naunyn-Schmiedeberg's Arch. Pharmacol., 284, 319-337.

Przybyla, A.C., and S.C. Wang (1968). Locus of central depressant action of diazepam. J. Pharmacol. exp. Ther., 163, 439-447.

Raabe, W., and R.J. Gumnit (1977). Anticonvulsant action of diazepam: increase of cortical postsynaptic inhibition. Epilepsia, 18, 117-120.

Schallek, W., W.D. Horst, and W. Schlosser (1978). Mechanisms of action of benzodiazepines. Advances in Pharmacology and Chemotherapy, Academic Press, New York. In press.

Schallek, W., W. Schlosser, and L.O. Randall (1972). Recent developments in the pharmacology of the benzodiazepines. Advances in Pharmacology and Chemotherapy, Vol. 10, Academic Press, New York. pp. 119-183.

Schallek, W., F. Zabransky, and A. Kuehn (1964). Effects of benzodiazepines on central nervous system of cat. Arch. int. pharmacodyn., 149, 467-483.

Schmidt, R.F., M.E. Vogel, and M. Zimmermann (1967). Die Wirkung von Diazepam auf die präsynaptische Hemmung und andere Rückenmarksreflexe. Naunyn-Schmiedeberg's Arch. Pharmacol., 258, 69-82.

Tsuchiya, T. (1977). Effects of 1,4-benzodiazepines with a long side chain in position 1 on the evoked potentials recorded in the limbic system and hypothalamus. Neuropharmacology, 16, 259-266.

Tsuchiya, T., and H. Fukushima (1977). Effects of benzodiazepines on PGO firing and multiple unit activity in the midbrain reticular formation in cats. EEG clin. Neurophysiol., 43, 700-706.

Tsuchiya, T., and H. Fukushima (1978). Effects of benzodiazepines and pentobarbitone on the GABA-ergic recurrent inhibition of hippocampal neurons. Europ. J. Pharmacol., 48, 421-424.

Wolf, P., and H.L. Haas (1977). Effects of diazepines and barbiturates on hippocampal recurrent inhibition. Naunyn-Schmiedeberg's Arch. Pharmacol., 299, 211-218.

Zakusov, V.V., R.U. Ostrovskaya, S.N. Kozhechkin, V.V. Markovich, G.M. Molodavkin, and T.A. Voronina (1977). Further evidence for GABA-ergic mechanisms in the action of benzodiazepines. Arch. int. Pharmacodyn., 229, 313-326.

Diazepam Metabolism in Healthy Subjects and Patients with Heart Failure, Renal Failure and Hepatic Cirrhosis

L. HILLESTAD* and T. HANSEN**

*Medical Department, Telemark Sentralsykehus, Porsgrunn, Norway
**Biological Department, Dumex Ltd., Copenhagen, Denmark

ABSTRACT

Following intravenous, oral and intramuscular administration of diazepam, the serum concentrations of diazepam and its metabolite as well as the concomitant clinical effects were studied. Sedation was marked, and accompanied by amnesia and paralleled serumconcentrations, while the clinical effects were comparably stronger in patients with failure of kidneys and liver. In patients with myocardial infarction, diazepam reduced effectively the stress reaction.

Key words: Diazepam, N-desmethyldiazepam, healthy subjects, patients, serum concentrations, metabolism, clinical effects, acute myocardial infarction, renal failure, hepatic cirrhosis.

The series of investigations were commenced in 1973 with the purpose of studying the effect of diazepam in acute myocardial infarction. This required some data on normal subjects which were not available in current literature, although diazepam at that time had been extensively used clinically for years. Therefore, studies had to be performed to ascertain the normal response to diazepam.

Figure 1 shows the serum concentrations of diazepam and its major metabolite, N-desmethyldiazepam, after 20 mg diazepam administered intravenously, orally and intramuscularly to healthy volunteers. The highest peak concentration was achieved after intravenous administration, occurring after 15 minutes. The infusion was done slowly over 5-7 minutes to avoid phlebitis. Next in order was the curve after oral ingestion, showing a much lower peak which occurred after 30 minutes. Surprisingly, the lowest peak level was measured after intramuscular administration, and also occurred most tardy, viz. after 1 hour. Repeated experiments confirmed the results. The formation of metabolite was small.

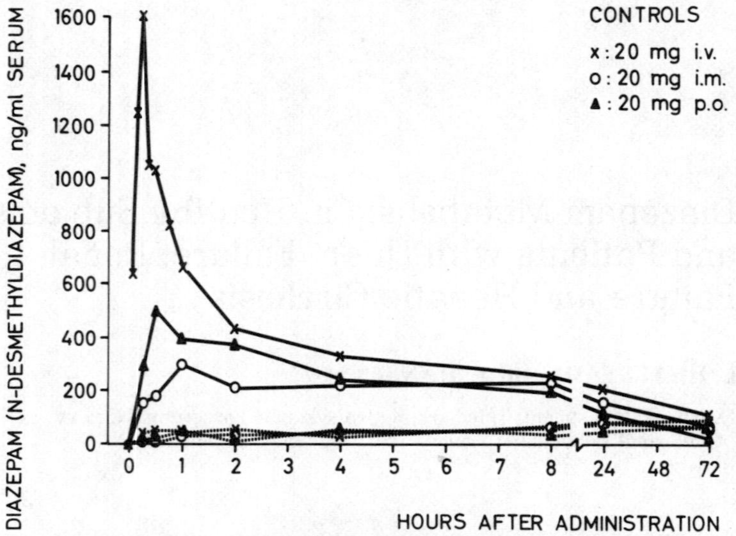

Fig. 1. Serum concentrations of diazepam and N-desmethyldiazepam following 20 mg diazepam administered intravenously, intramuscularly, and orally. Mean values in 6 healthy subjects.
——— Diazepam
------ N-desmethyldiazepam

The clinical effects were recorded by monitoring ECG, blood pressure, pulse rate, and respiration, and by means of rather crude tests which, however, were good enough to assess sleepiness and disclose mental deterioration, amnesia and dyscoordination. The results were scored according to an arbitrarily chosen system in order to quantitate the effects (Table 1).

TABLE 1 Clinical Effects of 20 mg Diazepam Administered Intravenously - Mean Values in 6 Healthy Subjects

Effects recorded	0 min	15 min	30 min	60 min	2 hrs	4 hrs	Total score
Sleepiness	0	2.5	1.1	0.5	0.2	0	4.3
Mental arithmetic	0	2.0	1.0	0.5	0.2	0	3.7
Blurred vision	0	1.0	1.0	1.0	0.5	0	3.5
Amnesia	0	3.0	2.0	1.0	0.5	0	6.5
Coordination	0	1.0	0.6	0.1	0.0	0	1.7
BP (mm Hg) - systolic	125	115	100	115	115	115	0.5
BP (mm Hg) - diastolic	80	75	75	75	75	75	0.5
Heart rate per min	69	78	80	70	74	73	0.5
Respiration rate per min	16	19	17	17	17	17	0.0
Diazepam in serum (ng/ml)	0	1607	1028	665	435	325	-

The investigations demonstrated that the clinical responses were consistent with the serum concentrations (Table 2), giving the highest scores after intravenous administration, lower after oral and lowest after intramuscular administration.

Table 2 Relationship between Mode of Administration and Clinical Effect - Mean Values in 6 Healthy Subjects

Diazepam Administration	Number of Subjects	Clinical effects (score)
20 mg i.v.	6	21.2
20 mg p.o.	6	8.0
20 mg i.m.	6	2.0
20 mg i.v.	2	21.0
10 mg i.v.	2	5.5

Another experiment showed that the lowering of the dose from 20 mg to 10 mg resulted in three times lower serum concentrations and nearly four times lower clinical scores (Figure 2 - Table 2).

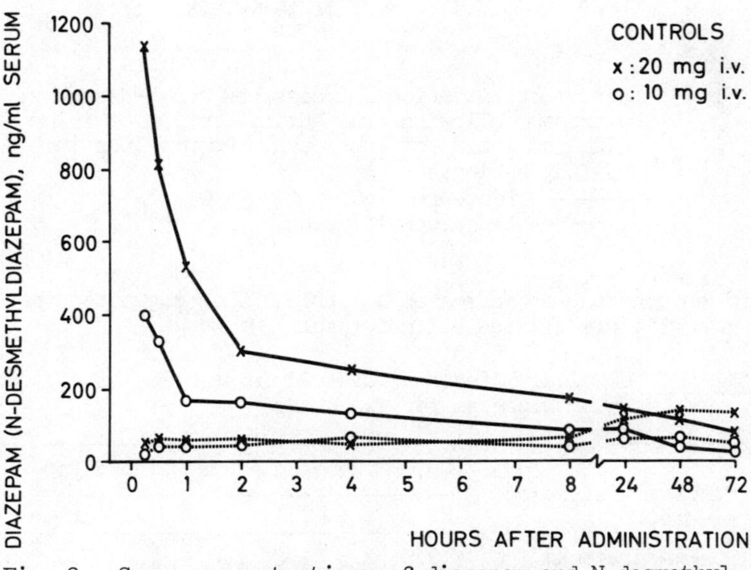

Fig. 2. Serum concentrations of diazepam and N-desmethyldiazepam following intravenous administration of 20 mg and 10 mg diazepam.
——— Diazepam
------ N-desmethyldiazepam

It must be added that throughout the trials the clinical effects were bound up with the initial high level of the serum concentration curves. Beyond four hours only some weak sedation could be demonstrated (Hillestad and co-workers, 1974).

Furthermore, cumulation after oral administration was examined and found to be marked. The diagramme in Figure 3 illustrates the findings after administration of 15 mg diazepam daily for two weeks. It shows that a balance between cumulation and elimination was reached during the second week. Formation of the major metabolite, N-desmethyldiazepam, increased rapidly and surpassed its parent substance about the fifth day. The clinical effects rose successively until the sixth day

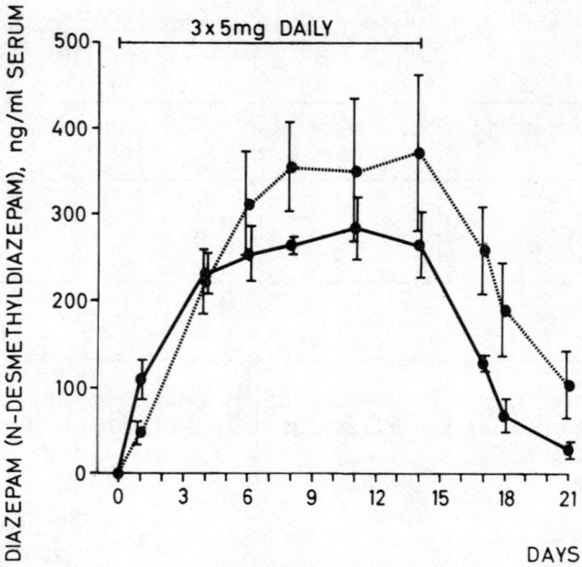

Fig. 3. Serum concentrations of diazepam and N-desmethyl-diazepam following oral administration of 15 mg diazepam daily for two weeks. Mean values in 3 healthy subjects.
——— Diazepam
-------- N-desmethyldiazepam

and then remained constant or decreased a little. This suggested that the metabolite exerted a negligible clinical effect (Table 3).

TABLE 3 Clinical Effects of Oral Administration of 15 mg Diazepam for Two Weeks

Oral Administration per day	Score on consecutive days						
	2	4	6	8	10	12	14
15 mg diazepam	0.5	0.5	1.0	1.0	1.0	0.5	0.5

The biological half-life of diazepam in healthy volunteers was calculated to be 54 hours, while the corresponding value (apparent biological half-life) for the major metabolite, N-desmethyldiazepam, was 92 hours (Figure 4) (Hillestad, Hansen and Melsom, 1974).

The initial studies on diazepam in healthy volunteers were followed by an investigation on patients with myocardial infarction. Thirty-eight male patients with proven acute myocardial infarction were used and randomly divided into a diazepam group and a control group. On admission, patients in the diazepam group immediately received 10 mg diazepam intravenously. One hour later they received an oral dose of 15 mg diazepam and this dose was repeated every 8 hours for the first three days.

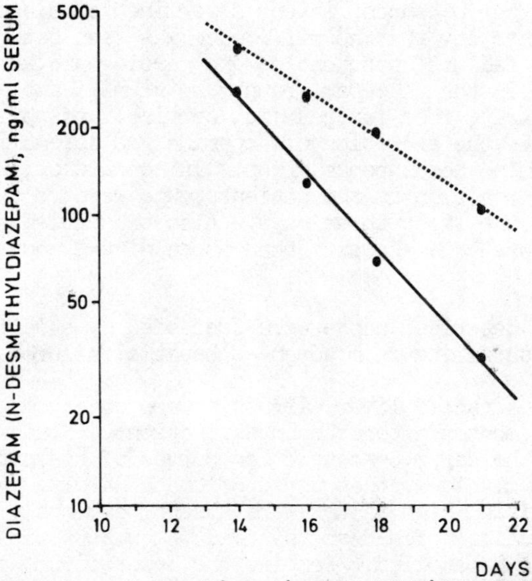

Fig. 4. Estimation of the biological half-life of diazepam and the apparent biological half-life of N-desmethyldiazepam with actual serum concentrations plotted in a semilogarithmic scale. Mean values in 3 healthy subjects.
——— Diazepam
----- N-desmethyldiazepam

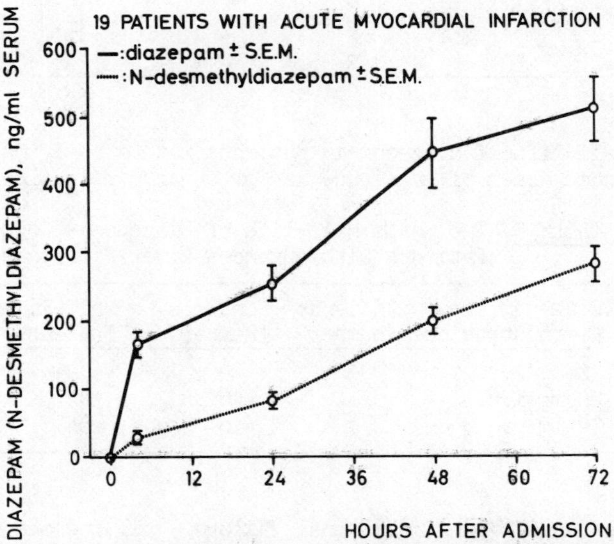

Fig. 5. Mean serum concentrations of diazepam and N-desmethyldiazepam in 19 patients with acute myocardial infarction treated with diazepam (a loading dose of 10 mg i.v. followed by a 15 mg oral dose three times daily for three days).

Figure 5 shows the serum concentrations determined of diazepam and N-desmethyldiazepam. Suffice it to say that no difference was seen between the groups in the incidence of heart failure, hypotension and cardiogenic shock. Malignant arrhythmias did not occur in the diazepam group. No significant effects upon aspartate aminotransferase (AST), free fatty acids, cortisol and noradrenaline excretion were observed, while the excretion of dopamine and adrenaline was found to be significantly lowered in the diazepam group. In conclusion, diazepam effectively reduced the stress reaction in the patients, who were relaxed and comfortable, having amnesia for the first three days. Also the patients in the diazepam group required less amounts of analgetics than those of the control group. (Melsom and co-workers, 1976).

The investigations described above were succeeded by studies on the effect of diazepam in patients suffering from advanced hepatic failure and renal failure.

Five patients with advanced liver cirrhosis were observed, three of whom died of their disease some months after the investigations. Following intravenous injection of diazepam, the serum concentration curves of the patients with hepatic failure were uniformly lower than those of the controls. After oral administration of diazepam the initial high values were absent, obviously owing to impaired absorption. The formation of N-desmethyldiazepam was retarded and subnormal, indicating altered drug metabolism. Despite the lower serum concentrations determined, the clinical responses observed (Table 4) were abnormally strong as compared with the control group.

TABLE 4 Clinical Effects of Diazepam - Comparison between Patients with Advanced Liver Cirrhosis and Controls

Diazepam Administration	Patients (number)	Controls (number)	Clinical effects (scores) Patients	Controls
10 mg i.v.	3	2	20.1	6.5
20 mg i.v.	1	6	45.0	21.2
20 mg p.o.	1	6	35.0	8.0

The serum half-life of diazepam in patients with grossly depressed liver function was in the same order of magnitude as for the controls (Table 5).

TABLE 5 The Serum Half-life of Diazepam - Comparison between Patients with Advanced Liver Cirrhosis and Controls

Diazepam Administration	Patients (number)	Controls (number)	Half-life of diazepam (hours) Patients	Controls
10 mg i.v.	3	2	37	36
20 mg i.v.	1	6	42	48
20 mg p.o.	1	6	44	27

Twelve patients suffering from renal failure - all but one with uremia - were observed. Three of these patients later on succumbed to their disease, whereas four were given kidney transplants. Largely, the serum concentration curves after intravenous injection of diazepam were of normal shape, though somewhat lower than those of the controls. As for patients with hepatic failure, oral administration yielded concentration curves deprived of the initial high values. Poor absorption is the obvious cause which is to be expected in uremic patients with gastritis and gastric fluid retention. The formation of N-desmethyldiazepam was retarded and subnormal, indicating altered drug metabolism in uremia. Table 6 shows the exaggerated clinical responses observed in the patients with renal failure as compared with those of the controls. The abnormally strong clinical responses bore no relationship to the levels of serum albumins.

TABLE 6 Clinical Effects of Diazepam. Comparison between Scores of Patients with Renal Failure and Controls

Diazepam Administration	Patients		Controls	Clinical effects (scores)	
	Number	Creatinine in serum, mg%	Number	Patients	Controls
10 mg i.v.	3	2 - 5	2	4.3	6.5
10 mg i.v.	2	5 - 15	2	22.0	6.5
20 mg i.v.	2	5 - 15	6	43.5	21.2
20 mg p.o.	2	2 - 5	6	25.5	8.0
20 mg p.o.	3	5 - 15	6	12.6	8.0

The serum half-life of diazepam in the patients with advanced renal failure was in the same order of magnitude as for the controls (Table 7).

TABLE 7 Serum Half-life of Diazepam in Patients with Renal Failure and Controls

Diazepam Administration	Patients		Controls	Half-life (hours)	
	Number	Creatinine in serum, mg%	Number	Patients	Controls
10 mg i.v.	3	2 - 5	2	38	36
10 mg i.v.	2	5 - 15	2	22	36
20 mg i.v.	2	5 - 15	6	37	48
20 mg p.o.	2	2 - 5	6	22	27
20 mg p.o.	3	5 - 15	6	41	27

The abnormally strong clinical responses in the presence of subnormal serum concentrations of diazepam (Hillestad, Hansen and Flaaten, 1978a; 1978b) may have several explanations. One of them could be that these very ill patients are abnormally susceptible to effects of drugs. Another more plausible explanation may be that the serum protein binding of diazepam in hepatic failure and renal failure is decreased, thus leaving a larger fraction of free diazepam in the serum, which permits a faster and greater influx of free agent into the CNS-system. Thiessen and co-workers (1976) have shown that diazepam is principally bound to serum albumin, and that this binding is significantly reduced in alcoholics, leading to stronger effects of the drug.

There is probably a situation analoguous to that of diphenylhydantoin, which Letteri and co-workers (1971) have shown provides subnormal serum levels in uremic patients, although the effects are normal. Reidenberg and co-workers (1971) have demonstrated decreased protein binding of the drug in uremia, and Blum and Riegeman (1972) have shown the level of free diphenylhydantoin in plasma of uremic patients to be two to four times above normal. Kangas and co-workers (1976) have shown a deficient ability of serum proteins to bind diazepam in poor renal function.

Andreasen (1973) has demonstrated that the serum proteins show a decreased binding capacity for several drugs in acute renal failure and ascribes this to a qualitative defect of the serum proteins.

The findings of the above studies support strongly the existence of a deficient binding of diazepam in advanced hepatic and renal failure, leaving more free drug in the serum, thereby augmenting the clinical effects.

REFERENCES

Andreasen, F. (1973). Protein binding of drugs in plasma from patients with acute renal failure. Acta pharmacol. toxicol., 32, 417-429.

Blum, M.B. and S. Riegeman (1972). Altered protein binding of diphenylhydantoin in uremic plasma. New Engl. J. Med., 286, 109.

Hillestad, L., T. Hansen, H. Melsom, and A. Drivenes (1974). Diazepam metabolism in normal man. I. Serum concentrations and clinical effects after intravenous, intramuscular, and oral administration. Clin. Pharmacol. Ther., 16, 479-484.

Hillestad, L., T. Hansen, and H. Melsom (1974). Diazepam metabolism in normal man. II. Serum concentrations and clinical effect after oral administration and cumulation. Clin. Pharmacol. Ther., 16, 485-489.

Hillestad, L. T. Hansen, and B. Flaaten (1978). Diazepam metabolism in hepatic failure. Observations of serum concentrations and clinical effects. (In press).

Hillestad, L., T. Hansen, and B. Flaaten (1978). Diazepam metabolism in renal failure. Observations of serum concentrations and clinical effects. (In press).

Kangas, L., J. Kanto, J. Forsstrøm, and E. Iisalo (1976). The protein binding of diazepam and N-desmethyldiazepam in patients with poor renal function. Clin. Nephrology, 5, 114-118.

Letteri, J.M., H. Mellk, S. Louis, H. Kutt, P. Durante, and A. Glazko (1971). Diphenylhydantoin metabolism in uremia. New Engl. J. Med., 285, 648-652.

Melsom, M., P. Andreassen, H. Melsom, T. Hansen, H. Grendahl, and L.K. Hillestad (1976). Diazepam in acute myocardial infarction. Clinical effects and effects on catecholamines, free fatty acids, and cortisol. Br. Heart J., 38, 804-810.

Reidenberg, M.M., I. Odar-Cederlöf, C. von Bahr, O. Borgå, and F. Sjöqvist (1971). Protein binding of diphenylhydantoin and desmethylimipramine in plasma from patients with poor renal function. New Engl. J. Med., 285, 264.

Thiessen, J.J., E.M. Sellers, P. Denbeigh, and L. Dolman (1976). Plasma protein binding of diazepam and tolbutamide in chronic alcoholics. J. Clin. Pharmacol., 16, 345-351.

The Differentiation Between Neurotic Depression and Anxiety and Drug Treatment

K. RICKELS, R. DOWNING and M. STEIN

Department of Psychiatry, University of Pennsylvania, 203 Piersol Building, Hospital of the University of Pennsylvania, 3400 Spruce Street, Philadelphia, PA. 19104, U.S.A.

ABSTRACT

Nine hundred thirteen anxious patients treated with chlordiazepoxide or placebo and 928 depressed patients treated with amitriptyline or placebo, who had participated in one of a series of double-blind drug trials of 4-6 weeks duration conducted by this research group over several years, were compared in terms of demographic factors, illness history, presenting symptomatology and response to treatment in an effort to explore group differences in these factors. Discriminant function analyses of physician ratings of symptomatology assessed with the Physician Questionnaire (PQ) revealed that nearly all the diagnostic discrimination between anxious and depressed patients is contained in physician estimates of the severity of the two cardinal symptoms of anxiety and depression. Results from analyses of patient-rated symptom dimensions of the Hopkins Symptom Checklist (HSCL) were similar in that again the two largest discriminators are anxiety and depression. In evaluating change produced by drug and placebo over a 4 week treatment period, it was found that all groups (active drugs and placebo) improved significantly but that improvement produced by active drugs was significantly greater than that produced by placebo.

INTRODUCTION

Anxiety and depression occur frequently as concurrent symptoms in neurotic disorders. At a theoretical level, this has generated discussions concerned with the possibility that one of these two symptoms may be the cause of the other and the possibility that both may result from a common causative factor (Derogatis, Klerman, and Lipman, 1972; Mendels and Weinstein, 1972). At a practical level, the concurrence of the two symptoms has led the clinician to utilize "mixed anxiety depression" as a kind of working diagnosis, although such a diagnosis is not included in any formal diagnostic system.

The present authors had for some time employed such an "unofficial" diagnosis, at least as a convenient description of a symptom configuration frequently encountered among neurotic outpatients participating in double-blind drug trials. However, when data concerning presenting symptomatology were subjected to statistical analysis (Downing and Rickels, 1974), they found that either anxiety or depression was clearly the dominant symptom in at least 85% of the patients who had been assigned a "mixed" diagnosis. It was also noted that when treating physicians had to choose between anxiolytics and antidepressants for the treatment of patients suffering from mixed anxiety depression, they typically prescribed anxiolytics for patients in whom anxiety was the dominant symptom and antidepressants for patients in whom depression was dominant. It was also the case that patients for whom antidepressants were prescribed had received a greater number of previous psychotropic drugs and, on the average, had responded less well to such treatment. Prusoff and Klerman (1974) also noted that depressed patients reported more severe psychic distress than did anxious patients, not only in depression, but also in many other emotional and somatic symptoms including several psychic components of anxiety.

The present study attempts a more broadly based comparison of large groups of anxious and depressed patients. Two patient groups are compared in terms of demographic factors, attributes of illness history, features of presenting symptomatology and response to treatment. Available for these comparisons is a group of 913 anxious patients treated with either chlordiazepoxide or placebo and a group of 928 depressed patients treated with either amitriptyline or placebo. These patients had participated in one of a series of double-blind drug trials of 4 to 6 weeks duration carried out over the past several years by this research group. Data from these trials have been collated and assembled into a series of computer disc files to make them accessible for exploratory studies in which large samples are required.

METHOD

Measuring Instruments

Assessments of symptom severity were made by both physician and patient at onset and after 4 weeks of treatment. Physician ratings employed the Physician Questionnaire (PQ) (Rickels and Howard, 1970), a questionnaire on which 10 symptoms indicating neurotic symptomatology are rated on 7-point scales, ranging from "not present" [1] to "extremely severe" [7]. Patient ratings employed the 35-item version of the Hopkins Symptom Checklist (HSCL) (Derogatis and colleagues, 1974) which provides 5 factors with scores ranging from "not present" [1] to "severe" [4]. A listing of the PQ items and the HSCL factors will be found in Table 1. Demographic data and information about illness history were originally recorded on standard forms prepared for that purpose.

Statistical Analyses

The significance of group differences in demographic and illness history attributes, transformed to categorical form when necessary, was assessed by chi square. Both univariate and multivariate procedures were employed to assess the significance of group differences in presenting sypmtomatology as well as four week clinical improvement.

RESULTS

Demographic and Illness Characteristics

Seventy-seven percent of the depressed and 70% of the anxious group ($p < .01$) were female, and 48% of the depressed but only 38% of the anxious patients were over 40 years of age ($p < .01$). In addition, compared to the anxious group, the depressed group was slightly less well educated (58% vs. 63% had at least high school education, $p < .05$), contained a smaller proportion of patients who had never been married (15% and 20%, respectively, $p < .05$), and was slightly more chronically ill (67% vs. 63%, $p < .05$). Although these differences reach statistical significance, they are small in size and unlikely to have any major responsibility for observed differences in either presenting symptomatology or in symptom change between the two groups. Both groups did not differ in number of previous psychotropic drugs and response to previous psychiatric treatment. Seventy-five percent had received prior psychotropic drug treatment.

TABLE 1 Presenting Psychopathology

	Depressed Sample		Anxious Sample		Univariate p	Discriminant Function Weights[1]
	M	SD	M	SD		
	(N=911)		(N=855)			
Physician Questionnaire Items (Range 1-7)						
Anxiety	4.42	1.07	4.84	1.02	.001	-.96
Depression	4.90	1.15	3.36	1.29	.001	1.25
Irritability	3.97	1.37	3.82	1.46	.07	-.12
Hostility	2.98	1.49	2.62	1.53	.001	-.003
Phobia/Obsession	2.74	1.59	2.73	1.65	n.s.	.05
Hypochondriasis	2.85	1.74	3.01	1.68	.09	-.05
Somatization	3.10	1.64	3.23	1.59	n.s.	.07
Insomnia	3.59	1.74	3.32	1.80	.01	.05
Appetite Disturbance	2.65	1.56	2.43	1.57	.01	.05
Headaches	2.90	1.62	2.96	1.66	n.s.	-.09
	(N=497)		(N=832)			
Hopkins Symptom Checklist Factors (Range 1-4)						
Somatization	1.94	.55	1.93	.58	n.s.	-.33
Performance Difficulty	2.24	.72	2.02	.67	.001	.24
Interpersonal Sensitivity	2.49	.72	2.27	.73	.001	-.15
Depression	2.45	.56	2.13	.59	.001	1.29
Anxiety	2.30	1.07	2.23	1.02	.10	-.44

[1] All multivariate tests are highly significant, $p < .001$

Presenting Psychopathology

Assessment of group differences in the severity of individual symptoms or symptom dimensions (Table 1) reveals the following: In terms of physician ratings, depressed patients were rated significantly more severe in depression, hostility, irritability, insomnia and appetite disturbance, while anxious patients were rated significantly more anxious and hypochondrical. Both groups did not differ in severity of phobic-obsessive symptomatology, somatization, and headaches. In terms of HSCL patient self-assessment, depressed as compared to anxious patients obtained significantly higher scores in performance difficulty, interpersonal sensitivity and depression factors and even show a trend ($p < .10$) toward having higher scores on the anxiety factor.

Results from a discriminant function analysis (as reflected in the discriminant function weights given in Table 1) indicate that there are 2 major independent contributors to group discrimination when all PQ symptom ratings are considered jointly: the higher anxiety of the anxious group and the higher depression of the depressed group. In other words, virtually all of the diagnostic discrimination between anxious and depressed patients is contained in physician estimates of the severity of these two cardinal symptoms.

Discriminant function results for the patient-rated symptom dimensions of the HSCL are essentially similar to those for the PQ based physician ratings. The two largest discriminators are depression and anxiety with scores for depression weighted in the direction of depression group membership and those for anxiety weighted in the direction of anxiety group membership.

Four Week Clinical Improvement

Results given in Table 2 clearly indicate that over a 4 week treatment period, anxious and depressed patients treated with active agents or with placebo, improve to a highly significant degree as seen in the "4 week change scores" reported for active drugs and for placebo.

In addition, univariate tests comparing change on active drug with change on placebo (Table 2) indicate that at a very high level of significance active drugs produce more improvement than placebo. Amitriptyline is superior to placebo in decreasing severity of all PQ rated symptoms except phobia-obsession, hypochondriasis and somatization. A discriminant function analysis shows that the major non-redundant contributors to this drug effect are insomnia and depression. Chlordiazepoxide is superior to placebo in reducing the severity of all PQ symptoms except hostility and appetite disturbance. Discriminant function weights indicate that the major non-redundant contributors to this drug effect are anxiety, phobia-obsession, somatization and insomnia.

For the HSCL patient measure, the only significant amitriptyline-placebo difference is found for the depression factor, a finding also reflected in the discriminant function analysis by a large positive weight only for depression. Significant chlordiazepoxide-placebo differences are found in somatization and anxiety factors, a finding again reflected in the results of the discriminant function analysis. Thus, largest differences in clinical change produced by active drug over placebo occur in those dimensions of psychopathology considered cardinal for the depressed and the anxious samples.

CONCLUSIONS

Anxious and depressed primarily neurotic outpatients, who participated in controlled clinical trials, differed only slightly in demographic characteristics. For example, depressed patients include a slightly higher percentage of female than male patients and are slightly older than anxious patients. In terms of initial psychopathology, depressed patients are consistently sicker than anxious patients, a finding also observed by others (Derogatis, Klerman and Lipman, 1972; Prusoff and Klerman, 1974). At the same time, among anxious patients initial anxiety was more severe than initial depression, and among depressed patients initial depression was more severe than initial anxiety.

Evaluating change produced by drug and placebo over a 4 week treatment period, we found that all groups, active drugs as well as placebo groups, improved significantly, but that improvement produced by active drug was significantly and consistently greater than that produced by placebo.

TABLE 2 Four Week Clinical Improvement (Change Scores)

	DEPRESSED SAMPLE				ANXIOUS SAMPLE			
	AMT Mean Δ+	PBO Mean Δ+	AMT VS. PBO Uni-Variate p	AMT VS. PBO Function Weight	CDZ Mean Δ+	PBO Mean Δ+	CDZ. VS. PBO Uni-Variate p	CDZ. VS. PBO Function Weight
	(N=287)	(N=307)			(N=338)	(N=226)		
Physician Questionnaire Items (Range 1-7)								
Anxiety	1.53	.93	.001	-.03	2.01	1.72	.001	.37
Depression	2.19	1.48	.001	.35	1.04	0.76	.05	-.28
Irritability	1.39	.83	.001	.25	1.37	1.24	.02	-.02
Hostility	.92	.49	.001	.04	.64	.66	.17	-.20
Phobia/ Obsession	.92	.64	.06	-.15	.94	.61	.001	.37
Hypochondriasis	.91	.63	.14	-.18	1.08	.67	.005	-.10
Somatization	.94	.77	.17	-.21	1.27	.88	.001	.45
Insomnia	1.85	.83	.001	.68	1.63	.97	.001	.62
Appetite Disturbance	.91	.57	.003	.02	.49	.55	.656	-.36
Headaches	1.22	.72	.001	.21	1.16	.89	.009	.12
Multivariate Test, p <			.001				.001	
	(N=179)	(N=126)			(N=293)	(N=257)		
Hopkins Symptom Checklist Factors (Range 1-4)								
Somatization	.27	.27	.76	-.40	.42	.24	.001	1.17
Obsessive-Compulsive	.31	.38	.73	-.62	.30	.25	.65	-.66
Interpersonal Sensitivity	.50	.48	.32	.09	.44	.36	.38	-.16
Depression	.63	.48	.04	1.53	.43	.33	.27	-.30
Anxiety	.44	.42	.97	-.48	.56	.42	.01	.48
Multivariate Test, p <			.03				.001	

+ All change scores (pre-post difference scores) are significantly greater than zero (p <.001) for active drugs and for placebo.

Amitriptyline was found to produce significantly more improvement than placebo in 7 of 10 PQ dimensions but only one of 5 HSCL dimensions, the depression factor. Similarly, chlordiazepoxide produced significantly more improvement than placebo in 8 of 10 PQ dimensions and in the somatic and anxiety HSCL factors. Multivariate analysis indicated considerable redundance in drug produced symptom change in terms of PQ-assessed psychopathology but not in terms of HSCL self-assessments. Thus discriminant analysis revealed that those seven rated symptoms from the PQ for which drug was superior to placebo in effecting improvement could be reduced to two non-redundant components represented by drug-placebo differences in change in depression and insomnia. Similarly, the 8 PQ symptoms for which chlordiazepoxide produced significantly more improvement than placebo could be expressed in terms of drug-placebo differences in four non-redundant components: Anxiety, Phobia-Obsession, Somatization and Insomnia. In contrast, for the patient-rated HSCL, those components contributing most to drug-placebo differentiation in the univariate analyses also do so in the multivariate analyses. This finding of less redundancy in the HSCL than the PQ analyses may be explained by the fact that originally orthogonal factors were used in the HSCL but items were used in the PQ analyses.

REFERENCES

Derogatis, L.R., Klerman, G.L. and Lipman, R.S. (1972). Anxiety states and depressive neuroses. J. Nerv. Ment. Dis., 155, 392-402.

Derogatis, L.R., Lipman, R.S., Rickels, K., Uhlenhuth, E.H. and Covi, L. (1974). The Hopkins Symptom Checklist (HSCL): A self-report symptom inventory. Behav. Sci., 19, 1-15.

Downing, R.W. and Rickels, K. (1974). Mixed anxiety-depression: Fact or myth? Arch. Gen. Psychiatry, 30, 312-317.

Mendels, J. and Weinstein, N. (1972). The relationship between depression and anxiety. Arch. Gen. Psychiatry, 114, 1549-1554.

Prusoff, B. and Klerman, G.L. (1974). Differentiating depressed from anxious neurotic outpatients. Arch. Gen. Psychiatry, 30, 302-309.

Rickels, K. and Howard, K. (1970). The Physician Questionnaire: A useful tool in psychiatric drug research. Psychopharmacologia, 17, 338-344.

The Phenomenological, Pharmacological and Psychophysiological Characteristics of Neurotic Outpatients to whom no Diagnosis has been Applied

C. D. FRITH*, EVE C. JOHNSTONE*, D. OWENS* and K. McPHERSON**

*CRC Division of Psychiatry, Watford Road, Harrow, England
**Dept of Social & Community Medicine, 8 Keble Road, Oxford, England

ABSTRACT

240 neurotic outpatients with moderate to severe symptoms of anxiety and/or depression were randomly and blindly assigned to four treatment regimes: Amitriptyline, Diazepam, Amitriptyline and Diazepam, Placebo. The patients were rated on a number of scales of anxiety and depression at the beginning and the end of the four week treatment period. In addition psychophysiological measures were taken. In terms of initial symptoms there was no evidence for the separate existence of anxiety states and neurotic depressions. However predominantly depressed patients showed more rapid skin conductance habituation than predominantly anxious patients. There were no differential effects of the different treatment regimes on the different symptoms. Amitripytyline was marginally better than the other treatments for both symptoms of anxiety and depression. The group receiving Diazepam showed no more improvement in symptoms than the group receiving placebo.

INTRODUCTION

Neurotic illness is normally subdivided into various categories. The most commonly diagnosed conditions are anxiety states and neurotic depressions. Where the boundary between these conditions lies is by no means clear. Attempts have been made to show that populations diagnosed and treated as anxiety states differ from populations diagnosed and treated as neurotic depressions and some of these have been successful. The situations in which these differential diagnoses have been made tend to differ substantially from the frequent clinical practice whereby a patient is placed in a category of anxiety, depression or anxiety/depression at or around his first outpatient visit and treated on this basis. It is generally considered that depressed patients should be treated with antidepressants and anxious patients with anxiolytics. We present here some preliminary results of a large scale study of the extent to which these beliefs and practices are justified.
We set out to examine the following questions:

1) Do anxiety states and neurotic depressions exist as separate entities in a group of neurotic outpatients?

2) Do the symptoms of anxiety and depression respond differentially to treatment with Amitriptyline and Diazepam?

Although anxiety states and neurotic depressions are conditions which are usually diagnosed purely upon a clinical basis psychophysiological measures may be changed in these disorders. These measures were therefore included in the study to see if they could be used to support the differential between anxiety states and neurotic depression.

METHOD

The study concerns 240 nonpsychotic psychiatric outpatients in whom depression, anxiety or both were thought to be present to a morbid degree. These patients were included in a four week study in which no diagnostic categories were applied all patients being rated on the same measures. To see to what extent the symptoms of depression and anxiety respond differentially to different kinds of treatment the patients were randomly and blindly assigned to one of four treatment groups:- placebo, diazepam, amitriptyline and diazepam plus amitriptyline all treatments appearing the same. After an initial assessment week treatment lasted for a further 4 weeks during which time a number of ratings were made of clinical features and other factors thought to be relevant. The clinical ratings were as follows:

1) The Goldberg observer rating scale of overall symptom severity
2) The Hamilton observer rating scale of depression
3) The Hamilton observer rating scale of anxiety
4) The Leeds self rating scale of depression
5) The Leeds self rating scale of anxiety
6) The Spielberger self rating scale of state anxiety

In the presentation that follows I shall report in detail only the Hamilton depression and anxiety scores. The results using the other scores do not differ materially from these.

RESULTS

The strongest evidence for the independent existence of anxiety and depression would be provided if the scores on the two scales were not only independent in the patient population but also were distributed in two discrete groups one of 'anxious' patients and one of 'depressed' patients.

In our sample this was clearly not the case. There was no evidence for two discrete groups of patients and furthermore anxiety and depression scores were significantly related ($r=0.47$, $p<.001$). Thus people who were deeply depressed tended to be highly anxious while people who were mildly depressed tended to be mildly anxious. The major source of variation in this population was thus severity of illness. Predominance of anxious or depressive symptoms had a relatively minor role. Thus if this distinction is an important one we shall have to find evidence for it elsewhere.

An additional measure relating to the distinction between depression and anxiety was taken before treatment began and after four weeks of treatment. This was the habituation of the skin conductance response.

A novel stimulus, usually a fairly loud noise will elicit in normal subjects a transient increase in skin conductance probably reflecting changes in the activity of the autonomic nervous system. If the same stimulus is repeated then the following skin conductance responses will decrease in size and after about 6 or 7 presentations cease to occur. In highly anxious subjects this habituation of the skin conductance response is greatly delayed and indeed the response may persist throughout the sequence of tones. In addition there are many spontaneous fluctuations, that is, responses unrelated to any stimulus being presented by the experimenter. An index of rate of habituation or skin conductance responsitivity was found for each of our neurotic patients by counting the number of responses elicited by a sequence of 14 85 decibel tones. Initial skin conductance responsivity was then related to the initial depression and anxiety scores: there was no relation at all between responsivity and severity of symptoms.

TABLE 1 Skin conductance and symptom severity

responses	>10	< 10	<5
severe	46	39	27
mild	42	36	30
$chi^2 = 0.4$, df = 2, ns			

There was however a relationship between responsivity and whether the symptoms were predominantly anxious or predominantly depressed.

TABLE 2 Skin conductance and symptom type

responses	>10	<10	<5
dep.	35	45	37
anx.	53	30	21
$chi^2 = 10.4$, df = 2, $p < .01$			

There was a strong tendency for the anxious patients to show many responses while the depressed patients showed rather fewer responses. These results suggest that symptoms of anxiety and depression in this population do reflect some genuine underlying difference which can be independently found in psychophysiological measures.

Evidence for a distinction between anxiety and depression of more practical relevance would be demonstrated if the different treatment regimes were found to affect different symptoms. In the extreme we would expect depression to be affected only by amitriptyline while anxiety would be affected only by diazepam.

The mean changes in the various symptom scores give little evidence for the distinction between anxiety and depression.

TABLE 3 Change in symptoms during 4 weeks of treatment
Mean (SE)

	Amitriptyline	Diazepam	A + D	Placebo
Goldberg	17.4 (1.85)	11.7 (1.75)	13.6 (1.55)	12.1 (1.75)
Hamilton depression	20.4 (2.20)	14.8 (2.00)	15.5 (2.05)	12.8 (2.00)
Hamilton anxiety	9.4 (1.00)	8.8 (0.85)	7.8 (0.90)	6.4 (1.10)
Leeds depression	3.8 (0.70)	3.0 (0.60)	2.8 (1.20)	1.7 (0.78)

TABLE 3 (continued)

	Amitriptyline	Diazepam	A + D	Placebo
Leeds anxiety	3.1 (0.30)	2.8 (0.60)	2.4 (0.50)	1.6 (0.30)
Spielberger anxiety	12.1 (1.35)	4.6 (2.00)	8.6 (1.90)	2.1 (2.25)

It is certainly the case that amitriptyline gives a greater improvement in depression scores than the other treatments but it is also the best treatment for the various measures of anxiety as well. On the basis of these results then there is no evidence that anxiety and depression respond differently to treatment. For either symptom amitriptyline seems to be more effective than diazepam although the former does seem to be more effective for depressive symptoms. It would be reasonable to think that the differential effects of the treatments would be apparent if we looked at patients rather than symptoms. In other words patients who were predominantly depressed might respond better to amitriptyline while patients who were predominantly anxious would respond better to diazepam. For the predominantly depressed there was no change in the total pattern. For the predominantly anxious patients diazepam did seem to be effecting some improvement, but it was never better than amitriptyline. Thus on the basis of their initial symptoms there seems to be no justification for assuming that some patients will benefit from amitriptyline while others will benefit from diazepam.

Perhaps if we take into account initial psychophysiology as well as initial psychophysiology as well as initial symptoms than more specific treatment effects will be revealed.

There was a marked effect of treatment upon skin conductance responsivity.

TABLE 4 Skin conductance and treatment

responses	decrease	increase
placebo	22	16
diazepam	38	4
amitriptyline	25	8
d and a	35	7

$chi^2 = 13.3$, $df = 3$, $p < .01$

Patients treated with diazepam in particular showed a marked reduction in responsiveness in many cases ceasing to respond to any of the tones.

Amitriptyline, on the other hand, had relatively little effect on skin conductance responsivity. Thus diazepam is certainly markedly reducing one of the peripheral signs of anxiety, namely skin conductance responsivity, but is apparently having relatively little effect on more complex behavioural manifestations. Initial skin conductance responsivity does however seem to have some success in predicting effects of treatment.

TABLE 5 Skin conductance and treatment effect

amitriptyline and depression			
improvement	good	mild	poor
high scr	8	0	8
low scr	9	6	1
$chi^2 = 11.5$, df = 2 $p < .01$			

There was a significant relationship between improvement in depression scores and initial skin conductance responsivity for patients treated with amitriptyline. Patients with low initial skin conductance responsivity were more likely to improve than those with high skin conductance responsivity. Such a relationship was not found for the placebo group or for the group treated with diazepam.

Similarly there was a significant relationship between improvement in anxiety scores and initial skin conductance responsivity for patients treated with diazepam but this time it was patients with high skin conductance responsivity who were most likely to improve.

TABLE 6 Skin conductance and treatment effect

diazepam and anxiety			
improvement	good	mild	poor
high scr	17	5	8
low scr	3	6	6
$chi^2 = 5.8$, df = 2, $p < .05$			

This relationship was also specific to the group treated with diazepam. These results are consistent with the previous observation that anxious patients are characterised by high skin conductance responsivity while depressed patients are characterised by low skin conductance responsivity.

Thus when we take psychophysiological measures into account there is some evidence that depression and anxiety do respond differently to different kinds of treatment. However although these results are of theoretical interest they have little practical relevance. The relationships are far too weak to make useful predictions at the level of a single case. If our results have any practical relevance then, rather unexpectedly, they suggest that there is little value in distinguishing between symptoms of anxiety and depression since both symptoms are likely to be improved rather more by treatment with amitriptyline than by treatment with diazepam.

Biological and Psychopharmacological Predictors of Drug Response

Prediction of Response to Anti-Anxiety Agents

C. HALLSTRÖM and M. LADER

Institute of Psychiatry, De Crespigny Park, Denmark Hill, London, SE5 8AF, England

ABSTRACT

The prediction of response to anti-anxiety agents is of clinical and theoretical importance. It has not been systematically studied. The distinction between depressive and anxiety states can act as a prognostic indicator, as can the phenomenology of the anxious patient. Doctor-patient variables significantly affect the response to minor tranquillizers in conditions that have a 25-50% placebo response. This makes any specific pharmacological assessment difficult. Benzodiazepine pharmacokinetics are of theoretical interest in the prediction of outcome and the new technique of salivary drug estimation may prove of practical use, enabling an estimation of the plasma unbound, and active, drug to be made. The individual's ability to acetylate sulphapyrimidine can act as an indicator for effective phenelzine dosage. In an assessment of therapeutic benefit one must also take into account the hazards of treatment.

Keywords - Anxiety, prediction, diagnosis, patient variables, pharmacokinetics, monoamine oxidase inhibitors, benzodiazepines

INTRODUCTION

The very use of the word practice as the conduct of our art implies experimentation with every patient and some uncertainty as to the outcome of treatment. This conference stands for the scientific approach to our work, that part in which we attempt to understand and quantify the problems and changes of our patients. Associated with the improved standing of our discipline should be an interest in the prediction of outcome to our therapies. This is fraught with many problems, none the least that we still have difficulty in retrospective assessment of outcome let alone prospectively.

The issue is important, however, not only from the aesthetic point of view, but also from a practical standpoint. If the patient starts effective medication sooner rather than later, an earlier resolution of symptoms should ensue; not only will this reduce the patient's suffering but it will increase his confidence in his doctor making the therapeutic relationship more fruitful facilitating psychotherapeutic and behavioural change. It is also important to avoid unnecessary and potentially harmful medication, and rapid resolution of symptoms means a quicker return to a full life with an equivalent reduction of the social and economic burden of illness.

Surprisingly, there has been little systematic work into the prediction of response to anxiolytic agents, probably because this superficially obvious problem is really very complex.

EFFECT OF DIAGNOSIS

Diagnosis presents the first problem. Clinicians can readily recognise anxiety states, but with respect to formal diagnosis, concordance between clinicians is low, especially when sub categories of anxiety states are concerned (American Psychiatric Association, 1952, 1968; Feighner, 1972; Spitzer, Endicott and Robins, 1975; Klein, D. 1964, 1974). Practically, it is important to distinguish between depression and anxiety as there do seem to be differences of some importance. Roth (1972) in the U.K. compared clinicians' diagnoses with structured ratings of anxiety and depression, and subjected the data to factor analysis. Two main clusters of symptoms emerged, one associated with anxiety, the other with depression (Table 1). The method and results can be interpreted in several ways but in general accord with currently held concepts. Prognostic differences exist as the outcome for depressive illness is far brighter than for anxiety states.

TABLE 1 MAJOR FACTORS ASSOCIATED WITH ANXIETY AND DEPRESSION

ANXIETY FACTORS	Factor Loading	DEPRESSION FACTORS	Factor Loading
Panic attacks	.6	Early waking	- .5
Increased vasomotor response	.5	Retardation	- .5
Dependence	.5	Depression worse a.m.	- .4
Age of onset < 35	.6	Duration < 1 year	- .4
Agoraphobia (marked)	.6		
Derealization	.5		

Spitzer (1970) found that the diagnostic groups remained distinct after a mean follow up of 3.8 years. The more favourable prognosis of the depressed patients could stem from the better response to imipramine than to diazepam or placebo, as shown by Covi (1974), and also the more favourable intrinsic natural history of the condition.

There is often some clinical difficulty in distinguishing between an anxiety state and a depressive one, yet in defining the distinction and acting on it one can predict therapeutic outcome in response to an anxiolytic.

Many depressive states are associated with anxiety, and these mixed syndromes respond better to tricyclic antidepressants than to anxiolytics especially to 'tertiary' compounds such as amitriptyline with sedative properties.

It is also important not to mistake organic pathology or schizophrenia for an affective disorder, since a different approach is indicated.

The Symptom Pattern

The phenomenology of the anxiety state repays careful study since by applying a rational therapy to the patient's symptoms or symptom complex we move away from the Kraepelinian view of disease entities towards a more individualised approach to the patient's symptoms. The patient may complain predominantly of somatic manifestations of the condition or of the psychological ones, or most commonly from a blend of the two.

TABLE 2 Common Symptoms of Somatic and Psychic Anxiety

Psychic Anxiety	Somatic Anxiety
Worry	Palpitations
Fearful anticipation	Muscular pains
Phobias	Tinnitus
Insomnia	Blurring of vision
Poor memory and concentration	Tightness in chest
Irritability	Butterflies in stomach
	Frequency of micturition

Work done by Tyrer and Lader (1974) in our department showed diazepam to be more effective than propranolol in a group of patients with chronic anxiety, nevertheless benefit was derived from propranolol alone, mainly by the patients who suffered from somatic anxiety. One could identify the characteristics of a small group of patients who suffered essentially from the peripheral symptoms of anxiety and treat these with β-blockers. This would have the advantage of allowing symptomatic relief without the central unwanted effects of tranquillisers such as drowsiness, disinhibition and dependence. We are conducting further studies of whether a group of patients can be identified who respond better to propranolol and diazepam in combination rather than to either alone. Predictive factors we shall explore include not only the demographic details and symptom profiles but also whether pre-treatment catecholamine urinary and plasma concentrations can predict the outcome of pharmacotherapy.

PATIENT DOCTOR VARIABLES

The personal characteristics of doctor and patient are more important in psychiatry than in any other branch of medicine in affecting outcome of treatment. Rickels (1978) has investigated the field estensively, and has outlined features that affect the therapeutic outcome with tranquillisers. He applied multiple regression analyses to his data from several studies of anxiolytics, mainly given to outpatients. Occupation, age, education, sex, race and marital status modified drug response to anxiolytics. The more socially advantaged patients had less placebo response than the less advantaged ones. Contributary life events also blurred the difference between responses to diazepam and to placebo. Rickels found that a short term response to anxiolytic therapy in chronically anxious people often heralded a relapse in a matter of months. In anxious outpatients the outcome was not related to a placebo response but was drug specific. Thus, factors associated with a good outcome were: the patient was employed, married, more educated, expected drug treatment and acknowledged he had an emotional problem; the illness had an acute onset precipitated by a life stress and was associated with depression or was of a longer duration but not vigorously treated by drugs; and the patient reported side effects after two weeks and had no other medical illness.

A poorer response tended to occur in menopausal women and in patients with mild obsessional disorders; in those with greater anxiety and those with problems in interpersonal relationships. Hypochondriacal patients were less likely to take their medication as were those who were depressed and hopeless.

TABLE 3 Factors that Influenced Outcome Favourably

Good prognosis generally
High income
Good education
Preference for pharmacotherapy
Seeing problems as emotional
Few previous drugs

25-50% of patients were placebo responders and improved non-specifically to care and attention. Because of this many patients apparently responding to active medication may well be showing non-specific improvements.

TABLE 4 Factors that Influenced Placebo Response

Time spent with patient
Race
Treatment setting
Duration of illness
Initial depression

It is worth emphasizing the characteristics of the doctor that are associated with good response. He works in a family practice, feels comfortable with patients with psychological problems and is familiar with the prescription of drugs. He also devotes more time to the initial interview.

It can be seen that whereas some of these predictors are drug specific, many of the predictors of good outcome are very similar to those for psychotherapy or are associated with a good prognosis whatever the therapy.

PHARMACOKINETIC CONSIDERATIONS

Because of the inherent shortcomings of the factors so far reviewed, interest is shifting from patient phenomenology to pharmacokinetic considerations. Pharmacokinetic factors are essentially those of the effects of the body on the drug. In simple terms if a drug cannot reach its site of action in adequate amounts at the right time, then it cannot exert its influence. Also the ultimate benefit of the drug is a function not only of its therapeutic action but also of its negative and unwanted effects.

Benzodiazepines

The benzodiazepines and the two common problems of chronic anxiety and insomnia provide an example. Since the symptoms of anxiety are present through most of the day, it would seem pharmacokinetically rational to prescribe a preparation with a relatively long half life so that the plasma concentrations do not fluctuate widely. For example nordiazepam has a half-life of about 72 hours so that the therapeutic effect should be constant. This contrasts with the situation with insomnia where the ideal drug would reach high plasma and brain concentrations rapidly after administration, but would have a short half life and no active metabolites so it is substantially removed from the brain by the time the patient needs to wake up, thus minimizing the hangover effect. For example, loreazepam has a half life of about 12 hours, as shown by Greenblatt (1976). Unfortunately clinical practice in England commonly uses nordiazepam (as Clorazepate) as a night time sedative and lorazepam as a day time anxiolytic. The problem is further conpounded by the generally poor relationship between plasma concentrations of and clinical response to benzodiazepines (Bond, Hailey and Lader, 1977). The evidence for the selection of a suitable benzodiazepine for a syndrome is also inconclusive but theoretically interesting.

Bianchi (1974) as a prognostic test gave a single oral dose of diazepam to 25 anxious neurotic patients before a three-week course of the drug and took blood 2 hours after the initial test dose. He found a statistically strong link between a low plasma concentration at 2 hours and improvement after the first week of treatment. A higher 2 hour concentration was found in patients who later complained of side effects. The 2 hour blood level correlated well with the steady state plasma level after one week. No attempts have been made to replicate this interesting study.

It is important not to confuse prediction of response with the monitoring of ongoing treatment. However, there has been considerable interest in plasma benzodiazepine concentrations and their significance (Gott Shalk and Kaplan, 1972; Bianchi, 1974; Hillestad, 1974; Bond, 1977). In general the higher the plasma concentration the greater the drug effects, but the results are inconclusive. Part of the problem may lie in the high level of protein binding of benzodiazepines in the plasma. Our preliminary findings (Hallstrom, in Press) agree with those authors who quote figures of about 99± 0.6 per cent. This standard deviation implies several-fold variations from patient to patient in the free (and hence biologically active) drug concentration. An estimate of total plasma concentration alone might account for the variability in the relationship between plasma concentration and clinical effect. We propose in our unit to re-examine the problem by looking at salivary benzodiazepine concentrations to seek a relationship between them and physiological, psychological and clinical variables. Saliva is an interesting body fluid to examine since drugs such as the benzodiazepines should theoretically be in equilibrium between the saliva and unbound plasma concentration (Giles, 1977).

Our preliminary data show a close correlation between salivary drug concentrations and both the plasma free and total plasma diazepam concentration. The results look promising but are not yet conclusive.

Monoamine Oxidase Inhibitors

Interest in the therapeutic properties of the monoamine oxidase inhibitors has been rekindled in recent years following the early observations of Sargant and Dally (1962), in which they describe the particular efficacy of phenelzine in the 'atypical depressions', those associated with high measures of anxiety. Tyrer (1973) suggested that phenelzine acts as an anxiolytic in patients with phobic anxiety and Lipsedge (1973) showed that iproniazid reduced anxiety ratings but not behavioural avoidance in severe agoraphobics.

Much work suggests that whilst these drugs are of dubious efficacy in the amelioration of depression they have a clear beneficial action in the treatment of phobic anxiety Several studies (Ravioni, 1976; Robinson, 1973) of the therapeutic activity of phenelzine have agreed that improvement is generally associated with an 80 per cent inhibition of platelet monoamine oxidase activity. This fits well with the work of Eve Johnson (1973) which showed that despite adequate dosage with phenelzine clinical improvement was greater in patients who were slow acetylators of sulphapyridine than fast acetylators. Acetylator status is an inherited quality and phenelzine is extensively metabolised by acetylation. The determination of sulphapyridine acetylator status should qualify for one of the few examples of a prognostic test for phenelzine treatment but only with respect to choice of dose.

PREDICTION OF COMPLICATIONS

In prediction of response to pharmacotherapy one must also catalogue the hazards of therapy. The risk of hypertensive crises and liver damage with phenelzine are known as are the cardiac complications associated with tricyclic antidepressants and the pulmonary problems of some β-blockers.

The problems of habituation to the benzodiazepines are currently of interest. Maletzy (1976) studied 50 medical and psychiatric patients taking diazepam at normal dose levels. Many suffered withdrawal symptoms when they tried to stop similar to symptoms occurring spontaneously in anxiety states. There are many reports in the literature of habituation and withdrawal symptoms, and it would seem that after a period of about one month on continuous benzodiazepine medication, many patients will suffer problems of withdrawal. It is not yet possible to characterise which patients will become habituated and possibly develop tolerance.

CONCLUSION

Some obvious predictors to pharamcotherapy exist. Response to the treatment during a previous exacerbation is a good predictor, as are the factors that are associated with a good prognosis whatever the treatment. Generalised anxiety will respond favourably to the benzodiazepines over the short term. More specifically, when the anxiety is associated with depressive symptoms, tricyclic antidepresants are of greater benefit and monoamine oxidase inhibitors are of value if the patients manifest phobic anxiety. β-blockers are indicated in those troubled specifically by the somatic aspects of anxiety.

In future studies we shall have to look more closely at the patients and their expectations. Also we must develop direct and indirect measures of drug activity in the patient not only to monitor treatment but to identify prognostic features.

REFERENCES

American Psychiatric Association (1952). Diagnostic and Statistical Manual. Mental disorders. A.P.A. Washington D.C.

American Psychiatric Association (1968). Diagnostic and Statistical Manual, Second Edition. A.P.A. Washington D.C.

Bianchi, Fennessy, Phillips and Everitt (1974). Plasma levels of diazepam as a therapeutic predictor. Psychopharmacologica, 35, 113-122.

Bond, Hailey and Lader (1977). Plasma concentrations of benzodiazepines. Brit.J.Clin.Pharmac., 4, 51-56.

Covi, Lipman, Derogatis, Smith and Pattison (1974). Drugs and group psychotherapy in neurotic depression. American Journal of Psychiatry, 131, 191-198.

Dasberg, Klein, Goelen and Van Praag (1974). Plasma concentrations of diazepam and of its metabolite N-desmethyldiazepam. Clinical Pharmacology and Therapeutics, 15, 473-483.

Feighner, Robins, Guze, Woodruff, Winokur and Munoz (1972). Diagnostic criteria for use in psychiatric research. Archives of General Psychiatry, 26, 57-63.

Giles, Zilm, Frecker, Macleod and Sellers (1977). Saliva and plasma concentrations of diazepam. Brit.J.Clin.Pharmacology, 4, 711-712.

Gottshalk and Kaplan (1972). Comprehensive Psychiatry, 13. 6, 519-527.

Greenblatt, Schilling, Kyriakopoulos, Shader, Sisenwine, Knowles and Ruelius (1976). Absorption and distribution of oral C^{14} Lorazepam. Clinical Pharmacology and Therapeutics, 20, 329-341.

Hallstrom, Lader and Curry. Salivary excretion of diazepam. In press.

Hillestad, Hansen, Melsom and Drivenes (1974). Diazepam metabolism in normal man. Clin.Pharm. and Therapeutics, 16, 479-489.
Johnson & Marsh (1973). Acetylator status and response to phenelzine in depressed patients. Lancet. I. 567-570.
Klein, D. (1964). Deliniation of two drug-responsive anxiety syndromes. Psychopharmacologica, 5, 397-408.
Klein, D. (1974). Endogenomorphic depression. Arch.Gen.Psychiatry, 31, 447-454.
Lipsedge, Hajioff, Huggins, Napier, Pearce, Pike and Rich (1973). The management of severe agoraphobic. A comparison of iproniazid and systematic desensitization. Psychopharmacologica, 32, 67-80.
Maletzy and Klolter (1976). Addiction to diazepam. Int.J.Addict. 11(1), 95-116.
Ravaris, Nies, Robinson, Ives, Lamborn and Korson (1976). A Multiple-Dose, Controlled Study of Phenelzine in Depression-Anxiety States. Arch.Gen.Psychiatry, 33, 347-350.
Rickels, K. (1978). Use of anti-anxiety agents in anxious outpatients. Psychopharmacology, 58, 1-17.
Robinson, Nies, Ravario, Lamborn and Burlington (1973). The monoamine oxidase inhibitor Phenelzine in the treatment of depressive anxiety states. Arch.Gen. Psychiatry, 29, 407-413.
Roth, Gurney, Garside and Kerr, (1972). Studies in the classification of affective disorders. Br. J.Psychiatry, 121, 147-161.
Sargent and Dally (1962). Treatment of anxiety states by antidepressant drugs. B.M.J. 1, 6-9.
Spitzer, Endicott, Fleiss and Cohn (1970). The Psychiatric status schedule. Arch.Gen.Psychiatry, 23, 41-55.
Spitzer, Endicott and Robins (1975). Research diagnostic criteria (R.D.C.) for a selected group of functional disorders. Manual prepared for C.R.B. - N.I.M.H. Collaborative Studies on depression.
Tyrer and Lader (1974). Response to Propranolol and Diazepam in somatic and psychic anxiety. B.M.J. 2, 14-16.
Tyrer, Candy and Kelly (1973). Phenelzine in Phobic Anxiety: A controlled trial. Psychological Medicine, 3, 120-124.

Provocative Pharmacological Agents for Psychiatric Diagnosis: Methylphenidate, Sodium Amobarbital and Physostigmine

J. JANOWSKY*, J. DAVIS, M. DYSKEN** and G. KILLIAN****

*Department of Psychiatry, University of California at San Deigo, School of Medicine

**The Research Service, Illinois State Psychiatric, with partial support from the Medical Research Service, Veterans Administration Hospital, San Diego

ABSTRACT

Although sedative and psychostimulant drugs have been used for many years to aid in the diagnostic and prognostic evaluation of psychiatric patients, few controlled studies of their efficacy exist. Recently, we have evaluated three pharmacologic agents, methylphenidate, physostigmine, and amobarbital, to further determine their diagnostic efficacy. This report briefly summarizes our observations concerning the differential effects of these agents in patients with various diagnoses.

INTRAVENOUS METHYLPHENIDATE

As reviewed previously (1) amphetamine-like psychostimulants have been observed to intensify psychotic symptoms in actively ill schizophrenics and to induce catharsis and talkativeness in normals, psychoneurotics and remitted schizophrenics. These observations recently have been extended by administering intravenous methylphenidate (0.5 mg/kg) to a variety of psychiatric patients and evaluating behavioral changes, using clinical ratings, as well as word association and projective psychological tests (1,2,3). Two such experiments are reported in the following paragraphs.

Method

The first set of experiments (1) utilized voluntary male and female psychiatric patients, having a variety of diagnoses, who ranged in age from 16 to 40 years. Diagnostic groups included: a) 22 actively ill schizophrenics, b) 3 remitted schizophrenics, c) 10 acutely ill manics, d) 4 acutely ill depressives, and e) 8 normals Following a series of placebo injections, a single intravenous injection of 0.5 mg/kg methylphenidate was administered to each subject over a 30-60 second period of time. Behavior was rated before and 15 minutes after injection of active methylphenidate. A trained nurse, blind to when and if active drug was being administered, evaluated the patients using a 15-point rating scale in which 0-5 represented mild symptoms, 6-10 represented moderate symptoms, and 11-15 represented extreme symptoms. Global psychosis and interactions were so rated.

A number of patients (13 actively ill schizophrenics, 7 acute manics, and 3 depressives) had the experimental sequence subsequently repeated, receiving a second infusion of methylphenidate after remission had occurred. This second infusion occurred no sooner than four weeks after the initial infusion.

In a second set of experiments (3), psychological tests were used to indirectly evaluate the psychosis activating effects of methylphenidate. This strategy was used to indirectly measure psychosis activation, so as to indicate whether or not "true" psychosis activation occurs following methylphenidate in schizophrenics, or whether patients merely become more trusting and talkative about their existing psychotic symptoms. Two groups, consisting of 16 actively psychotic schizophrenic inpatients, and 18 non-psychotic inpatients were utilized.

A design similar to the above described first set of experiments was used. 20 minutes before intravenous methylphenidate infusion (0.5 mg/kg), 20 minutes after infusion, and 24 hours after infusion, 15 of 16 schizophrenics, and 17 of 18 non-psychotic subjects were given the Kent-Rosanoff word association test(4), a 50 item standardized word association test designed to measure subjects' ability to give common word associations. This test was then scored for the number of common responses, this being defined as one of the five most frequent responses, according to published norms(4).

Furthermore, at 20 minutes before, 20 minutes after, and 24 hours after methylphenidate infusion, each subject was also given 3 different sets of projective ink blot tests, consisting of 5 Holtzman ink blots each(5). For each Holtzman card, each patient was asked to give one response, telling what the blot looked like. The responses to the Holtzman ink blots were then rated blindly by a clinical psychologist (Lowell Storms, Ph.D.) on four dimensions, using a 0-7 point scale. The dimensions were: 1) paranoid trends, 2) autism, 3) inappropriateness to the blot, and 4) thought disorder. The total number of responses given a rating of 6 or 7 (in the pathological range) was used as the pathological response score. All data was analyzed utilizing a Student's T test for paired results.

Results

In the 22 actively ill schizophrenic patients, there was a statistically significant and clinically dramatic intensification of pre-existing psychotic symptoms, including hallucinations, delusions, bizarre thinking and behavior, and catatonic posturing (baseline global psychosis score = 6.5 ± 0.4; + 15 minutes post-methylphenidate psychosis score = 10.5 ± 0.7, $p<.003$, students T test for paired results). Most schizophrenics changed from having active symptoms to moderate control to manifesting severe, florid psychotic symptoms. In most cases, symptom activation occurred within one or two minutes of injection and intensified to a peak within 15 to 30 minutes. Symptoms spontaneously decreased to their baseline level after a one to four hour period of time, as did increases in pulse rate and blood pressure. Interaction ratings also increased significantly after methylphenidate infusion in the actively ill schizophrenic patient group as a whole, although this phenomena did not occur in every patient(1).

For the 13 schizophrenic patients who had a second methylphenidate infusion, receiving a methylphenidate infusion while actively ill and later while in remission, methylphenidate increased psychosis ratings only while the patients were actively psychotic, but not while they were in remission. In contrast, methylphenidate increased the interaction ratings of these patients while they were actively psychotic, as well as after they had remitted.

Among both actively ill and remitted schizophrenic patients, no changes in global psychosis, or interaction ratings, depression or anxiety occurred following placebo administration during the baseline phase.

In the acutely ill manic patient group, as with the schizophrenics, interaction scores increased significantly following administration of methylphenidate. In addition, four of the ten manic patients showed obviously increased psychosis ratings after methylphenidate infusion. In these, the content of the psychotic material generally was grandiose, elated, or paranoid in nature. Overall, psychosis ratings did not increase significantly in the manic patient group.

In addition, of the ten acutely ill manic patients, 5 showed increased manic symptoms, 3 showed no change, and 2 showed decreased manic symptoms after receiving methylphenidate.

Furthermore, methylphenidate did not increase psychosis scores in any of those 7 manic patients given methylphenidate a second time after remission had occurred, although interaction scores again were significantly increased following the second methylphenidate infusion.

The depressed patient group showed no significant increase in psychosis scores following methylphenidate administration. Interaction scores consistently and significantly increased in these four cases. In two cases, depression was significantly and dramatically alleviated, and the patients entered a euphoric, hyperverbal state, which lasted from one to two hours. In the other two cases, dramatic catharsis, increased interactions, and increased talkativeness occurred.

The reaction of the 12 normal controls to methylphenidate infusion was similar to that of the remitted manic and schizophrenic patients and the depressives. No increase in psychosis ratings occurred. Most subjects showed increased talkativeness, catharsis, interactions, and thoughts.

For the second set of experiments(3) a significant decrease over baseline ($p<.05$) in common word associations occurred 20 minutes after, but not 24 hours after, methylphenidate infusion in the schizophrenic group only. This effect was not found for the non-psychotic patient group (mean number of appropriate responses: Schizophrenics-baseline = 23.8 $\pm$ 2.1, + 20 minutes = 18.3 $\pm$ 3.0, + 24 hours = 22.2 $\pm$ 2.0; Non-psychotics-baseline = 32.9 $\pm$ 1.3, + 20 minutes = 32.6 $\pm$ 2.1, + 24 hours = 34.0 $\pm$ 1.9). Furthermore, a significantly lower number of common word associations occurred overall at baseline, + 20 minutes, and + 24 hours after methylphenidate infusion, in the psychotic patients as compared to the non-psychotic patients.

A significant increase over baseline in pathologic projective responses to the Holtzman ink blot test occurred in the schizophrenic group 20 minutes after ($p<.05$), but not 24 hours after, methylphenidate intoxication (number of pathologic responses: Schizophrenics-baseline = 2.3 $\pm$ 0.5, + 20 minutes + 4.4 $\pm$ 0.9, + 24 hours = 2.2 $\pm$ 0.4). This statistically significant increase did not occur in the non-psychotic group of patients, although a slight increase in pathologic responses did occur.

Discussion

The above data are consistent with the assumption that methylphenidate significantly intensifies schizophrenic symptoms and activates the schizophrenic thought process in actively ill schizophrenic patients, but not in remitted or non-schizophrenic subjects; and that methylphenidate generally increases interactions, talkativeness, and catharsis in most subjects. The fact that the word association test scores of the schizophrenic patient group showed less commonality after methylphenidate infusion suggests that methylphenidate causes a loosening of associations in schizophrenic patients. The projective test results parallel the above observations, and indicate that the autistic and projective components of schizophrenic thinking are increased by methylphenidate. Since both of these tests are indirect measures of psychotic thinking, it is likely that methylphenidate increases psychotic symptoms, and it is unlikely that methylphenidate merely makes patients more trusting or talkative.

Thus, the administration of psychologic tests, plus a psychostimulant may have clinical usefulness in the rapid differential diagnosis of psychiatric patients beyond that of conventional interviewing or psychodiagnostic tests used alone. In addition, use of a methylphenidate interview at the end of a hospitalization may allow a clinician to tell whether the schizophrenic patient is clinically remitted and free of psychotic symptoms, or is merely withholding or suppressing information concerning his symptoms.

PHYSOSTIGMINE

Various cholinesterase inhibitors have been shown to induce depression, antagonize manic symptoms, and cause anergic effects in psychiatric patients, presumably by increasing central acetylcholine levels(6,7,8). The current study was conducted to determine whether or not physostigmine has a differential effect in causing depressive symptoms in groups of patients with and without affective symptoms respectively(6).

Method

Subjects studied consisted of: a) 8 floridly ill schizophrenic patients without marked affective symptoms, b) 6 acutely ill schizo-affective patients with notable affective symptoms, c) 8 manic-depressive patients, manic type, and d) 2 depressed patients, suffering from unipolar depression.

As described elsewhere(6), each patient participating in the study was pretreated with methscopolamine (0.75 - 1.0 mg, I.M.), so as to partially block peripheral cholinomimetic effects. A varying number of placebo injections were given, followed by intravenous injection of up to a total of 3.0 mg physostigmine or 1.5 neostigmine. Subjects were rated on a 0-5 point continuum scale for global depression and on a 0-5 point continuum scale for sadness by a nurse-rater who was blind to the type of drug infused and the timing of when active drug was infused. Increases over placebo-baseline scores for the sadness and global depression ratings in the manic depressive and schizo-affective groups were compared with increases in these variables in the schizophrenic group of patients who did not have significant affective symptoms. Comparison of groups occurred, using the Student T-Test (one tailed) for unpaired results.

Results

Most patients who received physostigmine exhibited symptoms of psychomotor retardation, similar to those observed in patients with retarded depression. Physostigmine did not produce marked sedation, slurred speech, or ataxia, although some patients became nauseated and/or vomited. Decreases in the subjects' levels of cheerfulness, friendliness, interactions, and talkativeness occurred. In contrast, neostigmine did not cause a significant change in behavior.

Physostigmine, appeared capable of inducing depressed mood and sadness in patients with an affective component to their illness. Six of the 8 manics and both depressives showed increased depressed mood after receiving physostigmine (manic group's increase in depression rating from baseline = $0.79 \pm .27$, significance = $p<0.02$; manics increase in sadness rating = $0.81 \pm .26$, significance = $p<0.01$). Likewise, 5 of the 6 schizo-affective patients showed depression after physostigmine infusion ($1.60 \pm .39$ = increase in depression rating, significance = $p<0.005$; increase in sadness rating = $1.48 \pm .40$, significance = $p<0.007$).

In contrast, physostigmine caused depression in only 1 of the 8 schizophrenics who did not show an affective component to their symptoms, and the increase in sadness and depression for this group was not significant. (Both sadness and depression increases = $0.23 \pm .48$).

Discussion

More recently, K.L. Davis, et al(8) administered physostigmine to 13 normal volunteers. Although a physostigmine inhibitory syndrome occurred frequently, depression was noted in only two subjects. Thus, there is evidence from the work of Davis et al(9), and Janowsky et al(6,7,8) to support the hypothesis that physostigmine may selectively cause a depressed mood in subjects with pre-existing affective disorder, in contrast to non-affective disorder patients.

Given that the above differentiation between physostigmine's effects on mood in patients with and without affective symptoms proves valid in larger samples, it is at least possible that physostigmine infusions might have some diagnostic potential.

AMOBARBITAL

There have been no placebo-controlled, double-blind studies evaluating the usefulness of barbituates, such as sodium amobarbital in uncovering schizophrenic or depressive symptoms, or indicating that barbituates improve diagnostic potential(10,11,12). The purpose of the present study is to compare sodium amobarbital and saline interviews in psychiatric inpatients to determine if this barbituate is effective in differentiating depressive from schizophrenic symptoms.

Method

Twenty psychiatric inpatients, including 11 schizophrenics, 5 affect disorder patients and four subjects with other psychotic and/or character disorder diagnoses, who had difficulty talking to their therapist during psychiatric evaluation, were studied. Subjects served as their own controls and were given two interviews on the same day. Sodium amobarbital was injected at a rate of 25 mg/min, and was stopped when sustained horizontal nystagmus developed (dosage ranged from 150 mg to 350 mg).

An interviewer conducted both sessions on each patient. The first session occurred in the late morning, while the second session occurred at least four hours later. The interviewer randomly administered intravenous saline solution during one session and intravenous sodium amobarbital during the other session. Following each session, the interviewer completed a Hamilton Depression Scale, a New Haven Schizophrenic Index (NHSI) and a Brief Psychiatric Rating Scale (BPRS). All interviews were audio-recorded, and also were rated blindly by another rater on the Hamilton Depression Scale, NHSI, and the BPRS.

In addition, the patient's regular therapist completed a pre-interview and a post-interview questionnaire. The pre-interview questionnaire was designed to measure the therapist's expectations and his diagnosis. The post-interview questionnaire was designed to measure his observation of the usefulness of each of the two interviews with respect to such components as a) new behaviors, b) information elicited, c) increased known information, d) diagnosis, e) treatment options, and f) psychodynamics elicited, on a scale ranging from 0-8. The therapists attended both interviews and were blind to the drug condition.

Results

On the basis of therapist ratings, there was no significant differences between the usefulness of the respective interviews. On the average, the therapists found both sessions moderately useful (range 3-4 out of 8), suggesting that neither the sodium amobarbital nor the interview sequence had a specific effect in facilitating diagnostic interviewing. In terms of eliciting new behaviors, new and known information, and clarifying diagnosis and psychodynamic formulations, there were no significant differences between the active and placebo sessions.

Furthermore, in comparing the Hamilton Depression Scale, the NHSI, and the BPRS for both sessions, no significant differences were found between placebo and active sessions, as noted by either the interviewer or the blind rater. Again, these results suggest that sodium amobarbital had no significant effect in unmasking repressed schizophrenic (psychotic) or affective symptoms.

Discussion

It should be recognized that sodium amobarbital interviews are used for other purposes, beyond those noted above (13,14). It has been reported, for example, that sodium amobarbital causes a lucid interval in catatonic patients (a finding we also observed in one catatonic), and barbituates may also be useful in clarifying a diagnosis of organicity.

However, our findings strongly suggest that sodium amobarbital is no more effective than placebo in eliciting new psychopathologic behaviors, or in eliciting new information or specific symptoms that would help in the differential diagnosis of schizophrenia versus affect disorder. Both the placebo and the active amobarbital condition moderately facilitated the acquisition of new information. Separate studies to verify the usefulness of barbituates in other situations need to be conducted to further explore their efficacy.

CONCLUSION

We have examined the use of physostigmine, methylphenidate and sodium amobarbital as provocative agents with potential to clarify diagnostic issues among hospitalized psychiatric patients. With the exception of catatonic schizophrenia, we conclude that sodium amobarbital does not have a specific pharmacological effect,compared to placebo, in uncovering material that might aid in the differential diagnosis between schizophrenia and depression. On the other hand, physostigmine may have some usefulness in identifying patients who have an affective component to their illness, by virtue of its possible ability to selectively increase depressive symptomatology. More research will have to be carried out before we can be certain that the risk/benefit ratio will justify physostigmine use as a diagnostic procedure in psychiatry, since physostigmine has numerous side effects and countraindications. Finally, methylphenidate administration exacerbates schizophrenic thought processes. This can be valuable in distinguishing schizophrenia (or other psychotic states) from non-psychotic syndromes. However, it must be noted that methylphenidate, like physostigmine, must be carefully evaluated as to its risk/benefit ratio in a given patient, since it also has a variety of side effects and several contraindications.

(1) Janowsky, D.S., El-Yousef, M.K., and Davis, J.M. Provocation of schizophrenic symptoms by intravenous administration of methylphenidate. Arch. Gen. Psychiatry 28:185-191 (1973).

(2) Janowsky, D.S. and Davis, J.M. Methylphenidate, d-amphetamine, and l-amphetamine: Effects on schizophrenic symptoms. Arch. Gen. Psychiatry 33(3):304-308 (1976).

(3) Janowsky, D.S., Huey, L., Storms, L. et al. Methylphenidate effects on psychological tests in acute schizophrenics and non-psychotics. Arch. Gen. Psychiatry 34:189-194 (1977).

(4) Palermo, D. and Jenkins, J. Word Association Norms: Grade School Through College. Univ. of Minnesota Press, Minneapolis (1974).

(5) Holtzman, W. Ink Blot Technique: Administration and Scoring Guide. Univ. of Minnesota Press, Minneapolis (1964).

(6) Janowsky, D.S., El-Yousef, M.K. and Davis, J.M. Acetylcholine and depression. Psychosom. Med. 36:248-257 (1974).

(7) Janowsky, D.S., El-Yousef, M.K., Davis, J.M., et al. Parasympathetic suppression of manic symptoms by physostigmine. Arch. Gen. Psychiatry 28:542-547 (1973).

(8) Janowsky, D.S., El-Yousef, M.K. and Davis, J.M. Antagonistic effects of physostigmine and methylphenidate in man. Am. J. Psychiatry 130:1370-1376 (1973).

(9) Davis, K.L., Hollister, L.E., Overall, J., et al. Physostigmine: effects on cognition and affect in normal subjects. Psychopharmacology 51:23-27 (1976).

(10) Pennes, H.H.: Clinical reactions of schizophrenics to sodium amytal, pervitin hydrochloride, mescaline sulfate, and d-lysergic acid diethylamide (LSD-25). J. Nerv. Ment. Dis. 119:95-112 (1954).

(11) Cohn, W.M., Speck, R.V. and Howard, W.J.: Sodium amytal as an aid in state hospital practice: single interviews with 100 patients. Psychiat. Quart. 31:289-300 (1957).

(12) Lindemann, E.: Psychological changes in normal and abnormal individuals under the influence of sodium amytal. Am. J. Psychiatry 88:1083-1091 (1932).

(13) Weinstein, E.A., Kahn, R.L., Sugarman, L.A., et al: The diagnostic use of amobarbital sodium ("amytal sodium") in brain disease. Am. J. Psychiatry 109:889-894 (1953).

(14) Thorner, M.W.: The psycho-pharmacology of sodium amytal in catatonia. J. Nerv. Ment. Dis. 82:299-303 (1935).

Neuropeptides and Psychiatry

Summary of Symposium on "Endorphins"

ERMINIO COSTA

Laboratory of Preclinical Pharmacology, N.I.M.H., Saint Elizabeths Hospital, Washington, D.C. 20032

The symposium on endorphins breached basic sciences with psychiatry and included presentations of the basic issues and of the first clinical trials with beta-lipotropin 61-91. This presentation was given by Dr. N.S. Kline (Rockland State Hosp. Orangeburg, N.Y.) who convinced the audience that there was some merit in continuing experiments on the effects caused by the administration of beta-lipotropin 61-91 to patients affected with psychoses. The reason for this therapeutic activity and the mechanisms that are operative in relieving the symptoms of psychoses were not elucidated by Dr. Kline and his associates.

Dr. H. Emrich (Max Planck Institute for Psychiatry, Munich, Germany) presented immunochemical studies of the endorphin content of spinal fluid and plasma of psychotics, but his data failed to reveal that in psychotics there are important changes in plasma and spinal fluid levels of immunoreactive material. He concluded that the use of beta-lipotropin 61-91 in psychaitry was not supported by these biochemical studies. Here, one should first consider whether it is justifiable to assume that a defect in the metabolism or storage of beta-lipotropin 61-65 or 61-91 in brain should be accompanied by a change in the spinal fluid or plasma content of beta-lipotropin 61-65 or 61-91-like immunoreactive material. First of all, it must be noted that the antibodies used by Dr. Emrich cross react with beta-lipotropin 61-91 and that this material reaches the blood following secretion from pituitary. However, as far as we know today, the brain pools of beta-lipotropin 61-91 and beta-lipotropin 61-65 are metabolically independent from the pituitary pool and presumably from the plasma levels of beta-lipotropin 1-91. However, it is possible that pituitary secretes beta-lipotropin into the spinal fluid and by this mechanism influences brain biosynthesis of beta-lipotropin 61-91 and 61-65. Of course, if the blood and spinal fluid levels reflect pituitary secretion, they could be in equilibrium and, therefore, blood levels could mirror the precursor concentrations reaching the brain. Indeed, we do not know what measurements can be made to evaluate the existence of a defect in the biosynthesis or utilization of beta-lipotropin 61-91 in the brain of psychotic patients. Actually, we are still unable to evaluate in vivo the synthesis rate of lipotropin 61-65 or 61-91 in the brain of rats. The report by Dr. W. Bunney, Jr. (Adult Psychiatry Branch, NIMH, Bethesda, Md) focussed again on clinical studies, dealt with the use of opiate receptor antagonists to alleviate the symptoms of schizophrenia. Essentially he presented negative results. Hence, he failed to support the contention that schizophrenia may reflect an excessive activation of endorphinergic transmission as suggested by the Swedish School.

A final attempt to relate psychoses to the changes in endorphin function could be based on the assumption that a deficit in endorphinergic transmission underlies psychoses. In support of this contention, Dr. J. S. Hong (Laboratory of Preclinical Pharmacology, NIMH, Washington, D. C.) reported that antipsychotic drugs increase beta-lipotropin 61-65 content in the N. accumbens and N. caudatus but not in the cortex, hippocampus, pons-medulla and pituitary. This increase appears only after repeated injections of antipsychotics and requires a treatment of at least one or two weeks to reach its peak. One injection is inactive and when the treatment is discontinued after two weeks of injections, it takes about ten days to attain normalization of the beta-lipotropin 61-65 content of striatum and N. accumbens. When a series of antipsychotics was compared for their potency to increase the beta-lipotropin 61-65 content the active dose of a given drug relates to its efficacy to limit the severity of certain symptoms of psychoses. For instance, the active dose of clozapine to increase the content of beta-lipotropin 61-65 in rat striatum and to overcome the symptoms of schizophrenia is about one-hundred times greater than that of haloperidol. Dr. Hong reported that preliminary results indicate that after chronic treatment the antipsychotics increase the synthesis rate of beta-lipotropin 61-65 in those brain structures that are innervated by dopamine. Moreover, he said that probably this increase was due to an increase in the number of molecules of a rate limiting enzyme. Finally, he showed that the antipsychotics increased the striatal content of a high molecular weight precursor of beta-lipotropin 61-65. This precursor is not an extension of the carboxy terminus of beta-lipotropin 61-65 such as beta-lipotropin 61-91 but an extension of the aminoterminus. This work could support the speculation that the involvement of dopaminergic transmission in schizophrenia relates to synapses between these neurons and enkephalinergic neurons. The increase in dopaminergic transmission may decrease the enkephalin available and this decrease would participate in causing certain symptoms in schizophrenia patients.

In view of the current uncertainties it was important to consolidate the picture of the current views on the role of beta-lipotropin derivatives endowed with opiate-like activity by listening to two reports from basic scientists: one was made by Dr. F. Moroni (Department of Pharmacology,University of Florence, Italy) and concerned the actions of beta-lipotropin 61-91 on the turnover of acetylcholine and GABA of various brain structures of rats and the other by Dr. Horace Loh (Department of Psychiatry, University of California, San Francisco, Cal.) and concerned basic pharmacological studies of beta-lipotropin activities. The data presented by Dr. Moroni can be interpreted to indicate that opiate receptors regulate the firing of neurons from the septal hippocampal cholinergic pathway. These neurons perform a number of important regulatory activities on the limbic system including an inhibitory role in the expression of emotional and aggressive behavior. It is possible to infer that if there is an insufficient occupancy of septal opiate receptor aggression and emotion are out of the septal control which is mediated by beta-lipotropin 61-91. This brings about an animal extremely aggressive and unable to respond with an intensity proportional to the stimulus. Dr. Moroni further showed that occupancy of striatal opiate receptors by beta-lipotropin 61-91 causes muscular rigidity. However, this extrapyramidal rigidity differs from that caused by a blockade of dopamine receptors. When dopamine receptors are blocked, the striatal acetylcholine turnover is decreased but the turnover of striatal GABA is unchanged, in contrast, the striatal opiate receptors are activated, the turnover of striatal GABA is increased but the turnover of striatal acetylcholine fails to change.

The present understanding of the secretion of beta-lipotropin 1-91 derivatives by various brain pathways suggests that there are two families of such neurons: those that secrete beta-lipotropin 61-91, and those that beta-lipotropin 61-65 together with leu-enkephalin. The latter is an analogue of beta-lipotropin 61-65 with leucine substituting methionine. Beta-lipotropin 61-91 is stored in a group of neurons with cell bodies in the hypothalamus and long projecting axons innervating among others structures medial septum, cortex and locus coeruleus. In contrast, neurons containing beta-lipotropin 61-65 and leu-enkephalin represent a diffuse system of interneurons which tend to establish axoaxonic contacts with postsynaptic elements. Such beta-lipotropin 61-65 secreting neurons are abundant in the N. accumbens and N. caudatus and project to the globus pallidus. Another long axon pathway of neurons containing beta-lipotropin 61-65 and leu-enkephalin has the cell bodies located in amygdala and the axons project to the stria terminalis.

Dr. Loh reported on the present understanding of the physiological role of these two families of neurons. Clearly little is understood: from pharmacological studies, it would appear that beta-lipotropin 61-91 might be the transmitter involved in pain reception regulation. However, it appears that many other functions are mediated in brain by this and the other family of neurons secreting opiate receptor agonists. These functions extend to the reward system; it might be that a defect in the latter function that is operative in the psychosis.

In conclusion, it is possible that like many other neuronal systems, also the endorphinergic neurons are malfunctioning in psychotic states. However, there is no compelling evidence available yet to support the view that a primary defect of schizophrenia is a dysfunction of these neuronal pathways.

Possible Function of β Endorphin

J. W. HOLADAY*, G. L. BELENKY*, A. I. FADEN* and H. H. LOH**

*Department of Medical Neurosciences, Walter Reed Army Institute of Research, Washington, D.C.
**Department of Pharmacology and Langley Porter Neuropsychiatric Institute, University of California, San Francisco

ABSTRACT

The pharmacological administration of endorphins as well as the specific opiate antagonist naloxone have been utilized to study the possible physiological and behavioral roles for endogenous opiates. While the most universally accepted function for endorphins involves their attenuation of the perception of painful stimuli, other important physiological roles for these substances have recently been suggested. Our research efforts have been focused upon the potential role of endorphins in heat adaptation and in shock states as well as in their effects on pituitary function and in electroconvulsive shock. These investigations are the primary focus of this review which also briefly examines the possible involvement of endorphins in such diverse functions as grooming behavior, memory, seizures, and sexual behavior.

INTRODUCTION

The possibility that the body can regulate its own perception of noxious stimuli through endogenous opiate systems has captured the imagination of biological scientists throughout the world. Many excellent reviews chronologically summarize the discovery of opiate receptors and the subsequent isolation and purification of their native ligands, generically termed endorphins (Goldstein, 1976; Guillemin, 1977; Snyder and Simantov, 1977; Li, 1977). Current interest is primarily focused upon two types of endorphins: the pentapeptide enkephalins which are distributed in proximity to opiate receptors in pain-modulating areas of the central nervous system and a larger hypothalamic-pituitary peptide, β endorphin, which may subserve a hormonal role and/or also affect the perception of pain.

Our own research over the past three years has been directed at establishing possible physiological and behavioral roles for β endorphin. This objective has been approached both through the pharmacological administration of β endorphin and through administration of naloxone, a specific antagonist of opiate compounds. Injections of β endorphin result in pharmacological effects which mimic those of morphine and other alkaloid opiates. However, due to differences between exogenously administered and endogenously released endorphin concentrations at receptor areas, the pharmacological effects of β endorphin may not reliably predict an endogenous physiological function. The use of naloxone may be of greater value in uncovering specific physiological endorphin involvement. Since naloxone blocks opiate receptors, its administration may produce effects which are predictive of a blockade of endorphin-mediated events. However, since naloxone is efficacious in blocking both enkephalin and β endorphin at the receptor level, one cannot use this tool per se to discriminate between the effects of these two endogenous opiate ligands.

We feel that the best evidence for an endorphin role in physiology and behavior would be obtained by using both the above techniques in conjunction with actual measurement of endorphin levels. However, radioimmunoassay techniques for these endogenous ligands are still fraught with difficulties and, for the moment, their routine usefulness is limited. The predominant problems facing investigators who are attempting to measure endorphin concentrations are these extremely low concentrations in biological tissues combined with extraction difficulties and antisera specificities.

In the following pages, we will only briefly mention the possible endorphin involvement in responses to pain since this subject is well reviewed in the cited literature. The focus of this manuscript is on other possible endorphin functions which we have studied in our laboratories. These include a possible role for endorphins in temperature regulation and in behavioral effects which follow electroconvulsive shock in rats. In addition, we present evidence which suggests that endorphins may be involved in the hypotension that occurs in shock states. Lastly, we briefly review the neuroendocrine effects of endorphins and naloxone followed by miscellaneous reports which implicate other possible endorphin functions.

PAIN PERCEPTION

The most universally accepted function ascribed to endorphins is their role in modulating responses to noxious stimuli (Terenius, 1978). In studies with rats and mice, β endorphin was shown to be more potent than morphine in its antinociceptive effects whether administered intraventricularly (ivt) or intravenously (iv) (Loh and colleagues, 1976; Tseng, Loh and Li, 1976). Moreover, evidence was obtained to suggest that β endorphin may result in analgesia in man as well (Catlin and coworkers, 1977).

The perception of noxious stimuli is enhanced following naloxone injections in mice and rats (Jacob, Tremblay, and Colombel, 1974). This would be expected if naloxone were antagonizing the antinociceptive effects of endogenous opiates. In humans, Buchsbaum, Davis and Bunney (1978) demonstrated hyperalgesic effects of naloxone in pain-insensitive individuals. In addition, Levine and colleagues (1978) reported that naloxone causes a significantly greater increase in reported pain intensity than placebo in patients following the extraction of impacted wisdom teeth. Even acupuncture analgesia in man is antagonized by naloxone preinjection (Mayer, Price, and Rafii, 1977). Taken together, it is apparent that endorphins may be important in decreasing the perceived intensity of painful stimuli. However, whether or not pituitary β endorphin subserves this role in a physiological sense remains to be firmly established.

TEMPERATURE REGULATION

The administration of alkaloid opiates and endorphins has been shown to alter body temperature (Lomax, 1970; Bloom and coworkers, 1976; Tseng, Loh and Li, 1977). Relatively low doses of opiates which result in only mild analgesia produce elevations in body temperature, whereas higher doses progressively lead to a lowering of body temperature (Lomax, 1970; Holaday and colleagues, 1977). We were curious as to why body temperature could both increase and decrease depending upon the dose of β endorphin injected. The possibility existed that β endorphin always lowered the body's central thermostat, however attempts to compensate for this perceived cooling could result in thermogenic behaviors that would initially, at lower doses, outweigh the ultimate _hypo_thermic effects of β endorphin.

Bloom and colleagues (1976) noted the occurrence of "wet-dog" shakes immediately following ivt β endorphin injections. We too noted this behavior (Holaday, Loh and Li, 1978), and found the number of "wet-dog" shakes to be positively correlated with increases in colonic temperature in rats. Temporally following the cessation of the thermogenic "wet-dog" shakes, β endorphin-injected rats developed copious salivation accompanied by a clonic, seizure-like behavior. The time of onset of this sialogogic effect coincided with increased body temperature. Parenthetically, salivation and saliva-spreading are the predominant cooling mechanisms in rats (Hainsworth, 1967). We found that the same dose of β endorphin produced greater salivation at elevated ambient temperatures, further suggesting that this effect of β endorphin is related to an alteration in thermoregulation. Thus, it appeared possible that the occurrence of initial "wet-dog" shakes may have resulted in an elevated body temperature which subsequently precipitated the excess salivation (Holaday, Loh and Li, 1978). Furthermore, following injection of higher doses of β endorphin, rats may be immobilized and therefore unable to elicit thermogenic behaviors. An actual fall in body temperature could then occur.

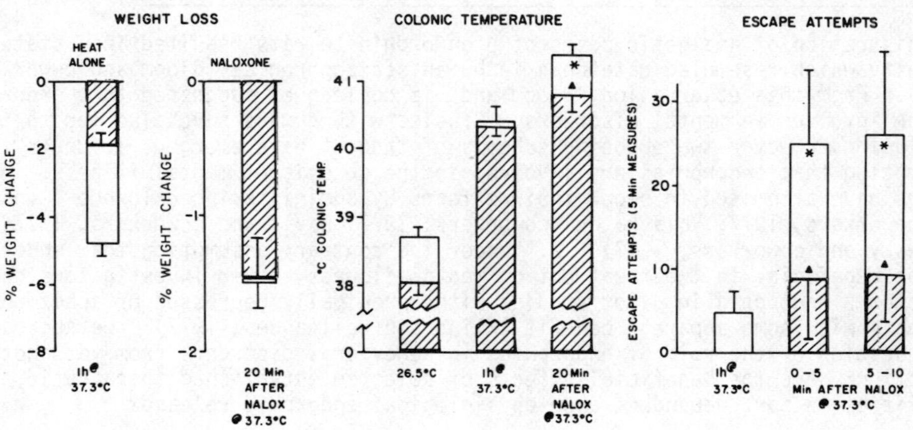

Fig. 1. Comparison of hypophysectomized rats (shaded bars) with sham-operated controls (clear bars) before and after 1 hr. exposure at 37.3°C and subsequent injection of 10 mg/Kg naloxone HCl. Vertical lines are SEM; statistical comparisons within surgical groups (n = 6/group). Asterisk denotes p < .05; triangle denotes lack of significance. Comparisons were made 20 min after naloxone injection.

If endorphins subserve a physiological role in the maintenance of normothermia, then their blockade by naloxone should produce an effect on body temperature. Naloxone injections in cold-exposed rats would be expected to lower body temperature if endorphins function as endogenous hyperthermic regulators. Goldstein and Lowery (1975), however, found no such effect of naloxone in cold-exposed rats.

From our prior work, we suggested the converse, ie that naloxone should elevate temperatures in heat-exposed rats if endorphins were endogenous hypothermic regulators. Indeed, we found that not only does naloxone elevate temperatures following heat-exposure, but other signs of hyperthermia were also observed (Holaday and colleagues, 1978a). This occurred after acute or chronic heat exposure.

To determine if pituitary endorphins were involved in these responses, we compared the effects of naloxone in hypophysectomized and sham-hypophysectomized control rats. The fact that naloxone was almost without effect in heat-exposed, hypophysectomized rats (Fig. 1) suggested to us that pituitary endorphins such as β endorphin may be important in the physiological regulation of body temperature.

Since pain and temperature sensations are known to be mediated through some common neuroanatomical pathways, it is not surprising that endorphins may play a dual role in regulating both body temperature and the perception of painful stimuli. Our evidence presented above suggests pituitary endorphins may modulate temperature (Fig. 1). Recently, Grevert, Baizman and Goldstein (1978) have used a similar paradigm to compare the efficacy of naloxone in producing hyperalgesia in hypophysectomized and sham-hypophysectomized control mice. In their study, naloxone did not reduce nociceptive latencies in hypophysectomized mice, only in the sham-control animals. Taken together, these findings may essentially suggest that pituitary endorphins are physiologically involved in temperature regulation as well as pain perception.

STIMULATED ENDORPHIN RELEASE - EFFECTS OF ELECTROCONVULSIVE SHOCK

Administration of analgetic doses of β endorphin to rats resulted in a state of rigidity which resembled catatonia in human schizophrenics (Bloom and coworkers, 1976). From this observation, Bloom and his colleagues suggested that endorphins may be involved in mental disorders. Studies with humans have also led to this conclusion, however two opposing schools of thought have emerged: 1. Under the assumption that endorphins are involved in the genesis of mental illness, investigators have attempted to block their effects by administering naloxone (Gunne and coworkers, 1977; Volavka and coworkers, 1977; Davis and coworkers, 1977; and Janowsky and coworkers, 1977). 2. Under the contrary assumption that endorphins may be beneficial in the treatment of mental illness, other investigators have injected β endorphin in pilot studies with chronically depressed or schizophrenic patients with some apparent benefit (Kline and colleagues, 1977). We approached the question of the role of endorphins in behavioral disorders from yet another direction: Are the beneficial effects of selected established therapeutic modalities in part dependent upon physiological endorphin release?

Electroconvulsive therapy (ECT), a technique that uses electroconvulsive shock (ECS) to induce a generalized seizure, is effective in treating severe depression and some cases of schizophrenia (Greenblatt, 1977). We wondered whether ECS would result in a functional release of endorphins in rats. We found that transauricular ECS in rats induced a state of catalepsy characterized by a loss of righting reflex

(Holaday, Belenky, Loh and Meyerhoff, 1978; Holaday and coworkers, in preparation). This treatment also resulted in an increase in nociceptive latencies. In fact, ECS treated rats closely resembled rats which we have observed following injections of morphine or β endorphin. These opiate-like effects of ECS appeared to be reduced when naloxone was injected prior to ECS (Fig. 2).

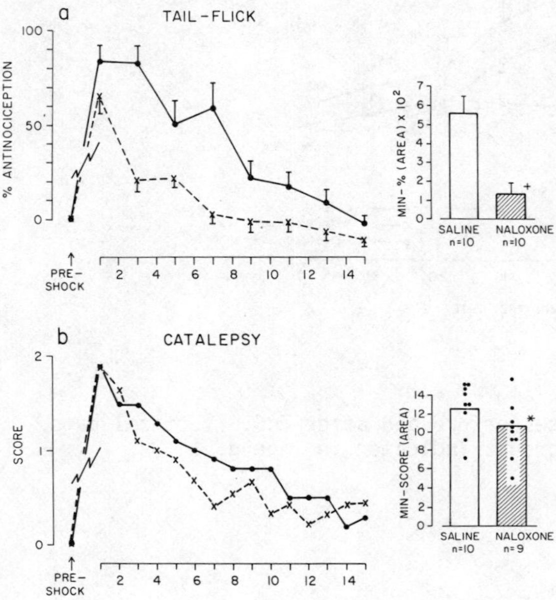

Fig. 2. Tail-flick latencies (top) and catalepsy (bottom) were measured following ECS. Solid lines and clear bars represent saline-pretreated rats, dashed lines and solid bars represent rats pretreated with 10 mg/Kg naloxone HCl. Drugs were injected ip 10 min. prior to ECS. Integrated response-areas over time for individual rats were averaged and shown on the right. Vertical lines (top) are + SEM; t = $p < .001$ (Student's t), * = $p < .05$ (Mann-Whitney U).

In an extension of these studies, we specifically focused upon respiratory rates and blood pressure changes following ECS (Holaday and Belenky, in preparation). The data in Fig. 3 demonstrate the effects of two different dosages of naloxone on respiratory rates in ECS-treated rats. We found respiratory rates post-ECS to be higher in those rats preinjected with naloxone, suggesting that endorphin release during ECS may serve to maintain normal respiratory rates following this procedure. Since ECT in humans is also known to produce transient hypertension, we characterized the ECS-induced changes in blood pressure in saline and naloxone-preinjected rats (Fig. 4). Peak elevations in mean arterial pressure (MAP) were the same in both groups of rats, however, naloxone-injected rats sustained a higher blood pressure for the first 20 seconds. Subsequently, these rats became significantly more hypotensive until 30 sec. following ECS.

Since ECS in rats produced a spectrum of opiate-like effects which were, to varying degrees, attenuated or modified by naloxone pretreatment, we suggest that ECS stimulates the functional release of endorphins. It is possible that such an endorphin release also occurs during ECT in humans and may contribute to the established therapeutic efficacy of that procedure. More conservatively, however, our data suggest that respiratory and cardiovascular changes following ECS may be related to endorphin release.

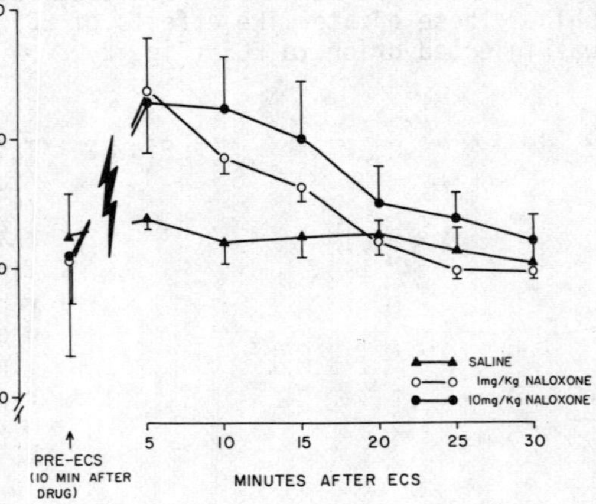

Fig. 3. Comparison of respiratory rates before and after ECS. Vertical bars represent ± SEM. Treatment groups indicated in legend.

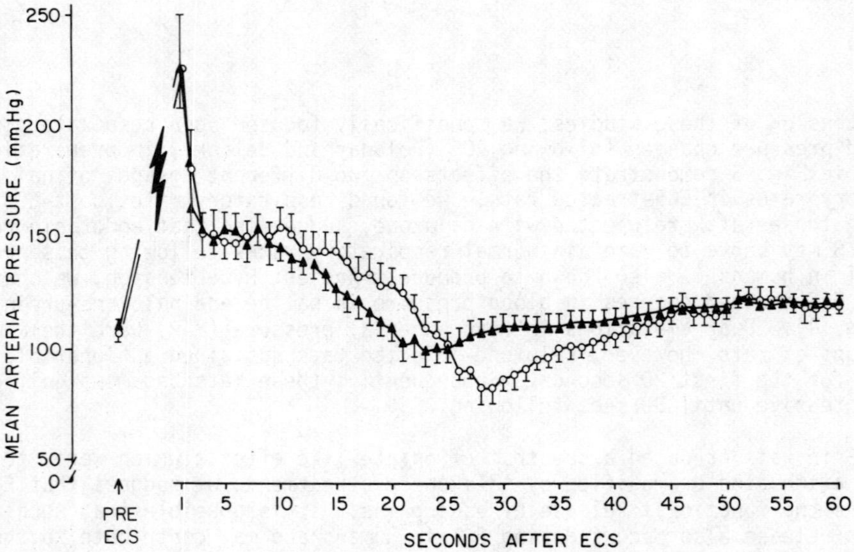

Fig. 4. Comparison of mean arterial pressure in saline-pretreated (triangles) and naloxone pretreated (10 mg/Kg; open circles) rats following transauricular ECS. Drugs were injected i.p. 10 min prior to ECS, vertical bars represent ± SEM.

ENDORPHINS IN THE PATHOPHYSIOLOGY OF SHOCK

The cardiovascular system is exquisitely sensitive to the effects of exogenous opiates (Evans, Nasmyth, and Stewart, 1952; Gokhale, Gulati, and Joshi, 1963). In rats, less than 1% of the morphine dose necessary to produce antinociception results in significant hypotension and bradycardia (Fennessy and Rattray, 1971). In addition, the endogenous opiate Met-enkephalin has been shown to have central hypotensive effects in rats (Florez and Mediavilla, 1977) and in dogs (Laubie and colleagues, 1977).

Intravenous β endorphin also produces hypotension in various animal models (Holaday and colleagues, in preparation). Since stressors result in the release of β endorphin from the pituitary gland (Guillemin and coworkers, 1977; Rossier and coworkers, 1978), it appeared possible that shock-induced stress could release β endorphin and thus result in a depression of blood pressure.

The administration of bacterial lipopolysaccharide endotoxin in animals has often been used as a model of human septic shock (Gilbert, 1960; Waisbren, 1964). It has been suggested that the profound hypotension induced by endotoxin is mediated through the release of endogenous substances (Gilbert, 1960; Waisbren, 1964). We hypothesized that if endorphins were functionally released by endotoxins and involved in the hypotensive effects produced by endotoxins, then blockade of endorphins should reverse such hypotension (Holaday and Faden, 1978; Faden and Holaday, in preparation). To test this hypothesis, we employed naloxone in studies of blood pressure changes following endotoxin administration to conscious rats. Out results demonstrated that naloxone not only rapidly reversed endotoxin-induced hypotension (Fig. 5), but also prophylactically blocked its occurrence (Holaday and Faden, 1978).

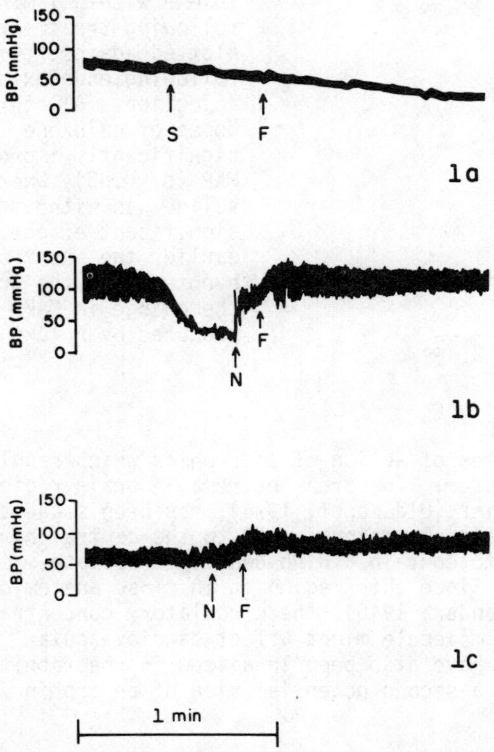

Fig. 5. Comparison of the effects of intravenous naloxone HCl [(N), 1 mg/Kg] versus saline (S) following endotoxin-induced hypotension in conscious rats. Cannulae were flushed (F) with 0.2 cc saline to ensure complete drug delivery. Fig. 1a represents the effects of saline following an early hypotensive episode, Fig. 1b represents the effects of naloxone on an equivalently early period of hypotension. Fig. 1c represents the effects of naloxone following a later hypotension that was more gradual in onset.

Further studies demonstrated that the more rapid and early the hypotension produced by endotoxin, the more rapid and complete the reversal of this effect by naloxone (Figs. 5 and 6). The important issue as to whether naloxone affects survival in endotoxin treated rats was also studied (Faden and Holaday, in preparation). We found that naloxone did not alter survival time in these rats, however the apparent cause of death was not a direct effect of lowered blood-pressure since naloxone treated rats had normal or elevated MAP at death whereas saline-control rats were significantly hypotensive at death.

From these data, we conclude that endorphins may play a pathophysiological role in shock states. We have also recently demonstrated a similar effect of naloxone in restoring blood pressure in a rat model of hemorrhagic shock (Faden and Holaday, in preparation). Thus, naloxone may be an important therapeutic drug in the treatment and management of a variety of shock syndromes.

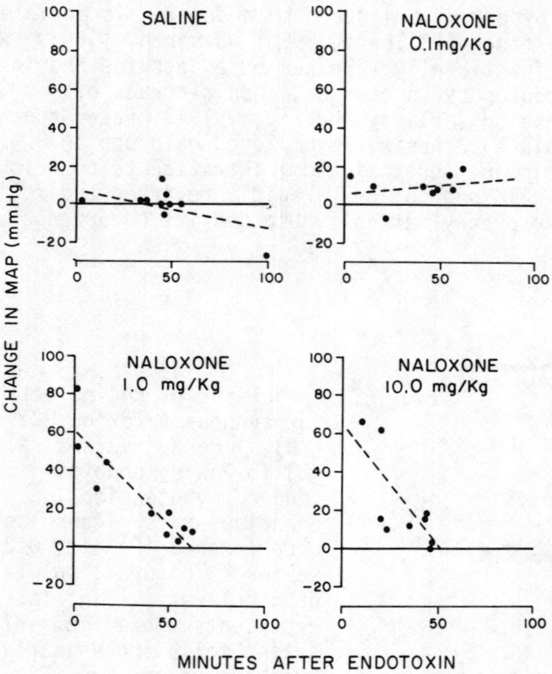

Fig. 6. The effects of saline and varying doses of naloxone HCl are compared following endotoxin-induced hypotension. Rats were not treated until mean arterial pressures (MAP) attained the low value of 65 mm Hg. Subsequent change in MAP within 1 min following treatment are plotted against time following endotoxin-injection. All three doses of naloxone significantly improved MAP ($p < .05$), whereas saline was without significant effect. The earlier the onset of hypotension, the greater the change in MAP produced by naloxone.

Once released, what are the possible sites of action of endorphins which result in alterations of the cardiovascular system? The area postrema, a brain region relatively devoid of a blood-brain barrier (Oldendorf, 1974), has been suggested to be a site where the polar morphine molecule gains access to the central nervous system. This area has also been shown to contain a high density of opiate receptors (Snyder and Simantov, 1977). Since this region is in close anatomical proximity to the vasomotor center (Alexander, 1946), the circulatory concentrations of the relatively large endorphin molecule might affect cardiovascular changes at this site. Opiate receptors have also been localized in the rabbit heart (Klee, 1977), possibly indicating a second potential site of endorphin action.

NEUROENDOCRINE EFFECTS OF ENDORPHINS AND NALOXONE

Pharmacological administration of alkaloid opiates is known to produce a spectrum of effects at the pituitary level (George, 1971; George and Lomax, 1972; de Wied, 1974). Recently, several investigators have studied such effects following pharmacological injections of enkephalins and β endorphin (see Holaday and Loh, 1978 for review). In general, if one restricts data to the acute effects of alkaloid or endogenous opiates, increases in adrenocorticotropin (ACTH), growth hormone (GH), prolactin (PRL), and anti-diuretic hormone (ADH) are seen. On the other hand, these opiates produce decreases or little change in circulating concentrations of thyrotropin (TSH), luteinizing hormone (LH), and follicle stimulating hormone (FSH). The great majority of studies indicate that isolated pituitary glands do not produce this spectrum of effects when directly exposed to opiates (Holaday and Loh, 1978). Thus, it seems probable that endorphins do not directly modulate pituitary function, but appear to affect the pituitary indirectly, possibly through hypothalamic neurotransmitter systems.

Again, since pharmacological injections of endorphins probably do not mimic the physiological state, caution must be exercised in interpreting the above results. The effects of naloxone on endocrine secretions may be more useful in this regard as well. Bruni and colleagues (1977) have reported that naloxone decreases PRL levels and increases LH and FSH in the plasma. Shaar and coworkers (1977) have also shown that naloxone decreases PRL and additionally decreases plasma GH. More recently, van Vugt, Bruni and Meites (1978) have shown that stress-induced increases in PRL secretion in rats were inhibited by naloxone. Therefore, evidence is accumulating to suggest that endorphins may function in the regulation of pituitary secretion.

MISCELLANEOUS EFFECTS OF ENDORPHINS

In addition to those already mentioned, the intense interest in endorphins has resulted in experimental evidence for a variety of other hypotheses regarding the possible function of these substances. Gispen and colleagues (1976) have found that β endorphin and other peptides that appear to originate from the same precursor (β melanocyte stimulating hormone and ACTH) produce excessive grooming behavior in rats upon intraventricular injection. Rigter (1978) proposes that the endorphins may subserve a role in memory since the systemic administration of enkephalins reduced experimentally induced amnesia in rats. It has also been suggested that endorphins may be involved in seizure disorders. Frenk, McCarty, and Liebeskind (1978) have found seizures and other pathological electroencephalographic changes following enkephalin injections into specific brain regions. We have observed overt behavioral seizures following intraventricular β endorphin administration (Holaday, Loh and Li, 1978). Lastly, the possibility that endorphins are involved in sexual behavior has been studied. Meyerson and Terenius (1977) report an effect of β endorphin on sexual behavior in the rat, although Goldstein and Hansteen (1977) found that naloxone produced no observable effects upon sexual arousal or orgasm in man.

Limitations of space and time have permitted but a brief discussion of some of the possible functions of endorphins. Further data are required to substantiate or refute the various potential roles ascribed to β endorphin in this manuscript. However, it is important to mention that endorphins are probably not ubiquitously involved as critical determinants in all of these systems which we have discussed. Instead, the variety of endorphin studies which have been performed reflects the diversity of interest their discovery has stimulated.

REFERENCES

Alexander, R.S. (1946). Tonic and reflex functions of medullary sympathetic cardiovascular centers. J. Neurophysiol., 9, 205-217.

Bloom, F., D. Segal, N. Ling, and R. Guillemin (1976). Endorphins: profound behavioral effects in rats suggest new etiological factors in mental illness. Science, 194, 630-632.

Bruni, J.P., D. van Vugt, S. Marshall, and J. Meites (1977). Effects of naloxone, morphine, and methionine enkephalin on serum prolactin, luteinizing hormone, follicle stimulating hormone, thyroid stimulating hormone and growth hormone. Life Sci., 21, 461-466.

Buchsbaum, M.S., G.C. Davis, and W.E. Bunney (1977). Naloxone alters pain perception and somatosensory evoked potentials in normal subjects. Nature, 270, 620-622.

Catlin, D.H., K.K. Hui, H.H. Loh, and C.H. Li (1977). Pharmacologic activity of β-endorphin in man. Commun. in Psychopharm., 1, 493-500.

Davis, G.C., W.E. Bunney, E.G. De Fraites, J.E. Kleinman, D.P. van Kammen, R.M. Post, and R.J. Wyatt (1977). Intravenous naloxone administration in schizophrenia and affective illness. Science, 197, 74-76.

de Wied, D., J.M. van Ree, and W. de Jong (1974). Narcotic analgesia and the neuroendocrine control of anterior pituitary function. In E. Zimmermann and R. George (eds.), Narcotics and the Hypothalamus. Raven Press, New York.

Evans, A.G.J., P.A. Nasmyth, and H.C. Stewart (1952). The fall of blood pressure caused by intravenous morphine in the rat and the cat. Brit. J. P'col., 7, 542-552.

Faden, A.I. and J.W. Holaday (1978). Naloxone treatment of endotoxin shock: physiologic, pharmacologic, and behavioral effects in the rat. (submitted).

Fennessy, M.R. and J.F. Rattray (1971). Cardiovascular effects of intravenous morphine in the anaesthetized rat. Eur. J. P'col., 14, 1-8.

Florez, J. and A. Mediavilla (1977). Respiratory and cardiovascular effects of met-enkephalin applied to the ventral surface of the brainstem. Brain Res., 138, 585-590.

Frenk, H., B.C. McCarty, and J.C. Liebeskind (1978). Different brain areas mediate the analgesic and epileptic properties of enkephalin. Science, 200, 335-337.

George, R. (1971). Hypothalamus: anterior pituitary gland. In D.H. Clouet (Ed.), Narcotic Drugs Biochemical Pharmacology. Plenum Press, New York.

George, R. and P. Lomax (1972). Hormones. In S.J. Mule and H. Brill (Eds.), Chemical and Biological Aspects of Drug Dependence. CRC Press, Cleveland.

Gilbert, R.R. (1960). Mechanisms of the hemodynamic effects of endotoxin. Physiol. Rev., 40, 245-279.

Gispen, W.H., V.M. Wiegant, A.F. Bradbury, E.C. Hulme, D.G. Smyth, C.R. Snell, and D. de Wied (1976). Induction of excessive grooming in the rat by fragments of lipotropin. Nature, 264, 794-795.

Gokhale, S.D., O.D. Gulati and N.Y. Joshi (1963). Effect of some blocking drugs on the pressor response to physostigmine in the rat. Brit. J. P'col., 21, 273-284.

Goldstein, A. and P.J. Lowery (1975). Effect of the opiate antagonist naloxone on body temperature in rats. Life Sci., 17, 927-932.

Goldstein, A. (1976). Opioid peptides (endorphins) in pituitary and brain. Science, 193, 1081-1086.

Goldstein, A. and R.W. Hansteen (1977). Evidence against involvement of endorphins in sexual arousal and orgasm in man. Arch. Gen. Psychiatry, 34, 1179-1180.

Greenblatt, M. (1977). Efficacy of ECT in affective and schizophrenic illness. Am. J. Psychiatry, 134, 1001-1005.

Grevert, P., E.R. Baizman, and A. Goldstein (1978). Naloxone effects on a nociceptive response of hypophysectomized and adrenalectomized mice. Life Sci., 23, 723-728.

Guillemin, R. (1977). Endorphins, brain peptides that act like opiates. New England J. Med., 296, 226-228.

Guillemin, R., T. Vargas, J. Rossier, S. Minick, N. Ling, C. Rivier, W. Vale, and F. Bloom (1977). β-endorphin and adrenocorticotropin are secreted concomitantly by the pituitary gland. Science, 197, 1367-1369.

Gunne, L.-M., L. Lindstrom, and L. Terenius (1977). Naloxone-induced reversal of schizophrenic hallucinations. J. Neural. Trans., 40, 13-19.

Hainsworth, F.R. (1977). Saliva spreading, activity, and body temperature regulation in the rat. Am. J. Physiol., 212, 1288-1292.

Holaday, J.W., P.-Y. Law, L.-F. Tseng, H.H. Loh and C.H. Li (1977). β-endorphin: pituitary and adrenal glands modulate its action. Proc. Nat'l. Acad. Sci. USA, 74, 4628-4632.

Holaday, J.W., H.H. Loh, and C.H. Li (1978). Unique behavioral effects of β endorphin and their relationship to thermoregulation and hypothalamic function. Life Sci., 22, 1525-1536.

Holaday, J.W., E. Wei, H.H. Loh, and C.H. Li (1978a). Endorphins may function in heat adaptation. Proc. Nat'l. Acad. Sci. USA, 75, 2923-2927.

Holaday, J.W. and A.I. Faden (1978). Naloxone reversal of endotoxin hypotension suggests role of endorphins in shock. Nature, 275, 450-451.

Holaday, J.W., G.L. Belenky, H.H. Loh and J.L. Meyerhoff (1978). Evidence for endorphin release during electroconvulsive shock. Neuroscience Abstracts, 4, #1292, 409.

Holaday, J.W., G.L. Belenky, H.H. Loh, and J.L. Meyerhoff (1978). Electroconvulsive shock in rats: evidence for endorphin release. (in preparation).

Holaday, J.W. and H.H. Loh (1978). Endorphin-opiate interactions with neuroendocrine systems. In H.H. Loh and D.H. Ross (Eds.), Neurochemical Mechanisms of Opiate Action. Raven Press (in press).

Jacob, J.J., E.C. Tremblay, and M.-C. Colombel (1974). Facilitation de reactions nociceptives par la naloxone chez la souris et chez le rat. Psychopharmacologia, 37, 217-223.

Janowsky, D.S., D.S. Segal, F. Bloom, A. Abrams, and R. Guillemin (1977). Lack of effect of naloxone on schizophrenic symptoms. Am. J. Psychiatry, 134, 926-927.

Klee, W.A. (1977). Endogenous opiate peptides. In H. Gainer (Ed.) Peptides in Neurobiology. Plenum Press, New York.

Kline, N.S., C.H. Li, H.E. Lehmann, A. Lajtha, E. Laski, and T. Cooper (1977). β-endorphin-induced changes in schizophrenic and depressed patients. Arch. Gen. Psychiatry, 34, 1111-1113.

Laubie, M., H. Schmitt, M. Vincent and G. Remond (1977). Central cardiovascular effects of morphinomimetic peptides in dogs. Eur. J. P'col., 46, 67-71.

Levine, J.D., N.C. Gordon, R.T. Jones, and H.L. Fields (1978). The narcotic antagonist naloxone enhances clinical pain. Nature, 272, 826-827.

Li, C.H. (1977). β-endorphin: a pituitary peptide with potent morphine-like activity. Arch. Biochem. Biophys., 183, 592-604.

Loh, H.H., L.-F. Tseng, E. Wei, and C.H. Li (1976). β-endorphin is a potent analgesic agent. Proc. Nat'l. Acad. Sci. USA, 73, 2895-2898.

Lomax, P. (1970). Drugs and body temperature. Int. Rev. Neurobiol., 12, 1-43.

Mayer, D.J., D.D. Price, and A. Rafii (1977). Antagonism of acupuncture analgesia in man by the narcotic antagonist naloxone. Brain Res., 121, 368-372.

Meyerson, B.J. and L. Terenius (1977). β-endorphin and male sexual behavior. Eur. J. P'col., 42, 191-192.

Oldendorf, W.H. (1974). Drug penetration of the blood-brain barrier. In E. Zimmermann and R. George (Eds.), Narcotics and the Hypothalamus. Raven Press, New York.

Rigter, H. (1978). Attenuation of amnesia in rats by systemically administered enkephalins. Science, 200, 83-85.

Rossier, J. E.D. French, C. Rivier, N. Ling, R. Guillemin, and F.E. Bloom (1978). Foot-shock induced stress increases β-endorphin levels in blood but not brain. Nature, 270, 618-620.

Shaar, C.J., R.C.A. Frederickson, N.B. Dininger, and L. Jackson (1977). Enkephalin analogues and naloxone modulate the release of growth hormone and prolactin-evidence for regulation of an endogenous opioid peptide in brain. Life Sci., 21, 853-860.

Snyder, S.H., and R. Simantov (1977). The opiate receptor and opioid peptides. J. Neurochem., 28, 13-20.

Terenius, L. (1978). Endogenous peptides and analgesia. Ann. Rev. Pharmacol. Toxicol., 18, 189-204.

Tseng, L.F., H.H. Loh, and C.H. Li (1976). β-endorphin as a potent analgesic by intravenous injection. Nature, 263, 239-240.

Tseng, L.-F., H.H. Loh, and C.H. Li (1977). Human β-endorphin: development of tolerance and behavioral activity in rats. Biochem. Biophys. Res. Commun., 74, 390-396.

van Vugt, D.A., J.F. Bruni, and J. Meites (1978). Naloxone inhibition of stress-induced increase in prolactin secretion. Life Sci., 22, 85-90.

Volavka, J., A. Mallya, S. Baig, and J. Perez-Cruet (1977). Naloxone in chronic schizophrenia. Science, 196, 1227-1228.

Waisbren, B.A. (1964). Gram-negative shock and endotoxin shock. Am. J. Med., 36, 819-824.

Beta-Endorphin Modulates Cholinergic and GABA-ergic Neurotransmission

F. MORONI[1]

Department of Pharmacology, University of Florence, Florence, Italy

ABSTRACT

The interactions of beta endorphin with the cholinergic and the gaba-ergic systems in the rat C.N.S. were studied by massfragmentographically monitoring the turnover rate (TR) of GABA and Acetylcholine in stereomicroscopically isolated brain nuclei after administration of this opioid peptide. Intraventricular beta endorphin is able to induce analgesia and catalepsy as well as a dose-dependent decrease of the TR_{Ach} in the hippocampus and in the globus pallidus. No change has been observed in n. caudatus. Intraseptal injection of beta-endorphin selectively decrease the TR_{Ach} in the hippocampus without causing analgesia or catalepsy. This finding supports the idea that opiate receptors may control neuronal activities unrelated to analgesia and catalepsy. In the GABA field, intraventricular and intra-caudatal injections of beta-endorphin decrease the TR_{GABA} of the caudate and increase that of the globus pallidus. No effects were observed in the hippocampus. These modifications of the GABA metabolism in the basal nuclei are probably correlated with the extrapiramidal effects of beta-endorphin.

INTRODUCTION

The existence of neuronal populations storing and releasing "opioid peptides" has been proposed by Hughes and others (1975) after the isolation and characterisation of the enkephalins,pentapeptides able of specifically binding with the "opioid receptors". Histochemical (Elde and others; 1976), biochemical (Yang and others, 1977), and electrophysiological (North and Williams, 1976; Bradley and others, 1976; Ziegliganzberger and others, 1976) evidence, all

[1]This work was performed in the Laboratory of Preclinical Pharmacology N.I.M.H. Washington D.C., U.S.A.

support this proposal and it is therefore widely accepted that "opioid receptor legands" may be neuromodulators or neurotrasmitters.
The acceptance of this idea implies that "opioid peptides", once released by neurons or exogenously administered, should specifically modifiy the functional activity of other neuronal populations.
Since the study of the interactions of opioid-peptides with other neurons may provide useful information on the physiology of the brain, on the mechanisms of tolerance and dependence on opioids, and on the mechanisms of the action of morphine, experiments were performed on these topics.
These studies may be carried out with electrophysiological or biochemical methods. Each method has inherent limitations.
The anatomical complexity of the brain and the lack of adequate histochemical controls make it difficult for the elctrophysiologists to be sure of the biochemical nature of the neurons they are recording.
Moreover, it is impossible to assess electrophysiologically, in the same animal, the global activity of a biochemically identified neuronal population. Biochemical techniques have, usually, a limited sensitivity in detecting instantaneous changes in neuronal activity, but sometimes can provide useful information about the global functionality of a neuronal population biochemically and anatomically identified.
Direct (Moroni and others, 1978a; Mao and others 1978) and indirect (Cheney and Costa, 1977) evidence supports the idea that the Turnover Rate (TR) of a neurotrasmitter is a good biochemical marker of the functional activity of the neurons storing and releasing that particular putative neurotransmitter.
Therefore, in the experiments here reported, we measured how the TR of Ach and GABA is modified in stereo-microscopically isolated brain nuclei after intraventricular or intranuclear administration of beta-endorphin.
Beta-endorphin is an "endogenous opioid peptide", containing in its molecule met-enkephalin, but probably stored in completely different neuronal populations from the enkephalins (Fratta and others, 1978; Bloom, 1978). We chose beta-endorphin as a prototype of opioid peptides in order to overcome the problems relative to the rapid metabolism of the enkephalins (Meek and others, 1977).
In fact, the metabolism of beta-endorphin seems to be relatively slow (Meek and others, 1977).

METHODS

Measurements of Ach and GABA "Turnover Rate"

The TR_{Ach} was measured in rats by intravenous infusion of Phosphoryl (d_9) choline (ammonium salt) (15 μmol min^{-1}) for 9 min beginning 21 min after intraventricular injection of beta-endorphin. Rats were killed with a high intensity microwave beam focussed on the head, (Guidotti and others, 1974). Brains were removed and sliced into 400 μm-thick coronal sections and punches were made (Koslow and others,

1974) using the atlas of Konig and Klippel (1963) as a general guide. From the brain punches, Ach and Ch were extracted and the percent of deuterium incorporation into Ach and Ch, as well as the Ach and Ch levels, were determined by G.C.M.S. (Zsilla and others, 1977).
From these data, the TR_{Ach} can be calculated (Racagni and others, 1974). The TR_{GABA} was determined by monotoring the ^{13}C-enrichment of GABA and glutamate during constant rate infusion of ^{13}C-glucose (50 µmol/Kg/min).
GABA, glutamate and their ^{13}C-analogues were measured by a sensitive and specific mass-fragmentographic technique. (Bertilsson and others, 1977).
As previously metioned, the measurements of the TR of Ach and GABA with our techniques, reflect the functional activity of the cholinergic and gabaergic neuronal population. (Moroni and others 1978a).

Canulae Implantation

In order to inject beta endorphin intraventricularly, polyetylene canulae were permanently implanted into the lateral ventricles (Robinson and others, 1969). The polypeptide was freshly dissolved in saline and injected in a volume of 10 µl. In other animals, beta-endorphin was directly injected in selected brain nuclei via chronically implanted canulae. To carry out these experiments, stainless-steel guide canulae (Plastic product Co., Roanoke, Va.) were stereotaxically implanted into various brain areas of "Equithesin"-anaesthetised rats (Konig and Klippel, 1963). Beta-endorphin was injected 2-3 days after surgery using a gear-driven syringe microburet connected through a P.E.20 polyetylene tubing, with an internal canula extending at least 0.5.mm beyond the tip of the guide canula. The volume of each injection was 1 or 2 µl.

RESULTS

Behavioural Effects of Intraventricular, Intraseptal and Intrastriatal beta-Endorphin.

Intraventricular injections of beta-endorphin induced a dose-dependent analgesia and catalepsy.
Table 1 reports the analgesic and cataleptogenic effects of beta-endorphin measured 30 min after intraventricular administration.
Naltrexone (15 µmol/Kg i.p., 15 min before beta-endorphin), completely prevented the beta-endorphin from inducing analgesia and catalepsy.
Injections of up to 2 nmol of beta-endorphin directly into the n.septi medialis, into the head of the caudate or into the globus pallidus did not produce any analgesia. Furthermore, little or no catalepsy was obeserved.

TABLE 1 The Analgesic and Cataleptogenic Effects of Intraventricular Administration of Beta-Endorphin

Dose of Beta-Endorphin nmol/brain	Catalepsy Scores	Analgesia % of Maximum
0.29	-	7±1.0
2.9	-	23±5.0
1.45	3.1±0.7	36±5.0
2.9	4.3±0.6	75±15
14.5	4.8±0.3	91±9.0

Analgesia was measured using the tail flick method of D'Amour and Smith (1942) as modified by Harris and Pierson (1964). The intensity of catalepsy was estimated by measuring the time the rats would remain with both limbs over a 10 cm bar as described by Costall and Olley (1971). The time was then converted to a numerical score from 0 to 5. The data are adapted from Moroni et al. (1978 b).

TR_{Ach} and TR_{GABA} in the Hippocampus after Intraventricular or Intraseptal Beta-Endorphin

The intraventricular injection of up to 2.9 nmol of beta-endorphin failed to modify the Ach or Ch content in the hippocampus (Table 2). However the TR_{Ach} decreased by approximately 70% after administration of as little as 0.29 nmol of beta-endorphin. Naltrexone (15 µmol/kg. i.p.) completely prevented the decrease if the TR_{Ach} alicited by the polypeptide (2.9 nmol) (Table 2). Since the cholinergic innervation of the hippocampus originates from the medial septal nucleus (Lewis and others, 1976), we investigated whether or not this impressive effect of beta-endorphin was due to a stimulation of opiate receptors located on septal neurons.

When beta-endorphin (0.7 nmol) was locally injected into the septum in a volume of 1 µl, the levels of Ach and Ch were not changed; however the TR_{Ach} in the hippocampus was significantly decreased (Fig.1). No changes were observed in other brain areas. These experiments suggest a direct or indirect interaction, at the septal level, between beta-endorphin and septal-hippocampal cholynergic system. In the GABA field, intraventricular administration of up to 2.9 nmol of beta-endorphin does not modify the hippocampal content of glutamate and GABA (87±5 and 21±2 nmol/mg/prot respectively) and the relative incorporation of labelling into these two putative neurotrasmitters. Unfortunately the calculations of the TR_{GABA} in this brain region are particularly troublesome, probably because in the hippocampus, a certain percentage of glutamate is directly used as neurotrasmitter and therefore the relationship between the precursor glutamate and the product (GABA) are not fully respected.

TABLE 2 Effects of Intraventricular Administration of beta-Endorphin on the Hippocampal Cholinergic System

Dose of Beta-Endorphin nmol/brain	Ach nmol/mg.prot.	Ch nmol/mg.prot.	TR_{Ach} nmol/mg.prot./hr
Saline	0.30±0.021	0.28±0.020	4.1 ±0.9
Beta-endorphin 0.29	0.33±0.023	0.25±0.020	1.0 ±0.15**
Beta-endorphin 2.9	0.31±0.020	0.30±0.030	0.65±0.09**
Beta-endorphin 2.9 +Naltrexone	0.20±0.021	0.28±0.020	4.9 ±1.2

Each value is the average ± SEM of at least 6 animals. $P < 0.01$
Data adapted from Moroni and others 1977.

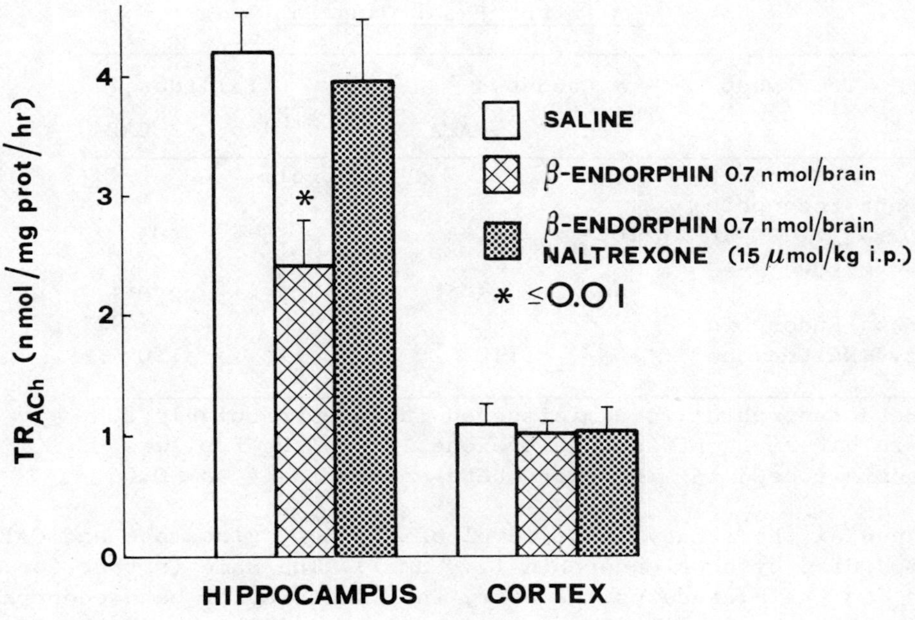

Fig. 1. The effects of intraseptal injections of beta-endorphin on the TR_{Ach}. Bars are the mean ± SEM of at least 6 experiments. Beta-endorphin was injected into the septum trough cronically implanted cannulae (Plastic Product co. Roanoke Va) 30' before the sacrifice. The volume of each injection was 1 μl which was delivered in approximately 1 min. Naltrexone was injected intraperitoneally 15' before beta-endorphin.

TR_{Ach} and TR_{GABA} in the Basal Ganglia after Intravetricular or Local Administration of beta-Endorphin

The concentration of endogenous opioid receptors and of "endogenous opioid receptor legands" is particularly high in the n.caudatus and in the globus pallidus (Simantov and others 1976; Hong and others, 1978; Yang and others, 1977). Thus the action of beta-endorphin on the metabolism of various putative neurotrasmitters in these brain areas may reflect a participation of opioid receptors in the physiological controls of the extrapiramidal motor function.

The intraventricular administration of beta-endorphin modifies the functions of cholinergic and gabaergic neuronal populations in the basal ganglia. Table 3 shows the effects of various doses of intraventricular beta-endorphin on the TR_{GABA} and on the TR_{Ach} in the caudate nucleus and in the globus pallidus.

TABLE 3 Differential Effects of Intraventricular Beta-Endorphin on the Turnover Rate of Acetylcholine and GABA in the Basal Ganglia

Treatment	N.Caudatus		G.Pallidus	
	TR_{Ach}	TR_{GABA}	TR_{Ach}	TR_{GABA}
	% of Controls			
Beta-Endorphin 0.29	102	60**	58**	205**
Beta-Endorphin 2.9	98	55**	52**	270**
Beta-Endorphin 2.9+Naltrexone	105	110	118	110

Beta-Endorphin was administered intraventricularly 30 min before sacrifice. Naltrexone 15 µmol/kg i.p. was administered 15 min before beta-endorphin. ** $p < 0.05$

In both nuclei the steady state level of Ch, Ach, glutamate and GABA is not modified by beta-endorphin (2.9 nmol). The same is true for the TR_{Ach} in the n.caudatus. However, intraventricular beta-endorphin significantly decrease the TR_{Ach} in the globus pallidus and the TR_{GABA} in the n.caudatus. On the contrary, the TR_{GABA} in the g.pallidus was significantly increased. (Table 2).

Since many electrophysiological data (Ziegleiganzberger and others, 1976; North and Williams, 1976; Bradley and others, 1976) suggest that activation of opiate receptors causes an inhibition of the firing rate of the neurons, we hypothesized that the increase GABA metabolism induced by beta-endorphin in the globus pallidus was due to a decrease of a tonic-inhibitory action in other brain areas. Therefore we locally injected beta-endorphin into various brain nuclei. Fig.2 shows that the administration of beta-endorphin through chronically implanted cannulae in the head of the n. caudatus resulted, not only in a decreased GABA utilization in this brain area, but also in an increased TR_{GABA} in the g.pallidus. These experiments suggest that the increase of the TR_{GABA} in the g.pallidus may be due to a decrease in a tonic gabaergic inhibition on GABA neurons whose cell bodies are in the caudate and whose terminals are located in the globus pallidus. (Moroni and others 1978c).

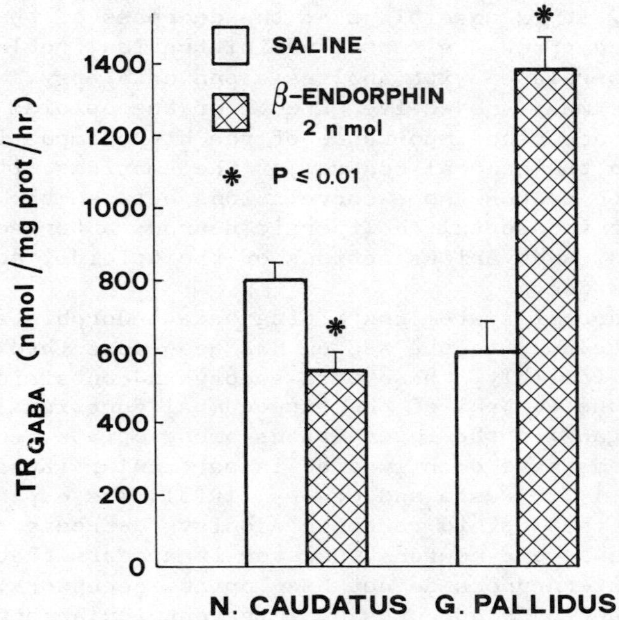

Fig. 2. Effects of intracaudatal administration of beta-endorphin on the TR_{GABA}. Bars are the mean ± SEM of at least 6 experiments. Beta-endorphin was freshly dissolved in saline and administered in the head of the caudate in a volume of 2 ul which were delivered slowly in approximately 1 minute. The rats were killed 30' min. after the injections.

CONCLUSIONS

The present experiments have shown that the activation of opioid receptors with an endogenous opioid receptor legand (beta-endorphin) specifically modifies the metabolism of various other putative neurotransmitters, in selected brain nulcei.
In this presentation, we have focussed our attention on the septal-hyppocampal cholinergic pathway and on the interactions among various putative neurotrasmitters in the extrapiramidal system. The stimul-

ation of opiate receptors decreases the firing rate of various neurons (North and Williams, 1976, Ziegleiganzberger and others, 1976) and our data demonstrate that the septal cholinergic neurons projecting to the hippocampus are inhibited by intraventricular and intraseptal administration of beta-endorphin. No changes were observed as far as the hippocampal gabaergic interneurons are concerned.
Since beta-endorphin injected into the septum fails to cause analgesia and catalepsy, it is possible that the decrease of the hippocampal TR_{Ach}, observed after its septal administration, reflects actions of opioids not correlated with analgesia and catalepsy.
In view of the many subjective effects of the opioids and in view of the generally accepted importance of the hippocampus in the learning process and in the central control of the emotions, it does not seem unreasonable to propose some correlations between the decrease in the firing rate of the septal cholinergic neurons after administration of beta-endorphin, and various actions of the opioids, not connected with the pain sensation.
Recently a neuronal system containing beta-endorphin and projecting from the hypotalamus to the septum has been described (Bloom and others 1978). Possibly, these beta-endorphin-containing fibers play some role in the control of the hippocampal functionality.
In the basal ganglia the interactions among opiate receptors and the dopamine systems have been studied in particular (Kuschinsky and Hornykiewicz, 1972; Costa and others, 1973). The experiments reported here indicate that opioid receptor agonists decrease the firing rate of caudatal gabaergic neurons. However it appears that the caudatal cholinergic interneurons do not bear opiate receptors. In fact, they are not affected by high doses of intraventricular beta-endorphin (Table 3). On the contrary, the TR_{GABA} and thus probably the firing rate of the gabaergic neurons projecting to the g.pallidus, is increased by intraventricular and intracaudatal beta-endorphin. It is possible that these effects are due to a decrease in gabaergic inhibition on GABA neurons projecting from the caudate to the g.pallidus. (Fonnum and others, 1977).
In the rat, high doses of beta-endorphin induce catalepsy (Table 1). The increase of the GABA metabolism in the g.pallidus has been associated with an akinetic status similar to the opioid-induced catalepsy. (Peacock and others, 1976; Moroni and others, 1978c).
Since the stimulation of opiate receptors may be operative either after a release of enkephalins at synaptic level, or after secretion of other endogenous "opioid-receptor legands" in the cerebrospinal fluid or in the blood, and since the active doses of beta-endorphin are particularly low (Moroni, Cheney and Costa, 1978b), it is possible that the modifications of the metabolism of various putative neurotransmitters induced by this opioid receptors agonist play an important part in the physiological control of various brain functions.

REFERENCES

Bradley, P.B., Briggs, I., Gayton, R.J. and Lambert-Lynn, A. (1976). Effects of microiontophoretically applied meth-enkephalin on single neorones in rat brain-stem. Nature, 261, 425-426.

Bloom, F. (1978). Is there a neurotrasmitter code in the brain? In 7th International Congress of Pharmacol., Paris.

Bertilsson, L., Mao, C.C. and Costa, E. (1977). Applications of principles of steady-state kinetics to the estimation of GABA turnover rate in the nuclei of rat brain. J.Pharmacol.Exp.Ther., 200, 277-284.

Cheney, D.L. and Costa, E. (1977). Pharmacological implications of brain Ach turnover measurements in rat brain nuclei. Ann.Rev. Pharmacol. Toxicol., 17, 369-386.

Costa, E., Carenzi, A., Guidotti, A. and Revuelta, A. (1973). Narcotic analgesic and the regulation of neuronal catecholamine stores. In E. Usdin and S. Snyder (ed.), Frontiers in Catecholamine Research. Pergamon Press, London. pp.1003-1010.

Elde, R., Hokfelt, T., Johansson, O. and Terenius, L. (1976). Immunohistochemical studies using antibodies of leu-enkephalin: Initial observations on the nervous system of the rat. Neuroscience, 1, 349-351.

Fonnum, F., Walaas, I. and Iversen, E. (1977). Localization of Gaba-ergic,cholinergic and aminergic structures in the mesolimbic system. J. Neurochem., 29, 221-239.

Fratta, W., Yang, H.Y.T., Hong J.S. and Costa, E. (1978). Studies on beta-endorphin. Soc. of Neurochem., Washington, D.C.

Guidotti, A., Cheney, D.L., Trabucchi, M., Doteuchi, M., Wang, C.T. and Hawkins, R.A. (1974). Focussed microwaye radiation: A technique to minimize post-mortem changes of cyclic nucleotides, dopa and choline and to preserve brain morphology. Neuropharmacology, 13, 1115-1122.

Hong, J.S., Yang, Y.T., Fratta, W. and Costa, E. (1978). Rat striatal met-enkephalin content after chronic treatment with cataleptogenic and noncataleptogenic antischizophrenic drugs. J.Pharmacol. Exp. Therap., 205, 141-147.

Hughes, J., Smith, T.W., Kosterlitz, H.W., Fothergill, L.A. Morgan, B.A. and Morris, H.R. (1975). Identification of two related pentaptides from the brain with potent opiate agonist activity. Nature, 258, 577-579.

Kuschinsky, K. and Hornykiewiecz, O. (1972). Morphine Catalepsy in the rat: relation to striatal dopamine metabolism. Eur.J.Pharmacol. 19, 119-122.

Koslow, S.H., Racagni, G. and Costa, E. (1974). Mass fragmentographic measurement of norepinephrine, dopamine, serotonin and Ach in seven dicreet nuclei of the rat tel-diencephamon. Neuropharmacology, 13, 1123-1130.

Konig, J.F.R. and Klippel, R.A. (1963). The rat brain: A stereotaxic atlas of the forebrain and lower parts of the brain stem. Williams and Wilkins, Baltimore.

Lewis, R.R., Shute, C.C.D. and Silver, A. (1967). Confirmation from choline acetylase of a massive cholinergic innervation to the rat hippocampus. J.Physiol., 191, 215-224.

Meek, K.J.L., Yang, H.Y.T. and Costa, E. (1977). Enkephalin catabolism in vitro and vivo. Neuropharmacology, 16, 151-154.

Mao, C.C., Peralta, E., Moroni, F. and Costa, E. (In the Press, 1978). The turnover rate of GABA in the substantia nigra following electrical stimulation or lesioning of the strio-nigral pathways. Brain Res.

Moroni, F., Cheney, D.L. and Costa, E. (1977). Beta-endorphin inhibits Ach turnover in rat brain. Nature, 267, 267-268.

Moroni, F., Malthe-Sorenssen, D., Cheney, D.L. and Costa, E.(1978a). Modulation of Ach turnover in the septal-hippocampal pathway by electrical stimulation and lesioning. Brain Res., 150, 333-343.

Moroni, F., Cheney, D.L. and Costa, E. (1978b).The turnover rate of Ach in brain nuclei of rats injected intraventricularly and intraseptally with alpha and beta-endorphin. Neuropharmacology, 17, 191-196.

Moroni, F., Cheney, D.L., Peralta, E. and Costa, E. (In the Press 1978c). Opiate receptors agonists as modulators of GABA turnover in the n. caudatus, globus pallidus and substantia nigra of the rat. J.Pharmacol.Exp.Ther.

North, R.A. and Williams, J.T. (1977). Enkephalin inhibits firing of myenteric neurones. Nature, 264, 400-461.

Pycock, C., Horton, R.W., and Marsden, C.D. (1976). The behavioural effects of manipulating GABA finction in the globus pallidus. Brain Res., 116, 353-359.

Racagni, G., Cheney, D.L., Trabucchi, M., Wang, C.T. and Costa, E. (1974). Measurement of acetylcholine turnover rate in dicreete areas of rat brain. Life Sci., 15, 1961-75.

Robinson, C.A., Hengerald, C.A. and De Balbian Vester, F. (1969). Improved polyethylene cannulation techniques. Physiol.Behav., 4, 123-124.

Segal, D.S., Browne, R.G., Bloom, F., Ling, N. and Guillemin, R. (1977). Beta-endorphin: Endogenous opiate of neuroleptic. Science, 198, 411-413.

Sethy, V.H., Kuhar, J.H., Roth, H.R., Van Woert, H.H. and Aghajanian, K.G. (1973). Cholinergic neurons: Effect of acute septal lesion on acetylcholine and choline content of rat hippocampus. Brain Res., 55, 481-484.

Simantov, R., Kuhar, H.J., Pasternak, G.W. and Snyder, S.H. (1976). The regional distribution of a morphin-like factor, enkephalin, in the monkey brain. Brain Res., 106, 189-197.

Yang, H.Y.T., Hong, J.S. and Costa, E. (1977). Regional distribution of met and leu-enkephalin in the rat brain. Neuropharmacology, 16, 303-307.

Zieliganzberger, W., Fry, J.P., Herz, A., Moroder, L. and Wivnsh, E. (1976). Enkephalin induced inhibition of cortical neurones and lack of this effect in morphine tolerant-dependent rats. Brain Res., 115, 160-164.

Zsilla, G., Racagni, G., Cheny, D.L. and Costa, E. (1977). Constant rate infusion of deuterated phosphorylcholine to measure the effects of morphine on acetylcholine turnover rate in specific nuclei of rat brain. Neuropharmacology, 16, 25-31.

ACKNOWLEDGEMENTS

We are grateful to Dr. G. Moneti from the Centre of Mass-spectrometry of the Faculty of Medicine of the University of Florence, for his aid in carrying out and interpreting the mass spectra, to Dr. Costa and Dr. Cheney for their continouus help, to Miss Susan Charlton and to Miss Roberta Ciampi for typing the manuscript.

Studies on a Possible Pathological Significance of Endorphins in Psychiatric Disorders

H. M. EMRICH*, V. HÖLLT*, H. LASPE, M. FISCHLER**, H. HEINEMANN***, W. KISSLING***, D. V. ZERSSEN*** and A. HERZ*****

*Max-Planck-Institut für Psychiatrie, Munich, F.R.G.
**Bezirkskrankenhaus Haar, F.R.G.
***Bezirkskrankenhaus Kaufbeuren, F.R.G.

INTRODUCTION

The hypothesis of a possible role of endorphins in the pathogenesis of psychotic disorders has been derived from 3 different observations:

1st is there a pronounced euphorogenic action of endorphins leading to the hypothesis that endorphins may play a role in the mood changes in affective psychoses (Kline and co-workers, 1977; Kline and Lehmann, 1978).

2nd partial agonists of opiates induce hallucinations and other psychotic experiences in normal probands leading to the idea that abnormal endorphins with a spectrum of action similar to that of partial agonists might induce psychotic symptoms in schizophrenia (Jasinski, Martin and Haertzen, 1967).

3rd some - though very weak - ameliorating effects of the specific opiate antagonist naloxone have been reported in schizophrenic patients (Emrich and co-workers, 1977; Watson and co-workers, 1978).

METHODS AND RESULTS

Two types of studies have been done: First the investigation of a possible antipsychotic action of a high dosage of naloxone in psychotic patients. Secondly, the attempt to measure actual levels of ß-endorphin in CSF and in plasma of patients with different types of neurological and psychiatric disorders.

In the naloxone study, 40 schizophrenic patients have been examined; 20 patients using a naloxone-dose of 4.0 mg (1.2 mg in 3 patients), 20 patients using a naloxone-dose of 24.8 mg. The type of the study in both cases was a double-blind placebo-controlled cross-over design. Only patients with frequent hallucinations and/or actual delusional experience were included in the study. Psychopathological changes

*Supported by the Fritz-Thyssen-Stiftung, Cologne.

were registrated by use of the IMPS-scale and by use of a self-constructed "VBS-scale" with 8 degrees of intensity which can especially be adapted to hallucinations and actual delusional experience. (For details see Emrich and co-workers, 1977).

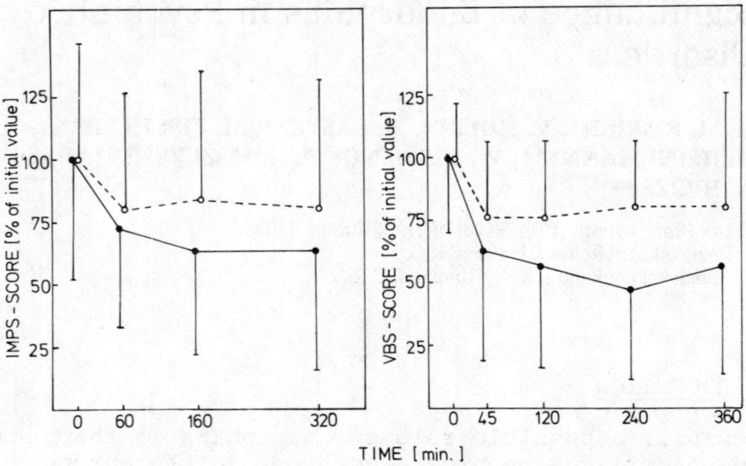

Fig. 1. Left: Mean IMPS-score (% of initial value; factors PCP + PAR + GRN + EXC + HOS) as a function of time in 20 psychotic patients with hallucinations and/or actual delusional experience.
Right: Mean VBS ("Verlaufs-Beurteilungs-Skala = course assessment-scale)-score (% of initial value; assessment of hallucinations and of actual delusional experience) as a function of time.
Open circles: placebo; dots: 4 mg naloxone (in 3 cases: 1.2 mg).

In the 4.0 mg study the amount of chronic cases was relatively low (20%). The results (Fig. 1) show a small but significant reduction of psychotic symptomatology if the average of the changes of these 20 patients is evaluated: on the left side the data of the IMPS-scale (here the sum score of acute psychotic symptoms is used: perceptual distortion, paranoid projection, grandiose expansiveness, excitement, hostile belligerence), on the right side the data of the VBS-scale, which especially reflect hallucinations and actual delusional experience. The open dots represent the mean placebo-data, the filled dots the mean naloxone-data, the bars standard-deviations. These effects are significant at the 1-4% level (t-test for intra-individual differences between changes under naloxone versus changes under placebo).

In the second part of the naloxone-study, the much higher naloxone-dose of 24.8 mg was used to find out if the small antipsychotic effect, seen in the 4.0 mg study can be increased with a higher dose, since it might be possible that in humans a dose of 4.0 mg is insufficient to antagonize special hypothetic endorphins possibly involved in the pathogenesis of schizophrenia.

In this second study, by chance, the amount of chronic cases was much higher than in the 4.0 mg study: it amounts to about 45% of the cases.

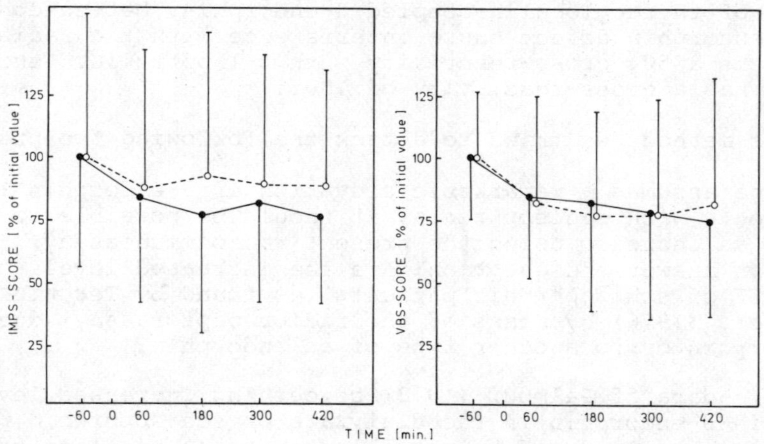

Fig. 2. Mean results after 24.8 mg naloxone/placebo in 20 patients with schizophrenia. The symbols are the same as in Fig. 1.

In Fig. 2, on the left side the IMPS-data are depicted, on the right side the VBS-data, especially reflecting hallucinations and actual delusional experience. The open dots again represent the mean placebo-data, the filled dots the mean naloxone-data. From these results we can derive that no increase in effect occurs with increasing naloxone-dose and that it is completely absent in the VBS-data. In the IMPS-data the effect is again a delayed one and is significant at the 4% level at 3h and 7h after injection. The discrepancy of the high-dosage study as compared with the 4.0 mg study in the VBS may be explained by the higher percentage of chronic cases who may respond at a lower extent to naloxone. However, from these findings with 24.8 mg naloxone one has to conclude that endorphins play no major role in the pathogenesis of schizophrenia.

On the other side, there are two hints from other experimental approaches indicating a possible role of endorphins in the pathogenesis of schizophrenic psychoses. One is the finding of Palmour (1978), that in the dialyzate of schizophrenic patients there exists a high amount of leucin-ß-endorphin. The other hint comes from measurements of endorphin-levels in the CSF.

Terenius and co-workers (1976), using the radioreceptorassay, studied two CSF-fractions and observed, especially in fraction I, an increase of endorphins in patients with schizophrenia, which was partially reversible by neuroleptic therapy.

However, by use of the radioreceptorassay it is not possible to determine the chemical nature of the opioid substance.

An approach to get some more information in regard of these findings has been performed by Höllt, Przewłocki and Herz (1978), using a radioimmunoassay of ß-endorphin.

Antibodies against human ß-endorphin which exhibit a high avidity for the C-terminal of the peptide were raised in rabbits following the injection of thyreoglobulin-coupled ß-endorphin. Met-enkephalin, and α- and γ-endorphin do not cause interference with the radioimmunoassay. But there is a 50% cross-reactivity with ß-lipotropin. Leucin-ß-endorphin has a cross-reactivity of 100%.

Using this method, we tried to attack the following two problems:

1st If one assumes a remarkable elevation of ß-endorphin in CSF of patients with schizophrenia, it should be possible to detect such an increase using the present radioimmunoassay. Especially we can answer the question: Are the increased levels of endorphins in CSF of schizophrenic patients (as found by Terenius and coworkers (1976) by means of the radioreceptorassay) due to ß-endorphin or to another type of an endorphin?

2nd If the data of Palmour (1978) concerning increased levels of leucin-ß-endorphin in the dialyzate of schizophrenic patients are valid, it should be possible to detect an elevated level of leucin-ß-endorphin <u>in plasma</u> of these patients.

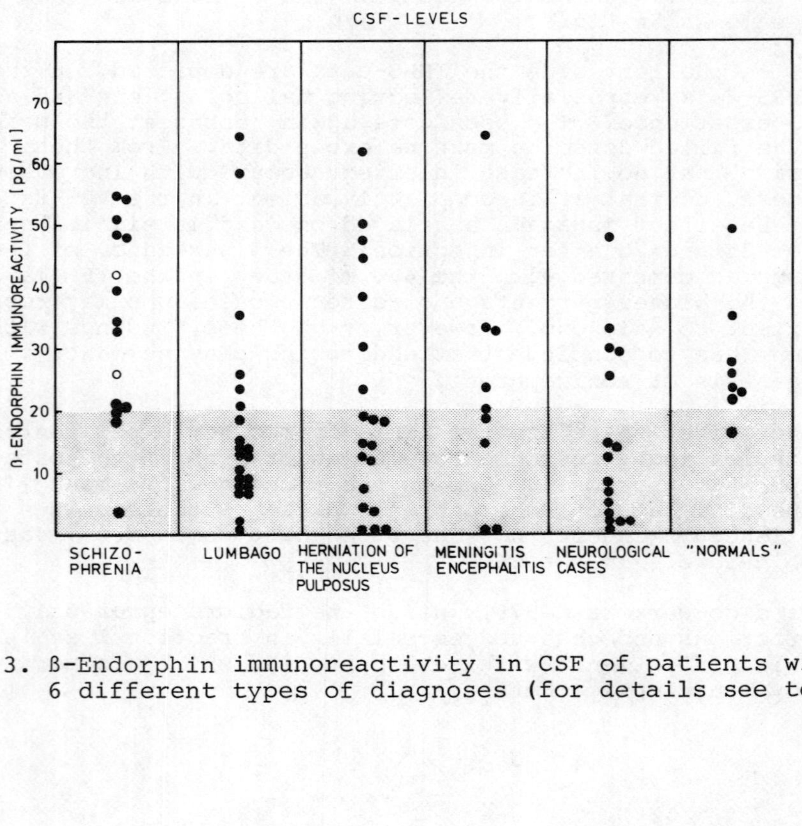

Fig. 3. ß-Endorphin immunoreactivity in CSF of patients with 6 different types of diagnoses (for details see text).

Fig. 3 shows CSF-levels of ß-endorphin immunoreactivity in 6 different diagnostic groups:

1. Schizophrenic patients (two of them without neuroleptic therapy, highly acute cases: open circles).

2. Patients with lumbago, punctured for myelography, pretreated with 10 mg diazepam.

3. Patients with a herniation of the nucleus pulposus of the vertebral disc, pretreated with 10 mg diazepam and operated later on.

4. Patients with meningitis/encephalitis.

5. Patients with mixed neurological diagnoses: multiple sclerosis, lateral sclerosis, cerebral atrophy, and so on.

6. Medical patients who were punctured because of the suspicion of a meningitis but the CSF was normal ("normals").

The grey zone in Fig. 3 represents the detection limit within which no reliable values can be measured. The values within this limit are only virtual and do not have a real significance.

If we compare the data of the schizophrenic patients with the data of the so-called "normal-group" there is practically no difference. There may be present a small tendency to lower values in the group of patients with lumbago and herniation of the nucleus pulposus. However, these patients were pretreated with a minor tranquilizer and we do not know the influence of these drugs on the endorphin-system. If ß-endorphin - like ACTH - is regarded as an indicator of stress-phenomena, one would suspect a lowering of values after pretreatment with a minor tranquilizer.

In the group of cases with meningitis/encephalitis there is no change at all, whereas in the mixed group of neurological patients there is also a small tendency to lower values.

From the normal findings in schizophrenic patients one may derive that the elevated values of Terenius and co-workers (1976) cannot be due to ß-endorphin.

Fig. 4 shows data of ß-endorphin immunoreactivity in plasma of patients with schizophrenia, different types of neuroses and affective psychoses (other patients than in Fig. 3). The grey zone again represents the region in which no reliable measurements are possible due to the limited sensitivity of the radioimmunoassay.

From the present preliminary data no conclusion should be drawn concerning possible <u>small differences between these groups</u>.

From these data one can derive that no increase of ß-endorphin immunoreactivity occurs in schizophrenics which should be present if an abnormally high amount of leucin-ß-endorphin would exist in the plasma of these patients, since the cross-reactivity of the radioimmunoassay with leucin-ß-endorphin is 100%. Thus, our data do not support the idea of a pathogenesis of schizophrenia by an abnormally high level of leucin-ß-endorphin.

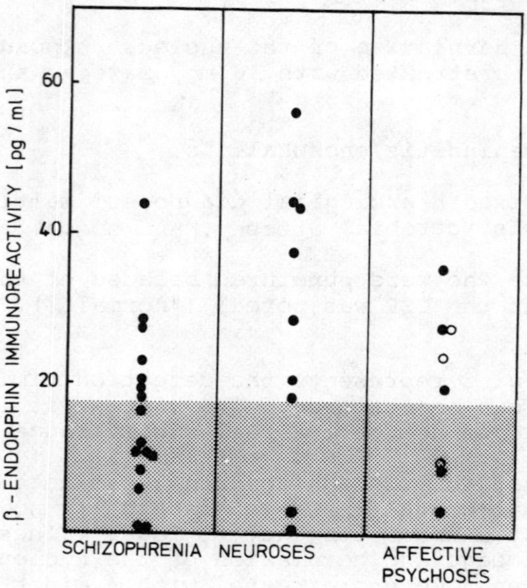

Fig. 4. ß-Endorphin immunoreactivity in plasma of patients with schizophrenia (acute and chronic cases), different types of neuroses and affective psychoses (open circles: mania, dots: endogenous depression).

In Fig. 5 data on plasma levels of ß-endorphin immunoreactivity before and after 9 electroconvulsive treatments (3 patients with endogenous depression) are presented. In the upper region in which reliable measurements are possible, 7 times an elevation after electroconvulsion was observed.

Since ß-endorphin immunoreactivity normally goes parallel with ACTH-values in response to electrically induced stress (Guillemin and co-workers, 1977) this finding is <u>in line</u> with data on an elevation of ACTH after electroconvulsion in humans (Allen and co-workers, 1974). On the other side, the possibility that electroconvulsion is effective via an endorphinergic mechanism has to be considered.

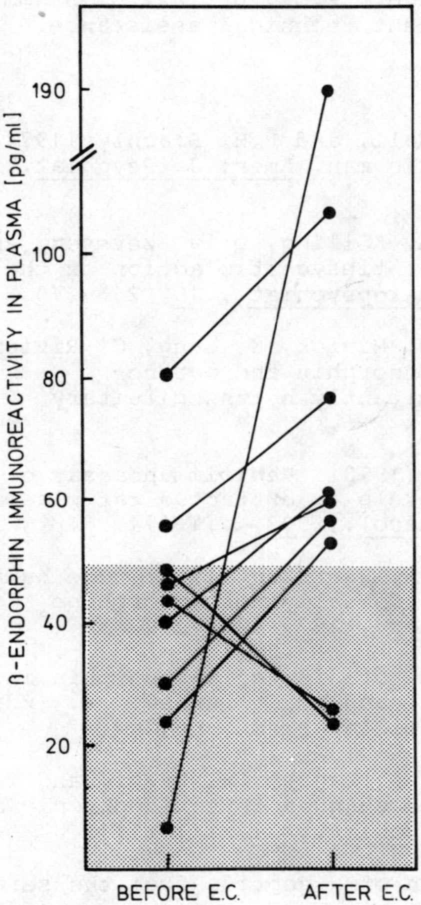

Fig. 5.
ß-Endorphin immunoreactivity in plasma of patients with endogenous depression before and 10 min. after electroconvulsive treatment.

Summarizing, our data from the naloxone studies and from the ß-endorphin studies are at variance with the assumption that endorphins play a central role in pathogenesis of schizophrenia.

ACKNOWLEDGEMENT

For the supply of CSF-samples thankful appreciation is given to: Prof. Dr. W. Krämer, Chief of the Dept. of Neurology, Bezirkskrankenhaus Haar; Dr. H. Dwinger, Dept. of Psychiatry, Bezirkskrankenhaus Haar; Dr. F. Schmidtberger, Chief of the Dept. of Neurosurgery, Krankenhaus München-Schwabing; Dr. E. Holzer, Chief of the 4th Dept. of Internal Medicine, Krankenhaus München-Schwabing; Dr. K. Einhäupl, Dept. of Neurology, Klinikum Großhadern, Munich and Dr. D. v. Cramon, Dept. of Neurology, Max-Planck-Institut für Psychiatrie, Munich. We thank director Dr. Dr. Chr. Schulz, Dr. L. Achner, Dr. I. Meisel-Kosik, Dr. J. Staudinger and Dr. R. Oechsner, Bezirkskrankenhaus Haar and their co-workers for their generous support of this study. The supply of naloxone by Dr. M. J. Ferster, Endo Laboratories, Inc., Garden City, N.Y., is thankfully appreciated. The authors wish to thank Mrs. F. Sailer and A. Wendl as well as the technical assistants in the Dept. of Clinical Chemistry (Chief: Prof. Dr. Dr. D. Stamm) and the nurses of our wards for excellent technical assistance.

REFERENCES

Allen, M. J. P., D. Denney, J. W. Kendall, and P.H. Blachly (1974). Corticotropin release during ECT in man. Amer. J. Psychiat., 131, 1225-1228.

Emrich, H. M., C. Cording, S. Pirée, A. Kölling, D. v. Zerssen, and A. Herz (1977). Indication of an antipsychotic action of the opiate antagonist naloxone. Pharmakopsychiat., 10, 265-270.

Guillemin, R., T. Vargo, J. Rossier, S. Minick, N. Ling, C. Rivier, W. Vale, and F. Bloom (1977). ß-Endorphin and adreno-corticotropin are secreted concomitantly by the pituitary gland. Science, 197, 1367-1369.

Höllt, V., R. Przewłocki, and A. Herz (1978). Radioimmunoassay of ß-endorphin. Basal and stimulated levels in extracted rat plasma. Naunyn-Schmiedeberg's Arch. Pharmacol., 303, 171-174.

Jasinski, D. R., W. R. Martin, and C. A. Haertzen (1967). The human pharmacology and abuse potential of N-allylnoroxymorphone (naloxone). J. Pharmacol. exp. Ther., 157, 420-426.

Kline, N. S., and H. E. Lehmann (1978). Studies of ß-endorphin in psychiatric patients. In E. Usdin, and W. E. Bunney, jr. (Eds.), Endorphins in Mental Illness, Macmillan Press, London.

Kline, N. S., C. H. Li, H. E. Lehmann, A. Lajtha, E. Laski, and T. Cooper (1977). ß-Endorphin-induced changes in schizophrenic and depressed patients. Arch. gen. Psychiat., 34, 1111-1113.

Palmour, R. M. (1978). Characterization of a peptide from the serum of psychiatric patients. In E. Usdin, and W. E. Bunney, jr. (Eds.), Endorphins in Mental Illness, Macmillan Press, London.

Terenius, L., A. Wahlström, L. Lindström, and E. Widerlöv (1976). Increased CSF levels of endorphins in chronic psychosis. Neurosci. Lett., 3, 157-162.

Watson, S. J., P. A. Berger, H. Akil, M. J. Mills, and J. D. Barchas (1978). Effects of naloxone on schizophrenia: reduction in hallucinations in a subpopulation of subjects. Science, 201, 73-76.

Beta-Endorphins and Naloxone in Psychiatric Patients: Clinical and Biological Effects

H. E. LEHMANN*, TH. COOPER, N.P.V. NAIR*** and N. S. KLINE****

*McGill University, Montreal, Quebec, Canada
**Rockland Research Centre, Orangeburg, New York
***Douglas Hospital Centre, Montreal, Quebec, Canada

ABSTRACT

In order to help clarify the mechanism of reported favorable therapeutic results with beta-endorphin injections in schizophrenics, anxiety neurotics, obsessive-compulsives and depressives, we have been investigating the effects of the morphine (beta-endorphin?) antagonist, naloxone. Since no adequate method of measuring beta-endorphin at endogenous levels has been reported, we have utilized an indirect method: beta-endorphin and ACTH are produced by a common precursor in a fixed proportion; thus, increases or decreases in ACTH (which can be measured) are assumed to reflect changes in beta-endorphin. Responses to 10 mg of naloxone measured at 1/2, 3 and 6 hours resulted in a statistically significant symptomatic improvement which was maximal at 6 hours. In this double-blind study there was also a relationship between ACTH (and thus beta-endorphin) levels and clinical response as measured by a rating scale.

KEYWORDS

Naloxone - ACTH - Schizophrenia - Endorphins - Peptides

INTRODUCTION

In a recent paper (Lehmann, Nair, Kline, 1978) we reported on an open trial with intravenous naloxone in a group of schizophrenic patients. In reviewing prior studies to our own, we noted that some were criticised for using too low a dose of naloxone and some were observed for too short a period of time. Last week (July 7, 1978) Watson and others from Stanford reported results similar to our own, but reports of the effect of naloxone were measured at the end of 1 1/2 to 2 hours.

By way of contrast, both our own work and other studies in the literature, suggest that maximal response requires at least <u>6</u> hours of observation. There seems to be now general agreement that at least 10 mg of naloxone should be used as a test dose. Our failure to use this high a dose in our beta-endorphin studies may account for the failure of naloxone to have any effect on most of beta-endorphin responses. On the other hand, there is still the possibility that naloxone has no role in the improvement resulting from beta-endorphin. These investigations need repetition with the higher naloxone dose.

In our previous open naloxone study we found significant improvement in a number of Brief Psychiatric Rating Scale (BPRS) items and factors. These findings were confirmed in our present double-blind controlled study in which each of 5 schizophrenic subjects were given placebo on one occasion and 10 mg of naloxone i.v. on another occasion. Informed consent to the investigation was obtained from the patients. Changes in the patients' status relative to pre-injection baselines were evaluated on the BPRS 1/2, 3 and 6 hours following injections of naloxone and placebo.

The <u>factors</u> which showed most improvement with naloxone as compared to placebo were:

1. Thought disturbance at .001 level (chi-square)
2. Activation at .01 level
3. Anxiety-depression at .05 level
4. Total BPRS at .05 level

Fig. 1, 2 and 3 illustrate these trends over time.

No significant changes between naloxone and placebo were observed in 1) anergia and 2) hostile suspiciousness.

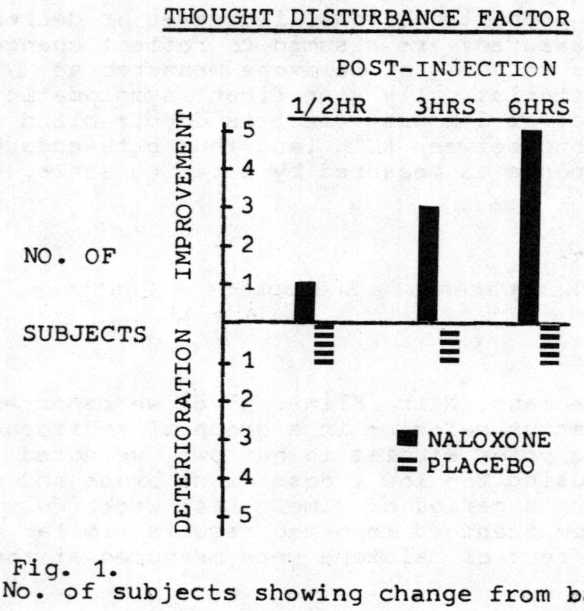

Fig. 1.
No. of subjects showing change from baseline.

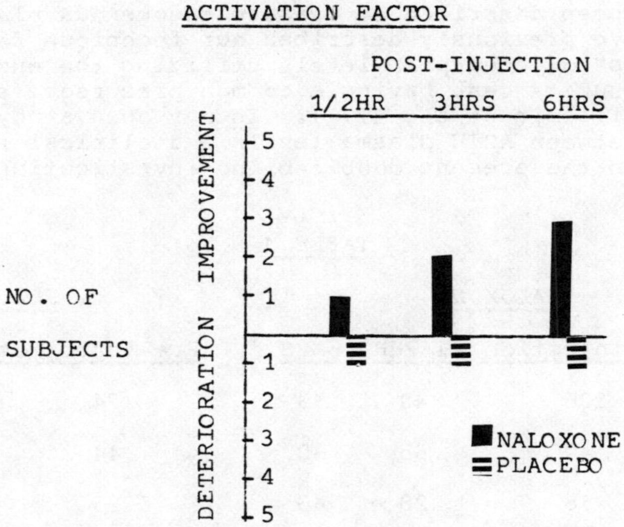

Fig. 2. No. of subjects showing change from baseline.

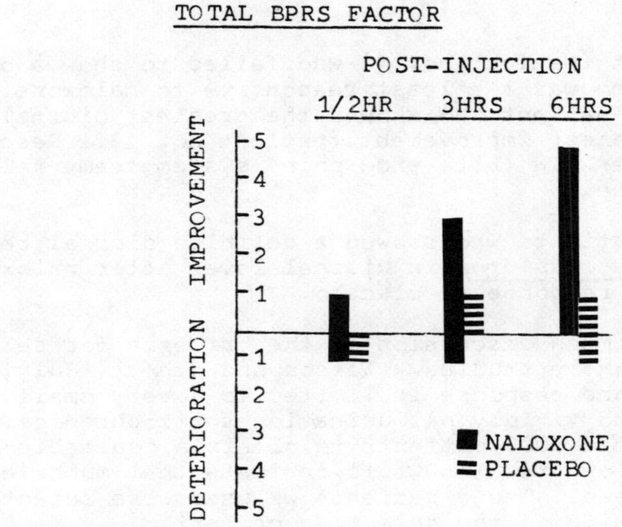

Fig. 3. No. of subjects showing change from baseline.

The individual <u>items</u> showing the greatest change were:

1. Hallucinatory behavior - .001
2. Conceptual disorganization - .05
3. Anxiety - .05
4. Tension - .05
5. Excitement - .05

No method has been described to measure endogenous plasma endorphin levels. We have previously described our technique for indirect "determinations" of endorphin levels utilizing the endorphin-ACTH yoke. (The 2 substances, having a common precursor, show parallel production (Guillemin et al, 1977). In our open study we found a relationship between ACTH plasma levels and clinical response. This is confirmed in the present double-blind investigation.

TABLE 1

Patient No.	NALOXONE			PLACEBO		
	Pre-injection	1/2HR	6HRS	Pre-injection	1/2HR	6HRS
1	106	41	33	74	39	28
2	40	85	60	44	54	31
3	38	28	40	25	5	18
4	61	59	56	58	53	64
5	32	28	24	-	-	-

ACTH plasma levels in picogms/ml

The one patient (patient no. 4) who failed to show a diurnal decrease while on placebo was the least responsive to naloxone. Along the same line, the patient who showed the greatest diurnal drop in ACTH showed the greatest improvement (patient no. 1). Responsivity-or-mobility of the ACTH (beta-endorphin) system seems related to favourable response.

Two of the 3 patients who showed a definite diurnal response also showed markedly less drop in diurnal level after naloxone when compared to their response to placebo.

There has been much discussion of the criteria for selection of patients for naloxone studies. Watson and others (July, 1978) state that the naloxone response is limited to a very small sub-group of continuously and vividly hallucination schizophrenics. His group actually screened 1000 patients to obtain a "suitable" sample of 11 subjects. Our own results would indicate that much less rigid criteria can be used. The 5 patients we used were selected from a group of 40, using as the selection criteria:

1. Hallucinations
2. Thought disorder
3. Dysphoria

We do not know what response would occur in the other schizophrenics. Perhaps they too would show improvement, and even our more liberal criteria are too restrictive. Future investigators might consider using random selection of schizophrenics, or perhaps of all psychiatric patients, to determine what limitations, if any, would apply.

REFERENCES

Guillemin, R., Vargo, T., Rossier, J., Minick, S., Ling, N., Rivier, C., Vale, W., Bloom, F. (1977). Beta-endorphin and adrenocorticotropin are secreted concomitantly by the pituitary gland. *Science*, *197*, 1367.

Lehmann, H.E., Nair, N.P.V. and Kline, N.S. (1978). Beta-endorphins and naloxone in psychiatric patients: clinical and biological effects. Presented at the Annual Meeting of the American Psychiatric Association, Atlanta, Georgia, May 12, 1978.

Watson, S.J., Berger, P.A., Akil, H., Mills, M.J. and Barchas, J.D. (1978). Effects of naloxone on schizophrenia: reduction in hallucinations in a sub-population of subjects. *Science*, *201*, 73.

The Interaction of Naloxone with Striatal Dopaminergic Mechanisms

JEFFEREY FEIGENBAUM, BYONG MOON and HAROLD KLAWANS

Departments of Neurology and Pharmacology, Rush Presbyterian St. Luke's Medical Center, Chicago, Illinois 60612, U.S.A.

ABSTRACT

An analysis was made of the interaction between naloxone (NX) and striatal dopaminergic (DA) mechanisms in an attempt to elucidate the complex action of this drug on behavior. In doses ranging from 0.20-0.80 mg/kg, NX inhibited the stereotyped behavior induced by the directly acting DA agonist apomorphine (AISB), in a dose-dependent manner. NX (0.40 mg/kg) also produced a sigmoidal inhibition of the stereotypy induced by successive low doses of apomorphine (0.10-0.25 mg/kg). Since the effect of NX on behavior has been shown to be species dependent, an identical study was also undertaken in the guinea pig. Though NX exerted similar effects on AISB in both the rat and guinea pig and the stereotypy curves plotted for both species were of nearly identical configuration, low doses of apomorphine produced considerably more stereotypy in the guinea pig than did identical doses in the rat. The concomitant administration of the indirect DA agonist d-amphetamine (0.50-5.0 mg/kg) resulted in an effect opposite to that seen with NX and apomorphine. NX potentiated amphetamine induced stereotypy (AmISB) with the amphetamine + NX curve significantly above and virtually parallel to the amphetamine + saline curve. To test the hypothesis that these effects were the result of an action exerted by NX on the release of striatal DA, the effect of NX on AISB was assessed in the presence and absence of drugs that inhibit DA release non-specifically (MPT) and specifically (-hydroxybutyric acid). Pretreatment with either drug significantly reversed the inhibitory effect of NX on AISB relative to saline pretreated animals. This was consistant with previous observations that drugs enhancing striatal DA levels also inhibit AISB in a dose-dependent manner, and potentiate AmISB. These results are also in agreement with our recent findings that NX (10^{-6} M) can significantly enhance the release of ^{3}H-DA stimulated by d-amphetamine (10^{-6} M) in rat striatal slices _in vitro_. NX appears to enhance striatal DA levels only if the nigrostriatal pathway is in a state of arousal (e.g. by amphetamine). This effect is probably not mediated by a direct action of NX on presynaptic DA receptors, but rather appears to be produced indirectly by an action on presynaptic opioid receptors localized on striatal DA nerve terminals.

INTRODUCTION

Seminal studies of the regional distribution of opiate receptor binding in the rat have revealed that those regions in the CNS containing the highest concentration of DA bodies and terminals are among those in which the greatest density of opiate receptors is found (1, 2). This suggested that opiate and dopaminergic agonists and antagonists might interact in either a synergistic or inhibitory manner, and prompted investigations into the behavioral interactions of morphine, endogenous opioid peptides, or NX, with central DA agonists or antagonists. Such studies revealed that NX does appear to interact with dopaminergic mechanisms (3, 4, 5) and that it may even be of benefit in the treatment of schizophrenia (6,7).

These reports are by no means consistant, however, and there consequently appeared to be a need for a systematic and quantitative investigation of this interaction. The present study was therefore undertaken in order to more fully and systematically observe, evaluate, and possibly explain the interaction of NX with striatal dopaminergic mechanisms. In the course of this study, both direct and indirect DA agonists were used in combination with NX. Since high doses of these drugs produce non-specific effects which could confound any results obtained, only low doses were used throughout. Finally, stereotypy was the only behavior observed, as interest was focused on the interaction of NX with the nigrostriatal pathway, which is thought to primarily if not exclusively mediate this behavior (8, 9, 10).

METHODS

Animals

Subjects were male Sprague-Dawley rats (ARS Sprague-Dawley Farms, Madison, Wisc.) 200-250 g, and male random-bred guinea pigs (Scientific Small Animal Farms, Arlington Heights, Ill.) 250-300 g. The animals were group housed in a large colony room in cages 50 cm x 20 cm, and were maintained at a constant room temperature of 23°C $\pm$1°C with a relative humidity of 55% and a 12 hour light-dark cycle (0600-1800 h off and 1800-0600 h on). All animals were given water and either Purina rat chow or Wayne lab blox *ad libitum*.

Drugs

Drugs used were apomorphine HCl (Merck), Naloxone HCl (NX; Endo), d-amphetamine sulphate (d-AM; Sigma), -hydroxybutyric acid (-HB; Sigma), DL- -methyltyrosine methyl ester HCl (MPT; Regis).

Following a thirty minute habituation period for each animal, 210 rats and 102 guinea pigs were divided into one of the following 12 groups:

Group	No. of Animals	Type of Animals	Pretreatment Drug (mg/kg)	Final Drug Treatment (mg/kg)
1	24	Rats	NX (.20, .40, .60, .80)	Saline
2	6	Rats	Saline	Apomorphine (.50)
3	24	Rats	NX (.20, .40, .60, .80)	Apomorphine (.50)
4	24	G.Pigs	NX (.20, .40, .60, .80)	Saline
5	6	G.Pigs	Saline	Apomorphine (.25)
6	24	G.Pigs	NX (.20, .40, .60, .80)	Apomorphine (.25)

Group	Animals	Type of Animals	Pretreatment Drug (mg/kg)	Final Drug Treatment (mg/kg)
7	24	Rats	NX (.40)	Apomorphine (.10, .15, .20, .25)
8	24	Rats	Saline	Apomorphine (.10, .15, .20, .25)
9	24	G. Pigs	NX (.40)	Apomorphine (.10, .15, .20, .25)
10	24	G. Pigs	Saline	Apomorphine (.10, .15, .20, .25)
11	24	Rats	γ-HB (200)+ NX (.20, .40, .60, .80)	Apomorphine (.50)
12	24	Rats	αMPT (400) + NX (.20, .40, .60, .80)	Apomorphine (.50)
13	30	Rats	NX (.80)	d-Amphetamine (.5, 1, 1.5, 3, 6)
14	30	Rats	Saline	d-Amphetamine (.5, 1, 1.5, 3, 6)

All drugs were dissolved in 0.9% saline in a volume of 1.0 ml/kg body weight, and administered subcutaneously. Drug doses are expressed in terms of the salt. When animals were pretreated with a given durg, (with the exception of αMPT) the subsequent injection occurred ten minutes later as this has been shown to be the time required for the mean peak brain levels of NX to be reached (11). αMPT was initially injected in a dose of 300 mg/kg followed 1 hour later by an additional injection of 100 mg/kg. These animals were subsequently injected with NX 4.5 hours later.

Following a 30 minute habituation period, each animal receiving apomorphine as a final drug treatment was observed continuously by 3 independent observers for 4 ten minute periods, with three observations made per interval. Animals receiving d-amphetamine as a final drug were observed for 15 ten minute periods. To make it possible to precisely discriminate among the various levels of stereotypy produced, an eleven point SB gradient was used. Modified from the 4 point scale of Costall and Naylor (1973; 12) the gradient contains mutually exclusive categories as shown in Table 1.

Since stereotyped behavior is comprised of several components which may be independent of each other, the use of a parametric statistical test such as the student T test did not seem justified in evaluating the statistical significance of the various treatments. Therefore, the Mann Whitney U test was used.

RESULTS

1. Dose Response Inhibition of AISB by Naloxone in the Rat

Relative to controls, NX (.20 - .80 mg/kg) produced a marked ($p<.001$) dose-response inhibition of the stereotypy induced by apomorphine (.50 mg/kg: Fig. 1). NX pretreated animals subsequently given saline exhibited a nearly total lack of stereotyped behavior (Fig. 1).

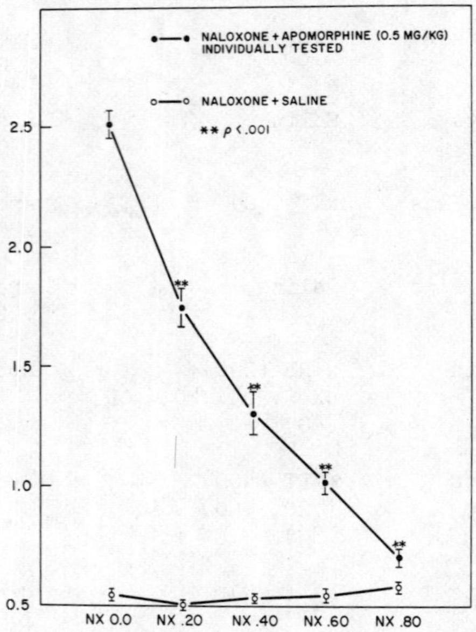

Fig. 1

2. <u>NS Elicited Inhibition of SB Induced by Increasing Doses of Apomorphine in the Rat</u>

After having obtained a dose related inhibition of AISB using varying doses of NX, an inhibition of the SB induced by progressively increasing doses of apomorphine (.01-.25 mg/kg) was undertaken using a low dose of NX (0.4 mg/kg). A significant inhibition of AISB was found ($p < .01$) with the curve of the saline pretreated rats almost perfectly parallel to the curve representing animals pretreated with NX (Fig. 2).

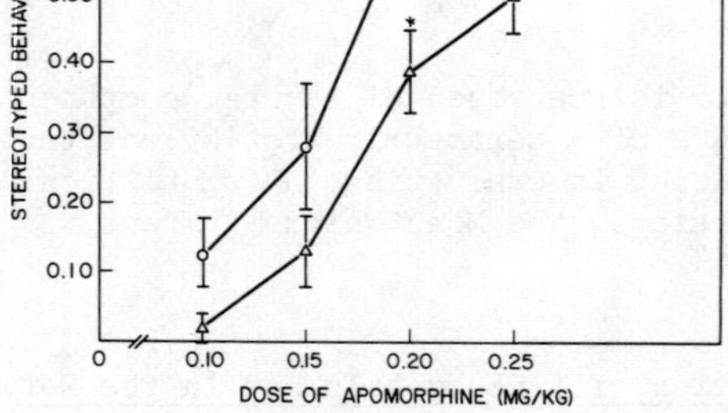

Fig. 2

3. Dose Response Inhibition of AISB by Naloxone in the Guinea Pig

NX (.20-.80 mg/kg) produced as marked ($p < .001$) a dose-response inhibition of AISB in the guinea pig (Fig. 3) as in the rat (Fig. 1 above). Apomorphine elicited a far more intense stereotypy response in the guinea pig in comparison to the rat, and consequently, to make the saline pretreated AISB produced in both species nearly equivalent, guinea pigs were administered only 0.25 mg/kg . At this dose, the guinea pigs exhibited nearly as much stereotypy as the rats injected with 2x this dose. The configuration of the curves in both species is quite similar. It should be noted however, that relatively low doses of NX (.20 mg/kg) have a greater inhibitory affect on AISB in the rat, while higher doses of NX (.60 mg/kg) are more inhibitory in the guinea pig (Fig. 3).

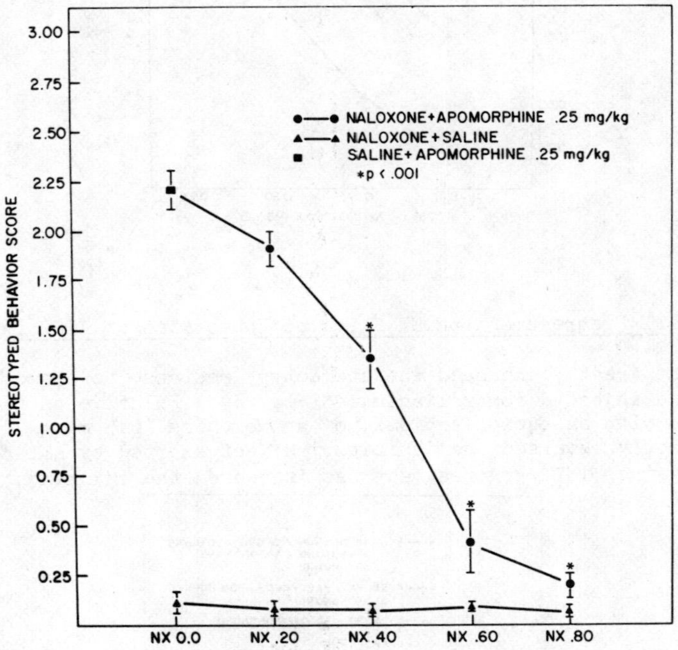

Fig. 3

4. NX Elicited Inhibition of SB Induced by Increasing Doses of Apomorphine in the Guinea Pig

As in the rat, progressively increasing doses of apomorphine (.10-.25 mg/kg) were inhibited by a low dose of NX (0.4 mg/kg) in a sigmoidal manner (Fig. 4). While the configuration of the curves generated by identical treatments in the rat and guinea pig are quite similar, it is again immediately apparent that at very low doses, apomorphine induces considerably more AISB in the guinea pig than in the rat. At the lowest doses (.10 and .15 mg/kg apomorphine) a 4-5 fold difference was seen. This diminished to approximately a 2.5-3 fold difference in the two species at the 2 highest doses of apomorphine administered (.20 and .25 mg/kg). Apparently this interspecies difference in stereotypy response to apmorphine varies in inverse proportion with dosage levels. Very likely because apomorphine exerted a greater arousal of AISB in the guinea pig than in the rat, NX (0.4 mg/kg) produced a greater inhibition of AISB in the former species (Fig. 4).

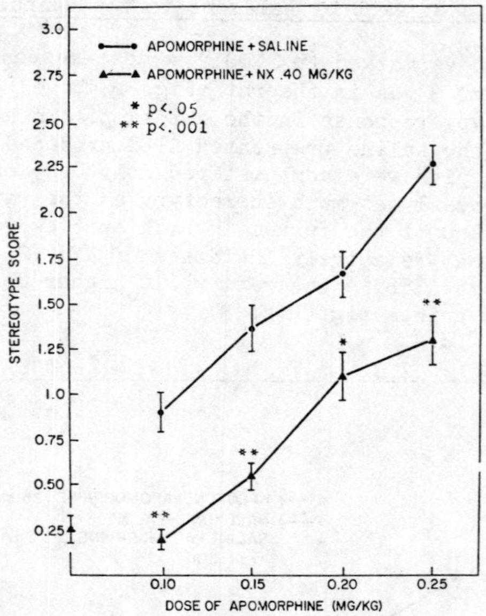

Fig. 4

5. Effect of AMPT Pretreatment on NX Elicited Inhibition of AISB in the Rat

AMPT pretreatment greatly enhanced the stereotypy response to apomorphine in comparison to saline injected control animals (Fig. 5). Relative to saline pretreated animals injected with an equivalent dose of apomorphine (0.5 mg/kg) the αMPT pretreatment completely reversed the inhibitory effect exerted by all doses of NX on AISB. However, since αMPT pretreatment has increased the stereotypy of control

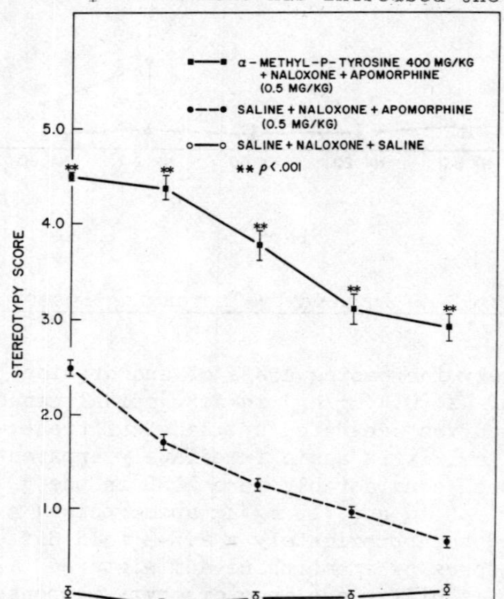

Fig. 5

animals receiving no NX, MPT pretreated animals administered NX and apomorphine should be more properly compared with αMPT pretreated animals injected with saline and apomorphine, as opposed to animals pretreated with only saline. In comparison with AMPT controls, NX still appears to exert a tonic inhibitory effect on AISB. As a consequence, the αMPT-NX-apomorphine curve is above and parallel to the saline-NX-apomorphine curve. Rather than abolishing the effect of NX on AISB, AMPT pretreatment appears to have merely shifted the entire curve upwards.

6. Effect of γ-Hydroxybutyric Acid Pretreatment on NX Elicited Inhibition of AISB in the Rat

Pretreatment with γ-hydroxybutyric acid produced an efffect on the AISB response that was somewhat similar (albeit less) to that produced by AMPT, i.e. it markedly enhanced it. Unlike AMPT pretreatment, however, γ-HB completely abolished the inhibitory effect of NX on AISB (Fig. 6).

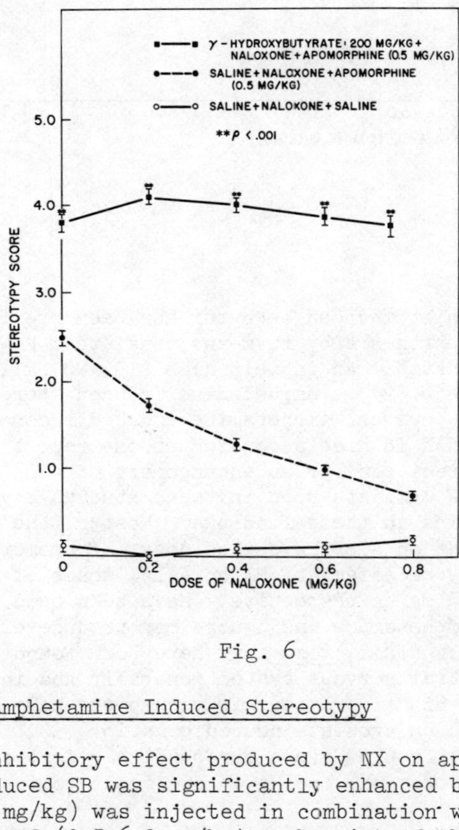

Fig. 6

7. Effect of NX on Amphetamine Induced Stereotypy

In contrast to the inhibitory effect produced by NX on apomorphine induced stereotypy, amphetamine induced SB was significantly enhanced by NX (0.8 mg/kg). As the same dose of NX (0.8 mg/kg) was injected in combination with the various doses of amphetamine administered (0.5-6.0 mg/kg) each point of the amphetamine + NX curve was shifted upward by equal increments for all doses of amphetamine + saline administered with the exception of 0.5 mg/kg amphetamine, which was unaffected by NX (Fig. 7).

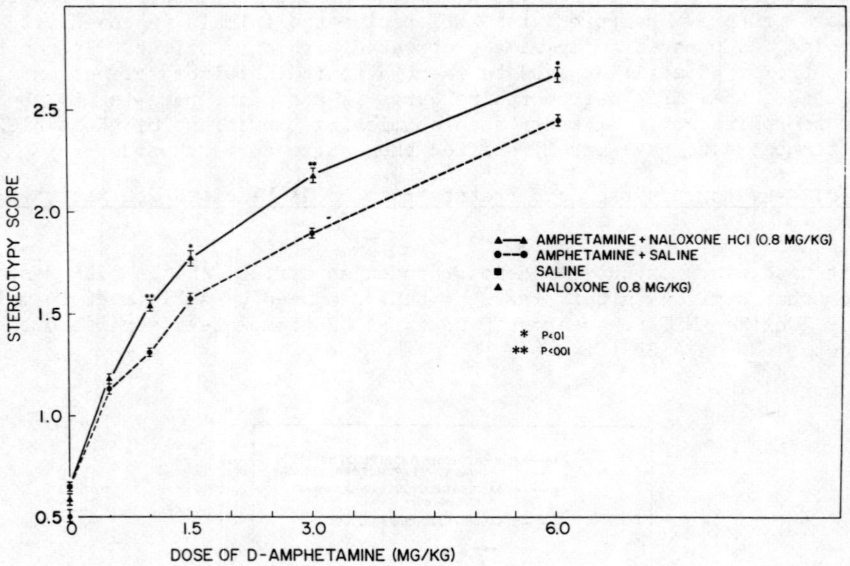

Fig. 7

DISCUSSION

The effect of NX on DA agonist induced behavior has been previously studied (13, 14, 15, 16, 17, 18). These reports are by no means consistent however. While some investigators have found that NX can inhibit AISB (19, 20, 21, 22), others have failed to observe this effect (23). Amphetamine induced stereotypy has been found to be enhanced by NX (24); however, amphetamine induced locomotor activity (AILA) is reportedly inhibited by NX in mice according to one report (25), though others have observed either no effect (26) or an enhancement of AILA by NX. Differences in the dosages of NX and DA agonists used in these studies may at least partially account for the discrepancies in these findings. Most of the studies that have been reported on the effect of NX on AISB have used doses of apomorphine no less than 10 mg/kg; while in studies of the effect of NX on AILA, doses of NX and d-amphetamine as high as 100 mg/kg and 10 mg/kg respectively have been used. High doses of the DA agonists apomorphine, amphetamine and l-dopa may produce effects that are non-specific relative to DA mechanisms, viz. they have been found to alter the level and release of 5-HT in the central nervous system generally and in the striatum specifically (26, 27, 28, 29). Since serotonergic mechanisms have been demonstrated to significantly interact with DA agonist induced behavior (30, 31, 32, 33, 34) high doses of central DA agonsits could have a confounding effect on the results obtained with concomitant NX administration, making it difficult to interpret these studies.

For this reason, only low doses of NX, apomorphine and d-amphetamine were used in the present study. Very wide dosages of NX were used initially varying from .01 to 50 mg/kg in combination with low doses of apomorphine, to determine whether NX could inhibit AISB and at what minimal doses of NX. From this preliminary study, low doses of NX varying from .20-.80 mg/kg were chosen for inclusion in the present study. Moreover, only very low doses of apomorphine (.10-.50 mg/kg) and amphetamine (.50-6.0) were used.

The present investigation was undertaken in order to more fully evaluate the interaction of NX with striatal dopaminergic mechanisms. We consequently sought to not only observe the stereotypy effects produced by this interaction, but to also explain these effects. It initially appeared possible that NX might exert an inhibitory effect on the binding of DA agonists to striatal DA receptors,in light of the marked inhibitory synergism produced by subthreshold doses of haloperidol and NX on AISB (35, 36). However, this possibility is precluded by reports that NX does not bind striatal dopamine receptors (37, 38, 39), and potentiates rather than inhibits amphetamine induced stereotypy (32; Fig. 7).

Recent evidence has been reported suggesting that apomorphine may be a more effective DA agonist than DA itself (40), binding striatal DA receptors at lower concentrations than DA (41, 42) and generally exhibiting an affinity for the dopamine receptor that is consistently higher than that of DA (40). As a behavioral consequence, drugs which increase DA levels in striatal synapses appear to inhibit AISB; while drugs inhibiting dopamine release increase AISB (43, 44, 45). It therefore seemed possible that NX might exert its inhibitory effect on AISB by releasing DA. This would also explain the observations of the present study that NX potentiates amphetamine induced stereotypy (Fig. 7), and further explain reports that NX enhances serum prolactin levels in rats (46, 47, 48). In support of this hypothesis, -hydroxybutyric acid which specifically inhibits DA but not norepinephrine, acetylcholine nor serotonin release (49, 50, 51) was able to completely reverse the effect of NX on AISB. It is interesting that MPT which inhibits newly synthesized DA release by blocking catecholamine synthesis should not exert the same effect. This may be due to an insufficient inhibition of striatal DA release by the dose of MPT used, or to an effect on a pool of presynaptic DA that is differently effected by -HB.

Additional evidence that NX can effect striatal DA release is provided by a recent report that NX (10^{-6}M) can significantly enhance the DA release stimulated by d-amphetamine (10^{-6}M) in striatal slices *in vitro*, but not in striatal homogenates (45).

Evidently, some structural integrity must be preserved for this effect to be seen. This may specifically involve presynaptic opioid receptors localized on striatal dopamine nerve terminals. The stimulation of these receptors by opiate agonists has been demonstrated to inhibit DA release (52, 53, 54). Apparently, an inhibition of these opioid receptors by NX produces the reverse effect, e.g. a stimulation of dopamine release. NX by itself exerts no affect on DA release in either striatal homogenates or slices (45). It would seem then, that the nigrostriatal pathway must be active for NX to produce any effects on DA agonist induced behaviors; particularly in light of the inability of NX to induce any of these behaviors on its own.

In summary, NX apparently does not directly interact with striatal DA mechanisms and therefore cannot by itself, induce those behaviors seen after the administration of DA agonists. NX can inhibit presynaptic opioid receptors localized on striatal DA boutons, but this has no behavioral consequence unless the nigrostriatal pathway is activated (e.g. by amphetamine). After such arousal resulting in the release of DA, NX induced inhibition of presynaptic opioid receptors may further enhance the DA agonist stimulated release of DA, resulting in a potentiation of AmISB and an inhibition of AISB.

TABLE 1 Stereotypy Rating Scale

RATING	BEHAVIORAL DESCRIPTION
0.0	Totally inert; asleep or catatonic
0.5	Extremely mild stereotypy interrupted by prolonged inactivity

RATING	BEHAVIORAL DESCRIPTION
1.0	Occasional SB other than licking and biting
1.5	Constant SB other than licking or biting (L or B)
2.0	Intense SB w/out L or B.
2.5	Intense SB with occasional licking
3.0	Constant licking; no locomotion or biting
3.5	Intense licking without B or with only very slight B
4.0	Licking and biting fairly frequent but not constant
4.5	Constant licking and biting; distractable (i.e. by noise)
5.0	Constant licking and biting; not distractable

The stereotypy gradient was defined by the behavior produced in the rat by progressive doses of most central dopamine agonists. As one increases the dosage of these agonists, the behavior induced in the rat changes as indicated. The gradient was also designed to represent the successive changes in behavior undergone as the behavioral arousal induced by a dopamine agonist increases or attentuates over time.

Quantitative terms appearing in the table are defined as follows:

Extremely mild; SB is very weak in intensity, brief in duration (5-10 seconds) and infrequent (=20 occurances of SB per interval).

Occasional: SB is seen at least every 30 seconds, with each occurance lasting a minimum of 10-20 seconds.

Constant: SB is fairly vigorous in intensity with less than 10 seconds intervening between stereotypies. The animals can be distracted by noise.

Intense: SB is very vigorous, and no more than a few seconds intervening between stereotypies. Each episode of SB lasts for at least a few minutes. LA is not seen, and it is difficult or impossible to distract the animals from their SB for more than a few seconds.

REFERENCES

1. M. J. Kuhar, C. B. Pert and S. H. Snyder, Nature 245, 447 (1973).
2. C. B. Pert and S. H. Snyder, Mol. Pharmacol. 10, 868 (1974).
3. B. Cox, M. Ary and P. Lomax, J. Pharmac. Exper. Ther. 196, 637 (1976).
4. G. Henderson and R. WestKaemper. Proc. West. Pharmacol. Soc. 18, 204 (1975).
5. J. J. Feigenbaum, B. H. Moon, W. Weiner, H. L. Klawans, J. Davis and P. E. Carson, Clin. Res. 26, 288A (1978).
6. L. Gunne, L. Lindstrom and L. Terenius, J. Neurotrans. 40, 13 (1977).
7. H. Emrich, A. Kolling, D. von Zerssen and A. Herz. Pharmokopsychiat. 10, 265 (1977).
8. N. Arden, A. Rubenson, K. Fuxe, T. Hokfelt J. Pharm. Pharmacol. 19, 627 (1967).
9. A. Ernst, Psychopharmacol. 10, 316 (1967).

10. T. Sourkes and S. Lal, Adv. Neurochem. 1, 247 (1975)
11. A.L. Misra, J. Pharm. Exp. 196, 257 (1976)
12. B. Costall and R. Naylor, Europ. J. Pharmacol. 24, 8 (1973)
13. B.H. Moon, J.J. Feigenbaum, W. Weiner and H.L. Klawans, VIIth Intl. Congress Pharmacol. Abstr. II, 193 (1978)
14. P. Dettmar, A. Cowan and D.S. Walter, Neuropharmacol. 17, 1041 (1978)
15. S. Holtzman, J. Pharmacol. Exper. Ther. 189, 51 (1974)
16. D.E. McMillian, Psychopharmacol. 19, 128 (1971)
17. N. Doggett, H. Reno and P. Spencer, Neuropharmacol. 14, 507 (1975)
18. W. Weiner, B.H. Moon, J.J. Feigenbaum, P.E. Carson and H.L. Klawans, Pharmacologist 20, 166 (1978)
19. G. Henderson and R. Westkaemper, Proc. West. Pharmacol. Soc. 18, 204 (1975)
20. B. Cox, M. Ary and P. Lomax, J. Pharmacol. Exper. Ther. 196, 637 (1976)
21. J. Buckett and R. Shaw, Psychopharmacol. 42, 293 (1975)
22. J.J. Feigenbaum, B.H. Moon, T. Cicero and H.L. Klawans, 11th CINP Congress Abstr. 387 (1978)
23. J.A. Gylys, K. Doran, and M. Szaraz, Fed. Proc. 33, 515 (1974)
24. D.S. Segal, R.G. Browne, A. Arnsten and D.C. Derrington in Developments in Neuroscience 4, J. van Ree and L. Terenius, eds., Elsevier, Amsterdam, 377-378 (1978)
25. P. Dettmar, A. Cowan and D.S. Walter, Neuropharmacol. 17, 1041 (1978)
26. S. Holtzman, J. Pharmacol. Exper. Ther. 189, 51 (1974). See also C.R. Rethy, C.B. Smith, and J.E. Villarreal, J. Pharmacol. Exper. Ther., 176, 472 (1971)
27. A.J. Vazquez and G. Krip, Biological Psychiat. 7, 11 (1973) ; see also G.M. Everett and T. Yellin, Res. Comm. Chem. Pathol. Pharmacol. 2, 407 (1971)
28. M. Grabowska, Psychopharmacol. 39, 315 (1974)
29. S. Algeri and C. Cerletti, Europ. J. Pharmacol. 27, 191 (1974); see also B.D. Hare, R. Neumayr and D.N. Franz, Nature 239, 336 (1972)
30. W.J. Weiner, C. Goetz, R. Westheimer, and H.L. Klawans, J. Neurol. Sci. 20, 373 (1973)
31. W.J. Weiner, C. Goetz and H.L. Klawans, Acta Pharmacol. et. Toxicol. 36, 155 (1975)
32. B. Costall and R. Naylor, J. Pharm. Pharmacol. 30, 257 (1978)
33. P. Mabry and B. Campbell, Brain Res. 49, 381 (1973)
34. W. Gumulka, W. Kostowski and A. Czlonkowski, Pharmacol. 10, 363 (1972)
35. B.H. Moon, J.J. Feigenbaum, W.J. Weiner and H.L. Klawans, 11th CINP Congress Pharmacol. Abstr. II, 193 (1978)
36. J.J. Feigenbaum, B.H. Moon and H.L. Klawans, MS submitted to Europ. J. Pharmacol. (1979)
37. J.J. Feigenbaum, B.H. Moon, T. Cicero and H.L. Klawans, 11th CINP Congress Abstr. 387 (1978)
38. D. Burt, S.J. Enna, I. Creese and S.H. Snyder, Proc. Natl. Acad. Sci. USA 72, 4655 (1975)
39. A. Czlonkowski, V. Höllt and A. Herz, Life Sci. 22, 953 (1978)
40. J.J. Feigenbaum, B.H. Moon and H.L. Klawans, Fed. Proc. In Press (1979)
41. L. Thal, I. Creese, and S.H. Snyder, Europ. J. Pharmacol. 49, 295 (1978)
42. D. Burt, S.J. Enna, I. Creese, and S.H. Snyder, Proc. Natl. Acad. Sci. USA 72, 4655 (1975)

43. C. Goetz and H. L. Klawans, Acta Pharmacol. et Toxicol. 34, 119 (1974)
44. S. Patni and P. Dandiya, Life Sci. 14, 737 (1974)
45. J. J. Feigenbaum, B. H. Moon, and H. L. Klawans, Fed. Proc. In Press (1979)
46. J. F. Bruni, D. van Vugt, S. Marshall and J. Meites, Life Sci. 21, 461 (1977)
47. C. J. Shaar, C. A. Frederickson, N. B. Dininger and L. Jackson, Life Sci. 21, 853 (1977)
48. C. Rivier, W. Vale, N. Ling M. Brown and R. Guillemin, Endocrinol. 100, 238 (1977)
49. G. L. Gessa, F. Crabai, L. Vargiu, and P. F. Spano, J. Neurochem. 15, 377 (1968)
50. N. Anden and G. Stock, Naunyn Schmeid. Arch. Pharmacol. 279, 89 (1977)
51. J. Walters, R. Roth and G. Aghajanian, J. Pharmacol. Exper. Ther. 186, 630 (1973)
52. N. Subramanian, P. Mitznegg, W. Sprügel, W. Domschke, S. Domschke E. Wünsch and L. Demling, Naunyn Schmeid. Arch. Pharmacol. 299, 163 (1977)
53. B. Celsens and K. Kuschinsky, Naunyn Schmeid. Arch. Pharmacol. 284, 159 (1974)
54. H. H. Loh, D. A. Brase, S. Sampath-Khanna, J. B. Mar and EL Way, Nature 264, 567 (1976). See also A. Bosse and K. Kuschinsky, Naunyn Schmeid. Arch. Pharmacol. 294, 17 (1976); C. Blundell, A. R. Crossman and P. Slater, Brit. J. Pharmacol. 31, 456P (1976) and K. Kuschinsky and O. Hornykiewicz, Europ. J. Pharmacol. 26, 41 (1974).

Biological Monitoring of Psychotropic Drugs Treatment

Chairman's Introductory Remarks

PAOLO L. MORSELLI

Department of Clinical Research, L.E.R.S.-Synthelabo, 58 rue de la Glacière, Paris Cédex 13, France

It is today a well accepted fact that responses to drugs depend on how much of the pharmacological agent reaches the sites of action, on how long the active concentration is maintained and on the sensitivity of the receptors to the drug. This means that the two main variables conditioning and determining the intensity and the duration of the response of the body to the drug are on the one side the sensitivity of the body to the drug and on the other the rate of disposition of the drug by the body.

Clinical pharmacology and pharmacokinetics have taught us that in many instances a drug has quite a long way to go before it reaches its main site of action. The amount of drug which reaches the receptors sites does in fact depends on several physiological variables such as absorption rate, protein binding, distribution in body fluids and tissues, metabolism and excretion rate.

Furthermore, it is well know, that all these variables, which because of genetic differences may vary considerably from one individual to another, may be further modified by other factors such as age, physiological and/or pathological status, pollutants, concomitant use of other drugs, levels of physical activity, etc.

Because of this interindividual variability in the pharmacokinetic profile of most drugs, everytime we administer a drug to a patient for the first time, we face three possibilities :

a) the drug dosage is correct and we obtain the "desired" response,
b) the dose is too high and together with the "therapeutic effect" we may obtain important adverse reactions,
c) the dose is too low and our patient appears as "unresponsive" to the treatment.

The same probabilities persist when we try to correct the dose in case of a wrong initial choice, and in many cases the process of defining the "correct dose" needed for a given individual may take several weeks with consequent discomfort for the patient and increased cost when caring for hospitalized cases.

Is there a way to overcome such an empirical approach ? Is there a means by which we can try to choose or to correct our dosing schedule in a more rational and faster way in order to assure each of our patients the maximum therapeutic benefit ?

In other branches of medicine, in parallel with the development of clinical pharmacology, we have learnt that in several instances therapeutic intervention may be improved if the concept of biological monitoring is applied.

What do we mean with such a term ? Biological monitoring is an integrated careful evaluation of several biological parameters which may be of relevance for : a) a better understanding of the disease ; b) a more rational therapy ; c) a better

differential diagnosis.
More specifically it means an integrated evaluation of blood levels of administered drugs, relevant biochemical parameters, endocrine responses, neurophysiological and cardiovascular variables as well as side effects, followed by a careful study of the possible relationships between the above mentioned variables and the clinical picture.
To be meaningful, such an evaluation should not be limited to a randomly chosen occasion, but all the mentioned parameters should be measured at regular intervals over several weeks or months with the specific aim of studying their mutual interrelationships within the individual patient (Morselli, 1976 ; 1978).
Examples of drugs or therapeutic areas where such an approach is or has already been usefully applied include antiepileptic drugs, anticancer drugs, antibiotics, antiarrhythmics, theophylline, salicylates, digoxin and hypoglycemics.
Now where do we stand in psychiatry ? The approach of biological monitoring is not only poorly developed but furthermore (with the exception of Lithium) is strongly questioned regarding its validity and usefulness. How has this come about ? Why do we have such a resistance to the acceptance of an approach which not only sounds logical and is based on correct pharmacological premises but in addition has also been proven useful in other areas for medicine ?
Reasons are multiple and too numerous to be fully discussed here. Among the principal ones which to me appear to be the major contributing factors for such a gap, can be quoted the following :
1. <u>The "natural" resistance</u> encountered <u>in most psychiatrists to fully accept the validity of the pharmacological approach</u>. Drugs are still used and considered as something "magic" and not as chemical entities which exert their actions by interacting with proteins of the body. Too often they are used with a very limited knowledge of their pharmacological spectrum and kinetic profile.
This leads frequently to an improper use with consequent poor results. The poor outcome or the variability of results reinforce a sceptical attitude towards pharmacological agents.
In other words there is a "refusal" to accept that the lack of a therapeutic response may have been due to our mistakes, and all the blaim is given to the patient who is either "unresponsive" or responding "paradoxically". There is really no attempt to try to understand which are the major causes for a poor response, but such a result is accepted as a part of the variability of human nature.
2. <u>The nature of the disease, or better, of the diseases</u>. Most of the syndromes treated with psychotropic drugs are not homogeneous ; despite our hope to be able to divide them into a rigid nosological classification, they are the expression of several pathological entities which are as different from one to the other as are the patients. When we proceed by giving them a vague "label" which only indicates a certain approximation, we surely cannot expect to observe homogeneous results.
Furthermore in most instances the pathological process proceeds by "poussées" and "phases" whose duration is unpredictable.
All these factors, the uncertainty in the diagnosis and the presence of phases in the evolution of the syndrome, make a precise evaluation of the "therapeutic results" very difficult.
3. <u>The lack of concordance among the data available</u> on the utility of monitoring. If we analyse very carefully what has been published on the topic, it is really not surprising to find a considerable disagreement. Because of the great dishomogeneity in most cases a comparison is impossible. Too often the clinical definition of the patient and the clinical evaluation is very poor, the observation period is too short, the analytical methodologies are questionable, the design is inadequate and the objectives very poorly defined.
Considering for instance the reports published on this topic for neuroleptic drugs from the year 1975 up to June 1978, we can find a careful differential diagnosis in less than 50 % of the studies while in the remaining reports the authors speak of psychotic patients or schizophrenic patients without any further specification.

In the majority of the studies, observation periods range from 2 to 4 weeks and only in a few studies have patients been monitored for 10-12 weeks.
The same can be said for antidepressants where, with the exception of 1 report, most of the data refer to observation periods of 2-6 weeks and a differential diagnosis is present only in less than 40 % of the reports.
Despite this considerable drawback, in about 60 % of the published reports, if we analyze them carefully, we can find (sometimes in disagreement with the conclusion of the authors) that there is a certain evidence of possible relationships between drug concentrations in plasma and therapeutic response or side effects.
For what concerns endocrine responses even if several studies have documented a rise in prolactin plasma levels after neuroleptic administration, as well as modification of other hormonal responses after both neuroleptics and antidepressants, the relationships between drug plasma levels and endocrine responses have not yet been clarified. The situation is even less encouraging concerning neurophysiological parameters, where if information is available on the relationships between EEG and drug plasma levels for volunteers and patients after a single dose, no data are available for patients following chronic treatment.
So even if some data point toward the usefulness of biological monitoring in psychiatry, for most of the drugs in use today we cannot still some of the question described in table 1.

TABLE 1 : Questions which if answered could help in better understanding the interindividual variability in response to psychotropic agents

1) Relationships daily doses-blood levels ?
2) Steady state levels ? Correct dose schedules ?
3) Causes of fluctuation of blood levels ?
4) Interactions with other drugs ?
5) Toxic thresholds ? (a) Acute ; (b) Chronic
6) Individual thresholds ?
7) Patient compliance ?
8) Compliance of paramedical personnel ?
9) Drug as a tool for differential diagnosis ?
10) Necessity of maintenance treatment ?
11) Active metabolites ?
12) Benefit of the individual patient ?

The fact that for most of these questions we are not yet capable to give a clear and comprehensive answer appears to me to be a good reason to support the necessity for the better integrated biological monitoring in psychiatry.
In other areas of medicine, answering these questions has not only helped us to gain more basic information about the drug under study but more importantly has helped to better understand the lack of response or adverse reactions of the individual patient giving him the possibility of rational and optimal therapy. I hope that the collegues who participate to this symposium will help, by analyzing more in detail the various aspects, to give an anwer at least to some of these questions so that we can shed more light on this very discussed topic.

REFERENCES

P.L. MORSELLI (1976) : Pediatric clinical pharmacology routine monitoring or clinical trials ? In Clinical Pharmacy and Clinical Pharmacology. B. Gouvei, G. TOGNONI & E. Van der Klein (eds), pp. 277-287. Elsevier/ North Holland Biomedical Press, Amsterdam, New York.

P.L. MORSELLI (1978) : Clinical significance of monitoring plasma levels of benzodiazepine tranquillizers and antiepileptic drugs. Neuropsychopharmacology. P. Deniker, C. Radouco-Thomas, A. Villeneuve (eds), pp. 877-888. Pergamon Press Oxford and New York.

Pharmacokinetics and Pharmacodynamics of Haloperidol in Man

A. FORSMAN and R. ÖHMAN

Psychiatric Department III, University of Göteborg, Lillhagen's Hospital, S-422 03 Hisings Backka, Sweden

ABSTRACT

The present paper is a review of the pharmacokinetics and pharmacodynamics of haloperidol in man. The background of interindividual differences in clinical response to the drug is discussed. Possible ways of monitoring antipsychotic drug dosage from assessment of drug and prolactin concentration in serum are presented.

KEYWORDS

Haloperidol, pharmacokinetics, prolactin, metabolism, protein binding, clinical effect, drug interaction, enzyme induction.

INTRODUCTION

Modern antipsychotic pharmacotherapy started in 1952 with the first report on the psychiatric use of chlorpromazine (Delay, Deniker and Harl, 1952). This revolutionized the treatment and the results achieved at psychiatric institutions. Chlorpromazine and other antipsychotic drugs, like for instance haloperidol, proved to have not only sedative effect but also a specific effect on psychotic symptoms. Still, several patients never obtained adequate relief. Side-effects were common and sometimes troublesome.

This paper is a compilation of several investigations, referred to in Table I, designed to elucidate the pharmacokinetic and pharmacodynamic background of such interindividual differences in clinical response to haloperidol, a low-dose neuroleptic of the butyrophenone type.

CLINICAL MATERIAL AND METHODS

Haloperidol was given orally or intravenously in single dose to healthy volunteers. The drug was also given <u>t.i.d.</u> to psychiatric in-patients. Blood samples were drawn repeatedly from an antecubital vein of the volunteers after the doses; and in a similar way from fasting patients in the morning before the first dose of drug, after at least one week of haloperidol treatment.

The concentrations of haloperidol and reduced haloperidol (a major metabolite)

TABLE I. Compilation of own Investigations summerized in this Review.

PHARMACOKINETICS	Dose of drug (Forsman, 1977d) Patient complicance.
	Bioavailability (Forsman and Öhman, 1976b; Drug distribution Forsman and Öhman, 1977b)
	Metabolism (Forsman and co-workers, 1977c; Excretion Forsman and co-workers, 1978c; Forsman and Larsson, 1978b).
	Steady-state serum concentration (Forsman and Öhman, 1977b; Forsman and Öhman, 1975)
	Free fraction of drug (Forsman and Öhman, 1977a; Rubin and co-workers, 1978)
	Interaction with other drugs (Forsman and Öhman, 1977b; Forsman and Öhman, 1977a)
PHARMACODYNAMICS	Varying pathogenesis of the diseases (Forsman, 1977d; Forsman, 1976a)
	Interindividual differences in responsiveness of central neurones (Forsman, 1977d; Forsman, 1976a; Forsman and Öhman, 1978a)

in serum and in various tissues were assessed with a gas-chromatographic method (Forsman and co-workers, 1974) or a high pressure liquid chromatographic method (Forsman and Öhman, 1978d); those of prolactin with a radioimmunoassay technique (Öhman and Axelsson, 1978).

RESULTS AND DISCUSSION

Amount of drug ingested

Only strictly controlled in-patients were included. The relationship between the steady-state serum concentration and the dose of the drug proved rectilinear in the individual patient. However, the correlation coefficient fell to approximately 0.6 ($p < 0.001$) in a group of patients. This was due to interindividual variation in pharmacokinetic parameters.

Bioavailability and drug distribution

Only 60 % of an oral dose of haloperidol finally reached the systemic circulation. The mean lag between ingestion of haloperidol and appearance of the drug in the blood was about one and a half hours. Maximal concentrations in serum were reached after five hours. The apparent distribution volume proved to be more than 1000 liters or around 25 liters per kg body-weight in most patients. Haloperidol was distributed rapidly to extravascular tissues, predominantly to the liver and adipose tissues, where the concentration was 1000 times and 20 times higher than in serum, respectively. Both bioavailability and distribution volumes varied less than two-fold from one individual to another.

Elimination of drug

After the distribution phase, the elimination was exponential, indicating first-order kinetics. The biological half-life, assessed mathematically or graphically from linear elimination curves, was around sixteen hours after intravenous administration, and about twentyfour hours after oral administration of drug. The elimination was slower during the night.

Haloperidol is eliminated by enzymatic degradation, mainly in the liver, but also to some extent in extra-hepatic tissues. Only minute amounts of haloperidol are excreted with the urine. There are indications of an entero-hepatic recirculation. Recent investigations have revealed a hydrated metabolite with a weak antipsychotic effect. Since it is present in serum at roughly the same concentration as the mother-molecule haloperidol itself, it is probably of minor clinical interest. As previously shown, haloperidol is degraded by oxidative dealkylation splitting the carbon-nitrogen chain necessary for an antipsychotic effect.

Free fraction of drug

Roughly 92 % of haloperidol is bound to serum constituents. The interindividual variation of this percentage is small. There is thus a wide variation also in the steady-state concentration of free and unbound drug, which is assumed to reflect closely the concentrations at the site of action, i.e. mainly dopamine receptors of the central neurons.

Interaction with other drugs

Haloperidol itself did not seem to enhance its own biodegradation. Nor did other neuroleptics, anti-Parkinsonian drugs, and carbamazapime influence the steady-state serum concentration following a given dose of haloperidol. On the other hand, well-known enzyme inducers, like diphenylhydantoin and barbiturates, lowered the concentrations of haloperidol in serum. Apparently, ethyl alcohol had a similar effect. No interference by other drugs was observed at binding sites of serum proteins.

Differences of the diseases of the patients studied

The mean total steady-state serum concentration was about 10 ng/ml (25 nM) in haloperidol-treated, chronically schizophrenic patients. The concentration of free drug was about 0.8 ng/ml (2 nM). This is close to the inhibition constant of haloperidol at the antagonist binding sites of calf striatal membranes estimated according to Creese, Burt and Snyder (1975). In patients suffering from senile dementia, the mean steady-state concentration was only 3.4 ng/ml (9 nM). Different diagnostic groups thus appeared susceptible to different concentrations of haloperidol. There was also an interindividual variation of effective drug concentrations within each diagnostic group, possibly indicating a variation in drug sensitivity of central neurons for reasons other than pathological, for instance in the genetically determined receptor sensitivity. It might also reflect that the diagnostic groups not were homogenous.

Interindividual differences in responsiveness of central neurons

It was not possible to use drug assessment only for the effective monitoring of haloperidol therapy since there was a wide range of therapeutically effective concentrations in serum from different patients. Consequently it proved impossible to define generally effective concentration ranges of haloperidol in serum. This prompted the search for a pharmacodynamic marker indicating optimal antipsychotic efficacy. Previous studies have failed to show a close relationship between extrapyramidal side-effects and antipsychotic effect. On the other hand, there was a close relationship in the rat between the concentration of dopamine receptor-blocking drug in the brain and several variables like the duration and amplitude of the metabolic response measured as DOPA turn-over, behavioural effects such as conditioned avoidance response, and prolactin concentration in serum (Öhman and co-workers, 1977). It was therefore concluded that prolactin response might reflect the degree of dopamine receptor blockade in the central neurons as well as behavioural effects induced by the drug. Provided that a similar relationship exists also in man, it would be possible to estimate not only the degree of dopamine receptor blockade in the central neurons, but also the antipsychotic effect of neuroleptic drugs by measuring the prolactin concentration in serum.

The prolactin response to haloperidol was studied in 12 chronic schizophrenics. There was a large interindividual variation in the amplitude of prolactin response within each sex. Women, as a rule, responded stronger than men. The serum prolactin concentration curve levelled off with a sufficiently large increase of drug dose (or drug concentration in serum). Some individuals reached this maximal response at low haloperidol levels, while others did so at higher levels. Preliminary results indicate that patients responding clinically only to high doses also reach their maximal prolactin response at higher doses than unselected patients.

Biomathematical model for prolactin response to neuroleptic drugs

The levelling off of the prolactin response to increasing steady-state serum concentrations of haloperidol closely resembles the kinetic situation of enzymatic saturation. Assuming that free drug and transmitter are competing for receptors of the central neurons, the law of mass action was applied. After introducing several assumptions (Axelsson and co-workers, 1978) it proved possible to deduce an equation closely related to that of Michaelis-Menten, providing the relationship between the dose or concentration of drug and the prolactin response. The applicability of the model was strongly supported by empirical data. In fact, it proved possible to predict the concentration or dose of drug to result in any fraction of maximal prolactin response from just two or more paired determinations of drug and prolactin in serum. If a favourable clinical outcome could be related to a certain fraction of the maximal prolactin response, it would thus be possible to monitor the drug dosage from such simple prolactin and drug assessments in serum.

Concluding remarks

Since the biological half-life of haloperidol is roughly 24 hours after oral doses, and since the half-life is even prolonged during the night, this drug might be administered only once or twice a day during maintenance treatment. The comparatively long half-life of haloperidol also implicates that steady-state serum concentrations of the drug are not achieved until at least five days after a dose change. A reduced bioavailability of oral doses of haloperidol and a lag between haloperidol ingestion as tablets and drug appearance in blood, should be borne in mind particularly in the acute situation. With the exception of enzyme inducers like barbiturates, diphenylhydantoin, and ethyl alcohol, interference by other drugs was not observed.

Since there was no simple relationsip between the pharmacokinetics of haloperidol and the clinical response, generally effective concentration ranges for haloperidol in serum could not be defined. Therefore, adjustment of dosage is still best achieved by clinical observations of the patients response to the drug. However, prolactin may be used as a pharmacodynamic marker, using the likely relationship between serum concentration of haloperidol, prolactin response, and a favourable clinical outcome.

REFERENCES

Axelsson, R., Forsman, A., Wendestam, C. and Öhman, R. (1978). A biomathematical model for prolactin response to dopamine-blocking agents in man. Pharmacol. Ther. Res. Submitted.

Creese, I., Burt, D. and Snyder, S.H. (1975). Dopamine receptor binding: differentation of agonist and antagonist states with ^{3}H-dopamine and ^{3}H-haloperidol. Life Sci. 17, 1715-1720.

Delay, J., Deniker, P. and Harl, J. (1952). Utilisation en thérapeutic psychiatrique d'une phenothiazine d'action centrale élective (4560 R.P.). Ann. méd. psychol. 110, 112-122.

Forsman, A., Mårtensson, E., Nyberg, G. and Öhman, R. (1974). A gas chromatographic method for determining haloperidol. Naunyn-Schmiedeberg's. Arch. Pharmacol. 286, 113-124.

Forsman, A. and Öhman, R. (1975). Some aspects on the distribution and metabolism of haloperidol in man. In:G. Sedvall, B. Uvnäs, and Y. Zotterman (Eds.), Antipsychotic drugs: pharmacodynamics and pharmacokinetics, Pergamon Press, Oxford and New York, pp. 359-365.

Forsman, A. (1976a). Individual variability in response to haloperidol. Proc. Soc. Med. 69 S, 9-13.

Forsman, A. and Öhman, R. (1976b). Pharmacokinetic studies on haloperidol in man. Curr. Therap. Res. 20, 319-336.

Forsman, A. and Öhman, R. (1977a). Studies on serum protein binding of haloperidol. Curr. Therap. Res. 21, 245-255.

Forsman, A. and Öhman, R. (1977b). Applied pharmacokinetics of haloperidol in man, Curr. Therap. Res. 21, 396-411.

Forsman, A., Fölsch, G., Larsson, M. and Öhman, R. (1977c). On the metabolism of haloperidol in man. Curr. Therap. Res. 21, 606-617.

Forsman, A. (1977d). Individual differences in clinical response to an antipsychotic drug. Thesis. Gotab, Göteborg.

Forsman, A. and Öhman, R. (1978a). On the objective evaluation of effects of neuroleptic drugs. Curr. Therap. Res. 24, 179-192.

Forsman, A. and Larsson, M. (1978b). Metabolism of haloperidol. Curr. Therap. Res. 24, 567-568.

Forsman, A., Larsson, M., Lundborg, H. and Renström, P. (1978c). On the distribution and elimination of haloperidol in cholecystectomized patients. Surgery. Submitted.

Forsman, A. and Öhman, R. (1978d). A high pressure liquid chromatographic method for the determination of haloperidol and reduced haloperidol in serum. To be published.

Öhman, R., Larsson, M., Nilsson, I.M., Engel, J. and Carlsson, A. (1977). Neurometabolic and behavioural effects of haloperidol in relation to drug levels in serum and brain, Naunyn-Schmiedeberg's Arch, Pharmacol. 229, 105-114.

Öhman, R. and Axelsson, R. (1978). The relationship between prolactin response and antipsychotic effect of thioridazine in psychiatric patients. Europ. J. Clin. Pharmacol. Accepted for publication.

Rubin, R.T., Forsman, A., Heykants, J., Öhman, R., Tower, B.B. and Michiels, M. (1978). Serum haloperidol determinations in psychiatric patients: Comparison of methods and correlation with serum prolactin. Arch. Gen. Psychiat. Submitted.

Monitoring of Phenothiazine Plasma Levels in Psychiatric Patients

SVEIN G. DAHL

Department of Pharmacology, Institute of Medical Biology, University of Tromsø, Tromsø, Norway

ABSTRACT

Up to now the levels of 10 different phenothiazines and some of their active metabolites have been measured in plasma from patients. A large number of different phenothiazine metabolites has been identified. Still, the number of active metabolites that contribute significantly to the effects of therapeutic doses is probably no more than 3 or 4 for each drug. Psychiatric patients treated with similar oral doses of phenothiazines show large interindividual variations in plasma drug levels. This is probably mainly due to variations in the extent of presystemic drug metabolism. Some studies have demonstrated a much smaller individual variation in plasma drug levels of patients who have had their phenothiazine doses adjusted to obtain optimal therapeutic effect. Patients who respond to phenothiazine treatment often have higher plasma levels of the drug and its active metabolites than non-responders, and certain side-effects seem to be more frequent at higher plasma levels. A clear-cut correlation between plasma levels and therapeutic effects of phenothiazines has, however, not been demonstrated so far. Neither have any definite toxic plasma level limits been established. Biological monitoring of phenothiazine plasma levels is therefore still of very limited value in clinical practice.

INTRODUCTION

Biological monitoring of plasma drug levels includes the chemical analysis of drugs and their metabolites in patient-plasma. This is performed to help the clinician to determine rational drug regimens for individual patients. As will be discussed later during this symposium, this implies both that a certain therapeutic plasma level range exists and is known for the drug, and that chemical methods for plasma level determination are available.

ANALYSIS OF DRUGS AND METABOLITES IN PLASMA

Sufficiently sensitive, specific and precise chemical methods for analysis of several phenothiazines in plasma have been developed during the last 10 years. The analysis usually includes one or several extraction steps, followed either by gas chromatography (GLC), gas chromatography combined with mass spectrometry (GLC-MS), spectrofluorimetry (SFL), measurement of radioactively labelled compounds (R),

TABLE 1 Phenothiazines Measured in Human Plasma

Drug	Number of metabolites quantitated separately	Methods based on
Butaperazine	-	SFL
Cyamepromazine	-	GLC
Chlorpromazine	18	GLC,GLC-MS,SFL,RIA
Fluphenazine	2	SFL,R,RIA
Levomepromazine	2	GLC
Mesoridazine	1	GLC,SFL
Perazine	1	SFL, TLC
Perphenazine	2	GLC
Promazine	1	GLC
Thioridazine	4	GLC,SFL

radioimmunoassay (RIA), or thin-layer chromatography and direct spectrodensitometry (TLC). As shown in Table 1, at least 10 different phenothiazine drugs and some of their metabolites have been measured in human plasma, by different chemical techniques. No metabolites of butaperazine and cyamepromazine have yet been quantitated in plasma, while 18 different chlorpromazine metabolites have been measured (Schooler and co-workers, 1976). For the next 6 drugs, fluphenazine, levomepromazine, mezoridazine, perazine, perphenazine and promazine, only one or two metabolites have been measured in addition to the parent drug, while 4 different thioridazine metabolites have been measured in plasma.

ACTIVE METABOLITES

Although the different phenothiazine drugs included in Table 1 have slightly different chemical formulas, their main pathways of metabolism in man are the same. These include demethylation, oxidation of the ring sulphur, nitrogen oxidation, and hydroxylation, which is often followed by a conjugation reaction. Thioridazine and mesoridazine may also undergo sulfoxidation at the side chain. By different combinations of these pathways, a large number of different metabolites may theoretically be formed. As many as 168 different metabolites of chlorpromazine have been postulated, and more than 30 of these have been identified in urine from different species (Usdin, 1971). The large number of possible phenothiazine metabolites has persuaded many pharmacologists to consider the establishment of plasma level-effect relationships for the phenothiazine drugs a hopeless task.

The contribution from a drug or some of its metabolites to the therapeutic effect and to the side-effects, depends on two main variables. One is the pharmacokinetics of the compound, which determines its plasma level at a certain dosage, and its distribution between the plasma and the tissues. The other is the pharmacodynamic properties, which are often expressed as the intrinsic pharmacologic activity of the compound. There are many papers in the literature showing that several different phenothiazine metabolites are biologically active. However, a further examination into which of the metabolites are both pharmacologically active, and achieve plasma levels in the same range as the parent compound, gives a very limited number of metabolites which may be considered as contributing significantly to the effects of the drug.

An example of this is shown in Table 2, which is reproduced from a recent paper by

TABLE 2 Striatal Dopamine Receptor Affinity

Compound	Relative potency
3- Hydroxychlorpromazine	2.3
Chlorpromazine	1.0
7- Hydroxychlorpromazine	0.7
Desmethylchlorpromazine	0.4
Didesmethylchlorpromazine	0.1
Chlorpromazine sulfoxide	< 0.01

Creese and others (1978). The affinity to dopamine receptors in rat brain has been used to predict clinical activity of neuroleptics, and Table 2 shows the relative activity of some chlorpromazine metabolites in this system. The 3-hydroxychlorpromazine showed higher activity than the parent drug. However, in pharmacokinetic studies this metabolite has not been found in measurable plasma concentrations. Chlorpromazine sulfoxide, which is one of the metabolites which reaches the highest plasma concentrations in patients, had virtually no activity in this system, and the same has been demonstrated with other biological systems. Both 7-hydroxychlorpromazine and desmethylchlorpromazine are active in this and in other test systems, and appear in relatively high plasma concentrations compared to chlorpromazine.

Also chlorpromazine N-oxide is considered as being active, and is found in relatively high plasma concentrations (Curry, 1978). Thus, a combination of the currently available information about both the pharmacokinetics and the pharmacodynamics of chlorpromazine and its metabolites, indicates that probably only three out of the large number of different chlorpromazine metabolites contribute significantly to the effects, and should therefore be included in a biological monitoring of this drug.

INTERINDIVIDUAL VARIATIONS IN PLASMA LEVELS

Plasma Levels after Similar Doses

Almost all studies have shown very large variations in phenothiazine plasma levels between patients receiving similar doses. An example of this is given in Fig. 1, which shows chlorpromazine plasma levels in a group of patients receiving 400 mg per day orally. The steady-state plasma levels in 26 patients varied between zero and 235 ng/ml. Variations of a similar magnitude have also been demonstrated for other phenothiazines which have been measured in plasma.

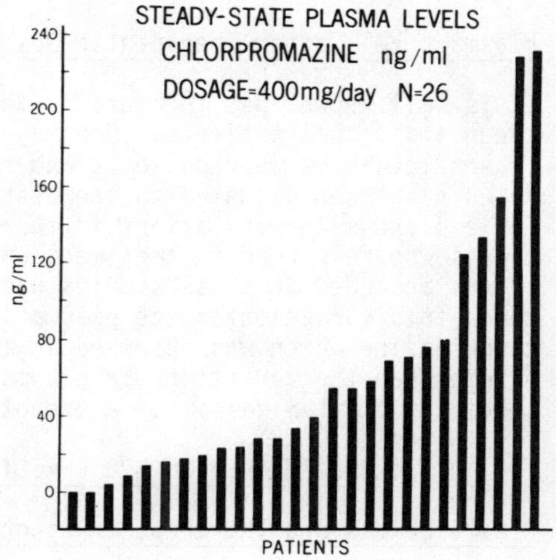

Fig. 1. Individual variations in chlorpromazine plasma levels. (Cooper and Simpson, 1976)

This raises two principal questions: What are the therapeutic consequences of this variation, and which factors are responsible for the variation? To answer the last question, let us look at the factors that determine the plasma levels of a drug after single doses as well as after repeated dosing. These are (1) the dose interval and size, and (2) the pharmacokinetics of the drug. Since the patients whose plasma levels are shown in Fig. 1 received similar doses at similar intervals, the variation in their plasma levels must have been due to individual variations in the pharmacokinetic factors. These are (1) The extent of biologic availability, (2) The distribution of the drug between the plasma and other parts of the body, which is measured by the apparent volume of distribution, and (3) The rate of elimination of the drug, which is measured by its biologic half-life.

TABLE 3 Interindividual Variations in Chlorpromazine Kinetics

	Range (N=8)	Highest / Lowest
Steady-state$^{(*)}$ plasma level (ng/ml)	16 - 124	8
Extent of biologic availability (%)	10 - 69	7
Apparent volume of distribution (L/kg)	10 - 35	3.5
Biologic $T_{1/2}$ (hr)$^{(*)}$	22 - 49	2

(*) After 33 d of chronic dosing, 100 mg x 2 P.O. (Dahl and Strandjord, 1977)

An analysis of the contribution of each of these factors to the variation in plasma levels is shown in Table 3, which summarizes some of the results of a pharmacokinetic study of chlorpromazine. The plasma levels after repeated dosing varied between 16 and 124 ng/ml in 8 patients. This is eightfold variation, as shown in the right column. The extent of biologic availability showed a 7-fold variation, while the variations in the apparent volume of distribution and the biological half-life were of a smaller magnitude. It has been demonstrated in this and in other studies that after oral administration the phenothiazines may undergo first-pass metabolism to a considerable extent (Curry, 1978; Dahl, 1976) and it is therefore not surprising to observe large interindividual variations in the fraction of oral doses entering the systemic circulation as unmetabolised drug. Similar variations in the extent of biologic availability have been demonstrated for other drugs that undergo first-pass metabolism, such many of the betablockers.

Plasma Levels after Therapeutic Doses

It is well known that therapeutic doses of neuroleptics vary over a wide range between individual patients. One may therefore ask how large are the variations in plasma levels between patients who respond to phenothiazine treatment, after the doses have been adjusted to the best attainable clinical result in each individual. Table 4 shows the variations in therapeutic doses and plasma levels in chronic patients who responded to treatment with a phenothiazine. Although the number of patients included in these studies was relatively small, it may be concluded that the three-fold variation in the plasma levels of chlorpromazine, levomepromazine and thioridazine which was observed in these studies, is of a considerably smaller magnitude than the variations in plasma levels usually observed in a panel of patients receiving similar doses of a phenothiazine.

PLASMA LEVELS AND EFFECTS

Plasma Levels and Therapeutic Response

The relationship between plasma levels and clinical effects in psychotic patients has been examined for 6 of the 10 drugs which are given in Table 1. Simpson and others (1973) and Garver and others (1977) found that there was some relation between plasma levels and the clinical effect of butaperazine. Out of 12 reports on the relationship between plasma levels and clinical effects of chlorpromazine,

TABLE 4 Variations in Plasma Level and Therapeutic Dose for "Chronic Responders"

DRUG	NUMBER OF PATIENTS	THERAPEUTIC DOSE		PLASMA LEVEL	
		Range (mg/d)	Largest / Smallest	Range (ng/ml)	Highest / Lowest
Chlorpromazine [1]	38	400 - 1000	2.5	18 - 51	3
Levomepromazine [2]	8	50 - 350	7	290 - 880	3
Thioridazine [3]	10	80 - 800	10	440 - 1180	3

([1] Rivera-Calimlim and co-workers, 1977; [2] Dahl, Strandjord and Sigfusson, 1977; [3] Axelsson, 1977).

6 concluded that there was some relation (Clark and Kaul, 1976; Curry, 1976; Rivera-Calimlim and Castaneda, 1973; Rivera-Calimlim and others, 1976; Sakalis and others, 1973; Sakurai and others, 1975). The other 6 concluded there was not (Kolakowska and others, 1976; Loga, Curry and Lader, 1975; Mackay, Healey and Baker, 1974; Phillipson and others, 1977; Sakalis and others, 1972; Wiles and others; 1976), but 2 of these did find some relation between the therapeutic effect of the drug and the ratio between the levels of active and inactive metabolites (Mackay, Healey and Baker, 1974; Phillipson and others, 1977). Almost all studies where chlorpromazine sulfoxide was measured, report of higher plasma levels of this relatively inactive metabolite in non-responders than in patients responding to the treatment.

Smulevitch and others (1973) reported that a therapeutic response to fluphenazine treatment was observed when the plasma levels were above a certain value, and Gottschalk and others (1976) found that the plasma levels of mesoridazine after a single intramuscular dose were higher in responders than in non-responders to the treatment. Breyer and others (1976) reported that responders to perazine treatment tended to have higher plasma levels than non-responders, while another study concluded with no such relationship (Hadass and others, 1974). Among 4 studies of the plasma level/effect relationship for thioridazine, 3 concluded with no relationship (Bergling and others, 1975; Sakalis, Traficante, and Gershon, 1977; Vanderheeren and Muusze, 1977), and one concluded that therapeutic response was observed when the plasma levels were within a certain range (Klein, Chandra and Matussek, 1975).

None of the studies where some relationship between plasma drug levels and effect was found have, however, demonstrated a clearly defined therapeutic plasma level range, or a direct correlation between plasma levels and the clinical outcome of the treatment.

Let us now look in more detail at one of the studies of butaperazine, which is shown in Fig. 2. The left curve shows a plot of clinical rating versus plasma drug level. Although no direct correlation is evident, a therapeutic benefit of the treatment appears to occur when plasma drug levels are within a certain range. This study also included assesment of drug levels in the red blood cells, as shown on the right curve. A curvilinear relationship between clinical rating and drug levels in the erythrocytes is demonstrated, and in spite of the preliminary nature of these data, this highly interesting finding certainly deserves further study.

Plasma Levels and Side-Effects

The relationship between side-effects and plasma levels of phenothiazines have also

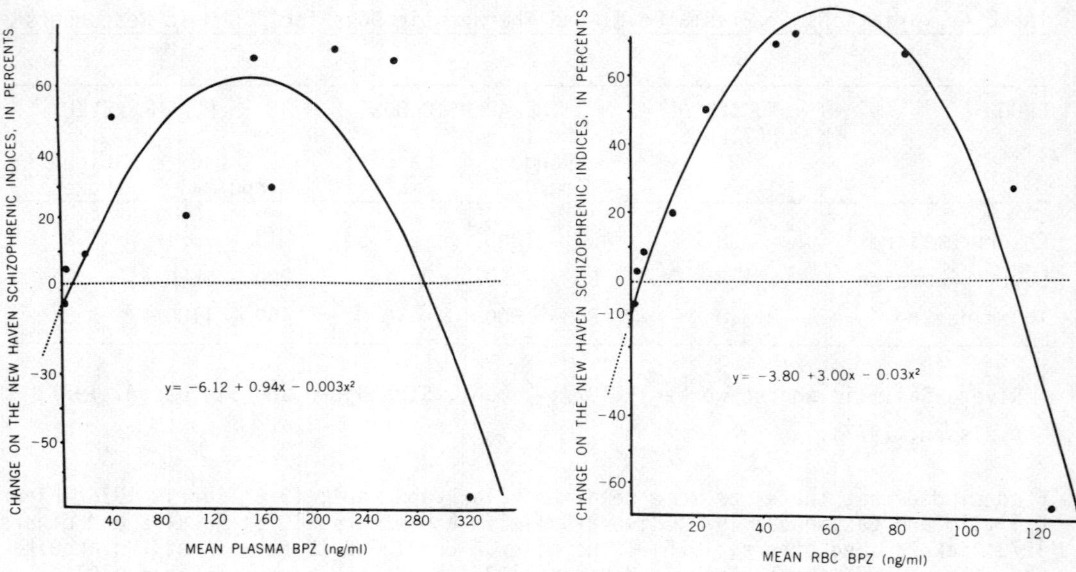

Fig. 2 Therapeutic Response as a Function of Plasma and Red Blood Cell (RBC) Concentrations of Butaperazine (BPZ). (Garver and others, 1977)

been examined for 5 of the 10 drugs which are given in Table 1. One study concluded that there was no such relationship for butaperazine (Garver and others, 1976), one arrived at the same conclusion for chlorpromazine (Sakurai, Nakahara and Takahasi, 1975), while 4 concluded that extrapyramidal (Kolakowska and others, 1975; Wiles and others, 1976) and other side-effects (Rivera-Calimlim and Castaneda, 1973; Dahl and Strandjord, 1977) were associated with high plasma levels of chlorpromazine. One study with fluphenazine (Smulevitch and others, 1973), and one with perazine (Hadass and others, 1974) concluded that extrapyramidal side-effects were associated with high plasma levels of the drug.

Two studies performed by the same group concluded that there was a certain degree of correlation between high plasma levels and side effects of perphenazine (Hansen and others, 1976; Hansen and Larsen, 1977). Bergling and others (1975) concluded with no such relationship for thioridazine, while two other studies reported that side-effects were associated with high levels of thioridazine and its active metabolites (Axelsson, 1977; Gottschalk and others, 1978).

However, nearly all these studies have shown that some patients have side-effects but relatively low plasma levels, while others have high plasma levels and no side-effects. And for none of these drugs has a well-defined and generally valid toxic plasma level limit been established.

REASONS FOR LACK OF CORRELATION

What then, are the reasons for the lack of correlation between plasma levels and effects of the phenothiazines? From the point of view of the pharmacologist, they may be divided into four groups: Analytical factors. These include (1) Unspecific methods where inactive metabolites may interfere. (2) Lack of precision in the assay, for instance due to the tendency of these compounds to adsorb to glass surfaces. (3) That one or several active metabolites which contribute to the effect are not measured. (4) Lack of precision in the evaluation of the clinical outcome of the treatment. Then we have the pharmacokinetic factors: (1) Individual variations in protein binding and distribution of the drug, and (2) Variation in the extent to which different metabolites with different activity are formed. The pharmacodynamic variables which may influence the concentration/effect relationship, can be summarized as being due to a heterogenous patient population. Finally we have the "therapeutic" factors: (1) The tendency of the disease to disappear without treatment, and (2) Interactions from concomitantly administered psychotropic or other drugs. I suppose we may take up the relative importance each of these and other factors during the discussion.

CONCLUSION

Although responders to phenothiazine treatment often have higher plasma levels of the parent drug and its active metabolites than have non-responders, there has not been demonstrated any direct correlation between plasma levels and therapeutic effects of these drugs. Certain side-effects of the phenothiazines appear to be more frequent at higher plasma levels of the drugs and their active metabolites, but definite toxic plasma level limits have not been established. Biological monitoring of phenothiazine plasma levels is therefore still of very limited value in clinical practice.

REFERENCES

Axelsson, R. (1977). On the serum concentrations and antipsychotic effects of thioridazine, thioridazine side-chain sulfoxide and thioridazine side-chain sulfone, in chronic psychotic patients. Curr. Therap. Res., 21, 587-605.

Bergling, R., T. Mjorndal, L. Oreland, W. Rapp and S. Wold (1975). Plasma levels and clinical effects of thioridazine and thiotixene. J. Clin. Pharmacol., 15, 178-186.

Breyer, U., F. Petruch, H. J. Gaertner,and B. Pflug (1976). Dünnschichtchromatographische Bestimmung von Plasmaspiegeln tricyclischer Psychopharmaka. Arzneim.-Forsch., 26, 1153.

Clark, M. L.,and P. N. Kaul (1976). A preliminary report on clinical response and blood levels of chlorpromazine and its sulfoxide during chlorpromazine therapy in chronic schizophrenic patients. In L. A. Gottschalk and S. Merlis (Eds.), Pharmacokinetics of Psychoactive Drugs, Spectrum Publ., New York 1976, p.191-197.

Cooper, T. B.,and G. M. Simpson (1976). Plasma blood level monitoring techniques in psychiatry. In L. A. Gottschalk and S. Merlis (Eds.), Pharmacokinetics of Psychoactive Drugs, Spectrum Publ., New York, p. 23-31.

Creese, I., A. A. Mamian, T. D. Prosser and S. H. Snyder (1978). ^{3}H-haloperidol binding to dopamine receptors in rat corpus striatum: Influence of chlorpromazine metabolites and derivates. Eur. J. Pharmacol., 47, 291-296.

Curry, S. H. (1976). Gas-chromatographic methods for the study of chlorpromazine and some of its metabolites in human plasma. Psychopharm. Commun., 2, 1-15.

Curry, S. H. (1978). Chlorpromazine: Pharmacokinetics, plasma levels and clinical response. In G. D. Burrows and T. Norman (Eds.), Plasma Levels of Psychotropic Drugs and Clinical Response, Marcel Dekker, London, in press.

Dahl, S. G. (1976). Pharmacokinetics of methotrimeprazine after single and multiple doses. Clin. Pharmacol. Ther., 19, 435-442.

Dahl, S. G., R. Strandjord, and S. Sigfusson (1977). Pharmacokinetics and relative bioavailability of levomepromazine after repeated administration of tablets and syrup. Eur. J. clin. Pharmacol., 11, 305-310.

Dahl, S. G., and R. Strandjord (1977). Pharmacokinetics of chlorpromazine after single and chronic dosage. Clin. Pharmacol. Ther., 21, 437-448.

Garver, D. L., J. M. Davis, H. Dekirmenjian, F. D. Johnes, R. Casper, J. Haraszti (1976). Pharmacokinetics of red blood cell phenothiazine and clinical effects. Arch. Gen. Psych., 33, 862-866.

Garver, D. L., H. Dekirmenjian, J. M. Davis, R. Casper, and S. Erichsen (1977). Neuroleptic drug levels and therapeutic response: Preliminary observations with red blood cell bound butaperazine. Am. J. Psychiat., 134, 304-307.

Gottschalk, L. A., E. Dinovo, R. Biener, H. Birch, M. Syben, and E. P. Noble (1976). Plasma levels of mesoridazine and its metabolites and clinical response in acute schizophrenia after a single intramuscular drug dose. In L. A. Gottschalk and S. Merlis (Eds.), Pharmacokinetics of psychoactive drugs, Spectrum publ., New York 1976, p. 171-189.

Gottschalk, L. A., E. Dinovo, R. Biener, and B. R. Nandi (1978). Plasma concentrations of thioridazine metabolites and ECG abnormalities. J. Pharm. Sci., 67, 155-157.

Hadass, H., H. Hippins, W. Maruschat, B. Müller-Oerlinghausen, and L. Rosenberg (1974). Multidimensionale pharmakopsychiatrische Untersuchungen mit dem Neuroleptikum Perazin. Pharmacopsychiat., 7, 17-30.

Hansen, C. E., T. R. Christensen, J. Elley, L. B. Hansen, and P. Kragh-Sørensen (1976). Clinical pharmacokinetic studies with perphenazine. Brit. J. clin. Pharmacol., 3, 915-923.

Hansen, L. B., and N.-E. Larsen (1977). Plasma concentrations of perphenazine and its sulphoxide metabolite during continous oral treatment. Psychopharmacology, 53, 127-130.

Klein, H. E., O. Chandra, and N. Matussek (1975). Therapeutische Wirkung und Plasmaspiegel von Thioridazin (Melleril[R]) bei schizophrenen Patienten. Pharmacopsych., 8, 122-131.

Kolakowska, T., D. H. Wiles, A. S. McNeilly, and M. G. Gelder (1975). Correlation between plasma levels of prolactin and chlorpromazine in psychiatric patients. Psychological Med., 5, 214-216.

Kolakowska, T., D. H. Wiles, M. G. Gelder, and A. S. McNeilly (1976). Clinical significance of plasma chlorpromazine levels. II. Plasma levels of the drug, some of its metabolites and prolactin in patients receiving long-term phenothiazine treatment. Psychopharmacology, 49, 101-107.

Loga, S., S. H. Curry and M. Lader (1975). Interactions of orphenadine and phenobarbitone with chlorpromazine: Plasma concentrations and effects in man. Brit. J. clin. Pharmacol., 2, 197-208.

Mackay, A. V., A. F. Healey, and J. Baker (1974). The relationship of plasma chlorpromazine to its 7-hydroxy and sulphoxide metabolites in a large population of chronic schizophrenics. Brit. J. clin. Pharmacol., 1, 425-430.

Phillipson, O. T., J. M. McKeown, J. Baker, and A. F. Healy (1977). Correlation between plasma chlorpromazine and its metabolites, and clinical ratings in patients with acute relapse of schizophrenic and paranoid psychosis. Brit. J. Psychiat., 131, 172-184.

Rivera-Calimlim, L., and L. Castaneda (1973). Effects of mode of management on plasma chlorpromazine in psychiatric patients. Clin. Pharmacol. Ther., 14, 978-986.

Rivera-Calimlim, L., H. Nasrallah, J. Strauss, and L. Lasagna (1976). Clinical response and plasma levels: Effect of dose, dosage schedules, and drug interactions on plasma chlorpromazine levels. Am. J. Psychiat., 133, 646-652.

Rivera-Calimlim, L., H. Nasrallah, T. Gift, B. Kerzner, P. H. Griesbach, and R. J. Wyatt (1977). Plasma levels of chlorpromazine: Effect of age, chronicity of disease, and duration of treatment. Clin. Pharmacol. Ther., 21, 115-116.

Sakalis, G., S. H. Curry, G. P. Mould, and M. H. Lader (1972). Physiologic and clinical effects of chlorpromazine and their relationship to plasma level. Clin. Pharmacol. Ther., 13, 931-946.

Sakalis, G., T. L. Chan, S. Gershon, and S. Park (1973). The possible role of metabolites in therapeutic response to chlorpromazine treatment. Psychopharmacologia, 32, 279-284.

Sakalis, G., L. J. Traficante and S. Gershon (1977). Thioridazine metabolism and clinical response: A pilot study. Curr. Therap. Res., 21, 720-724.

Sakurai, Y., T. Nakahara, and R. Takahashi (1975). Prediction of response to chlorpromazine treatment in schizophrenics. Psychopharmacologia, 44, 195-203.

Schooler, N. R., G. Sakalis, T. L. Chan, S. Gershon, S. C. Goldberg, and P. Collins (1976). Chlorpromazine metabolism and clinical response in acute schizophrenia: A preliminary report. In L. A. Gottschalk and S. Merlis (Eds.). Pharmacokinetics of Psychoactive Drugs, Spectrum Publ., New York, p. 199-219.

Simpson, G. S., R. Lament, T. B. Cooper, J. H. Lee, and R. B. Bruce (1973). The relationship between blood levels of different forms of butaperazine and clinical response. J. Clin. Pharmacol., 13, 288-297.

Smulevitch, A. B., E. I. Minsker, N. A. Mazayeva, R. P. Volkova, and S. K. Lukanina (1973). The problem of clinical activity of long-acting neuroleptics. Comprehensive Psychiatry, 14, 227-233.

Usdin, E. (1971). The assay of chlorpromazine and metabolites in blood, urine,and tissues. CRC Crit. Rew. Clin. Lab. Sci., 2, 347-391.

Vanderheeren, F. A. J., and R. G. Muusze (1977). Plasma levels and half-lives of thioridazine and some of its metabolites. I. High doses in young acute schizophrenics. Eur. J. clin. Pharmacol., 11, 135-140.

Wiles, D. H., T. Kolakowska, A. S. McNeilly, B. M. Mandelbrote, and M. G. Gelder (1976). Clinical significance of plasma chlorpromazine levels. I. Plasma levels of the drug, some of its metabolites and prolactin during acute treatment. Psychological Med., 6, 407-415.

Plasma Level Monitoring of Tricyclic Antidepressants: Usefulness and Limitations

LARS F. GRAM[1]

Western Psychiatric Institute and Clinic, University of Pittsburgh School of Medicine, Pittsburgh, Pennsylvania 15261, U.S.A.

ABSTRACT

The evidence of a relationship between steady state plasma levels and therapeutic effect of tricyclic antidepressants (TCA) has accumulated rapidly in recent years. Three independent groups have in six studies found optimal therapeutic effect of nortriptyline when plasma levels were 100-150µg/L, and poor effect when levels were above 150-200µg/L. Two larger independent studies on imipramine showed optimal therapeutic effect when plasma levels of imipramine+desipramine were above 200-250µg/L and no upper critical limit. Three studies on amitriptyline indicated a lower critical plasma level limit of about 80-120µg/L (amitriptyline+nortriptyline), and a recent study indicates that there is no upper critical limit. Before plasma level monitoring of TCA can be recommended for more general clinical use, more research on clinical variables such as depressive typology, duration of therapy, and kinetic variables as active metabolites and plasma protein binding needs to be done. Such research should also include a cost benefit analysis of the clinical use of plasma level monitoring of TCA.

INTRODUCTION

The development of techniques for plasma level monitoring in many fields of drug therapy has been followed by an increased understanding of the theoretical and practical basis for using this potentially useful tool clinically (Sheiner and Tozer, 1978). Tricyclic antidepressants (TCA) are one of the pharmacokinetically most extensively studied groups of drugs (Gram, 1974, 1977a), and during the recent 8-10 years several groups have attempted to relate the acquired pharmacokinetic knowledge to the clinical use of these drugs (Gram, 1977b). These studies have pointed out that plasma level monitoring of TCA may be potentially useful, and in particular the theoretical and practical basis and limitations of such procedure have become clear.

---

[1]Present address:
Department of Clinical Pharmacology,
Institute of Pharmacology, Odense University,
J.B. Winsløws Vej 19, DK-5000 Odense C,
Denmark.

THEORETICAL AND PRACTICAL BACKGROUND

The theoretical criteria for recommending plasma level monitoring as listed in Table 1 generally apply to TCA.

TABLE 1

Theoretical and Practical Basis of Therapy Control by Plasma Level Monitoring

1. Therapeutic effect not immediately observable, and no intermediate effect measurement available.
2. Wide interindividual variability in pharmacokinetics.
3. Therapeutic index small.
4. Therapeutic effect is obtained by maintaining a certain drug concentration for a relatively long time.
5. Correlations between plasma concentrations and therapeutic and toxic effects have been established.
6. Assay procedures meet certain requirements for sensivity, specificity, reproducibility, applicability, and economy.
7. Clinical pharmacokinetics of the compounds are known.

The insidious onset of the effect of the tricyclic antidepressants has been well recognized since the first trials with imipramine 20 years ago. The appropriate dose thus can not be titrated by the therapeutic effect. Further, there are no good biological measurements that could predict the therapeutic effect and possibly replace plasma level monitoring. The wide interindividual variability in pharmacokinetics such as metabolite elimination and steady-state plasma levels was observed more than 10 years ago (Christiansen and others, 1967; Hammer and Sjöqvist, 1967), and such variability has later been shown for many of the TCA in current use. For imipramine (IP) there is pronounced variation in the levels of parent compound IP and the demethylated metabolite desipramine (DMI) and no correlation between the levels of the two compounds (Gram and others, 1977).

Before plasma level monitoring was taken into use, our information on the therapeutic index of TCA was relatively inaccurate. It was known that single doses 10-20 times larger than the usual daily maintenance dose could cause severe intoxication, and also that serious toxicity occasionally was seen in patients on therapeutic doses. The data from plasma level studies brought some clarification on this. For IP and nortriptyline (NT), the therapeutic index thus appears to be about 3-4, for NT determined by the unfavorable therapeutic effect of higher levels, and for IP by the risk of toxic reactions (see below).

Our knowledge about the time factor involved in the therapeutic effect of TCA mainly stems from studies before plasma level monitoring became feasible. The time it takes to achieve full antidepressive effect appears to be individually variable from 2-8 weeks, and a correlation between plasma level and effect will only be meaningful if the plasma level is kept constant throughout this time period.

STUDIES ON PLASMA LEVEL-EFFECT RELATIONSHIP

Through the last 8-9 years about 20-30 studies have been published where attempts have been made to establish a correlation between plasma levels of presumed active compounds and antidepressive effect. In a smaller number of studies, plasma levels have also been related to side effects or toxic reactions. There are now six controlled studies on NT from three different groups describing the so-called curvilinear relationship (Kragh-Sørensen and others, 1973; Kragh-Sørensen and others, 1976; Montgomery and others, 1978; Ziegler and others, 1976b; Ziegler and others, 1977; Åsberg and others, 1971). In essence, all these studies conclude that patients with high NT levels in plasma respond poorly or not at all. The critical level above which this is seen appears to be slightly different in different studies varying from 140 to 200 µg/L. Patients with lower levels generally responded well, but the lower critical limit, below which the levels are too low and ineffective, have not been clearly defined in any of these studies. The mechanism behind the paradoxical reaction on high level is not clear.

For IP, two large studies (Glassman and others, 1977; Gram and others, 1976; Reisby and others, 1977) have shown a simpler direct relationship between the total concentration of IP + DMI and antidepressive effect. These studies indicate a lower critical plasma level limit of about 200-250 µg/L. Above this limit the therapeutic effect is good, whereas patients with lower levels show only partial or no response. Very high levels were not associated with particularly good or poor effect. Amitriptyline (AT) has been studied by several groups. When a plasma level/effect relationship has been found this has been a positive correlation as for IP, but most of the studies have indicated the critical limit to be somewhat lower (about 100-120 µg/L) (Braithwaite and others, 1972; Ziegler and others, 1976a; Ziegler and others, 1977). The recent study by Kupfer and others (1977) clearly indicates that high levels of AT and/or NT are not associated with unfavorable therapeutic effect. The present data on AT are, however, less consistent than those on NT and IP, and further studies are needed. For NT, IP and AT there are studies that have shown only a weak or no correlation between plasma levels and therapeutic effect (Burrows and others, 1972; Coppen and others, 1978; Davies and others, 1975; Muscettola and others, 1978).

There is probably no single clear-cut explanation of these negative findings, but to some extent they may relate to methodological factors. The diagnostic selection and stratification of patients thus is important, since TCA only have a true drug-related effect in endogenous depressions (Bielski and Friedel, 1976; Gram, 1977b, Reisby and others, 1977). Pharmacokinetic factors may be of some importance and for a drug like AT, one may speculate if the combination of two compounds with possibly different or even opposite plasma level/effect relationship may create particular problems. Also the dominant sedative-anxiolytic effect of AT may cause problems by being confused with the antidepressive effect.

There has recently been a tremendous interest in developing assay techniques for TCA in plasma, and a variety of methods of sufficient quality are now available for research in this field. The applicability in clinical practice and the economy involved in their use, has only been established in a few cases.

CONCLUSION AND FUTURE DEVELOPMENT

The development in this field has been rapid in recent years both technically and clinically, and the potential usefulness of plasma level monitoring has been quite well documented (Gram, 1977b). Plasma level monitoring therefore has a clear place in future research on TCA, but there is a need for further clinical research, before plasma level monitoring of TCA can be recommended for general clinical use.

(Table 2).

TABLE 2

Plasma Level Monitoring of Antidepressants in Future Research:

General and Theoretical Issues:

- Effect of antidepressants in different types of depressions.
- Time factor in therapeutic action of antidepressants.
- Significance of active metabolites.
- Significance of variations in plasma protein binding.
- Biological effects of antidepressants in man.
- Effective levels of antidepressants in man and in animal models.

Practical Applications:

- Monitoring in special risk groups (children, elderly, physical diseases).
- Plasma level/effect relationship of antidepressants in current use.
- Clinical testing of new antidepressants.
- Monitoring in treatment of intoxications.
- Cost-benefit analyses of the clinical use of plasma level monitoring.

The research fields listed in Table 2 relate to the use of antidepressants in the treatment of depressive episodes. However, other possible indications of these drugs, in particular their use in prophylaxis against recurrent depressive or manic episodes as an alternative to lithium, also deserve more attention.

Since plasma levels of TCA seem to be an important variable determining their clinical effect, this variable should be controlled when studying the influence of other variables such as diagnostic classification and time factor. Pharmacokinetically, there are several unanswered questions: the significance of metabolites and and variability in plasma protein binding being some of the most important ones (Gram, in press). Very little is known so far about how therapeutic and side effects are related to the parent compound and the various metábilites formed in the body. The practical significance of the observed 2-3 fold variability in plasma protein binding has still not been definitely established.

In the research on the mode of action of TCA and the biological effects of TCA, it is important that such effects are related to drug and metabolite concentrations in body fluids rather than to the dose. A given effect in a valid experimental model should be related to the therapeutic drug concentrations seen in patients. For this transition from patient levels to animal model levels, it is probably necessary to calculate the free water concentrations of drug, rather than using tissue and total plasma concentrations. A recent study on the effect of IP on brain histamine receptors illustrates how such considerations may be applied (Kanof and Greengard, 1978).

For the practical application of plasma level monitoring more research is required in several fields. Most plasma level effect studies have been carried out in physically healthy adults, and little is known about how plasma level monitoring may improve the efficacy and safety of TCA treatment in patients at possible special risk.

Plasma level/effect relationship has only been reasonably well established for a few TCA (NT, IP) and more research is needed on other TCA on the market. Further, it seems self-evident that plasma level monitoring ought to be part of the clinical as well as the experimental testing of new antidepressants. Although we have data showing a certain correlation between plasma levels of TCA and toxic symptoms (Petit and others, 1977; Spiker and others, 1975), we still need an evaluation of the practical usefulness of plasma level monitoring in the treatment of these often very severe intoxications. This evaluation indeed relates to the ability of the laboratories to carry out the assay on an emergency basis.

Finally, by having the various methodological factors better elucidated and having more practical clinical data on plasma level monitoring available, it should be possible to carry out cost-benefit analyses in a scientific way. Such analyses then would permit us to give proper recommendations for the more general use of plasma level monitoring of TCA in future clinical practice.

REFERENCES

Åsberg, M., B. Cronholm, F. Sjöqvist, and D. Tuck (1971). Relationship between plasma level and therapeutic effect of nortriptyline. Brit. Med. J., 3, 331-334.

Bielski, R. J. and R. O. Friedel (1976). Prediction of tricyclic antidepressant response. A critical review. Arch. Gen. Psychiatry, 33, 1479-1489.

Braithwaite, R. A., R. Goulding, G. Theano, J. Bailey, and A. Coppen (1972). Plasma concentration of amitriptyline and clinical response. Lancet, 1, 1297-3000.

Burrows, G. D., B. Davies, and B. A. Scoggins (1972). Plasma concentration of nortriptyline and clinical response in depressive illness. Lancet, 2, 691-723.

Burrows, G. D., B. A. Scoggins, L. R. Turecek, and B. Davies (1974). Plasma nortriptyline and clinical response. Clin. Pharmacol. Ther., 16, 639-644.

Christiansen, J., L. F. Gram, B. Kofod, and O. J. Rafaelsen (1967). Imipramine metabolism in man. Psychopharmacologia, 11, 255-264.

Coppen, A., S. Montgomery, K. Ghose, V. A. Rama Rao, J. Christiansen, P. L. Mikkelson, H. M. van Praag, F. van de Poel, and A. Jørgensen (1978). Amitriptyline plasma concentration and clinical effect. Lancet, 1, 63-66.

Davies, B., G. D. Burrows, and B. Scoggins (1975). Plasma nortriptyline and clinical response. Aust. N. Z. J. Psychiatry, 9, 249-253.

Glassman, A. H., J. M. Perel, M. Shostak, S. J. Kantor, and J. L. Fleiss (1977). Clinical implication of imipramine plasma levels for depressive illness. Arch. Gen. Psychiatry, 34, 197-204.

Gram, L.F. (1974). Metabolism of tricyclic antidepressants. A review. Dan. Med. Bull., 21, 218-231.

Gram, L. F., N. Reisby, I. Ibsen, A. Nagy, S. J. Dencker, P. Bech, G. O. Petersen, and J. Christiansen (1976). Plasma levels and antidepressive effect of imipramine. Clin. Pharmacol. Ther., 19, 318-324.

Gram, L. F. (1977a). Factors influencing the metabolism of tricyclic antidepressants. Studies on interactions and first pass elimination (Thesis). Dan. Med. Bull., 24, 81-89.

Gram, L. F. (1977b). Plasma level monitoring of tricyclic antidepressants. Clin. Pharmacokinet., 2, 237-251.

Gram, L. F., I. Søndergaard, J. Christiansen, G. Odden Petersen, P. Bech, N. Reisby, I. Ibsen, J. Ortmann, A. Nagy, S. J. Dencker, O. Jacobsen, and O. Krautwald (1977). Steady state kinetics of imipramine in patients. Psychopharmacology, 54, 255-263.

Gram, L. F. (in press). Plasma level monitoring of tricyclic antidepressants: Methodological and pharmacokinetic considerations. Commun. in Psychopharmacology.

Hammer, W. and F. Sjöqvist (1967). Plasma levels of monomethylated tricyclic antidepressants during treatment with imipramine-like compounds. Life Sci., 6, 1895-1903.

Kanof, P. D. and P. Greengard (1978). Brain histamine receptors as targets for antidepressant drugs. Nature, 272, 329-333.

Kragh-Sørensen, P., M. Åsberg, and C. Eggert Hansen (1973). Plasma nortriptyline levels in endogenous depression. Lancet, 1, 113-115.

Kragh-Sørensen, P., C. E. Hansen, P. C. Baastrup, and E. F. Hvidberg (1976). Self-inhibiting action of nortriptyline's antidepressive effect at high plasma levels. Psychopharmacology, 45, 305-316.

Kupfer, D. J., I. Hanin, D. G. Spiker, T. Grau, and P. Coble (1977). Amitriptyline plasma levels and clinical response in primary depression. Clin. Pharmacol. Ther., 22, 904-911.

Montgomery, S., R. A. Braithwaite, S. Dawling, and R. McAuley (1974). High plasma nortriptyline levels in the treatment of depression. Clin Pharmacol. Ther., 23, 309-314.

Muscettola, G., F. K. Goodwin, W. Z. Potter, M. M. Claeys, and S. P. Markey (1978). Imipramine and desipramine in plasma and spinal fluid. Arch. Gen. Psychiatry, 35, 621-625.

Petit, J. M., D. G. Spiker, J. F. Ruwitch, V. E. Ziegler, A. N. Weiss, and J. T. Biggs (1977). Tricyclic antidepressant plasma levels and adverse effects after overdose. Clin. Pharmacol. Ther., 21, 47-51.

Reisby, N., L. F. Gram, P. Bech, A. Nagy, G. O. Petersen, J. Ortmann, I. Ibsen, S. J. Dencker, O. Jacobsen, O. Krautwald, I. Søndergaard, and J. Christiansen (1977). Imipramine: Clinical effects and pharmacokinetic variability. Psychopharmacology, 54, 263-272.

Sheiner, L. B. and T. N. Tozer (1978). Clinical pharmacokinetics: The use of plasma concentrations of drugs. In K. L. Melmon and H. F. Morrelli (Eds.), Clinical Pharmacology, Basic Principles in Therapeutics, 2nd ed. Macmillan Publishing Co. Inc., New York. pp. 71-109.

Spiker, D. G., A. N. Weiss, S. S. Chang, J. F. Ruwitch, and J. T. Biggs (1975). Tricyclic antidepressant overdose: Clinical presentation and plasma levels. Clin. Pharmacol. Ther., 18, 539-546.

Ziegler, V. E., B. T. Co, J. R. Taylor, P. J. Clayton, and J. T. Biggs (1976a). Amitriptyline plasma levels and therapeutic response. Clin. Pharmacol. Ther., 19,

Ziegler, V. E., P. J. Clayton, J. R. Taylor, B. T. Co, and J. T. Biggs (1976b). Nortriptyline plasma levels and therapeutic response. Clin. Pharmacol. Ther., 20, 458-463.

Ziegler, V. E., P. J. Clayton, and J. T. Biggs (1977). A comparison study of amitriptyline and nortriptyline with plasma levels. Arch. Gen. Psychiatry, 34, 607-612.

Biological Monitoring of Psychotropic Drug Treatment: Usefulness and Limitations

MALCOLM LADER

Institute of Psychiatry, Univeristy of London, England

ABSTRACT

The problems of clinical management of psychiatric patients using psychotropic drugs have led to search for biological monitoring of drug response. The requirements of such a monitor are that it should be relevant, reliable, linear in relationship, easy to measure and acceptable to the patient. We are still some way from developing such useful practical indicators but several measures, physiological, endocrinological and biochemical, promise well.

INTRODUCTION

My challenging task is to review the biological measures that are available to monitor clinical effects of psychotropic drugs. The almost complete absence of routine monitoring variables testifies to the research status of this entire topic. As such, there are many measures available of varying degrees of reliability and validity. A comprehensive review is thus impossible and I shall concentrate on the principles involved with appropriate examples. Other speakers are dealing with the correlations, or lack of them, between plasma drug concentrations and clinical response.

THEORETICAL BACKGROUND

The prime goal of the prescribing physician is to attain as great a clinical response as possible commensurate with few side-effects. The monitoring of psychotropic drug usage with biological measures has two main objectives : to maximize clinical response and to minimize unwanted effects. In general, the former is more important. Accordingly, if the clinician is satisfied with his patient's response, he will not feel any need for monitoring his therapy. It is the drug-unresponsive patient who presents the problems.

The questions to be asked stem from the fundamental pharmacological relationship : $E \int CxS$. The clinical effect is some function of the concentration of drug at the site of action and the sensitivity of that site of action to the drug. Lack of response can be examined under three headings derived from this equation:

Firstly, the function relating the effect to the concentration-sensitivity combination may be a complex one. One example concerns the parabolic relationship between clinical response and plasma nortriptyline concentrations, as claimed by several groups of investigators. Both low and high concentrations are associated with lack of response. However, this relationship reflects the complexity of the

$\int$ component. At high drug concentrations, sensitivity seems to fall off, perhaps because of post-synaptic receptor blockade. Such problems reflect the complexities of drug actions on receptors, mixed agonist-antagonist properties being common.

Secondly, lack of response can be due to insufficient drug concentrations at the receptor sites. The measurement of plasma concentrations of drugs is an attempt to detect such insufficiency. Such estimations are only an approximation to receptor-site concentrations with complicating factors such as plasma binding, active metabolites, penetration and binding in the brain. Some systems, e.g. the sedative actions of glutethimide, are more related to the rate of change of drug concentrations than to absolute levels (Curry and Norris, 1970).

Thirdly, lack of response can be due to insensitivity of the response system which can be assessed, at least in theory. In practice, there is no way by which the sensitivity of the response system in man to any psychotropic drug can be directly estimated. This reflects the lack of knowledge of the precise biological mechanisms of action underlying the clinical properties of psychotropic drugs, most of which were discovered serendipitously. Also the accessibility of human brain response systems is almost zero. Attempts to assess responsiveness, e.g. giving test doses of methamphetamine to depressives or measuring the Ki values for MAO inhibitors on blood platelets are only very indirect estimates of S.

PROPERTIES OF A BIOLOGICAL MONITOR

The alternative and most parsimonious approach is to seek an easily quantifiable measure which correlates clearly and cleanly with the clinical response. Of course, to obtain a high correlation, each variable must be capable of reliable and accurate estimation. This is a problem with clinical ratings which tend to be less precise than we might wish. Consequently, the correlation with other measures will fall short of those acceptable for between-biological-measure correlations. An alternative approach is to validate the biological measure concurrently to a definable behavioural response. For example MAO inhibition assessed on blood platelets should be related to extinction of phobic object avoidance behaviour, if claims for antiphobic anxiety properties following MAO inhibition are to be substantiated (Tyrer, Candy and Kelly, 1973).

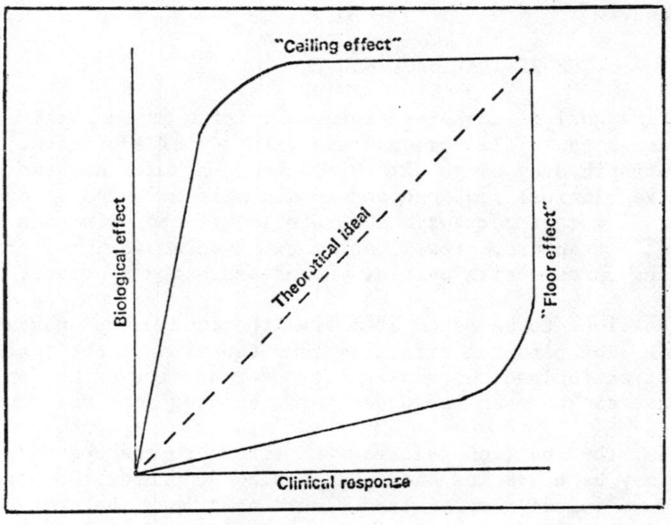

Fig. 1.

However, 'ceiling' and 'floor' effects may limit the usefulness of a concomitant biological variable (Fig. 1). The ceiling effect refers to the biological measure reaching its maximum at subtherapeutic clinical levels. For example, prolactin levels in the blood rise rapidly after the administration of an antipsychotic agent. However, maximum secretion, i.e. secretion following complete removal of dopaminergic inhibition mediated via the tubero-infundibular tract, occurs before therapeutic concentrations of the drug are reached (Gruen et al., 1978). Therefore, this 'ceiling' effect precludes the use of prolactin levels to estimate the dose at which therapeutic levels have been attained. However, if prolactin levels are not elevated, then it is highly unlikely that any therapeutic effect is being exerted.

The 'floor' effect works the other way. Here, the measure is insensitive to therapeutic drug concentrations but only alters at supratherapeutic levels. The assessment of nystagmus with barbiturate usage is a case in point. Many estimates of toxicity fall in this category.

Another limitation is that of temporal dissociation. Thus, clinical response to the MAO inhibitors is generally associated with inhibition of blood platelet MAO of at least 85 per cent (Robinson et al., 1978). Such inhibition is attainable within one or two doses of tranylcypromine (Gentil, Alevizos and Lader, 1978) and yet clinical response may not be apparent for four to six weeks. Furthermore, the MAO inhibitors are an example of irreversible antagonism and such systems are less easy to monitor than competitive ones.

To summarise, the main properties of a useful biological monitor are that it should be assessing some relevant aspect of the drug's action, wanted or unwanted; that it should bear a rectilinear relation to that drug action, and be sensitive at both subtherapeutic and supratherapeutic levels. Other considerations include reliability, ease of measurement, acceptability to the patient and cost. Specific examples from several areas will now be discussed under four headings: a) primary response monitors; b) secondary response monitors; c) non-specific response monitors; d) empirical response monitors.

PRIMARY RESPONSE MONITORS

There are no true primary response monitors in the sense of being able to quantify a biological measure which is intrinsic to the clinical response. What are available are several indicators of other parts of the same system in some functional relationship.

The best example is the estimation of monoamine oxidase inhibition in patients treated with MAO inhibitors. Measures of brain inhibition are not available and measures of total body inhibition such as urinary tryptamine excretion seem inaccurate. Other MAO systems have been explored and platelet MAO is the most popular choice. Even so there are relatively few studies attempting to correlate clinical response with platelet MAO inhibition, perhaps reflecting the unpopularity of these drugs. Various centres tend to agree that platelet MAOI inhibition of 85 per cent or more is associated with clinical response whereas patients with less than this degree of inhibition respond no better than to placebo. Our own data are in broad agreement with this. Nevertheless, there are complications. Tryptamine as MAO substrate provides an estimate of MAO inhibition whereas benzylamine does not (Robinson et al., 1978). Also, platelet MAO inhibition is apparent after the first few doses of the MAOI yet clinical response may be delayed for several weeks. Nevertheless, the figure of 85 per cent corresponds with that known to be associated with elevation of brain amines in animal experiments (Gey and Pletscher, 1961). It has also become apparent that the usual dosage of phenelzine may be too low in many patients and that 60 mg/day or more may be necessary. The further development of this technique may yet enable these drugs to be used more rationally in those untypical, phobic, hypochondriacal depressives where the MAOI's are often useful.

In a similar fashion, blood platelets provide a model for the tricyclic antidepressants. Serotonin is actively taken up by platelets but dopamine uptake probably utilises the serotonin pump and noradrenaline merely diffuses passively (Sneddon, 1973). Even so, an estimate of tricyclic action is obtainable. We have also examined this technique using it to monitor a trial of various antidepressants. Blockade of uptake follows administration of a tricyclic antidepressant. This blockade is further enhanced if the tricyclic drug is combined with an MAOI (Dawes and Lader, unpublished data).

Another estimate of tricyclic action, this time of an in vivo noradrenaline pump, is the blockade of tyramine pressor activity. For example, desipramine (50 mg single dose) increased the amount of infused tyramine needed for an elevation of 30 mm systolic blood pressure about threefold in 10 volunteers (Ghose, Gifford, Turner and Leighton, 1976). This action is directly relevant to the interactions between tricyclics and some anti-hypertensive agents but its relationship to clinical response is unclear.

Another type of monitor is one which involves the same neurotransmitter as the putative main action but at a different site. An early example was the suggestion that extrapyramidal actions were essential for a clinical response to antipsychotic medication. Although this is not strictly true, extrapyramidal effects do at least show dopamine-receptor blockade in the corpus striatum. If this has not occurred then dopamine-receptor blockade at the antipsychotic site of action, presumably mesolimbic or mesocortical regions, maynot have occurred either. However, this relationship has never been clearly established and the clinical consensus now is that extrapyramidal effects may supervene at supratherapeutic levels or not be closely related to clinical effects.

The quantification of some extrapyramidal effects can be surprisingly easy. Haase and Janssen (1965) have long advocated handwriting length as a measure of bradykinesia. In one of our studies, we found that the length of a line of handwriting easily detected the parkinsonian effects of chlorpromazine, 100 mg 8 hourly, and the antiparkinsonian effects of adding orphenadrine, same dose (Loga, Curry and Lader, 1975).

The other dopaminergic system which has been closely studied is the tubero-infundibular pathway which is one control of prolactin release, inhibitory in nature. Administration of antipsychotic drugs results in a release of inhibition so that plasma prolactin concentrations rise markedly and very promptly. The Oxford group have shown a useful relationship between prolactin increase and extrapyramidal effects. Thus, all patients with extrapyramidal signs had prolactin levels over 35 ng/ml; but none of the patients with low prolactin levels had extrapyramidal effects (Kolakowska, Wiles, McNeilly and Gelder, 1975). However, there was no correlation with clinical response. This is probably because of a 'ceiling' effect. The release of inhibition of prolactin release reaches its maximum at drug concentrations below or just at the lower limit of the clinical range as mentioned earlier (Gruen et al., 1978). Moderate or high clinical concentrations produce no further elevation. A normal prolactin level in a patient suggests that no dopamine blockade whatsoever has occurred and clinical response is unlikely - the patient is not taking his medication, or he is metabolising the drug too rapidly, or his effector systems are insensitive. Conversely, elevated prolactin does not indicate a probable clinical response, merely that dopaminergic blockade has occurred in the pituitary.

SECONDARY RESPONSE MONITORS

These measures are manifestly of less interest as they relate to secondary effects, mainly side- or unwanted effects. Most psychotropic drugs have a plethora of actions so there are many measures available. Of these, autonomic variables have been widely studied, especially as a range of techniques can be borrowed from cardiovascular and gastro-intestinal medicine, ophthalmology, etc.

One example must suffice. In the study mentioned earlier (Loga et al., 1975), pupil size under standard dim illumination was measured in 12 acute schizophrenic patients using a simple disc-comparison method. Chlorpromazine 100 mg 8-hourly produced a marked constriction (from 7.5mm to 4.5mm on average); this suggests that alpha-adrenergic blockade predominated over anticholinergic effects. The addition of orphenadrine, 100 mg 8-hourly, almost completely reversed the effects of chlorpromazine, the pupil dilating back to a mean of 7mm. A low but significant correlation ($r=0.33$; $p<0.001$) *within-patient* was found between IMPS scores and pupil size. *Between-patient* correlations were not significant.

This finding illustrates a general point which it is now appropriate to interpolate. It may be too ambitious a strategy to seek correlations between a biological measure of drug effect and a clinical measure among a *group* of patients. Individual variability in both baseline levels and responsivity and inaccuracies of measurement may be too great. However, monitoring a measure *within-individual* may be more useful. In this way, a 'calibration curve' can be constructed for each patient and clinical improvement should parallel changes in the measure. Test doses of medication are one way of attempting to calibrate the individual's responsivity. Nevertheless, it must be emphasised that substantial correlations (above 0.8) are necessary before such monitoring would prove useful.

NON-SPECIFIC RESPONSE MONITORS

In these measures, inferences are made concerning the nature of the function being monitored. Instead of the measure being left in physiological terms, prolactin levels, blood-pressure, and so on, with direct pharmacological interpretations, dopamine blockade, anticholinergic effects etc., the variables are interpreted in psychological terms. The most widely used system is the psychophysiological where autonomic and other measures are employed, not as direct pharmacological monitors, but as indirect reflections of central constructs such as arousal, attention and vigilance. This immediately places a restriction on the drugs which can be monitored. If one is interpreting pupil size, sweat-gland activity or catecholamine excretion in terms of central activation, then drugs which alter these measures peripherally are inadmissible. Thus, a drug like amitriptyline with anticholinergic properties will lessen sweat-gland activity. It is then impossible to deduce whether central arousal as monitored by sweat-gland activity has altered or not. However, the barbiturates and the benzodiazepines which do not have peripheral actions of this sort can be successfully monitored (Lader and Wing, 1966).

Somewhat surprisingly, urinary catecholamine excretion which should provide a semi-quantitive integrated measure of central activation and stress response has not been used very much in the clinical context. We have carried out a series of studies which I have not time to detail now. As a rule, noradrenaline is a more sensitive indicator of stress response than adrenaline (Al-Aslan, Nelson, Carruthers and Lader, unpublished data).

EMPIRICAL RESPONSE MONITORS

Finally, there are measures which can be established as empirical correlates of clinical effects but which cannot be easily interpreted in either pharmacological or psychological terms. The electroencephalogram is the best example. The work of Fink (1975), Itil and others has established the utility of the EEG as an empirical screening test in humans: a drug which gives an imipramine-like profile of EEG changes is likely to be an antidepressant, and so on. These changes can be monitored during drug treatment. For example, benzodiazepines increase the proportion of fast-wave activity and decrease the proportion of alpha waveband activity (Bond, James and Lader, 1974). Patients whose EEG's showed little or no change reported no clinical improvement. Note that the benzodiazepines and barbiturates increase fast wave activity which is more or less what is seen under conditions of psychological activation. Yet subjects may feel drowsy on the drugs. The direct effects of the drug on the EEG outweigh the indirect effects

REFERENCES

Bond, A.J., C.D.James and M.H.Lader (1974). Sedative effects on physiological and psychological measures in anxious patients. _Psychological Medicine_, _4_, 374-380.

Curry, S.H. and H.Norris (1970). Acute tolerance to a sedative in man. _British Journal of Pharmacology_, _38_, 450-451.

Fink, M. (1975). Prediction of clinical activity of psychoactive drugs: application of cerebral electrometry in phase-1 studies. In A. Sudilovsky, S.Gershon and B.Beer (Eds.), _Predictability in Psychopharmacology : Preclinical and Clinical Correlations_, Raven Press, New York. pp. 65-82.

Gentil, V., B. Alevizos, and M. Lader (1978). Effects of single doses of tranylcypromine on platelet MAO and amine uptake in normal subjects. _Biochemical_ Pharmacology, in Press.

Gey, K. F. and A. Pletscher (1961). Activity of monoamine oxidase in relation to the 5-hydroxytryptamine and norepinephrine content of the rat brain. _Journal of Neurochemistry_, _6_, 239-243.

Ghose, K., L. A. Gifford, P. Turner and M. Leighton (1976). Studies of the interaction of desmethylimipramine with tyramine in man after a single oral dose, and its correlation with plasma concentration. _British Journal of Clinical Pharmacology_, _3_, 334-337.

Gruen, P. H., E.J. Sachar, G. Langer, N. Altman, M. Leifer, A. Frantz and F.S. Halpern, (1978). Prolactin responses to neuroleptics in normal and schizophrenic subjects. _Archives of General Psychiatry_, _35_, 108-116.

Haase, H. J. and P. A. Janssen (1965). The Action of Neuroleptic Drugs : A Psychiatric, Neurologic and Pharmacological Investigation. North-Holland, Amsterdam.

Kolakowska, T., D. H. Wiles, A. S. McNeilly and M. G. Gelder (1975). Correlation between plasma levels of prolactin and chlorpromazine in psychiatric patients. _Psychological Medicine_, _5_, 214-216.

Lader, M. H. and L. Wing (1966). _Physiological Measures, Sedative Drugs and Morbid Anxiety_. Oxford University Press, London.

Loga, S., S. Curry and M. Lader (1975). Interactions of orphenadrine and phenobarbitone with chlorpromazine : plasma concentrations and effects in man. _British Journal of Clinical Pharmacology_, _2_, 197-208.

Robinson, D. S., A. Nies, C. L. Ravaris, J. O. Ives and D. Bartless (1978). Clinical psychopharmacology of phenelzine : MAO activity and clinical response. In M. A. Lipton, A. DiMascio and K. F. Killam (Eds.), _Psychopharmacology : A Generation of Progress_. Raven Press, New York. pp. 961-973.

Sneddon, J. M. (1973). Blood platelets as a model for monoamine-containing neurones. _Progress in Neurobiology_, _1_, 151-198.

Tyrer, P., J. Candy and D. Kelly (1973). Phenelzine in phobic anxiety : a controlled trial. _Psychological Medicine_, _3_, 120-124.

Quantitative EEG, Drug Levels and Clinical Effects

P. ETEVENON

Section d'E.E.G. Quantitative du S.H.U. de Santé Mentale et de Thérapeutique
du Centre Hospitalier Sainte-Anne, 1 rue Cabanis, F. 75674 Paris, Cédex 14

ABSTRACT

Methodological problems are first presented : interactions between factors influencing psychotropic drug administration and the subject, choice of EEG measurements and difficulties of assessing behavioral or clinical changes.

A short review is then presented of the few published articles correlating drug levels, EEG measurements and/or clinical rating scales. Anxiolytics usually enhance EEG beta activity. Thymoleptics enhance slow and fast activities and we have correlated this EEG profile with chlorimipramine plasma level. Neuroleptics enhance slow activities. In six schizophrenic patients being treated by increasing doses of haloperidol, plasma levels were correlated with left/right ratio of fast EEG beta activity recorded from posterior areas.

Challenge and difficulties of such multicentric and interdisciplinary studies are discussed.

KEYWORDS: Quantitative EEG, drug levels, clinical effects, cerebral dominance in schizophrenia.

METHODOLOGICAL PROBLEMS

A number of methodological problems involved by the administration of a psychotropic drug are represented schematically on figure 1.

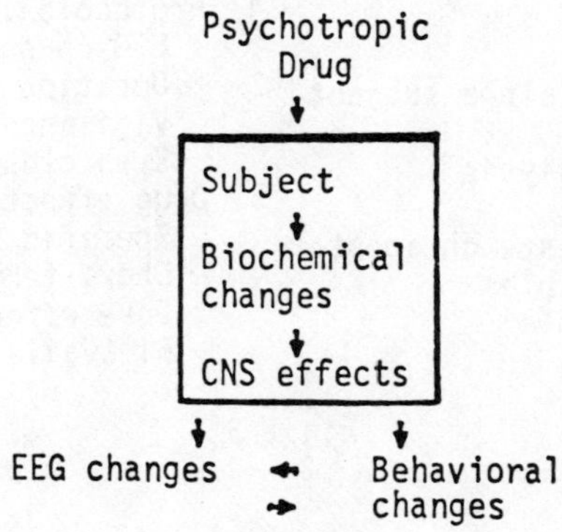

Fig. 1

Usually it is assumed that when CNS effects are occuring, they are concomitant with EEG changes as well as behavioral changes (Fink, 1978 ; Mucciardi, 1974 ; Shapiro and Glasser, 1974). But it is not the case when induced biochemical changes are slowly appearing during the course of a chronically administered treatment.

On figure 2 are represented some of the major variables involved in the interaction of a specific psychotropic drug administered to a human subject. Trials of different doses are very important (Matejcek and Devos, 1976). Ethnopharmacological research has also recently brought forward the importance of race as a specific response factor to the treatment.

PSYCHOTROPIC DRUG :

Form
Dose
Administration
Rate
Acute or chronic

↓

SUBJECT :

Age, Sex, Race
Control group

Normal :	Patient :
Volunteer	Illness
Placebo reactor	Duration
Genuine	Therapy resistant

Fig. 2

On figure 3, we have represented some of the problems involved in the appraisal and quantification of EEG changes following psychotropic effects. The effects may be dependent on the previous base-line of the subject, either a high alpha or a low alpha subject. The subject can also react positively or negatively to a placebo, with an excited or a depressed reaction, and this should be taken into consideration for the assessment of psychotropic effects. Depending on the method of EEG analysis: amplitude histograms, integrated amplitude analysis, period analysis (zero-crossing), spectral analysis, the results by one method may not be comparable with the results obtained by another method (Etevenon, 1977 ; Etevenon and Pidoux, 1977). For instance, the time window analysis should be the same when comparing two different techniques of EEG analysis. The protocole may also involve different EEG channels, different recorded sequences with or without sustained vigilance, during eyes closed or eyes open recording conditions.

EEG CHANGES :

1 High alpha or low alpha subject
2 Placebo effect
3 Method of data analysis :
  goal directed
  easiest, quickest, cheapest
  most comprehensible
  most interpretable
4 Protocole :
  EEG channels
  Duration
  Vigilance controlled EEG
  Eyes closed or Eyes opened
5 Drug effects :
  Specific Drug profile
  Short term or long term
  Dose effects curve
  Bioavailability study

Fig. 3

On figure 4 we have represented for a chosen technique of EEG analysis, what are the main choices of data analysis (Etevenon, 1977 ; Etevenon et al., 1978).

QUANTITATIVE EEG ANALYSIS

1 Method : Amplitude histograms
- Integrative method
- Zero-crossing
- Spectral analysis
- Other

2 Choice of data analysis :
- Longitudinal study
  - Evolutive spectra
  - Averaged spectra
  - Data reduction - Parameters
  - Drug profile
- Transversal study
  - Classical statistics
  - Multivariate analysis
- Sophisticated analysis
  - Multiple channel analysis
  - Modulation analysis

Fig. 4

However, further data reduction is needed for transversal group studies of quantified EEGs. Mean variables together with standard deviations are usually good EEG descriptors. A set of 20 parameters are sufficient to quantify one EEG channel and provide enough variables for later multivariate statistical analysis. Such parameters are listed on figure 5.

EEG DATA REDUCTION

Statistical Spectral Parameters:
- Alpha intensity $\pm$ s
  - absolute or relative
- Alpha dominant frequency $\pm$ s
- Averaged amplitude (RMS) $\pm$ s
  - activity
- Averaged frequency N
  - mobility
- Resonance coefficient k
- Complexity coefficient
- Spectral frequency bands $\pm$ s
  - Delta, theta
  - alpha, sigma
  - beta 1, beta 2

Fig. 5

PSYCHOTROPIC DRUG LEVELS VERSUS QUANTITATIVE EEG

Up to now, relatively few studies have been conducted relating psychotropic drug levels and quantitative EEG effects. Still fewer are studies which take into account behavioral and clinical changes quantified by rating scales.

1. Anxiolytics

Dumermuth et al. (1976) have reported the effects of clonazepam administration in children, over 30 weeks of administration. Some positive correlations between plasma levels and the amount of EEG beta fast waves activity were reported. The anxiolytic EEG profile (Fink, 1961, 1969 ; Itil, 1972, 1974, 1977) of increasing beta activity has also been correlated with plasma levels of triflubazam (Fink et al., 1976 a), diazepam and bromazepam (Fink et al., 1976 b), dipotassium chlorazepate (Marjerrison et al., 1973) and chlordiazepoxide (Whitman and Stern, 1966). Antihistaminics can also present the same pattern (Matejcek, 1978).

2. Thymoleptics

The antidepressive EEG drug profile (Fink, 1969 ; Itil, 1972, 1974, 1977 ; Itil et al., 1973) is an increase of slow delta activity together with an increase of fast beta activity. Recently, we have correlated chlorimipramine plasma levels (administered to 7 depressed patients over 3 weeks), with EEG spectral parameters. On figure 6 we present for one patient the linear increase of delta and beta activity together with an increase of chlorimipramine blood plasma levels (in ng/ml). These increased low and fast activities were matched by a quadratic decrease of the alpha spectral intensity.

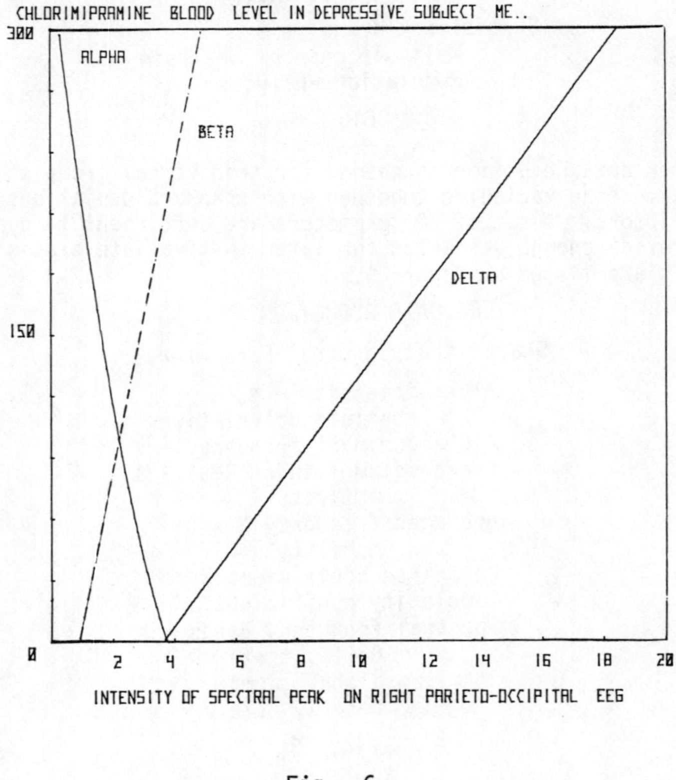

Fig. 6

3. Neuroleptics

The EEG profile of neuroleptic compounds correspond in general to an increase of slow and a decrease of fast activity. In schizophrenia (Itil, 1977) and in psychotic children (Itil et al., 1976), increase of delta and beta activity has also been observed, similar to the EEG effects of haloperidol (Itil et al., 1970). A new problem has also recently appeared : a dysfunction in cerebral dominance observed in schizophrenic patients and quantified by left/right EEG amplitude or variance ratios (d'Elia et al., 1971 ; Goldstein, 1975 ; Pidoux et al., 1978).

However, few studies have been conducted, measuring blood plasma levels and EEG parameters. The effects of one year of chronic treatment by clopenthixol have been reported by Saletu et al. (1973) and following penfluridol or thiothixene treatments by d'Elia et al. (1977).

We have recently completed a study of 6 therapy-resistant schizophrenic patients, treated by increasing doses of haloperidol. Haloperidol drug plasma levels, spectral EEG analysis, BPRS clinical rating scales were measured every week over two months. As an example of our results (to be published), we present on figure 7 the positive correlation between haloperidol plasma levels (in ng/ml) and the EEG left/right ratio of fast waves beta 1 activity recorded over parieto-occipital areas. This appears to be the first effect on cerebral dominance, related to haloperidol treatments in schizophrenic patients.

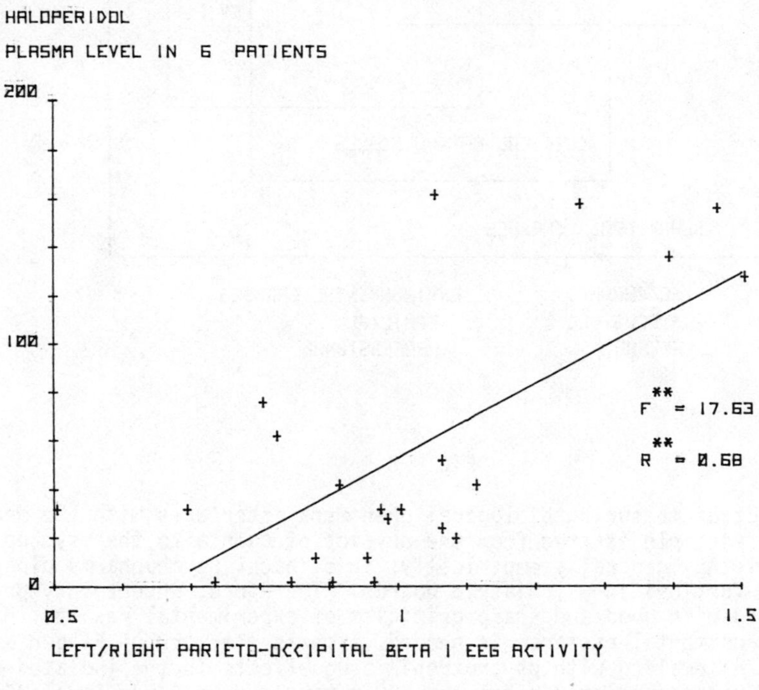

Fig. 7

CHALLENGE AND DIFFICULTIES

Fink (1974, 1978), Fink and Irwin (1976), Fink et al. (1976a, b) and Itil (1972, 1974, 1977), Itil et al. (1971, 1973), Saletu et al. (1973, 1976, 1977), have already presented bioavailability studies of psychotropic compounds and predictive studies of new compounds, based on EEG profiles used for the classification of psychoactive drugs. This area is a growing research and will involve correlations with pharmaco-kinetics, biochemical measurements (prolactine, growth hormone, ACTH, etc.), electrophysiological measurements (quantitative EEG, evoked potentials, CNV response, etc.) together with clinical rating scales. Such multiple interactions are represented on figure 8. However, behavioral changes encompass these physico-physiological and clinical measurements and they are themselves submitted to time-bounded biological rythms and to environmental changes. The reality is far more complex than experimental conditions.

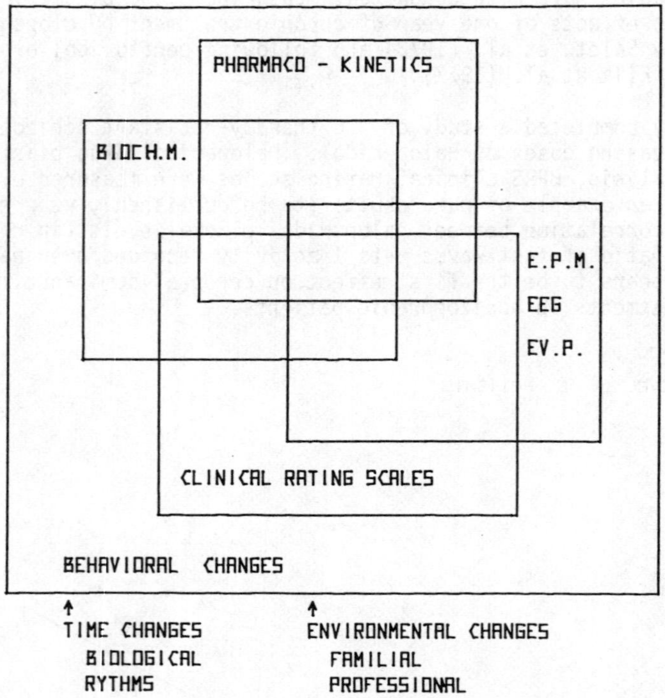

Fig. 8

Moreover, the act of measuring biological phenomena interferes with the measured subject. This principle is true from the physics of quanta to the psychophysics that we are applying, generally empirically, in clinical psychopharmacology settings and at fortiori in psychiatric boards. Therefore, uncertainty principles should be matched with good and sharp criticism of experimental results. However, basic or more fundamental research is needed, such as the work of Rieger and Krieglstein (1974) dealing with psychotropic drug effects in the isolated perfused rat brain, measuring correlations between EEG parameters and drug levels.Cerebral blood flow changes, EEG correlates and drug levels, can also be highly valuable to correlate together in the future. Finally, pathological metabolism correlated with EEG changes and drug plasma levels appear to be also an important new trend of research. For Branch et al. (1976), the increase in albumine level is correlated with the increase of slow EEG activity. For Donker et al. (1978), the increase of phenylalanine is parallel to the increase of EEG theta activity.

ACKNOWLEDGEMENTS

The new results illustrating this report are coming from interdisciplinary studies : Dr. PIDOUX for the quantification of EEG, Dr. COTTEREAU for clinical rating scales. For the pharmacokinetics, we have greatly appreciated the help of Dr. MORSELLI and Dr. ZARIFIAN, the chlorimipramine dosages were made by Dr. ROVEI and the haloperidol dosages by Dr. BIANCHETTI, using LERS-Synthelabo facilities.

This work was supported by French INSERM grants 39-76-71, 65-78-97, and UER Cochin Port Royal.

REFERENCES

Branch, R.A., M.H. Morgan, J. James and A.E. Read (1976). Intravenous administration of diazepam in patients with chronic liver disease. Gut,12, 975-983.

D'Elia, G., L. Jacobsson, J. von Knorring, B. Matsson, T. Mjörndal, L. Oreland, C. Perris and W. Rapp (1977). Changes in psychopathology in relation to EEG variables and visual averaged evoked responses (V. AER) in schizophrenic patients treated with penfluridol or thiothixene. Acta Psychiatr. Scand., 55, 309-318.

Donker, D.N.J., D. Reits, W. Storm Van Leeuwen, F.J. Van Sprang and S.K. Wadman (1978). Analyse d'EEG par calculateur pour définir l'arrêt du traitement diététique des phénylcétonuries. Rev. EEG Neurophysiol., 8, 55-60.

Dumermuth, G., T. Gasser, A. Hecker, M. Herdan and B. Lange (1976). Exploration of EEG components in the Beta Frequency Range. In P. Kellaway and I.Petersen (Eds.), Quantitative Analytic Studies in Epilepsy, Raven Press, New York, pp. 533-558.

Etevenon, P. (1977). Etude méthodologique de l'électroencéphalographie quantitative. Application à quelques exemples. Thèse D. Sc., Paris, Faculté des Sciences, Université de Paris VI, pp. 1-303.

Etevenon, P. and B. Pidoux (1977). From biparametric to multidimensional analysis of EEG (1977). In A. Remond (Ed.), EEG Informatics. A didactic review of methods and applications of EEG data processing, Elsevier/North Holland, Amsterdam, pp. 193-214.

Etevenon, P., B. Pidoux, P. Peron-Magnan, P. Rioux, G. Verdeaux, J.R. Boissier and P. Deniker (1978). Electroencephalography statistical spectral analysis of quantitative electroencephalography. In P. Deniker (Ed.), Proc. Xth Intl. Congress C.I.N.P., Pergamon Press, Oxford, pp.1141-1150.

Fink, M. (1961). Quantitative electroencephalography and human psychopharmacology. I. Frequency spectra and drug action. Med. exp., 5, 364-369.

Fink, M. (1969). EEG and human psychopharmacology. Ann. Rev. Pharmacol., 9, 241-258.

Fink, M. (1974). EEG Profiles and Bioavailability Measures of Psychoactive Drugs. In T.M. Itil (Ed.), Psychotropic Drugs and the Human EEG, Mod. Probl. Pharmacopsychiat., Karger, Basel, pp. 76-98.

Fink, M. (1978, in press).Classification of psychoactive drugs : Quantitative EEG Analysis in Man. In H.M. Van Praag, M.H. Lader, O.J. Rafaelson and E.J. Sachar (Eds.), Handbook of Biological Psychiatry, vol. 4, New York, Marcel Dekker Inc.

Fink, M. and P. Irwin (1976). Relation of EEG to blood levels of psychoactive drugs. In L. Gottschalk, S. Merlis (Eds.), Pharmacokinetics, blood levels and clinical responses, New York, Spectrum Pub., pp. 243-250.

Fink, M., P. Irwin, M. Schwartz, A. Conney and R. Weinzfeld (1976) (a). Plasma levels and EEG effects of Benzodiazepines. Clin. Pharmacol. Ther., 20, 184-191

Fink, M., P. Irwin, R.E. Weinfeld, M.A. Schwartz and A.M. Conney (1976) (b). Blood levels and electroencephalographic effects of diazepam and bromazepam. Clin. Pharm. Therap., 20, 184-191.

Goldstein, L. (1975). Time Domain Analysis of the EEG. The integrative method. In G. Dolce, H. Kunkel (Eds.), CEAN.Computerized EEG Analysis, G. Fischer, Stuttgart, pp. 251-270.

Itil, T.M. (1972). Quantitative Pharmaco-Electroencephalography in the Discovery of a New Group of Psychotropic Drugs. Dis. Nerv. Syst., 33, 557-559.

Itil, T.M. (1974). Psychotropic drugs and the human EEG. Mod. Probl.Pharmacopsychiat., vol. 8, Karger, Bâle.

Itil, T.M. (1977). Qualitative and quantitative EEG findings in schizophrenia. Schizophrenia Bulletin, 3, 61-79.

Itil, T.M., P. Gannon, W. Hsu and H. Klingenberg (1970). Digital computer analyzed sleep and resting EEG during haloperidol treatment. Amer. J. Psychiatry, 127, 462-471.

Itil, T.M., F. Güven, R. Cora, W. Hsu, N. Polvan, A. Sanseigne and G.A. Ulett (1971). Quantitative pharmaco-electroencephalography using frequency analyzer and digital computer methods in early drug evaluations. In Smith (Ed.), Drugs, development and brain functions, Thomas, Springfield,pp 145-166

Itil, T.M., B. Saletu, P. Gannon, M. Arat and W. Hsu (1973). Clinical and EEG investigations with CI-579 and CI-600 (quantitative Pharmacoelectroencephalography and "sleep prints"). Behavior. Neuropsych., 4, 11-12 and 5, 1-6, 61-68.

Itil, T.M., J. Simeon and C. Coffin (1976). Qualitative and quantitative EEG in Psychotic children. Dis. Nerv. Syst., 37, 247-252.

Marjerrison, G., A.H. Neufeld, V. Hosmes and T. Ho (1973). Comparative psychophysiological and mood effects of diazepam and dipotassium chlorazepate. Biol. Psychiatry, 7, 31-41.

Matejcek, M. (1978). Quantitative EEG plasma levels of BC 105, an antihistaminic agent (unpublished results and personal communication).

Matejcek, M. and J.E. Devos (1976). Selected methods of quantitative EEG analysis and their applications in psychotropic drug research. In P.Kellaway I. Ingemar (Eds.), Quantitative Analytic Studies in Epilepsy, Raven Press, New York, pp. 183-205.

Mucciardi, A.M. (1974). New Computational Techniques in the Evaluation of Drug-Induced EEG Changes. In T.M. Itil (Ed.), Psychotropic Drugs and the Human EEG, Mod. Probl. Pharmacopsychiat., Karger, Basel, pp. 350-377.

Pidoux, B., P. Etevenon, G. Verdeaux and P. Deniker (1978 in press). L'activité alpha dans un groupe de schizophrênes : Analyse spectrale et comparaison avec un groupe têmoin. Rev. EEG Neurophysiol. clin.

Rieger, H. and J. Krieglstein (1974). Quantitative Analysis of the EEG Effects Produced by Imipramine, Desipramine, Promazine and Monodesmethyl Promazine in the Isolated Perfused Rat Brain. Psychopharmacologia (Berl.), 39, 163-179.

Saletu, B., J. Grünberger and L. Linzmayer (1977). Classification and determination of cerebral bioavailability of psychotropic drugs by quantitative "pharmaco-EEG" and psychometric investigations (studies with AX-A411-BS). Int. J. Clin. Pharmacol., 15, 449-459.

Saletu, B., T.M. Itil, M. Arat and S. Akpinar (1973). Long term clinical and quantitative EEG effects of clopenthixol in Schizophrenics : clinical-neurophysiological correlations. Int. Pharmacopsychiat., 8, 193-207.

Saletu, B., M. Matejcek, K. Knor, U. Ferner and U. Schneewind (1976). Assessing the psychoactivity of cloxazolam (MT 14-411) by quantitative EEG and psychological studies. Curr. Ther. Res, 20, 510-528.

Shapiro, D.M. and M. Glasser (1974). Measurement and Comparison of EEG-Drug Effects. In T.M. Itil (Ed.), Psychotropic Drugs and the Human EEG, Mod. Probl. Pharmacopsychiat., 8, Karger, Basel, 1974.

Whitman, E.N. and M.M. Stern (1966). Correlation of serum levels with EEG effects of chlordiazepoxide in man. J. Newark City Hosp., 3, 3-10.

Concluding Remarks

PIERRE DENIKER

Service Universitaire de Santé Mentale et de Thérapeutique, 100-102 rue de la Santé, 75014 Paris, France

After this session, I think that everybody would agree that the time is now arrived where the use of psychotropic drugs in man as to be monitored and controlled, especially for drugs used in long term chemotherapies.

In view to develop some monitoring techniques for current practice selected from the research field that we have reviewed this morning, we have to keep in mind not only their relevance and fiability but also their ability to be learned and accepted by residents and practicionners. In addition we have to consider its cost to the community or to social security charges.

Blood level of drugs or metabolites appears to be primary data indicating what's happened after the patients have taken their medication and before that the drug should develop its action on CNS. Especially we can know if patient has really taking his drug and if he takes enough of it, which is very important. But the plasma level of drugs is different from the tissue level and from the active portion of drug in the site of action. It is known from the lithium-therapy that the quantity of lithium in plasma and in blood cells can differ in certain conditions. In the future we have to know what's happened in neurones and in specific receptors for each kind of drug. In this way, research developped in plattelets seems to be promising but may be other models can be used. The neuro-endocrinal response of prolactin secretion seems to be a faithfull index to verifie the neuroleptic activities but in our experience it is limited to a certain blood level of drug upon it the neuroendocrine response as the same.

An other unsolved question concerns the problem of patients' therapeutic reactivity. In particular with antidepressant agents and more with phenothiazines it seems that the therapeutic activity is not directly correlated with the blood level of drug, with the exception that the lowest level are generally, in relation with an insufficient response. Same thing appears in schizophrenic psychoses which do not respond to any compound at any dosage.

The different biological changes which can be directly observed in body by clinical monitoring have been reviewed by Prof. Lader. In this very simple and usefull field, it is necessary to determine which changes are directly related to the true therapeutic action and which are secondary or side-effects. By example, the method of mesuring the hand-scripture, proposed by Hase,is only able to indicate that a minimal akineto-hypertonic syndrom is present and, in fact, it is an indicator of slight neurologic side-effects more than a proof of therapeutic action.

It is possible that vegetative changes like pupil size, pulse rate, blood-pressure modification and temperature variation, etc..., considered in whole, should be more relevant. I remember that in the very first trials of chlorpromazine and reserpine we have been impressed by the symetric modification induced by the drugs in temperature curve and in blood pressure index : with CPZ they become more instable and with reserpine variations are much reduced. It is possible to imagine a system of polygraphic integration which can show the principal changes of these types. But we know that patients who are under a recording apparatus system can show some changes produced not by the drug studied but from the restraint induced by the recording system that is also the true for the EEG monitoring methods.

I am not in agreement with Malcolm Lader when he said that EEG are giving "empirical" data, if I understood well. On the contrary from the classical EEG pattern we have the ability to differentiate the principal types of psychotropic drugs : by example neuroleptics induce slow waves, minor tranquilizers produce rapid rythms, antidepressants desynchronise the EEG etc. It is possible that the EEG could be the best relevant method to the drug therapy monitoring. Matejcek shows that quantitative EEG its able to differentiate the different route of administration of the same drug. But the different methods of quantitative EEG are perhaps to much sensitive to explore some very active drugs.

In conclusion, I assume that now and especially from this symposium it is not possible to ignore pharmacokinetic and other monitoring methods in psychopharmacology. If possible we have in the future to simplify the established data in a didactic purpose. First of all the psychiatrist in charge of a clinical research has to know the basic rules of pharmacokinetic in general, and not only for psychotropic drugs.

Circadian Rhythms and Psychotropic Drugs

Introduction

RYO TAKAHASHI and HARUO NAGAYAMA

Department of Neuropsychiatry, Nagasaki, University School of Medicine,
Nagaski, 852, Japan

ABSTRACT

A review of past works on circadian susceptibility rhythm to psychotropic drugs was made. The fluctuation of lethality rate according to the difference in time of administration was shown with all the drugs tested like pentobarbital, phenobarbital, ethanol, amphetamine, chlordiazepoxide, chlorpromazine and lithium. Depending on the dose, considerable differences in the time of appearance of a peak are reported, even when the same drug was administered. In view of the existence of fluctuation of toxicity, it seems necessary to adopt the concept of time for the determination of LD_{50}.

The circadian fluctuation in effect of psychotropic drugs has also been demonstrated in the effects of barbiturates, ethanol, p-chlormethamphetamine, amphetamine, tetrabenazine, chlorpromazine and haloperidol. Various studies have been made on the influence of factors from outside and inside the living organism on the fluctuation of effect of drugs. It was suggested that the light-dark rhythm of the environment might act as a synchronizer of the rhythm of the effect. With sleep drugs, it is assumed from the results of studies on plasma level and intracerebral concentration of the drugs, that the circadian fluctuation in the effect might be induced by the circadian rhythm of drug sensitivity of the brain. (The content of this paper is derived from a part of the original paper by Nagayama, Takagi and Takahashi(1978)).

Keywords : Circadian rhythm — Psychotropic drugs — Chronopharmacology — Sleep drugs — Chronotoxicology — Brain susceptibility

INTRODUCTION

It has been considered that when the same dose of a drug is administered to a given living organism, the drug will always exert the same action upon the organism, and give rise to the same response, regardless of the time of administration. This understanding, however, may be much too simple, since the living organism itself is continuously displaying various types of circadian rhythm (biological rhythm having a period of about 24 hours). It can be assumed that the response of the organism to a drug may also fluctuate in concomitance with these biological fluctuations. Many drugs have been examined on the basis of this assumption. As a result, it has been shown that there is a circadian fluctuation in the effects of many drugs, depending upon the time of drug administration (TODA). So far as psychotropic drugs are concerned, studies have just been started on the above-mentioned subject. The clarification of this subject may lead to a better understanding of the mechanism of action of these drugs and of the function of the brain. Moreover, it may also bring about the development of a new method of treatment, including the determination of the single daily doses of drugs in the clinical practice. The present paper deals with the circadian fluctuation in the effect of psychotropic drugs or in the susceptibility of the living organism to these drugs.

There are at least three main issues in the study of the relationship between drugs and biological rhythms. The first issue is the toxicity of a drug as it varies with TODA, or the fluctuation of lethality rate due to the difference in TODA (circadian chronotoxicology). The second issue is the fluctuation of the drug effects depending on the TODA. The third issue is concerned with the influence of the drug upon the various rhythms of the living organisms. This paper will deal exclusively with the first and second issues.

CIRCADIAN FLUCTUATION OF PSYCHOTROPIC DRUG TOXICITY

Various experiments to study the lethality rate have been conducted on animals raised in environments where conditions of illumination and temperature were strictly controlled. The drugs used were pentobarbital, phenobarbital, ethanol, amphetamine, chlordiazepoxide, chlorpromazine, and lithium. All the drugs tested showed a significant circadian fluctuation of their lethality rate. The results of these experiments are summarized in Table 1. In each experiment, the day was divided equally into 12-hour light and dark periods, and the actual clock hour was converted into the time after the beginning of the light period.

In the conventional pharmacological research a method has extensively been applied in which LD_{50} is used as one of the indicators of the intensity of toxicity of a drug. As mentioned above, there is a circadian fluctuation in lethality rate, and the ratio of fluctuation has even reached 11.76 in a certain drug. Therefore, it seems necessary to adopt the concept of time for the determination of LD_{50}, so that LD_{50} may be indicated for a given time (LD_{50}/TODA). If this method turns out to be too complicated, it will be possible to replace it by a method in which LD_{50} is determined for the time when the toxicity of the drug is expressed to the largest extent.

Scheving (1968) and Nelson and Halberg (1973a) pointed out by their experiments with amphetamine and ethanol respectively that the light-dark rhythm of the environment might have acted as a synchronizer of the rhythm of lethality rate.

CIRCADIAN FLUCTUATION IN EFFECT OF PSYCHOTROPIC DRUGS

TABLE 1 Circadian Fluctuation of Lethality Rate Caused by Various Psychotropic Drugs

Drugs	Dose (mg/kg)	Species	Time showing the highest lethality rate: light period	Time showing the highest lethality rate: dark period	Ratio of crest to trough	References
pentobarbital	75	rat		↑	2.67	Pauly & Halberg, 1964
	85	rat		↑	5.00	
	90	rat		↑	3.00	
	130	mouse		↑	-	Lindsay & Kullman, 1966
phenobarbital		mouse	↑–↑		1.08	Walker & Owasoyo, 1974
ethanol	0.2ml	mouse		↑	7.02	Haus & Halberg, 1959
	6	mouse		↑	-	Nelson & Halberg, 1973a
D-amphetamine	26-30	rat		↑	11.76	Scheving, 1968, 1969
dl-amphetamine		mouse		↑–↑	1.20 1.97	Walker, 1974
chlordiazepoxide		mouse		↑	-	Marte & Halberg, 1961
chlorpromazine	74	rat		↑	2.25	Nagayama & coworkers, 1978
	250	mouse	↑		-	Hata & coworkers, 1975
lithium	940	mouse	↑		-	Hawkins & coworkers, 1978

TABLE 2 Circadian Fluctuation of Effectiveness Caused by Various Psychotropic Drugs

Drugs	Dose (mg/kg) & Species	Time of administration when the maximum response was shown to drug: light period	dark period	Ratio of crest to trough	References
Pentobarbital	35 rat		↑	1.71	Scheving & co-workers,1968
	50 rat	↑		1.47	Friedman & walker,1969
	50 rat	↑		1.99	
	60 mouse	↑		1.85	Davis,1962
	65 mouse	↑		-	
	71.5 mouse	↑		-	Nelson & Halberg,1973b
	78.7 mouse	↑		-	
	86.5 mouse	↑		-	
hexobarbital	40 rat	daily fluctuation (-)		-	Roberts & co-workers,1970
	125 mouse	↑		-	Vesell,1968
	125 mouse	↑		-	Holcslaw & co-workers,1975
	150 rat	↑		-	Müller,1971, 1974
	150 rat	↑		-	Nair & Casper, 1969;Nair,1974
phenobarbital	190 rat	↑		-	Muller,1971, 1974
ethanol	2 mouse	crest 12:00 (light 06:00-22:00)		-	Lagerspetz, 1972
p-chlorprometh -amphetamine	0.5 rat	↑		-	Evans & co-workers,1973
	4 rat	↑		-	
methamphetamine	0.2 rat		↑	-	Evans & co-workers,1973
	1.6 rat		↑	-	
d-amphetamine	1.5 rat	↑	↑	-	wolfe & co-workers,1977
	5 rat	crest 22:00-02:00 (light 08:00-17:00)		-	Urba-Holmgren & coworkers, 1977

As shown in Table 2, a circadian fluctuation has been demonstrated in the effects of pentobarbital, hexobarbital, phenobarbital, ethanol, p-chlormethamphetamine, amphetamines. Furthermore, Davies and Redfern (1973) reported results obtained from amphetamine, LSD, and mescaline. Tetrabenazine, chlorpromazine, and haloperidol has been also studied by Nagayama and coworkers. The data of these neuroleptics was excluded from Table 2. Almost all the data had a crest in the light period and only in the case of methamphetamine and d-amphetamine was a crest found in the dark period. From these results, it seems that, with a few exceptions, inhibitory drugs may exhibit a crest in the light period, and stimulative drugs in the dark period. Actually, however, the relationship between the character of a drug and the appearance of a crest is not so simple. Even when the same drug was administered, the time of appearance of a crest varied with the dose administered. For example, in the case of pentobarbital, when a small dose had been administered a crest appeared at the end of the light period or in the transitional stage from the light to the dark period. With an increase in the dosage, the crest shifted to the left-hand side of Table 2, or the beginning of the light period, regardless of the difference between investigators or between the species of experimental animals. As will be discussed in the following paper in the symposium by Dr.Nagayama, this phenomenon appeared also when neuroleptics had been administered, although in a different form.

Influence of Factors from Outside the Living Organism on the Fluctuation of Effect of Drugs

When the light-dark rhythm of the environment was modified to maintain a light period for a long time, the circadian fluctuation disappeared in the effect (duration of sleep) of pentobatbital (Davis, 1962; Scheving and coworkers, 1968) and hexobarbital (Holcslaw and coworkers, 1975). A circadian fluctuation in the effect of pentobarbital also disappeared from blinded animals (Scheving and coworkers, 1968). It is obvious that the light-dark rhythm of the environment exerted a decisive influence upon the circadian fluctuation of the effect of a drug. As an environmental condition other than light and dark, room temperature was examined. At a high temperature (36°C) a considerable levelling of the pattern was presented. When animals isolated at the time of experiment were compared with those grouped at that time, a circadian fluctuation of effect was exhibited by both groups of animals. When pentobarbital was administered, it was elucidated that the crest was significantly larger in value in the grouped animals than in the isolated ones (Davis, 1962).

Influence of Factors from Inside the Living Organism on the Fluctuation of Effect of Drugs

Many previous investigators have agreed that there is a circadian rhythm in the drug-metabolizing activity of the liver with hexobarbital (Radzialowski and Bousquet, 1968; Vesell, 1968; Nair and Casper, 1969; Roberts and coworkers, 1970; Jori and coworkers, 1971; Müller, 1971 and 1974; Holcslaw and coworkers, 1975). They have also reached an agreement to a considerable extent with regard to the wave pattern of this rhythm. The five groups of investigators agreed in finding a trough during the light period (Vesell,1968;

Nair and Casper, 1969; Jori and coworkers, 1971; Müller, 1974) or in the transitional stage from the light to the dark period (Roberts and coworkers, 1970). The wave pattern of this rhythm is the reverse of that of the rhythm of duration of sleep with the same drug (Vesell, 1968; Nair and Casper, 1969; Müller, 1974; Holcslaw and coworkers, 1975). That rhythm is related to changes in the ultrastructure of the liver (Nair, 1974). It is maintained, but shows a phase shift, in animals subjected to bilateral superior cervical ganglionectomy or regulated hourly feeding. It disappears in animals with medial or lateral hypothalamic lesions. Therefore, it has been reported that the rhythm is regulated by the hypothalamic centers and is partially dependent on the sympathetic innervation to the pineal gland (Nair and coworkers, 1970). In addition to hexobarbital, imipramine also gave rise to a circadian rhythm of metabolism. A trough appeared at the beginning of the light period, or at 3.5 hours of illumination. When the light and dark periods were reversed, this rhythm was also reversed (Jori and coworkers, 1971).

From what was mentioned above, it is considered that so far as hexobarbital is concerned, the rhythm of metabolism in the liver may be a cause of the circadian fluctuation of pharmacological effects. Actually, however, the situation is rather complicated. Studies have been made to develop another rather direct method to search for a cause of the circadian fluctuation of pharmacological effectiveness. Nelson and Halberg (1973b) selected two time points between which there was a significant difference in the duration of pentobarbital-induced sleep, and determined chronologically the serum level and the brain concentration of pentobarbital at these time points. They found no significant difference based on TODA in the serum level or the brain concentration of the drug during the time of drug-induced sleeping. There was, however, a significant difference in the serum level and the brain concentration of the drug at the time of awakening; both level and concentration of the drug were higher in animals showing the shorter sleep than in those showing the longer sleep.

All the data reported in the literature can be summarized in the following manner when the interpretation by the respective authors is disregarded. Namely, after administration with hexobarbital or pentobarbital, the metabolic rate was high when the duration of sleep was short, but there was no difference in chronological changes in the blood level or intracerebral concentration of the drug during the period of sleeping according to TODA. This result indicates that the concentration of a drug distributed in the brain was the same, regardless of TODA, although there was a difference in the rate of metabolism in the liver according to TODA. This latter difference seemed to be compensated eventually by the intervention of some other mechanism and failed to be reflected to the blood level or intracerebral concentration of the drug. Since the concentration of a drug distributed in the brain was same regardless of TODA, it is reasonable to assume that the difference in the duration of sleep between any two TODA's may have been induced by the circadian rhythm in the drug susceptibility of the brain. This assumption is also supported by the results that there was a difference based on TODA in the intracerebral concentration of the drug at the time of awakening, and that this concentration was significantly high when the duration of sleep was short.

REFERENCES

Davies,J.A., and Redfern,P.H.(1973). The effect of hallucinogenic drugs on maze exploration in the rat over a 24 hour period. Br.J.Pharmacol., 49, 121-127.

Davis,W.M.(1962). Day-night periodicity in pentobarbital response of mice and the influence of socio-psychological conditions. Experientia, 18, 235-237.

Evans,H.L., Ghiselli,W.B., and Patton,R.A.(1973). Diurnal rhythm in behavioral effects of methamphetamine, p-chloromethamphetamine and scopolamine. J.Pharmacol.Exp.Ther., 186, 10-17.

Friedman,A.H., and Walker,C.A.(1969). Rat brain amines, blood histamine and glucose levels in relationship to circadian changes in sleep induced by pentobarbitone sodium. J.Physiol., 202, 133-146.

Hata,T., Okage,T., Miyake,Y., and Kita,T.(1975). Relationship between administration time of drugs and acute toxicity in mice. Folia Pharmacol.Jpn., 71, 29-37.

Haus,E., and Halberg,F.(1959). 24-hour rhythm in susceptibility of C mice to a toxic dose of ethanol. J.Appl.Physiol., 14, 878-880.

Hawkins,R., Kripke,D.F., and Janowsky,D.S.(1978). Circadian rhythm of lithium toxicity in mice. Psychopharmacology, 56, 113-114.

Jori,A., Di Salle,E., and Santini,V.(1971). Daily rhythmic variation and liver drug metabolism in rats. Biochem.Pharmacol., 20, 2965-2969.

Lagerspetz,K.Y.H.(1972). Diurnal variation in the effect of alcohol and in the brain 5-hydroxytryptamine metabolism in mice. Acta Pharmacol.Toxicol., 31, 509-520.

Lindsay,H.A., and Kullman,V.S.(1966). Pentobarbital sodium : variation in toxicity. Science, 151, 576-577.

Marte,E., and Halberg,F.(1961). Circadian susceptibility rhythm of mice to librium. Federation Proceedings, 20, 305.

Müller,O.(1971). Circadian rhythmicity in response to barbiturates. Naunyn-Schmiedebergs Arch.Pharmacol., 270, suppl R 99.

Müller,O.(1974). Circadian rhythmicity in response to barbiturates. In L.E.Scheving, F.Halberg, and J.E.Pauly (Eds.), Chronobiology, Igaku Shoin, Tokyo. pp.187-190.

Nagayama,H., Takagi,A., Tateishi,T., and Takahashi,R.(1974). Studies on diurnal fluctuation of sedative effect of tetrabenazine. Jpn.J.Pharmacol., 24, 112.

Nagayama,H., Takagi,A., Tateishi,T., and Takahashi,R.(1977). Circadian susceptibility rhythm to neuroleptics : tetrabenazine. Psychopharmacology,55, 61-66.

Nagayama,H., Takagi,A., and Takahashi,R.(1978). Chronopharmacological study of neuroleptics. In W.B.Essman and L.Valzelli (Eds.), Current developments in psychopharmacology, Spectrum, in press.

Nair,V.(1974). Circadian rhythm in drug action; a pharmacologic biochemical, and electromicroscopic study. In L.E.Scheving, F.Halberg, and J.E.Pauly (Eds.), Chronobiology, Igaku Shoin, Tokyo, pp.182-186.

Nair,V., and Casper,R.(1969). The influence of light on daily rhythm in hepatic drug metabolizing enzymes in rat. Life Sci., 8, 1291-1298.

Nair,V., Casper,R., Siegel,S., and Bau,D.(1970). Regulation of the diurnal rhythm in hepatic drug metabolism. Federation Proceedings, 29, 804.

Nelson,W., and Halberg,F.(1973a). Effects of a synchronizer phase-shift on circadian rhythms in response of mice to ethanol or ouabain, Space Life Sci., 4, 249-257.

Nelson,W., and Halberg,F.(1973b). An evaluation of time-dependent changes in susceptibility of mice to pentobarbital injection. Neuropharmacology, 12, 509-524.

Pauly,J., and Scheving,L.E.(1964). Temporal variations in the susceptibility of white rats to pentobarbital sidium and tremorine. Int.J.Neuropharmacol., 3, 651-658.

Radzialowski,F., and Bousquet,W.(1968). Daily rhythmic variation in hepatic drug metabolism in the rat and mouse. J.Pharmacol.Exp. Ther., 163, 229-238.

Roberts,P., Turnbull,M.J., and Winterburn,A.(1970). Diurnal variation in sensitivity to and metabolism of barbiturate in the rat : lack of correlation between in vivo and in vitro findings. Eur.J. Pharmacol., 12, 375-377.

Scheving,L.E.(1968). Daily circadian rhythm in rats to d-amphetamine sulphate : effect of blinding and continuous illumination on the rhythm. Nature, 219, 621-622.

Scheving,L.E.(1969). Circadian variation in susceptibility of the rat to d-amphetamine sulfate. Anat.Rec., 160, 422.

Scheving,L.E., Vedral,D.F., and Pauly,J.E.(1968). A circadian susceptibility rhythm in rats to pentobarbital sodium. Anat.Rec., 160, 741-749.

Urba-Holmgren,R., Holmgren,B., and Aguiar,M.(1977). Circadian variation in an amphetamine induced motor response. Pharmacol.Biochem. Behav., 7, 571-572.

Vesell,E.S.(1968). Genetic and environmental factors affecting hexobarbital metabolism in mice. Ann.NY.Acad.Sci., 151, 900-912.

Walker,C.(1974). Implications of biological rhythms in brain amine concentrations and drug toxicity. In L.E.Scheving, F.Halberg,and J.E.Pauly (Eds.), Chronobiology, Igaku Shoin, Tokyo, pp.205-208.

Walker,C.A., and Owasoyo,J.O.(1974). The influence of serotonin, GABA and L-dopa on the circadian rhythm in the toxicity of picrotoxin, pentylenetetrazol and phenobarbital in mice. Int.J.Chronobiol., 2, 125-130.

Wolfe,G.B., Bousquet,W.F., and Schnell,R.C.(1977). Circadian variations in response to amphetamine and chlorpromazine in the rat. Communications in Psychopharmacology, 1, 29-37.

The Influence of Dopaminergic Mechanism on 24-Hour Temperature and Activity Rhythms in Rodents

J. A. DAVIES

Department of Pharmacology, Welsh National School of Medicine, Heath Park, Cardiff, U.K.

ABSTRACT

In this experiment the effect of apomorphine alone and that of l-dopa in combination with a peripheral dopa-decarboxylase inhibitor was studied on 24-hour rhythms of core temperature in mice. Both treatments produced marked falls in temperature at all time intervals tested and the normal temperature rhythm was inverted. Pretreatment with pimozide, a specific dopamine receptor antagonist, prevented both the decreases in temperature and the inversion of the rhythm. The effect of manipulating dopaminergic mechanisms on locomotor activity in the rat was also investigated with γ butyro-lactone which has been shown to prevent the release of dopamine from the neurone. GBL has a biphasic action on activity, in that initially there is a period of hypoactivity followed by intense hyperactivity. When GBL was given intra-peritoneally during the light phase of the lighting cycle the onset of inactivity occurred rapidly (4m), while when GBL was given during the dark phase of the cycle the onset was delayed (16m). Duration of the inactive phase also varied with time of administration. GBL was also administered in the drinking water and total activity over 24 hours was recorded. Results showed that the amplitude of the activity patterns during the dark phase of the lighting cycle was greatly increased. The results of both the temperature and activity experiments are discussed in terms of a change in the sensitivity of dopaminergic receptors.

KEYWORDS 24-hour rhythms, temperature, activity, dopamine, apomorphine, l-dopa, γ butyro-lactone.

INTRODUCTION

Dopaminergic mechanisms have been shown to have a marked effect on both body temperature in the mouse (Kruk, 1972, Fuxe and Sjoqvist, 1972 and Davies and Redfern, 1973a), and also on locomotor activity in the rat (Kelly, Seviour and Iversen, 1975, Elkhawad and Woodruff, 1975). As both the parameters have a marked diurnal rhythm the experiments reported here investigated whether there was a 24-hour rhythm of response to the various dopaminergic drugs. We have previously shown (Davies, Ancill and Redfern, 1972) that amphetamine has a varying response over the 24-hour period on locomotor activity and also on maze exploration (Davies and Redfern, 1973b).

The effect of stimulation of central dopaminergic receptors in the mouse produces a marked hypothermia either by stimulation of the receptor directly, with, for example, apomorphine (Fuxe and Sjoqvist, 1972) or indirectly by administering amantadine which is thought to release endogenous dopamine (Davies and Redfern, 1973). The present study has investigated the effect of apomorphine and l-dopa on body temperature rhythms over a 24-hour period. The l-dopa was given in conjunction with a peripheral dopa-decarboxylase inhibitor, benserazide, in order to increase brain dopamine levels. The effect of the specific dopamine receptor blocker pimozide was also investigated.

To investigate the effect of dopaminergic mechanisms on locomotor activity over a 24-hour period γ butyro-lactone (GBL) was administered; GBL is a naturally occurring metabolite found in brain (Roth and Giarman, 1970). When administered parentally it produces a selective increase in brain dopamine levels (Gessa and others, 1966). Noradrenaline, 5 hydroxytryptamine (Gessa and others, 1966) or gamma-amino-butyric acids (GABA) levels are not affected (Giarman and Schmidt, 1963). Walters, Roth and Aghajanian (1973) have shown that this selective increase in brain dopamine levels is due to an inhibition of activity in the dopaminergic neurone. High doses of GBL (400 mg/kg) have been shown to produce a 'sleep-like' state (Roth and Suhr, 1970), while lower doses of GBL (100-200 mg/kg) have been shown to have a biphase action on locomotor activity, in that there is a period of hypoactivity lasting approximately 50 min followed by a period of intense activity (Davies, 1978). It has been suggested that this hyperactive state is due to the release of dopamine that accumulates in the neurone during the inactive phase as a result of the inhibition of neuronal firing (Davies, 1978).

The effect of GBL has been investigated both by administering the drug to different groups of rats at 6-hourly intervals and measuring locomotor activity, and also by administering the GBL in the drinking water and measuring the pattern and total 24-hour activity over prolonged periods of time. We have shown previously (Davies, Ancill and Redfern, 1972) that amphetamine administered to rats in the drinking water markedly affects locomotor activity, in that the animals are active throughout 24 hours even though they are housed under strict lighting conditions of 12 hours light/12 hours dark.

It is hypothesised that dopaminergic mechanisms may have an important role to play in maintaining both the body temperature and locomotor activity rhythms. The experiments reported here attempt to elucidate some of these mechanisms.

METHODS

Body Temperature

Male albino mice weighing 30-35g were used throughout. They were housed in cabinets which were ventilated, sound-proofed, temperature-controlled ($21^{o}\pm1^{o}C$) and light-controlled (Hillier, Davies and Redfern, 1973). The animals were adapted to a 24-hour light/dark cycle with the lights coming on at 0600 hours and going off at 1800. The animals were kept in these cabinets for at least 14 days prior to the experiment.

Core temperature was measured using a rectal probe, inserted to a depth of 2.5 cm connected to an electrical thermometer (Light Laboratories, Brighton, U.K.). Temperatures were measured at 3 hours and 9 hours into both the light and dark phases of the lighting cycle. The mice were only used once.

All injections were given intra-peritoneally (i.p.) in saline except for pimozide which was given sub-cutaneously (s.c.) in 5.5% glucose after being dissolved in 0.1ml glacial acetic acid. All injections in the dark phase were given under the illumination of a red photographic safe-light.

Statistical significance was calculated using Student's t-test and the level of significance is given in the appropriate figures.

Locomotor Activity

Male Wistar rats were used throughout these experiments; in the first series where activity was recorded for 2 hours, the animals weighed 210 ± 10g, in the second series where activity was recorded continuously, the rats weighed approximately 150g at the start of the experiment. The animals were housed in identical environmental cabinets as described for the mice, except that the lights came on at 0700 hours and off at 1900 hours.

Locomotor activity was recorded on Colombus Varimex meters (P.M.S. Slough, U.K.) with a remote print out which recorded counts every minute. The 2-hour activity recording was carried out in identical environmental cabinets to those in which the rats were housed, except that recording was always done under dark conditions.

GBL was injected at 200 mg/kg i.p. and activity recorded for 2 hours at 3 hours and 9 hours into both the light and dark phases of the lighting cycle.

Drinking water was supplied to the animals, where activity was constantly monitored, from a burrette mounted on the outside of the environmental cabinet. After a settling down period of about 6 days the drinking water was substituted with tap water containing 10 mg/ml of GBL. The daily consumption of water or drug solution was recorded throughout the experiment.

Statistical significance was calculated using Student's t-test and the level of significance is given in the appropriate Figures.

RESULTS

Temperature

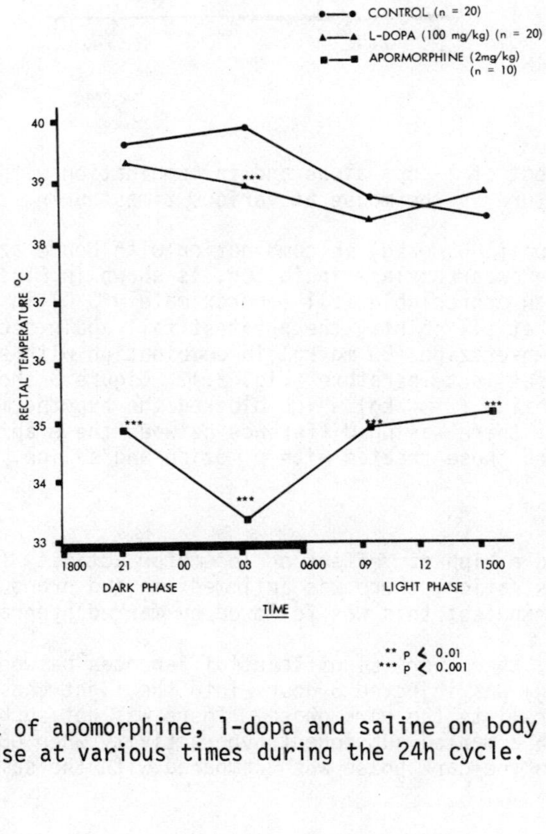

FIG. 1 The effect of apomorphine, l-dopa and saline on body temperature in the mouse at various times during the 24h cycle.

As can be seen from Fig. 1, control animals showed the expected 24-hour rhythm in body temperature. The highest temperature occurred at 9 hours into the dark phase (0300 hr) and the trough 12 hours later at 9 hours into the light phase (1500 h). The effect of apomorphine (2 mg/kg) is also shown in Figure 1 and there is a profound fall in temperature of approximately 6-7°C at all times measured. However, the greatest fall occurred at 9 hours into the dark phase where the peak in the control animals was converted into the trough in the apormorphine-treated animals. The only significant decrease with l-dopa also occurred at 9 hours in the dark phase (Fig. 1.).

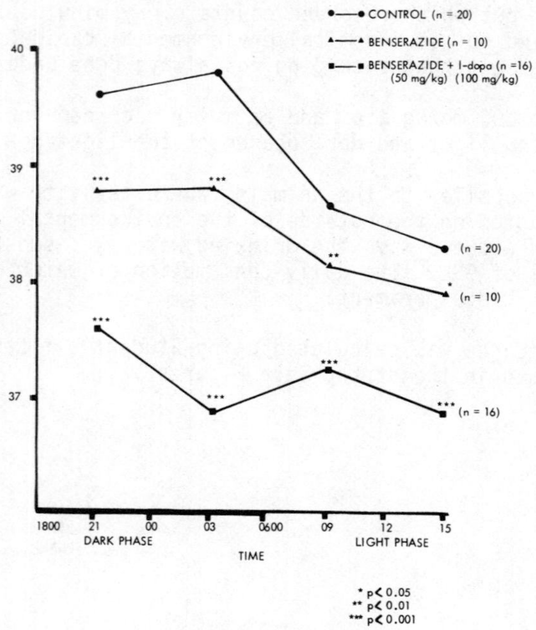

FIG. 2 The effect of l-dopa alone and in combination with benserazide on body temperature in the mouse at various times during the 24h cycle.

The effect of l-dopa (100 mg/kg) in combination with benserazide (50 mg/kg i.p.), a peripheral dopa - decarboxylase inhibitor, is shown in Fig. 2. The combination of drugs produced an appreciable fall (approximately 3°C) in temperature which was highly significant at all points, the greatest fall again occurred at 9 hours into the dark phase. Benserazide (50 mg/kg) in combination with saline also produced significant decreases in temperature (Fig. 2.). Figure 3 shows the effect of pretreatment with pimozide (2 mg/kg) which blocked the hypothermia produced by apomorphine (2 mg/kg); there was no difference between these animals given pimozide and apomorphine, and those treated with pimozide and saline.

Locomotor Activity

GBL (200 mg/kg) had a biphasic effect on locomotor activity (Fig. 4). Depending on the time of administration, there was an immediate and pronounced hypoactivity which lasted from 40-60 minutes; this was followed by marked hyperactivity.

As shown in Fig. 4, there were significant differences between the results obtained when GBL (200 mg/kg) was injected 3 hours into the light phase and when the drug was injected 9 hours into the dark phase. There was not such a profound decrease in activity or such a marked subsequent hyperactivity when GBL (200 mg/kg) was given at 9 hours in the dark phase when compared with the same dose 3 hours into

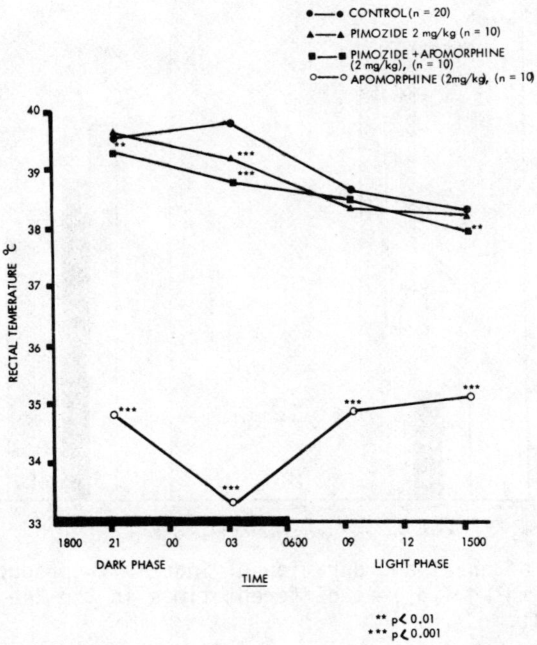

FIG. 3 The effect of pimozide on the hypothermia produced by apomorphine at various times during the 24h cycle.

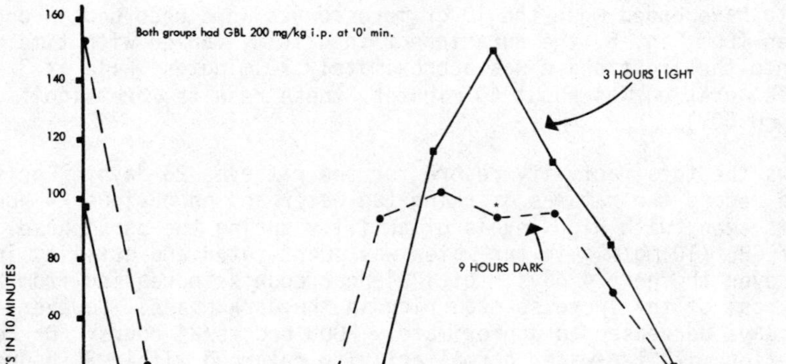

FIG. 4 The effect of GBL (200 mg/kg i.p.) on locomotor activity in the rat when given 3 hr into the light phase or 9h into the dark phase of the lighting cycle.

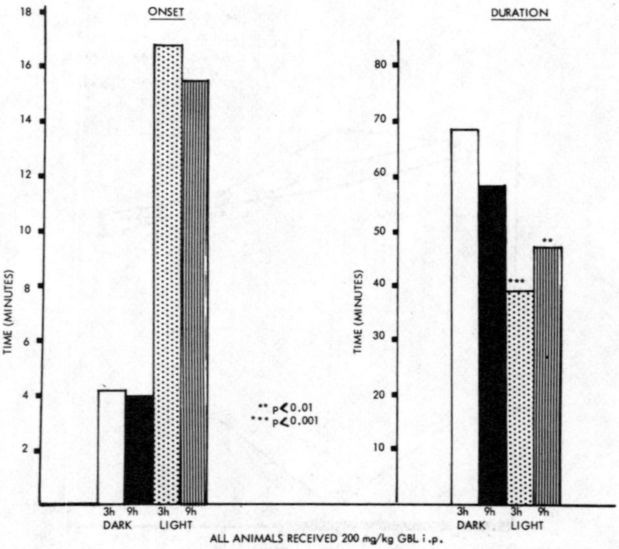

FIG. 5. The time of onset and duration of inactivity produced by GBL (200 mg/kg i.p.) at different times in the 24h cycle of the rat.

the light phase. These results were further analysed and shown in Fig. 5. The onset of the inactive period of the animals was defined as three consecutive zero scores (i.e. 3 minutes of inactivity) and it can be seen that GBL (200 mg/kg) had an onset time of about 4 minutes when administered during the light phase, whereas during the dark phase the onset was about 16 minutes. The duration of inactivity was defined to have ended when the 10 or more counts were recorded in one minute. As can be seen from Fig. 5, the duration of inactivity varied with time. Duration at 3 hours into the light phase was approximately 70 minutes while at 3 hours into the dark phase duration was about 40 minutes, these results were significantly different ($p<0.001$).

Figure 6 shows the total activity record for one rat over 25 days. For the first 6 days of the record the rat was drinking tap-water and an obvious 24-hour rhythm of activity is seen, with high levels of activity during the dark phase. On day 7 a solution of GBL (10 mg/ml) in tap-water was substituted and activity increased dramatically over the next 4 days, total 24-hour counts increasing from 21,000 to 41,000, with most of the increase occurring in the dark phase. However, activity on following days decreased to approximately 7000 counts/24 hours. On replacing the drug solution with tap-water normal activity returned within 24 hours. The total activity counts are presented in a different manner in Fig. 7. Here control levels are compared with the number of counts obtained after 3 days of GBL solution. As can be seen from Fig. 7 there are peaks of activity followed by inactive periods, the amplitude of these differences was far greater in the test animals than in the controls. A similar pattern, of activity followed by inactivity, was also found when the animals became hypoactive when compared with control after 8 days of GBL (10 mg/ml) in the drinking water (Fig. 8).

DISCUSSION

The results presented for the drug effects on body temperature support the hypothesis that dopamine produces hypothermia. Apomorphine, a specific dopamine receptor agonist, and l-dopa, in combination with benserazide, both produced marked hypothermia, the former by direct stimulation of the dopamine receptor and

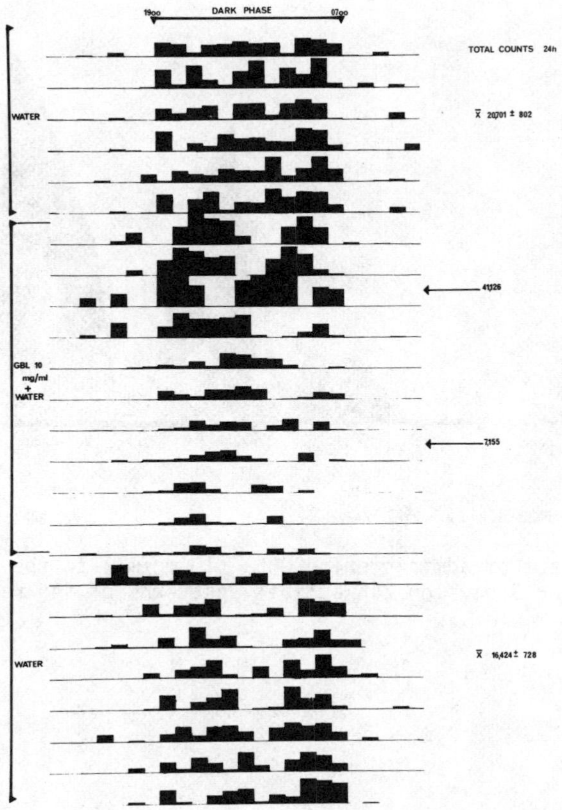

FIG. 6 The effect of administering GBL in the drinking water on total activity in the rat. Each horizontal band represents 24 h.

the latter, indirectly, by increasing the levels of endogenous dopamine in the central nervous system. Also, pimozide, a dopamine receptor antagonist, was very effective in blocking the hypothermia produced by apomorphine. However, the effect of these experiments was to investigate any rhythmical effects of dopamine receptor stimulation on the 24-hour rhythm of body temperature. The results obtained showed that the 24-hour temperature rhythm could be inverted by dopaminergic drugs. In the experiment with apomorphine the highest temperature in the control rhythm (9 hours into the dark) was converted, under the influence of apomorphine, to the lowest. As apomorphine is believed to act only on the dopaminergic receptor, one must assume that the sensitivity of the receptor changed, that is, became supersensitive during the dark period. Barnett, Taber and Peschel (1969) proposed that dopamine, in the mouse, acts to limit temperature increases. Thus, when the temperature of the control mice is high, at 9 hours into the dark phase, one might assume that there is little dopamine being released to limit the increase in temperature. If this is the case, the lack of dopamine at its post-synaptic receptor will result in supersensitivity of that receptor. A standard dose of apomorphine (in this experiment 2 mg/kg) would thus be expected to produce a greater fall in temperature if the receptor was supersensitive, as indeed it did. A similar, though less pronounced effect is seen with l-dopa in that the greatest fall in temperature occurred at 9 hours into the dark phase. There is considerable evidence that dopaminergic receptors become supersensitive following various

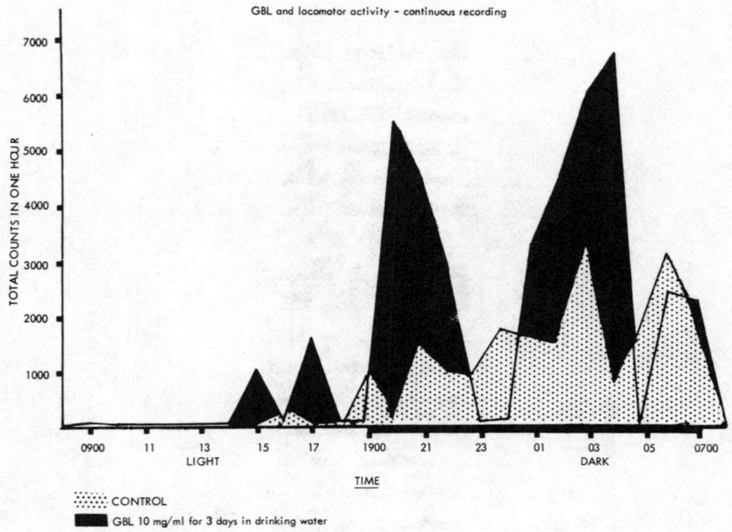

FIG. 7 The effect of administering GBL (10 mg/ml) in the drinking water for 3 days on 24h activity patterns of the rat.

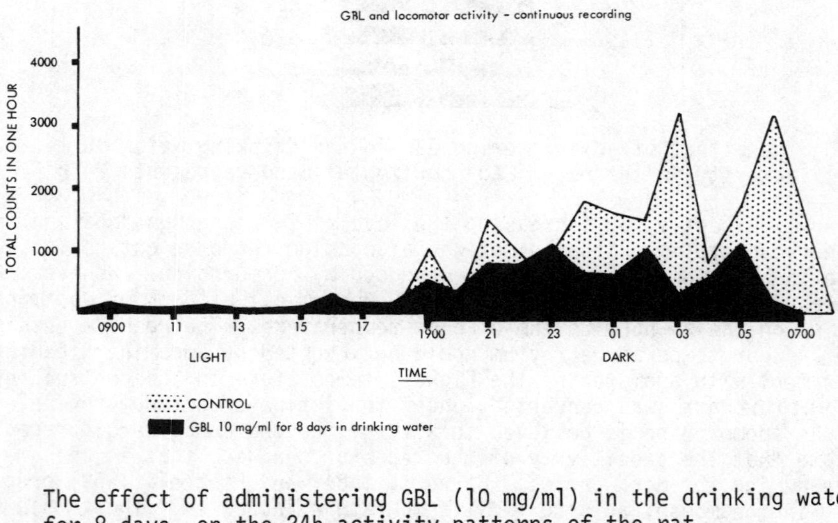

FIG. 8 The effect of administering GBL (10 mg/ml) in the drinking water for 8 days, on the 24h activity patterns of the rat.

experimental procedures such as 6-hydroxydopamine lesions (Ungerstedt 1971) pretreatment with morphine (Scheel-Kruger, Golembiowska and Mogilnicka 1977), and pretreatment with neuroleptics (Gianutsos and Moore, 1977). Whether the sensitivity of dopamine receptors changes over a shorter time e.g. hours instead of weeks, as is proposed in this paper, is not proven. If, however, this were the case the 'on-off' phenomenon found in the treatment with l-dopa of Parkinson's Disease could possibly be explained.

The effect of drugs and various lesioning studies on dopaminergic systems in the central nervous system have major effects on locomotor activity. Amphetamine, a drug which releases dopamine from the neurone, stimulates locomotor activity in the rat at low doses (1 mg/kg) whereas higher doses (5 mg/kg) produce stereotyped behaviour. Kelly, Seviour and Iversen (1975) showed that following 6.OH.DA lesions at the nucleus accumbens, low doses of amphetamine did not stimulate locomotor activity. However, higher doses in these nucleus accumbens-lesioned animals did produce stereotypy. The inference from this study being that dopaminergic mechanisms in the nucleus accumbens are essential for the maintenance of locomotor activity in the rat. Gamma-butyrolactone acts by preventing the release of dopamine from the neurone, and should thus have a marked effect on locomotor activity and may be useful in elucidating locomotor activity rhythms.

In the experiments reported in this present paper the effect of GBL on activity varied with time. Onset of inactivity was far shorter during the light phase than during the dark phase, while duration was shorter during the dark phase than the light phase. This finding was not unexpected in that rats during the light phase are normally inactive and the administration of a depressant drug would be expected to act sooner and last for longer than during the dark period. However, GBL, a drug known to affect dopaminergic mechanisms, shows a 24-hour rhythm of effect. When one examines the total activity over a two-hour period (Fig. 4) the increase in activity following the inactive phase was significantly higher during the light phase of the cycle (i.e. activity counts are high). This is a similar result to the one obtained with apomorphine on temperature and both may be explained by supersensitivity of receptors. If dopamine is the transmitter responsible for maintaining locomotor activity in the rat, the amount released during the light (inactive) phase should be low, thus resulting in the dopaminergic receptors becoming supersensitive.

The results obtained with GBL administered in the drinking water showed that the drug did not upset the 24-hour rhythm of activity, the rats were still inactive during the light phase of the cycle . This is not surprising in that over 90% of the daily fluid intake occurs during the dark phase of the cycle. However, GBL had marked effects on the pattern of activity during the dark phase of the lighting cycle. The main effect being an initial increase in the level of activity over the first few days of drug administration. The pattern of activity changed during the dark phase in that the amplitude of the peaks and troughs one normally finds in locomotor activity was very pronounced. This can be explained by the following sequence of events: ingestion of the drug solution followed by a period of inactivity due to the prevention of the release of dopamine by GBL, when the effects of the drug wear off the animal becomes hyperactive due to dopamine release, and also during this time it will eat and drink, thus leading to another hypoactive phase. This behaviour lasted for some days but was then followed by a marked decrease in activity to below control levels. This decrease is presumably due to a build-up of GBL in the central nervous system. However, even during this time there were pronounced active and inactive periods. Recovery of the animals was rapid when tap-water was re-introduced.

In conclusion, these results provide evidence that manipulation of dopaminergic mechanisms have a marked effect on temperature and locomotor activity rhythms.

The variation in effect at different times of the lighting cycle may well be due to a change in the sensitivity of the post-synaptic dopaminergic receptor.

REFERENCES

Barnett, A., R.I.Taber and E. Pesche (1969). A role for dopamine in temperature regulation of mice. *The Pharmacologist*. 11 255.

Davies, J.A. (1978). The effect of gamma-butyrolactone on locomotor activity in the rat. *Psychopharmacology*. In Press.

Davies, J.A., R.J. Ancill and P.H. Redfern (1972). Hallucinogenic drugs and circadian rhythms. *Prog. Brain. Res.* 36 79-95.

Davies, J.A. and P.H. Redfern (1973a). A note on the effect of amantadine on body temperature in mice. *J. Pharm. Pharmac.* 25 705-707.

Davies, J.A. and P.H. Redfern (1973b). The effects of hallucinogenic drugs on maze exploration in the rat over a 24-hour period. *Br. J. Pharmac.* 49 121-127.

Elkhawad, A.O., and G.N. Woodruff (1975). Studies on the behavioural pharmacology of a cyclic analogue of dopamine following its injection into the brain of conscious rats. *Br. J. Pharmac.* 54 107-114.

Fuxe, K. and F. Sjoqvist (1972). Hypothermic effect of apomorphine in the mouse. *J. Pharm. Pharmac.* 24 702-705

Gessa, G.L., L. Vargiv, F. Carbai, G.C. Coero, F. Caboni and R. Camba (1966). Selective increase of brain dopamine induced by gamma-hydroxybutyrate. *Life Sci.* 5 1921-1930.

Gianutsos, G. and Moore, K.E. (1977). Dopaminergic supersensitivity in striatum and olfactory tubercle following chronic administration of haloperidol or clozapine. *Life Sci.* 20 563-568

Giarman, N.J. and K.F. Schmidt (1963). Some neurochemical aspects of the depressant action of butyrolactone on the central nervous system. *Br. J. Pharmac.* 20 563-568.

Hillier, J.G., J.A. Davies and P.H. Redfern (1973). An environmental cabinet for twenty-four hour rhythm research of small animals. *J. Interdiscipl Cycle Res.* 4 79-82.

Kelly, P.H., P.W. Seviour and S.D. Iversen (1975). Amphetamine and apomorphine responses in the rat following 6-OHDA lesions of the nucleus accumbens septi and corpus striatum. *Brain Res.* 94 507-522.

Kruk, Z.L. (1972). The effect of drugs acting on dopamine receptors on the body temperature of the rat. *Life Sci.* 11 845-850.

Roth, R.H. and N.H. Giarman (1970). Mechanisms of the γhydroxybutyrate-involved increase in brain dopamine and its relationship to "sleep". *Biochem. Pharmacol.* 19 3001-3012.

Scheel-Kruger, J., K. Golembiowska and E. Mognicka (1977). Evidence for increased apomorphine-sensitive dopaminergic effects after acute treatment with morphine. *Psychopharmacology.* 53 55-63.

Ungerstedt, U. (1971). Postsynaptic supersensitivity after 6-hydroxydopamine induced degeneration of the nigro-striatal dopamine system. *Acta Physiol Scand. Suppl.* 367 69-93.

Walters, J.R., R.H. Roth and G.K. Aghajanian (1973). Dopaminergic neurones. Similar biochemical and histochemical effects of γ hydroxybutyrate and acute lesions of the nigro-neostriatal pathway. *J. Pharmacol. Exp. Ther.* 186 630-639.

The Influnce of the 24-Hour Rhythm in Brain 5HT on Response to Tryptophan and NN-Diemethyltryptamine

F. BROWN, J. NICHOLASS and P. H. REDFERN

School of Pharmacy and Pharmacology, University of Bath, Claverton Down, Bath BA2 7AY, U.K.

ABSTRACT

In this paper the hyperactivity produced in rats by Tryptophan (TRY) and a MAO inhibitor, pargyline, is compared to that produced by 5-methoxydimethyltryptamine (DMT) and pargyline. It is shown that whereas there is a significant variation in TRY - hyperactivity over 24 hours, no such circadian rhythm exists for DMT - hyperactivity. It is concluded that 24 hour control of 5HT in brain involves presynaptic mechanisms, a conclusion supported by comparing the effects of chlorimipramine with those of nomifensine over 24 hours. Closer examination of presynaptic processes indicates that synthetic mechanisms are most likely responsible for ultimate control of the circadian rhythm of 5HT, but in vitro examination of both 5HTP decarboxylase and TRY-hydroxylase failed to show any significant circadian rhythm in enzyme activity.

INTRODUCTION

It is not difficult to identify variations of constant circadian frequency in biological systems. As Stroebel (1967) pointed out "virtually every physiologic variable which has been sampled longitudinally has demonstrated a 24 hour periodicity". Problems arise, however, when one attempts to identify the origin of these circadian rhythms.

It is well known, for instance that in the rat brain the concentration of 5-hydroxytryptamine (5HT) fluctuates by as much as 40% about the mean over each 24h period.

The factors responsible for this remarkably constant rhythm, and its pharmacological significance in terms of those centrally-acting drugs which affect tryptaminergic mechanisms are not clearly understood, and are the problems to which the work described here was addressed. Male C.F.Y. rats weighing 120 - 140g at the start of each experiment have been used throughout; for the bio-chemical estimations, animals were used in groups of 7 or 8, and estimations were carried out on whole brain, from which the pineal gland had been separated. For the behavioural experiments groups of 3 animals were used. Before each experiment all animals were exposed for at least 10 days to a controlled environment (Hillier, Davies and Redfern, 1973) and to a rigid light-dark cycle of 12 h. light: 12h dark.

RESULTS

Tryptophan Hyperactivity

We have examined the influence of endogenous 24h rhythms on the characteristic hyperactivity syndrome produced by adminstration of L-tryptophan (TRY) in combination with a monoamine oxidase inhibitor, and believed to be caused by excess 5HT at central synapses (Grahame-Smith 1971a) Tryptophan was injected i.p. 30 minutes after the i.p. injection of pargyline and the combined activity of the group of 3 animals was recorded remotely over the next 6 hours using 'Varimex' recorders (Columbus Instruments).

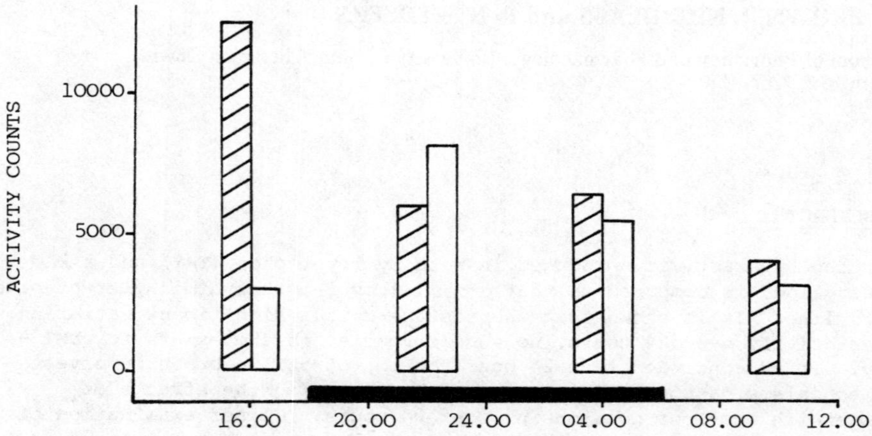

Fig. 1. Circadian variation in TRY-hyperactivity. Open columns-controls; hatched columns-drug treated.

In fig. 1. the effect of TRY 50 $mg.kg^{-1}$ and pargyline 50 $mg.kg^{-1}$ is shown. It should be emphasized that, because of the nature of the experiments, it was not possible to observe the animals, nor therefore, to analyse the type of behaviour exhibited; only total activity scores are shown. It can be seen that the activity of control animals shows the expected circadian rhythm, with greatest activity during the dark period. After TRY, no significant increase in activity was observed in the dark period or at the beginning of the light period, but a significant increase was seen between 16.00h and 22.00h after TRY injected at 1600h. As expected, it was possible to produce hyperactivity irrespective of the time of TRY administration, simply by increasing the dose of either TRY or pargyline. However, any given combination of TRY and pargyline always produced significantly greater activity at the end of the light phase. These results showed first that this particular behavioural response was subject to a significant degree of circadian variation and further suggested a relationship between the observed variation and the known rhythm of brain 5HT concentration, in that the greatest behavioural activity was consistently coincident with the highest levels of brain 5HT.

Many possible reasons could be advanced why this apparent relationship should be more than coincidence. The high levels of endogenous 5HT could be associated, for instance, with facilitated uptake or increased availability of TRY in central neurones, with increased synthesis of 5HT, with an increased rate of 5HT release or with saturation of intraneuronal storage sites for 5HT, allowing greater quantities of that 5HT synthesised from exogenously-administered TRY to spill over from the vesicles.

All these mechanisms imply changes in presynaptic mechanisms. Equally the possibility exists of a circadian rhythm in post-synaptic mechanisms.

DMT Hyperactivity

In order to investigate this possibility, the effect of TRY was compared to that of 5-methoxy-NN-dimethyltryptamine (DMT), an hallucinogenic drug which produces a hyperactivity syndrome like that associated with TRY, but by direct stimulation of post-synaptic receptors. This difference in mechanism may be inferred, for example, from the fact that whereas TRY-hyperactivity is prevented by pretreatment with p-chlorophenylalanine (PCPA) the response to DMT is unaffected (Grahame-Smith 1971b).

After DMT, 2.5 $mg.kg^{-1}$ i.p. combined with pargyline, 75 $mg.kg^{-1}$ i.p., the hyperactivity was rapid in onset, of shorter duration than that produced by TRY but essentially similar in character. As fig. 2 shows, there is no evidence of circadian variation in the size of response to DMT.

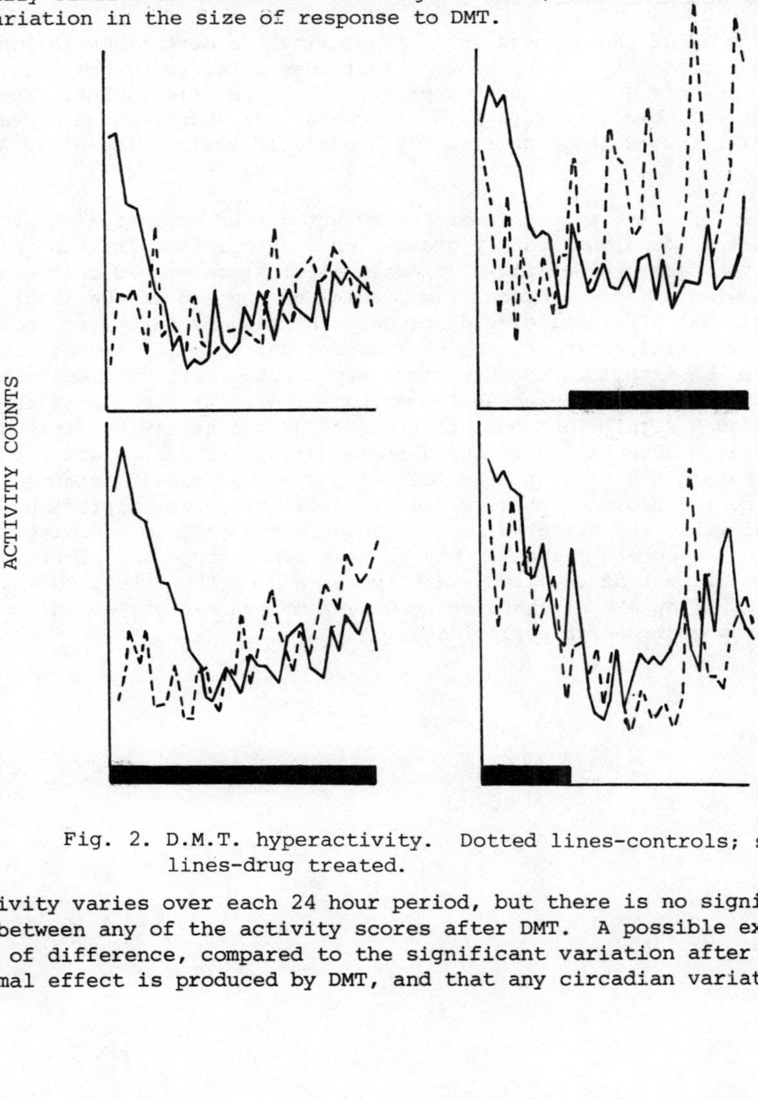

Fig. 2. D.M.T. hyperactivity. Dotted lines-controls; solid lines-drug treated.

Control activity varies over each 24 hour period, but there is no significant difference between any of the activity scores after DMT. A possible explanation of the lack of difference, compared to the significant variation after TRY, is that a maximal effect is produced by DMT, and that any circadian variation in receptor sensitivity is obscured by a change in behavioural response i.e. an increased incidence of stereotyped movements not necessarily reflected in an increase in total activity recorded.

Such an explanation, which seems unlikely in view of the fact that the activity scores after 2.5 $mg.kg^{-1}$ DMT are less than those after TRY 50 $mg.kg^{-1}$, is rendered untenable by the observation that an increase in the dose of DMT to 10 $mg.kg^{-1}$ i.p. produced a significant increase in activity scores. Again the hyperactivity was the same, irrespective of the time of day at which DMT was administered.

These experiments therefore clearly demonstrate a difference in response to TRY and DMT. Assuming that DMT acts post-synaptically, it must be concluded that any circadian variation in response to TRY is due to 24h variation in presynaptic mechanisms and not to changes in sensitivity of 5HT receptors or to 24-fluctuations involving neuronal events remote from but consequent on 5HT-receptor activation.

The Effect Of Uptake Inhibition

Further evidence of the importance of tryptaminergic mechanisms in controlling the 24-hour periodicity of TRY hyperactivity was obtained by comparison of the effects of two uptake inhibitors, nomifensine and chlorimpramine. Nomifensine, which selectively blocks reuptake of catecholamines (Hunt, Kannergiesser and Raynard, 1974) failed to potentiate TRY-hyperactivity in doses up to 20 $mg.kg^{-1}$ i.p.

It is also interesting to note that the extent of the potentiation after chlorimipramine was significantly greater when chlorimipramine was injected at the end of the dark phase, (fig 3). Again it might be argued that the lack of effect following injection of chlorimipramine at the end of the light phase is because a maximal effect is already produced by TRY and pargyline, so that addition of chlorimipramine to the pharmacological cocktail causes free-running locomotion to be displaced by more stereotyped behaviour. Since administration of a high dose of chlorimipramine (25 $mg.kg^{-1}$ i.p.), at the end of the light phase produced a significant potentiation of TRY hyperactivity, this appears not to be the case. Observation of the animals during the period did not disclose any difference in the type of behaviour displayed by animals injected with TRY and pargyline and those which received, in addition, chlorimipramine. Only the degree of activity was different. We are therefore left to speculate on the extent to which the 5HT-uptake mechanism may be less susceptible to chlorimipramine at this particular part of the light-dark cycle, and on the extent to which the influence of 5HT-uptake blockade on resultant concentrations of 5HT in the synaptic cleft may show a circadian periodicity.

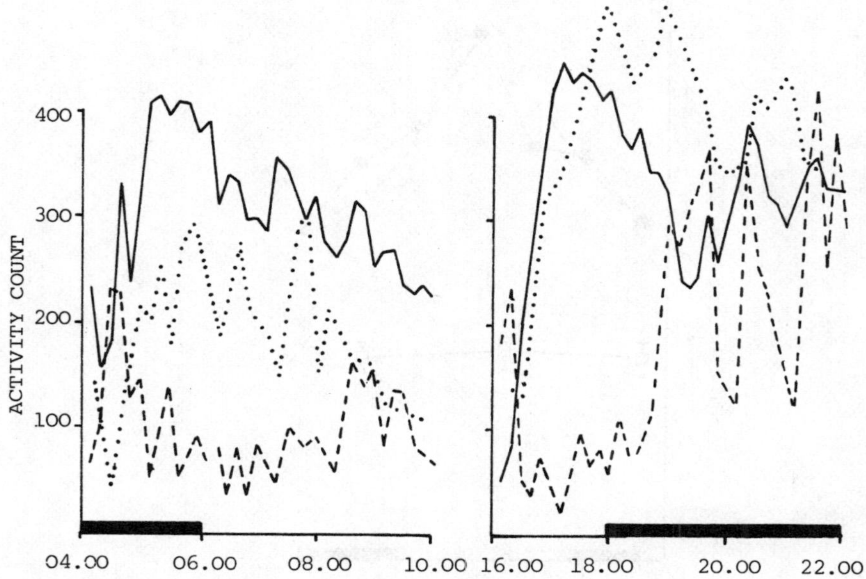

Fig. 3. Chlorimipramine on TRY-hyperactivity. Dashed line-pargyline alone. Dotted line-pargyline + TRY. Solid line-pargyline + TRY + chlorimipramine.

The Control of 5HT over 24-hours

The general conclusion to be drawn from these results is that when considering which factors were responsible for the 24-hour variation in brain 5HT concentrations, and which are in consequence likely to influence pharmacological responses to drugs acting through tryptaminegic mechanisms, we should concentrate primarily on presynaptic mechanisms. In doing so, some further assumptions may be made. First, if 5HT concentrations are low during the dark phase because release and metabolism of 5HT outstrips synthesis, then the concentration of 5-hydroxyindoleacetic acid (5HIAA) in brain tissue should be higer during the dark phase than during the light phase. Experimental evidence shows that, on the contrary, 5HIAA concentrations follow exactly the pattern of 5HT concentrations, peaking at the end of the light phase (Hillier & Redfern 1977). Irrespective of whether the 5HIAA is derived from 5HT released directly into the synaptic cleft or from 5HT overflowing from vesicles into the cytoplasm of the presynaptic nerve ending, the observed correlation between 5HT and 5HIAA levels over 24 hours must suggest that 5HT is synthesised most rapidly during the light phase. Support for this conclusion may be gained from observing the effect of PCPA, which prevents 5HT synthesis by inhibiting TRY-hydroxylase.

As would be expected, the 5HT concentration in the brain of animals three days after PCPA, 316 mg.kg^{-1} p.o., was significantly lowered irrespective of the clock hour at which the animals were killed. The salient point in terms of the present discussion is that after PCPA, 5HT concentrations were the same in the brains of animals killed in the middle of the dark phase and in the middle of the light phase, that is, the proportional decrease in 5HT was much greater in the light phase. Thus inhibition of 5HT synthesis effectively abolishes the circadian rhythm in brain 5HT concentrations (fig 4) and provides evidence that in seeking to identify controlling influences of this 24h periodicity, we should concentrate on the synthetic pathway.

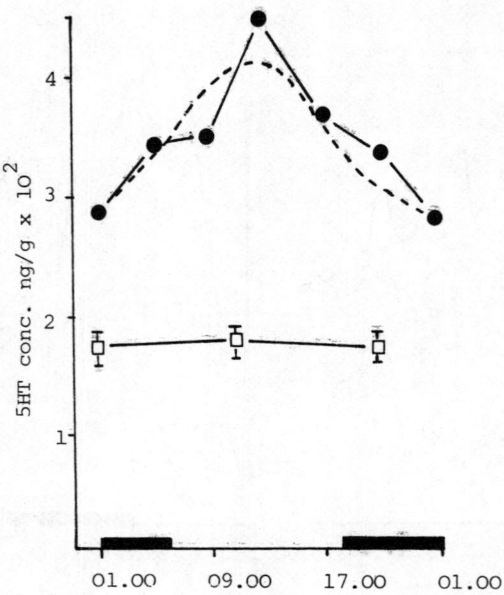

Fig. 4. PCPA on 5HT over 24 hours. Circles-control levels (with best fit sine curve). Squares-levels 3 days after PCPA 316 $mg.kg^{-1}$ p.o.

The rate-limiting step in 5HT synthesis is generally held to be hydroxylation of TRY to produce 5-hydroxytryptophan (5HTP). This would also seem to be a likely point at which the rate of synthesis might be most easily controlled, although previous experiment in our laboratories had indicated a possible 24-hour variation in 5HTP decarboxylase activity (Hillier and Redfern 1976). In these earlier experiments the amount of 5HT produced by incubation of 5HTP with crude homogenates of rat brain was estimated isotopically. More recent experiments, in which, after incubation, the newly synthesised 5HT was separated and assayed fluorimetrically, did not show a difference in 5HTP decarboxylase activity large enough to account alone for the 24 hour variation in 5HT concentrations (Brown, Nicholass and Redfern 1977).

TRY-Hydroxylase

Earlier experiments, in which TRY-hydroxylase activity was measured by a modification of the method of Grahame-Smith (1964) had also showed no significant variation in enzyme activity over 24 hours (Hillier and Redfern 1977). More recently, further experiments have been performed in which TRY-hydroxylase activity has been estimated by the method of CO_2-trapping (Ichiyama and others 1970). Tryptophan hydroxylase was prepared from sucrose homogenates of whole brain and was incubated at 37° and pH 8.1 with TRY labelled with ^{14}-C on the carboxyl group. After 30 min, incubation was stopped, and the labelled carbon dioxide formed during conversion of TRY, through 5HTP to 5HT was released by addition of perchloric acid, collected in hyamine solution, and counted (Brown, Nicholass & Redfern, in preparation).

Using this method the Km and Vmax of TRY hydroxylase were calculated to be 61.5 μM and 0.125 μmol/g/hr respectively. The concentration of TRY used to assay the enzyme activity over 24h was 5 67 x 10^{-6}M; at this concentration the amount of labelled CO_2 likely to arise from tryptamine production is insignificant (Ichiyama and others 1970) and does not interfere with the assay. Table 1 shows that when TRY hydroxylase is estimated by this method in homogenates from animals killed at different clock hours, there is no discernable rhythm in enzyme activity during the 24 hour period.

TABLE 1 24Hour Variation in Tryptophan Hydroxylase Activity

	Clock hour	nmol $^{14}CO_2$ produced/g/hr
	12.00	8.56 ± 0.24
18.00	16.00	8.21 ± 0.16
↑	20.00	7.42 ± 0.28
dark	24.00	8.45 ± 0.31
↓	04.00	7.64 ± 0.22
06.00	08.00	7.17 ± 0.31
	12.00	8.84 ± 0.18

(n = 8)

CONCLUSIONS

So, although there is a well-defined and well-documented 24-hour rhythm in brain 5HT concentration, a rhythm apparently controlled through the synthetic pathway for 5HT, variation in enzyme activity does not hold the key to the circadian regulatory mechanism. It has been clearly demonstrated that under certain circumstances, manipulation of TRY concentrations in blood or brain can affect brain 5HT concentration (Fernstrom and Wurtman, 1971). It seems doubtful whether this mechanism can account for the circadian rhythm of brain 5HT concentration since under physiological conditions, the 24h rhythm of TRY in blood and brain is approximately 12 hours out of phase with that of 5HT (Morgan and others 1975, Hillier and Redfern 1977).

Perhaps there is a sub-compartment of TRY in brain, not differentiated in measurement of total brain TRY, which is important in controlling the rate of 5HT synthesis. Perhaps the rate of uptake of TRY into the tryptaminergic nerves is important in regulating 5HT synthesis. Most likely, many interlocking elements are involved, including elements of neuronal circuitry and feed-back mechanisms which are destroyed by the in vitro methods used here to examine single isolated facets of the system. These possibilities await further examination. It is clear that, whatever the underlying control mechanisms, the physiological circadian rhythm in brain 5HT concentration can be demonstrated to produce significant variation in pharmacological responses involving tryptaminergic mechanisms.

REFERENCES

Brown, F., J. Nicholass and P.H. Redfern, (1977). A circadian rhythm in 5HTP-decarboxylase. J. Pharm. Pharmac., 29 56P

Fernstrom, J.D. and R.J. Wurtman. (1971). Brain serotonin content : physiological dependence on plasma tryptophan levels. Science, 173, 149-151.

Grahame-Smith, D.G. (1964). Tryptophan Hydroxylation in brain. Biochem. Biophys. Res. Commun., 16, 586-592.

Grahame-Smith, D.G. (1971a). Studies *in vivo* on the relationship between brain TRY, brain 5HT synthesis and hyperactivity in rats treated with a monoamine oxidase inhibitor and L-Tryptophan. J.Neurochem., 18, 1053-1066.

Grahame-Smith, D.G. (1971b). Inhibitory effect of chlorpromazine on the syndrome of hyperactivity produced by L-Tryptophan or 5-methoxy-N,N-dimethyltryptamine in rats treated with a monoamine oxidase inhibitor. Br.J.Pharmac., 43, 856-864

Hillier, J.G., J.A. Davies and P.H. Redfern (1973). An environmental cabinet for small animals. J.Int. Cycle Res., 4, 79-82

Hillier, J.G. and P.H. Redfern (1976). The 24-hour variation in 5HTP-decarboxylase activity in the rat brain. J.Neurochem., 27, 311-312

Hillier, J.G. and P.H. Redfern (1977). 24-hour rhythms in serum and brain indoleamine concentrations, TRY-hydroxylase and MAO activity in the rat. Int.J.Chronobiology, 4, 197-210

Hunt, P., M.H. Kannergiesser and J.P. Raynaud (1974). Nomifensine: a new potent inhibitor of dopamine uptake into synaptosomes from rat brain corpus striatum. J.Pharm.Pharmac., 26, 370-371

Ichiyama, A., S.Natamura, Y.Nishizutea and O.Hayaishi (1970). Enzymatic studies on the biosynthesis of serotonin in mammalian brain. J.Biol. Chem., 245, 1699-1709

Morgan, W.W., J.J. Saldama, C.A. Yndo and J.F. Morgan (1975). Correlations between circadian changes in serum amino acids or brain tryptophan and the contents of serotonin and 5-hydroxyindoleacetic acid in regions of the rat brain. Brain Res., 84, 75-86.

Stroebel, C.F. (1967). A biologic rhythm approach to psychiatric treatment. in Proceedings of the Seventh Medical Symposium. I.B.M. Corp. New York pp. 215-241

Chronobiology, A New Perspective for Biology and Medicine

LAWRENCE E. SCHEVING

Department of Anatomy, University of Arkansas for Medical Sciences, Little Rock, Arkansas 72201, U.S.A.

ABSTRACT

This paper is based on a presentation given as the opening address before a symposium on Chronobiology held during the 11th Collegium Internationale Neuropsychopharmacologicum Congress in Vienna, Austria, 9-14 July 1978. The author discusses the ubiquitous nature of rhythms, current terminology, the different frequencies found, and the current methods used for analyzing time-series data. Rhythms having frequencies of about a day, the circadian, are emphasized throughout the paper; the different properties of circadian rhythms are described; and examples are given of a number of diverse circadian rhythms in rodent and man. Finally, some potential applications of chronobiological principles to medicine are suggested.

KEYWORDS

Circadian, man, rodent, drug susceptibility rhythms, cancer chronochemotherapy.

INTRODUCTION

It is a pleasure for me to have been invited to give a talk at this symposium on chronobiology. Professor Ryo Takahashi, the symposium organizer, had asked me to present at the beginning some concepts developed in recent years relating to the science of chronobiology, especially as they relate to man and to the subject matter to be presented by my colleagues during this symposium. To begin with a definition of chronobiology seems appropriate - "Chronobiology is defined as that branch of science that explores mechanisms of biological time structure including the important rhythmic manifestations of life" (Halberg and others, 1977).

The past three decades have been a period of rapid proliferation of data documenting rhythms in plants, experimental animals and human beings. Rhythms of many frequencies and at all levels of plant and animal life, as well as all levels of biological organization have been demonstrated. Oscillation has become firmly established as a fundamental property of all life. Because of the regularity of these rhythms, some refer to them as biological or physiological clocks. The range of frequencies that have been found in the living system extends from cycles of less than a second - as in nerve cells - to cycles of a year or more (Halberg and others, 1977). There is evidence that some rhythms are adaptive and serve to adjust the organism to periodic changes in the environment; on the other hand it becomes difficult to ascribe adaptive significance to some other rhythms.

Enthusiasm or recognition, among the majority of the medical profession, for the idea that it may be worthwhile to consider seriously the temporal structure of man in the over-all basic research or in the scheme of prevention, diagnosis and treatment of disease has not always been as high as it is today (Scheving, 1974). There are many reasons for this and a few of these deserve comment

The time-honored concept of "milieu interieur constant", as put forth by Claude Bernard (1865), or William Cannon's concept of "homeostasis" are taught in medical school physiology courses and are interpreted by many as being contradictory to the concept of rhythmicity as it has developed. A great number of rhythms become overt only when they are properly measured and plotted; thus one is not apt to be aware of such oscillation unless the oscillating variable is first carefully investigated. Of course there are well-known, overt rhythms which include the high-frequency rhythms characterizing the heart and respiratory systems as well as the well-known circadian rhythm in oral or rectal temperature which characterizes man. Also well known is the lower frequency menstrual rhythm which fortunately is characterized by several markers including the prominent one of periodic bleeding; without such overt markers one wonders whether even today our understanding of the menstrual rhythm would be as good as it is. Thus the mapping or exposure of the covert rhythms was an essential step; and it was while this mapping was being done that ambiguity arose. In retrospect, the cause of this ambiguity was usually poorly designed studies. For example, the data from a well-designed study on standardized animals with frequent intervals of sampling might demonstrate a rhythm. Another investigator attempting to reproduce the data might not pay sufficient attention to experimental design and obtain conflicting results. In his design, for instance, he might have paid too little attention to the standardization of the animals, or he might have sampled only once during the day and once during the night (under the mistaken idea that rhythms are strictly a day-night affair). The end result frequently was confusion.

During the period of the mapping of the rhythmic structure of different organisms, it was found that some rhythmic variables are characterized by high-amplitude rhythms whereas other rhythms were of low amplitude. Thus among some scientists a notion developed that rhythms represented no more than minor fluctuations around a 24-hr mean and probably were not worth the expense necessary to measure them (Scheving, 1974). Others thought that rhythms were probably no more than a response to getting up or to going to bed or to the ingestion of a meal, etc. For reasons that are difficult for the chronobiologist to accept, it became (and still is) popular to sample at only one time of day; ostensibly this somehow would take care of the rhythm problem - of course it does no such thing.

One of the greatest impediments to carrying out chronobiological research by those who fully appreciate its potential merit involves logistical problems. For example, if one wishes to evaluate properly the circadian rhythm in a particular variable, one must sample around the clock. The conventional social cycle of the scientist and his staff does not make this easy to accomplish. Normally the working day is 8 hr; and that period is usually the time when samples are obtained. In fact, most often the sampling is done during the first part of the working cycle; thus at best only a small segment of the circadian system is being explored. With the strict labor laws found in many countries, it is difficult to get work done at "odd hours" without special arrangements and compensation, and on a limited budget this is not always easily done. To further compound this problem it is not uncommon in many laboratories to find that those who care for the animals, cleaning their cages, etc., do so at night; this subjects the animals to light and other disturbances which well may confound the results from one laboratory as compared with another. The United States Food and Drug Administration has thus far chosen not to include in their widely recognized guidelines, the "Good Laboratory Animal Practices Guide", the necessity of controlling rhythms - this is done in spite of a plethora of data indicating that such an approach is wrong and perhaps even dangerous.

As to the merits of giving serious consideration to the temporal organization of man, we still find skeptics and those who choose to ignore the problem. Fortunately they are becoming a minority among the scientific community, but that is not to say that they have not impeded progress in the past. Those who still espouse the idea that rhythms are of little consequence usually lack sufficient knowledge of at least the more recent developments. The point to be emphasized is that we no longer can consider chronobiological studies as esoteric. The time is coming when study groups, review committees and advisory panels must insist upon the awareness of circadian strategies in research protocols.

It is the objective of this symposium to call your attention to the fact that a critical mass of data does exist which demonstrates the biological time structure is indeed important. The more specific objectives will be (1) to give a few illustrative examples of rhythms, (2) to comment briefly on the properties of rhythms, (3) to mention methods for analyzing time-series data so that the reader can have an understanding of how some of the data to be presented has been analyzed, (4) to discuss briefly the mechanism of rhythms, and (5) to call attention to a limited amount of data which illustrates the potential application of chronobiology to medicine. In doing so, I will avoid covering material which will be presented by other participants in this symposium.

ILLUSTRATIVE EXAMPLES OF RHYTHMS

As mentioned above, there are rhythms of many frequencies; however, my presentation will deal primarily with those rhythms having a frequency of approximately or exactly 24 hr, or the circadian period. Figure 1 illustrates the well-documented rhythm in body temperature of man. The chronogram illustrates a group rhythm for 14 individuals (7 blinded males and 7 blinded females) over a 72-hr period. Each point represents the group mean and standard error (SE) of the mean. Obviously temperature is a variable which has a very low amplitude rhythm; however, no physiologist would deny that the 1.5° to 2°F change found in body temperature along the 24-hr time scale is important in the regulation of metabolism in man or any other homeothermic organism. Figure 2 demonstrates still another rhythmic variable, the cortisol rhythm of man, as well as the corticosterone rhythm in the rodent (both steroids represent the predominant serum steroid of that species). Note that there is a 180° difference in the phasing of the rhythm in diurnally active man as compared to that in the nocturnally active rodent (Scheving and Pauly, 1974). We have found that not all rhythmic variables characterizing man and rodent are 180° out of phase, and for this we have no explanation. However, it does point out that one must be very careful when extrapolating from the rodent to man (Scheving and Dunn, 1974).

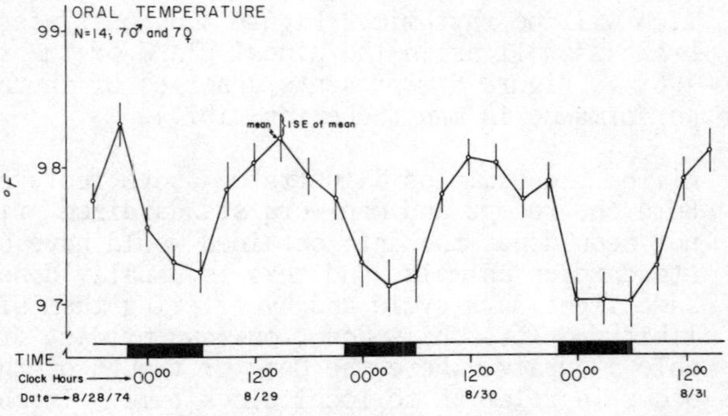

Fig. 1. Circadian fluctuation in oral temperature of blinded human beings. The dark bar on the abscissa represents rest and/or sleep (Pauly and others, 1977).

Figure 3 illustrates a rhythm in the amylase found in the saliva of man (Scheving and others, 1976).

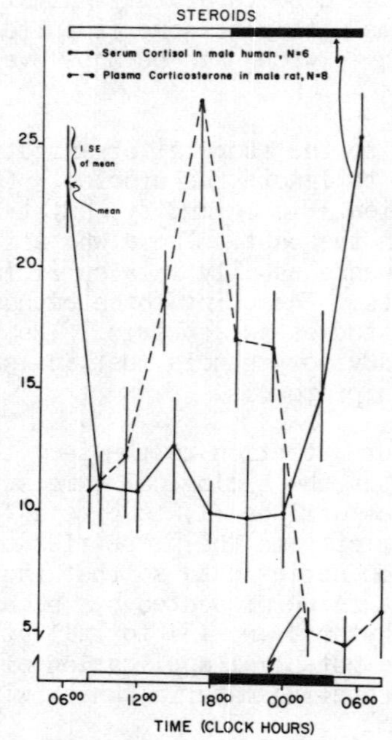

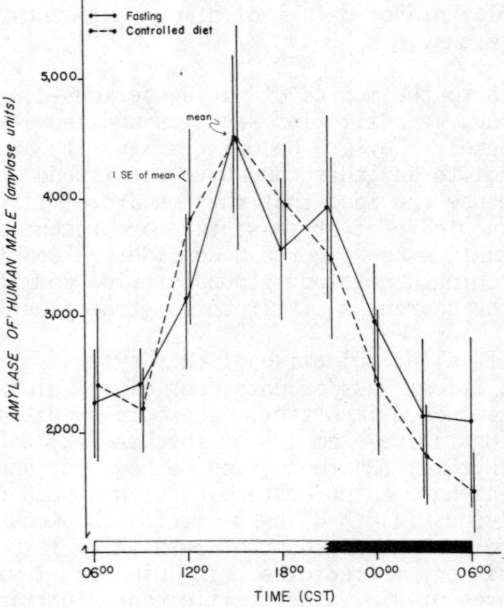

Fig. 2. Corticosterone level in rats standardized to a light-dark cycle and fed ad libitum (12 hr light alternating with 12 hr darkness). Cortisol levels in presumably healthy young males. Meal times: 0700, 1245 and 1645; rest or sleep time: 2100-0600, however the subjects were awakened for sampling at 2400 and 0300 (Scheving and Pauly, 1974; Scheving and Dunn, 1974).

Fig. 3. The chronograms demonstrate the group rhythm seen in the saliva of presumably healthy young men. The data have not been published previously, but the details of the overall study have been described in relation to other rhythmic variables (Scheving and others, 1976).

It must be emphasized that it makes little difference whether one measures variables in a tissue, urine, blood, or saliva (Fig. 3), the variable under consideration will be rhythmic. Figure 4 demonstrates the level of serotonin in the whole brain as well as in the pineal gland of the rat (Quay, 1963; Scheving and others, 1968). Figure 5 represents a series of rhythmic variables related to behavior and performance in man (Scheving, 1977).

All of the examples illustrated above represent data obtained on rodents or man. Both the rodent and man were standardized prior to collection of data; if this had not been done, the data obtained would have been much "noisier". It is easy to standardize animals, and this is usually done by subjecting all animals to the same light-dark cycle and by offering them similar feeding schedules, such as ad libitum. If such is done, one can predict from one study to another, with reasonable accuracy, where the peak or trough of the rhythm (or any other phase) will occur in relation to local clock time. It should be noted that for most variables the phasing may vary somewhat from day to day, but usually not dramatically. However, for some metabolic variables, strong seasonal influences may alter rhythms even in experimental animals that are rigidly standardized from season to season (Mayersbach, 1967). For man, standardization involves subjecting all subjects to

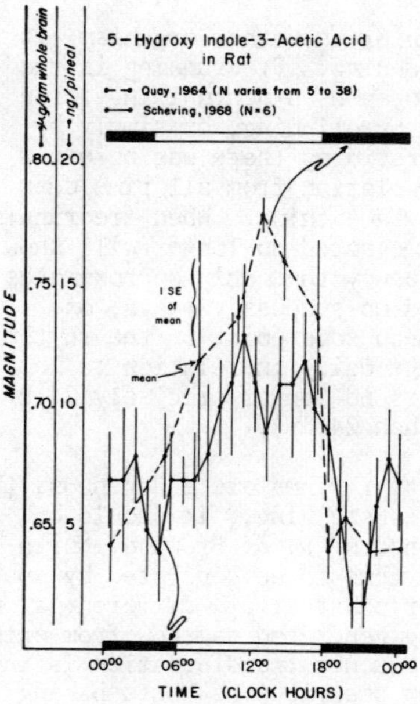

Fig. 4. Circadian rhythm in pineal serotonin of adult male rats. The daily change is nearly 900%. The circadian rhythm in whole brain serotonin is of relatively modest amplitude (18%). Both have similar phasing. For details of pineal serotonin study, see Quay (1963); for brain serotonin study, see Scheving and others (1968).

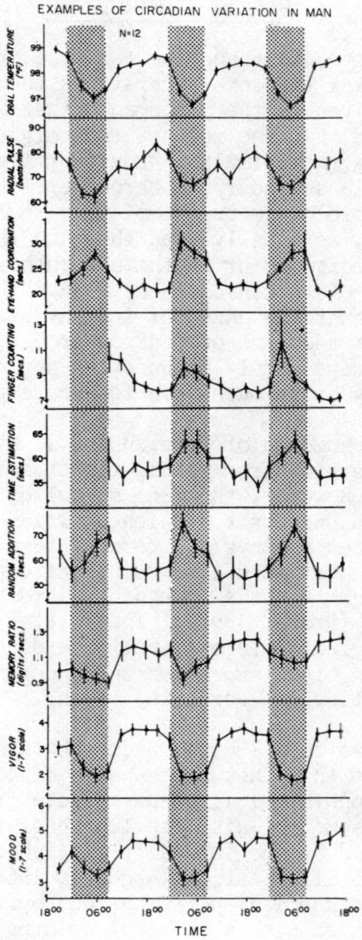

Fig. 5. Rhythmic variation in diverse variables in a group of 12 presumably healthy young men over a 72-hr period (sampled at 3-hr intervals). Note that the time of poorest performance represents the crest of the rhythm. Meal times: 0615, 1215 and 1630 hr; rest or sleep time: 2100-0600, however subjects were awakened for sampling at 2400 and 0300 hr (Scheving, 1977).

similar hours of sleep and wakefulness and similar meal times. Thus one can conclude that the dominant synchronizer of rhythms of certain frequencies, such as the circadian, in the rodent is the light-dark cycle, whereas in man the dominant synchronizer is the social cycle. We expect that the light-dark cycle also can have a strong influence, under certain circumstances, in the synchronization of even man. The point to be emphasized, however, is that if one wishes to obtain data which is likely to display a prominent group rhythm, one must pay attention to standardization and must be aware of seasonal influences.

FREERUNNING RHYTHMS

To fully understand the temporal organization of man or any other organism, it is essential that one understands the concept of freerunning. Freerunning is the name given to the phenomenon that occurs when an exogenous synchronizing force is removed. In the rodent, this might be accomplished by blinding, or simply by keeping the animals in constant light or darkness providing there was no other possible secondary synchronizer. For man, strict isolation from all time cues for a prolonged period of time would accomplish the same thing. When freerunning occurs, we usually find that any rhythmic variable measured no longer will show the precise 24-hr rhythm but rather one with a frequency that only approximates 24 hr. As a consequence, when a rhythm is monitored on successive days, one finds that the phase of the rhythm (by "phase" we mean some point on the rhythm such as the time of peak or trough, etc.) will change daily in relation to local clock time simply because the period of the rhythm is no longer precisely 24 hr (it may be as much as a few hours greater or less than 24 hr).

The phenomenon of freerunning is strong evidence that rhythms are endogenous, that is generated from within the organism, and are self-sustaining. It should be noted, however, that one school of thought, championed by F. A. Brown of Northwestern University, Chicago, Illinois, considers rhythms to be generated by subtle exogenous geophysical forces. Brown views those periods that are different from 24 hr under so-called "constant conditions" as being generated somehow from external 24-hr signals. In other words, some kind of frequency transformation is involved (Brown, 1965). This latter concept, which he describes as "autophasing", is of great interest, but time does not permit its full discussion. Perhaps in the long run, exogenous and endogenous factors both may be found to be at work in generating a freerunning rhythm.

Much has been learned about the properties of freerunning rhythms (Wever, 1974). We know that they are capable of being synchronized to periodic stimuli such as the geophysical light-dark cycle or the social cycle in the case of man. In at least some animals, the length of the period of the freerunning rhythm may be influenced by the intensity of light, providing the animals are maintained in continuous illumination (Aschoff, 1966). Freerunning rhythms are remarkably resistant to chemical perturbation; by this we mean that if an experimental animal is challenged with a chemical or drug, the frequency of a particular rhythm may remain remarkably unchanged while the amplitude of the rhythm or the over-all mean level of the variable measured may change significantly. It should be mentioned that certain chemical substances have been shown to be capable of perturbing the freerunning rhythm; among these are alcohol, valinomycin, heavy water (D_2O), and lithium (Bunning, 1973).

In summary, one can think of rhythms of being (1) generated from within; (2) innate, that is genetically determined and not learned; (3) capable of being synchronized; (4) capable of freerunning; and (5) dependent, in some cases, upon light intensity but at the same time remarkably resistant to chemical perturbation. Furthermore, when we consider rhythm behavior, we must think of four different parameters of a rhythm - its wave form, its phasing, the over-all mean level, and the wave form.

TECHNIQUES FOR ANALYZING TIME-SERIES DATA

As chronobiology developed, it became increasingly evident to some workers that classic statistical procedures, such as analysis of variance, were not adequate because they did not provide the desired quantitative numerical endpoints for the different parameters of a periodic function, such as the period length, phase or amplitude. A number of mathematical models for evaluating and quantifying time-series data have been developed. Among them was the periodogram introduced by Schuster (1900) for the detection and analysis of geophysical time series. A periodogram provides quantitative estimates for both period and amplitude of a given periodicity. It can be an appropriate means for the detection of periods of sufficiently long series with a consistant rhythm overlain by noise; but its indiscriminant use in the study of biological time series may lead to the description of spurious as well as real periods, and real periods sometimes may not be revealed. For a more detailed treatment of the computational aspects of this method and its usefulness and limitations for describing biological time-series data, see Koehler and others (1956).

Generalized harmonic or power spectral analysis also has been used for the study of periodic phenomena. Spectrum analysis is based upon the assumption of a time series representing the sum of infinite or sinusoidal functions, the so-called "harmonics" with different periods. The "variance spectrum" or so-called "power spectrum", which may be obtained by electronic computer methods, shows the contribution of different oscillations with various periods to the total variance. This method was made practical for application to the limited, noisy time series found in biological material by the development by Tukey (1949) of methods for determining the statistical reliability of spectral estimates. The variance spectrum method was adapted for use in biological time series by Halberg and Panofsky (1961) and Halberg, Panofsky and Mantis (1964). This method detects rhythms in noisy time series and evaluates their statistical significance; such may be particularly useful if a biological variable exhibits changes from several frequencies, some of which may be ill-defined. It does not, however, give any phase information on the rhythms detected, nor does it provide a numerical endpoint for the amplitude. Another shortcoming is that the technique requires sampling at regular intervals over a relatively long time span.

Because of the limitations of the above techniques, it was necessary to develop better methods of analyzing biological time-series data. One such method is the so-called "cosinor". This technique frequently is employed by chronobiologists and has been the method chosen to analyze data by several at this symposium; thus one should be familiar with the method if the data are to be fully appreciated. Originally, the cosinor method was described by Halberg, Tong and Johnson (1967), and recently some modifications were reported (Halberg and others, 1972). A brief explanation of what the cosinor is and what it does follows.

Let us assume that over a single (or several) 24-hr period we have collected data at regular intervals on a particular variable such as deep body temperature. If the animal is standardized and the data obtained appears to show a rhythm with a period of 24 hr, as is illustrated in Fig. 6, it simply would be enough to fit a 24-hr cosine curve to the sequential data by the statistical method of least squares. The cosinor program (performed readily by a computer) objectively determines the following information:

(1) a probability or P value which indicates the significance of the fit of the cosine curve to the data; if the P value is 0.05 or less, the fluctuation of the variable studied is presumed to be cyclic and not random; and
(2) three rhythmic parameters and their dispersions; these are designated as the acrophase (ϕ, ♭, Φ), mesor (M) and amplitude (A).

The acrophase represents the crest of the fitted cosine curve in relation to some arbitrarily selected reference point along the 24-hr time scale. Usually the acrophase corresponds to the time when the data values are, on the average, highest; however it should be noted that the acrophase is not necessarily identical to the time when the "peak" value is recorded. The mesor is the cosinor-determined overall 24-hr mean; this is equivalent to the 24-hr arithmetical mean only if the data points are equidistant. The amplitude is defined as one-half the total cosine

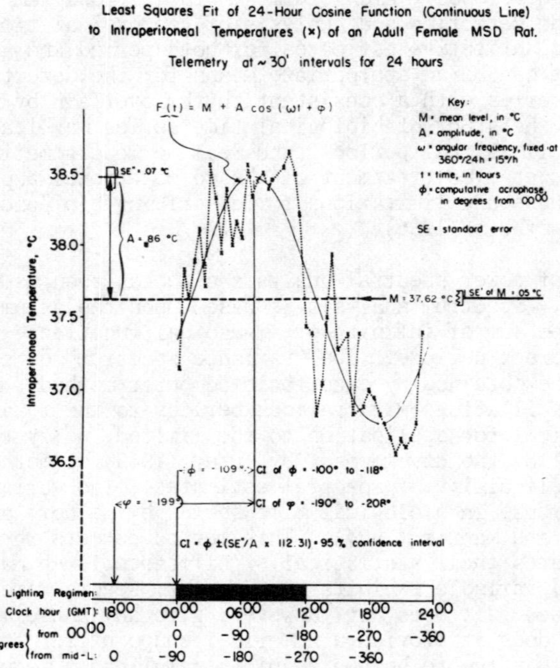

Fig. 6. Scheme of quantitative rhythm characteristics. Illustrates a circadian rhythm in deep body temperature in the rat and demonstrates a fit of a 24-hr cosine curve to the data by the least squares method. Serves to show how the mesor (mean), amplitude and acrophase are determined. (Courtesy of Halberg, Halberg and Montalbetti, 1969.)

excursion best approximating the rhythm; it represents the distance between the mesor and the crest of the cosine function used to approximate the rhythm. Both amplitude and mesor are expressed in the original units of the variable analyzed, e.g., degrees of temperature, mg/ml, etc. It is also important to know that since the amplitude value represents only one-half of the total cosine excursion, it is not necessarily equivalent to the difference between the actual peak and trough values of the raw data as plotted on a typical chronogram (the latter we refer to as the range of change).

The above description will become clear from a study of the data plotted on Fig. 6 as a chronogram. These data represent intraperitoneal temperature obtained from an adult female rat at about 30-min intervals over a single 24-hr period. Also shown on Fig. 6 is the superimposed fit of a 24-hr cosine curve to the sequential data by the method of least squares. Had there been any reason to suspect that a freerunning circadian period was involved, additional cosine periods at 10-min intervals ranging from 20 to 28 hr would have been fitted to determine which one demonstrated the best fit to the data.

In brief, the least-squares analysis and the cosinor program determine how effectively the cosine curve of a particular frequency fits the data and ascertain the degree of statistical significance. If the variable under study is characterized by a good fit to a specific frequency from one one study to another, one decides that the variable is indeed rhythmic; however, if the data do not show a good fit, they are not necessarily arhythmic. The waveform of a rhythm can take a wide variety of shapes, but in the rat and in man a great many variables fluctuate in a sinusoidal manner. In summarizing the data presented in Fig. 6, it is seen that the amplitude and SE is 0.86 ± 0.07°C, and the mesor (M) and SE is 37.62 ± 0.05°C. The designation of acrophases is somewhat more complicated as it depends upon the selection of some fixed arbitrary reference point. Local midnight frequently is used and is designated by the non-standard phi symbol, ϕ. If the midpoint of the light span on the synchronizing environmental cycle is selected as the reference, the acrophase is designated by the small Greek phi, φ. A third reference point may be located on some phase of another rhythm having the same frequency. For example, body core temperature acrophase could be the phase reference; in such an instance, the acrophase is designated by the large Greek phi, Φ. Thus one can expect to find all three symbols used to distinguish the acrophase in the literature.

In further summarizing the data of Fig. 6 relative to acrophases, note that if midnight is the selected reference point the acrophase is -109° (0000 Greenwich meridian clock time; 1800 if converted to CST) with confidence intervals extending from -100° to -118°. If the reference point selected is mid-light, the acrophase is -199° (1800 GMT) with confidence intervals extending from -190° to -208°. We have not attempted in Fig. 6 to illustrate the acrophase Φ, which would use some point such as the acrophase of some other rhythm as a reference point.

One way frequently used to portray cosinor-quantified data is on a polar coordinate system such as that seen in Fig. 7. In such a display time is usually expressed in degrees; if for this purpose 360° ≡ 24 hours, then it follows that each 15° = 1 hour. Figure 7 illustrates oral and urine temperature data collected on groups of leprosy patients at 3-hr intervals, except during their period of rest and sleep. Each point represents the mean and SE of oral temperature for the group; thus we

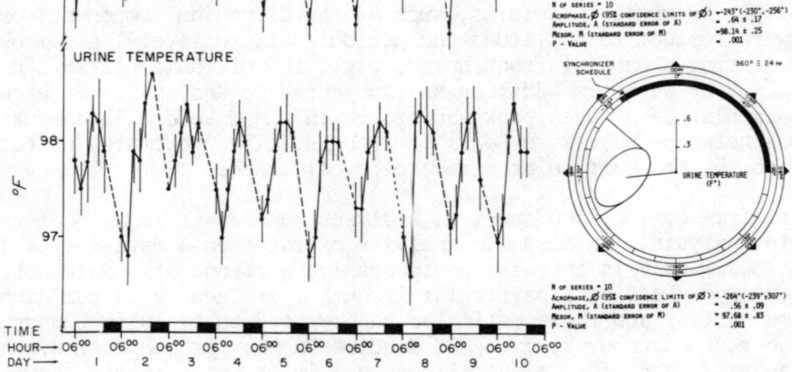

Fig. 7. Oral and urine temperatures over a 10-day span for a group of 10 patients with lepromatous leprosy. Samples were collected at 3-hr intervals. All subjects ate an identical 3 meals/day diet; sleep/rest time was from 2200-0600 hr. Also shown is polar plot of same data (Scheving and others, 1975).

speak of such as a group rhythm. In addition to the 10-day chronogram display, we also have summarized the data by cosinor analysis. A 24-hr time scale is equated to a 360° circle. The amplitude is presented as a line starting from the center and directed to the point on the periphery representing the time from midnight (the symbol ϕ informs the reader that midnight was the reference point chosen) to the computed time of the acrophase (in this case -243° or 1612 hr CST). The amplitude is $0.64 \pm 0.17^{o}C$. The mesor and SE is $98.14 \pm 0.25^{o}F$, and the fit is highly statistically significant ($P < 0.001$). Note that a 95% confidence ellipse is constructed (usually by computer) and is centered on the end of the vector. The ellipse is an expression of statistical error, computed by comparing the deviations of the actual data from the fitted mathematical curve. Lines (radii) are then drawn tangentially from the periphery to the ellipse to show the confidence arc of the acrophase. If the ellipse were to cover the center of the circle (usually called the pole), the fit would not be considered as being statistically significant. Note that the synchronizing schedule tells us that rest and sleep occurred between 2200 and 0600 hr. No sampling was performed at 1200 or 0300 hr, thus the 0600 collection time represented a 6-hr span. The cosinor summary, once understood, can be read quickly. This speaker prefers to see the data displayed as both chronogram and polar plot whenever possible. However, those knowledgeable of the polar plot presentation do not need the chronogram to properly interpret the data.

A major requirement for using the cosinor analysis is that the data being analyzed fluctuate in a sinusoidal manner. This assumption is met often, and the cosinor analysis remains a broadly useful technique. However, there are instances in which the parameters of biological rhythms are themselves dynamic. Periods, amplitudes and mean levels change as a function of endogenous and exogenous factors. The frequency structure of a biological time series may be complex, with some components representing multiple rhythms and others reflecting the waveform of the time series. To the extent that these factors are non-random, i.e., not attributable to "noise", they merit quantitative attention.

Multiple complex demodulation (MCD) provides one approach to these problems (F. W. Hegge, personal communication). MCD is accomplished by synthesizing a series of narrow digital bandpass filters ranging from 1 to 36 cycles/day in 1 cycle/day (CPD) steps. An objective amplitude criterion is applied to the output of each filter, and those frequencies whose amplitudes meet the criterion are selected for further analysis. At this juncture, a variety of options are open to the investigator. Single frequency waveforms, such as the circadian component, may be examined with respect to amplitude and period. Alternatively, a composite waveform representing a band of frequencies, e.g., the ultradian 12-20 CPD band, can be constructed by waveform addition and subjected to analysis. In each case the timing and amplitude of each peak and trough in the waveform is computed as are the periods between successive peaks or troughs. The proportion of total variance accounted for by the particular waveform is calculated.

MCD differs from cosinor and spectral analyses in that it is a local rather than an ensemble analysis. An ensemble analysis operates on a data set as a whole, whereas a local analysis operates on successive portions of a data set. Estimates of amplitude and phase at a particular frequency are generated for each data point in the time series, and these estimates can be used to evaluate the dynamic properties of the rhythms under study. MCD requires a heavier computer overhead than the cosinor analysis; and, for technical reasons, it is not suitable for short time series. Therefore, it should not be employed indiscriminantly. The indications for the use of MCD are: (1) interest in complex rhythm structures, and (2) rhythm parameter variation. In this context, MCD analysis opens new avenues of approach to the role of biological rhythms in health and disease.

FURTHER EXAMPLES OF RHYTHMS

Figure 8 represents an acrophase "map" of several variables of healthy young men. The acrophase is represented by a dot which approximates the peak of the circadian cycle in the clinically important variables measured. The horizontal bar represents the 95% confidence intervals. Non-overlapping bars roughly indicate statistically significant differences in timing. Absence of a bar indicates that the fitted 24-hr cosine curve did not describe a statistically significant fit to the data, which could mean that there was no rhythm in the data or that the waveform of any rhythm present was not sinusoidal. Note that the peaks for memory and performance tests represent the times of poorest performance. The center column in Fig. 8 gives the average 24-hr range of change for the group - that is, the percent difference between the lowest and highest recorded means (temperature range is an exception; the change is shown in °F, degrees Fahrenheit) (Kanabrocki and others, 1973, 1974).

Averaging data may be misleading simply because any of the estimated parameters may vary greatly from individual to individual; this is especially true for the amplitude and mesor. For example, the average range of change for all temperature over the 24-hr period was 2°F. For pulse, the range of change averaged 30% for the group; but the change was as great as 81% and as small as 21% for single individuals within the group. The range of change for systolic blood pressure was 15% for the group, but for the single individual it was as great as 57% and as small as 10%. Diastolic blood pressure changes for the group averaged 14%, but were as great as 78% for a single individual and as small as 13% for another. At one phase of the circadian cycle, 2 of the 13 men had blood pressure readings that might suggest at least diastolic elevation (150/108 and 148/96); the lowest readings recorded for these men were 122/68 and 120/70 respectively. One could cite similar variation among individuals for each of the 41 variables listed in Fig. 8. Figure 9 illustrates the extremes of variation in urine sodium and potassium in two individuals, and compares them to the group rhythm. All subjects consumed an identical diet (Kanabrocki and others, 1973, 1974).

It is noteworthy that a National Center for Health Statistics survey (1964) reports that, on the average, human blood pressure varies during the day by no more than 3-4 mm Hg. Although undoubtedly the statement can be made for a particular set of averaged data, the variation for individuals is artificially reduced. Such statistics can be very misleading, especially when it can be demonstrated that diastolic blood pressure in a presumably healthy resting subject can vary as much as 10 times the amount mentioned in the survey report.

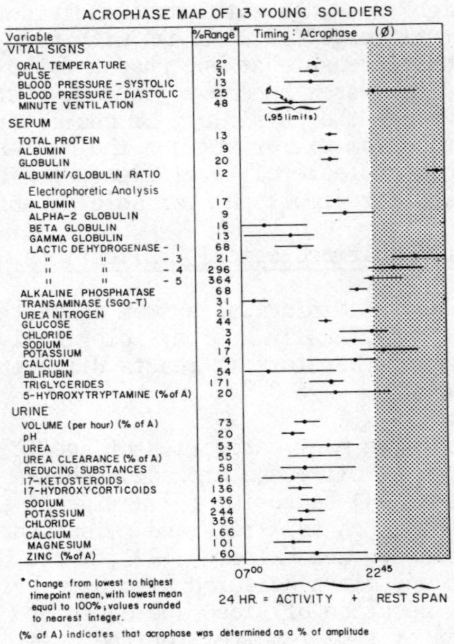

Fig. 8. Acrophase (represented by dot) approximating the peak of circadian cycle in variables measured, shown with reference to activity-rest schedule of subjects (Kanabrocki and others, 1973, 1974).

From our own studies on several different populations, including the elderly (Scheving and others, 1974b) and patients with leprosy (Scheving and others, 1975), it seems evident that individuals fall into one of three categories: (1) those having a high range of change for particular variables, (2) those having a low range of change, and (3) those (possibly the largest group) who fall in between these extremes. What, if anything, do these differences imply as far as health is concerned? It is conceivable that the amplitude of a rhythm may be important in evaluating the physiology of man. Some variables in presumably healthy individuals do indeed have so-called "unusual values" at certain time points in the circadian cycle, whereas at other times they are well within conventional, "normal" ranges. This raises such questions as: Will the younger individual who shows high blood-pressure readings (near the currently postulated limits of hypertension) only during the acrophase become hypertensive at all phases of his or her circadian cycle with increasing age? Or, are these "high" readings within the <u>individual's</u> normal range? Will a man with high intraocular pressure at one phase of the circadian system become a glaucoma victim? How does the physiology of cholesterol metabolism differ between the man who has a fluctuation of 6% daily and another whose cholesterol level fluctuates as much as 100%. Similar questions may be asked for almost any variable measured.

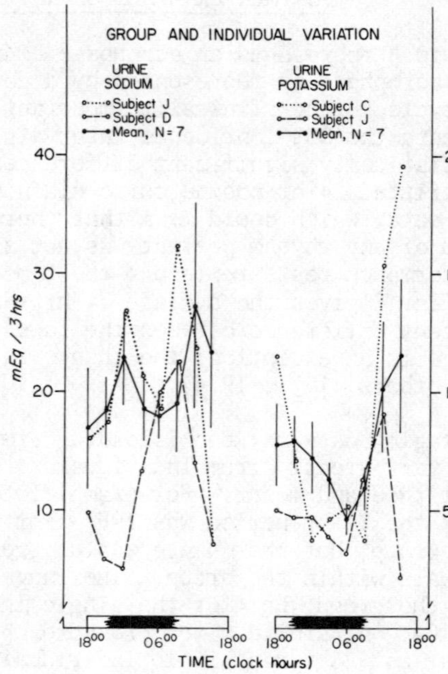

Fig. 9. Individual and group variation in urine sodium and potassium (Kanabrocki and others, 1973, 1974).

Chronopharmacological Implications

Since the biological system is rhythmically changing, it follows that the organism is biochemically and physiologically a different entity at different circadian phases; therefore it reacts differently to an identical stimulus at different times.

Among the many categories of agents reported to elicit differing responses when given at different circadian phases are: (1) carcinogens; (2) tumor cells; (3) viruses; (4) bacteria; (5) antigens, such as sheep red blood cells; (6) physical agents such as X-rays and noise; and (7) a host of poisons, chemicals and drugs (Reinberg and Halberg, 1971; Moore Ede, 1973; Scheving, Mayersbach and Pauly, 1974). The endpoints measured also have been diverse and have included: (1) mortality rate; (2) duration of sleep subsequent to a fixed dose of an anesthetic agent; (3) duration of time required for the onset of tremor subsequent to giving a drug capable of inducing them; and (4) survival time and "cure" rate subsequent to treating L1210 leukemic mice on a therapeutic protocol designed to exploit the circadian system. We and others have recently reviewed this general phenomenon in some detail (Scheving, Mayersbach and Pauly, 1974).

Three examples of such a response are illustrated in Fig. 10. It is evident that these responses vary dramatically. For example, the mean duration of sleep resulting from an identical dose of pentobarbital sodium given to different groups of rats at different times during the rat's circadian cycle averaged 91 minutes when the dose was given at one phase of the cycle and only 53 minutes when given at another time (Scheving, Vedral and Pauly, 1968a). This same figure shows that whether or not an animal survives a potentially lethal, fixed dose of amphetamine may be circadian-phase dependent; for at one phase 76.6% died and at another time only 6.6% died (Scheving, Vedral and Pauly, 1968b). The third example demonstrates that a carcinostatic drug, cytosine arabinoside (ara-C), is far more toxic at one phase of the mouse circadian system than at others (Scheving and others, 1974a).

Most of the other agents mentioned above are capable of eliciting equally dramatic circadian variation in response. Clearly the pharmacological response is circadian-phase dependent (Reinberg and Halberg, 1971; Moore Ede, 1973; Scheving, Mayersbach and Pauly, 1974). Evidence now exists which challenges any pharmacokinetic study done without the consideration of circadian variation. For example, ethanolemia studies suggest that pharmacokinetic rates and rate-constants cannot be considered a priori to be unchanging through the 24-hr period (Sturtevant and others, 1976). The possibility obviously should be investigated if pharmacokinetic results are intended to be used in calculating therapeutic doses of a drug. It may be inappropriate to administer a drug repeatedly over a 24-hr period on the basis of a single pharmacokinetic study performed at only one time of day.

The above-mentioned variation in toxicity suggests that such could have a profound effect on therapy. Halberg, a leading pioneer and major contributor to this field, has written extensively on the urgency of exploring timed treatment according to body rhythms (Halberg and others, 1973). To date, little has been done on a large scale. Among those drugs whose effectiveness has been shown to depend on the phase of the circadian system when administered are the corticosteroids. For example, Moore-Ede (1973) using oxymethalone reported that he could better manage calcium loss in his paraplegic patients by timing the administration of the drug. In this case, the drug was dramatically more effective if given just before the peak in calcium-urinary excretion; this was, as might have been predicted from Fig. 8, during the morning hours. Most clinicians accept the idea that a prime understanding of the basic circadian rhythmicity of adrenal physiology is essential to routine steroid therapy, and many symposia have been held and papers reported on this subject (Scheving, Mayersbach and Pauly, 1974). Admittedly, significant advantages have been gained, but there still exists a tremendous potential for realizing even greater benefits from timed steroid therapy. To achieve this goal, one must recognize the importance of understanding the phasing of each individual patient's steroid rhythm, or indeed if

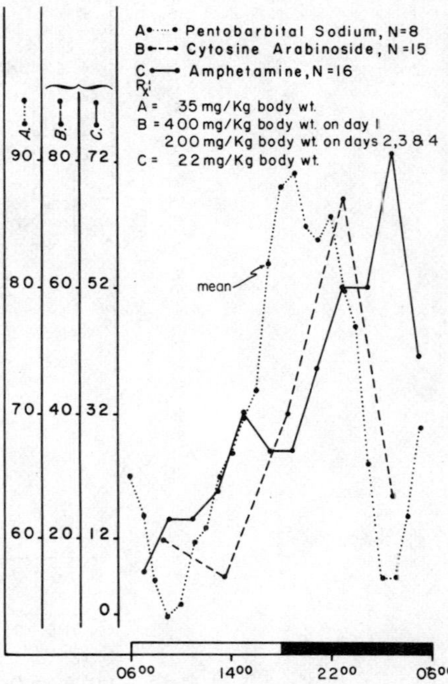

Fig. 10. Circadian variation in susceptibility of rodents to 3 drugs. For details, see Scheving, Vedral and Pauly (1968a, 1968b), and Scheving and others (1974a).

his steroids are fluctuating in a rhythmic manner.

Recently it has been demonstrated that timed treatment according to body rhythms, especially in the Lewis lung tumor (Burns, Scheving and Tsai, 1978) or mouse L1210 leukemia systems (Haus and others, 1972; Kühl and others, 1974; Scheving and others, 1977), increases survival time as well as "cure" rate. Although cancer chemotherapy might not be considered relevant to this symposium, we feel that it might be of interest to give one example of what has been accomplished in this field with the view that it might serve to stimulate attempts to design protocols for the treatment of mental illness. Thus in Fig. 11, we show the optimization of the treatment of mouse leukemia by a chronobiological approach (Scheving and others, 1977). Each mouse was injected with 1.2 x 10^6 leukemia cells 44 hr prior to the initiation of treatment. The triangles on Fig. 11 indicate that each mouse in those groups received 4 courses of cytosine arabinoside (ara-C) with a 3-day rest period between courses; each course consisted of a total of 150 mg/kg of ara-C administered in 8 injections, at 3-hour intervals over a single 24-hr span. The dosage administered at each of the 8 time points varied so that the greatest amount of the drug was administered at a time when the mouse was known to be most resistant to it, and the smallest dosage at a time when the host was known to be most resistant. In addition to the ara-C, each of these mice received 50 mg/kg of cyclophosphamide (Cyto) once per course; this is indicated by the dot within the triangle. As controls, other groups of mice received the same total amount of ara-C, but it was administered in 8 equal-dose injections; these mice, indicated by the square, also received the 50 mg/kg of cyclophosphamide.

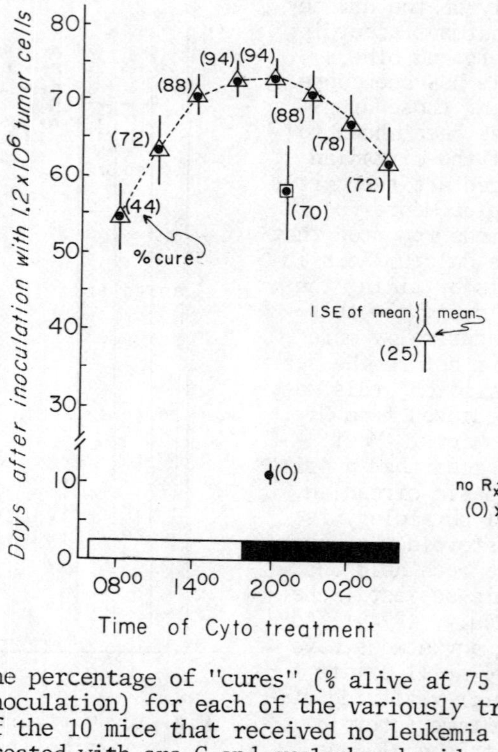

Fig. 11. The percentage of "cures" (% alive at 75 days after tumor inoculation) for each of the variously treated groups. All of the 10 mice that received no leukemia cells but were treated with ara-C and cyclophosphamide were alive at 75 days; these results were omitted from the figure. Horizontal scale, time when cyclophosphamide (Cyto) was administered (Scheving and others, 1977).

An important observation was that all groups receiving the chronobiological treatment schedule suffered only 2 deaths out of 140 animals, which may have been accidental or from acute drug toxicity. On the other hand, those animals receiving the non-chronobiological schedule suffered a mortality rate of 30% which was clearly due to drug toxicity, thus making it a non-satisfactory treatment protocol. Attempts to lower the conventional dosage of either or both drugs to avoid the 30% toxicity resulted in a large number of animals dying from leukemia. Thus the data clearly indicate that there is a right and a wrong chronobiological time to administer the drug. All animals receiving no treatment died within 7.1 ± 0.4 days; those receiving ara-C alone (open triangle) had a mean survival time of 28.2 ± 0.6 days; and those receiving cyclophosphamide alone (solid circle) had a mean survival time of 11 ± 0.8 days.

We and others have been exploring rhythms in various organs in both tumor-bearing and normal animals. High-amplitude circadian rhythms have been reported for the DNA synthesis of liver, bone marrow, gut, thymus and spleen of normal rodents; the presence of a tumor may dramatically alter the rhythm. Also these studies have led to the initiation of limited studies currently underway to apply this information to the treatment of cancer in humans. The task will not be easy because of logistical and technical problems, but the benefits may make such an endeavor very worthwhile.

Certain drugs have been known to phase-shift rhythms (Scheving and others, 1976). The degree and direction of phase shifting depends on when the drug is given. For example, if ara-C is given at 0900 hr (when the mitotic index is high), no effect is seen on the subsequent mitotic cycle. If, however, the drug is given at the time of minimum mitotic activity, the next day the expected peak at 0900 hr is delayed for several hours (Fig. 12). Recently it was demonstrated that the rhythm in

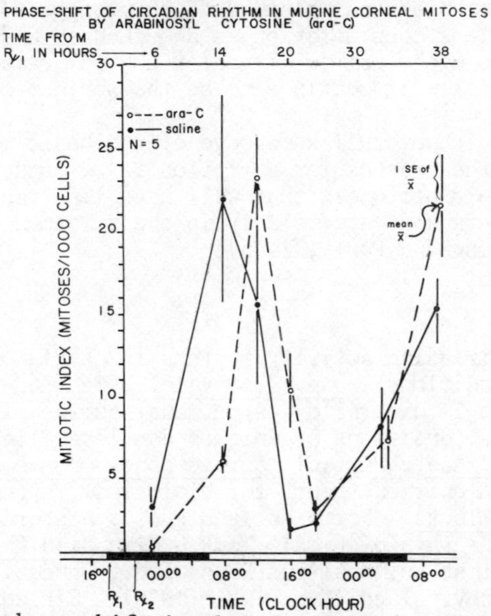

Fig. 12. A 4- or 5-hr phase-shift in the mitotic index rhythm of mouse corneal epithelium was observed when arabinosyl cytosine (ara-C) was injected during a phase of the mouse circadian system when the synthesis of DNA probably is minimal. Although not shown here, there was no such phase-shift when the drug was administered at a time when one would have expected a substantially higher rate of DNA synthesis or at the peak time of the mitotic-index rhythms (Scheving and others, 1976).

body temperature of the mouse could be delayed if theophylline or pentobarbital were given just before the daily rise in temperature. On the other hand, the rhythm is set ahead (advanced) if theophylline is given just after the daily high in temperature; but pentobarbital does not advance the rhythm (Ehret, Potter and Dobra, 1975). Thus, drugs can be thought of a chronobiotics and may be used to alter the biological time structure by rephasing the circadian rhythm - this too may be exploited in chemotherapy as well as radiotherapy.

Mechanism

After reviewing a number of the investigations designed to explore the mechanisms of rhythmic responses to drugs and toxic materials, we conclude that they have raised many cogent questions; but a discussion of this problem is beyond the scope of this talk. The subject has been treated more in detail elsewhere (Scheving, Mayersbach and Pauly, 1974). In general, such studies caution against generalizing about causative mechanisms of chronopharmacological variation. It seems clear that one cannot ascribe circadian variation and response to drugs as a simple reflection of the underlying circadian variation in hepatic drug-metabolizing enaymes or microsomal biotransformation enzymes; the enzyme or enzyme system of the target organ also may be rhythmic and must be considered (Scheving, Mayersbach and Pauly, 1974).

Many attempts have been made on mammals to elucidate the mechanism of rhythmicity. Among these were studies employing the classical endocrinologic approaches of adrenalectomy, hypophysectomy, cerebral ablation, pinealectomy, and more recently ablation of a suprachiasmatic nucleus. In spite of these studies and others, no single regulator has been found to account for the control of all rhythmic variables. Halberg and others (1951) have shown that certain aspects of 24-hr periodicity are controlled by the adrenal gland; and they suggest that the adrenal cortical cycle deserves serious consideration as a mechanism underlying adaptation to the daily routine. The mechanism of circadian control remains an important and fundamental question that will continue to be the subject of intense research.

It is hoped that even without full knowledge of the basic mechanisms of molecular control of rhythms or the reasons for variation in response to drugs, data can be produced by rather simple protocols that will have important practical applications in clinical matters and particularly in the treatment of mental disease (Scheving, 1976; Scheving and Pauly, 1976).

REFERENCES

Aschoff, J. (1966). Circadian activity rhythms in chaffinches (Fringella coelebs) under constant conditions. Jap. J. Physiol., 16, 363-370.

Bernard, C. (1865). De la diversité des animaus soumis a l'experimentation. De la variabilité des conditions organiques dan lesquelles ils s'offrent a l'experimentateur. J. Anat. Physiol. Norm. Pathol. Homme Anim., 2, 497-506.

Brown, F. A. (1965). A unified theory for biological rhythms. In J. Aschoff (Ed.), Circadian Clocks. North Holland Publ., Amsterdam. pp. 231-261.

Bünning, E. (1973). The Physiological Clock - Circadian Rhythms and Biological Chronometry. English Universities Press Ltd., London. p. 152.

Burns, E. R., L. E. Scheving and T. H. Tsai (1978). Circadian rhythms in DNA synthesis and mitosis in normal mice and in mice bearing the Lewis lung carcinoma. Europ. J. Cancer, (in press).

Ehret, C. F., L. R. Potter and K. W. Dobra (1975). Chronotypic action of theophylline and of pentobarbital as circadian zeitgebers in the rat. Science, 188, 1212-1215.

Halberg, F., and H. Panofsky (1961). II. Thermo-variance spectra; simplified computational example and other methodology. Exp. Med. Surg., 19, 284-309.

Halberg, F., E. Halberg and H. Montalbetti. (1969). Premesse e sviluppi della cronofarmacologia. Quadeini di Medicina Quantitativa, 7, 7-54.

Halberg, F., H. Panofsky and H. Mantis (1964). Human thermo-variance spectra. Ann. N.Y. Acad. Sci., 117, 254-270.

Halberg, F., Y. L. Tong and E. A. Johnson (1967). Circadian-system phase - an aspect of temporal morphology. In H. v. Mayersbach (Ed.), The Cellular Aspects of Biorhythms. Springer-Verlag, Berlin. pp. 20-48.

Halberg, F., M. B. Visscher, E. B. Flisch, K. Berge and F. Boch (1951). Diurnal rhythmic changes in blood eosinophil levels in health and in certain diseases. Lancet, 71, 312-319.

Halberg, F., E. A. Johnson, W. Nelson, W. Runge and R. Sothern (1972). Autorhythmometry procedures for physiological self-measurements and their analysis. Physiol. Teacher, 1, 1-11.

Halberg, F., E. Haus, S. S. Cardoso, L. E. Scheving, J. F. W. Kühl, R. N. Shiotsuka, G. Rosene, J. E. Pauly, W. Runge, J. F. Spalding, J. K. Lee and R. A. Good (1973). Toward a chronotherapy of neoplasia: tolerance of treatment depends upon host rhythms. Experientia, 29, 909-934.

Halberg, F., F. Carandente, G. Cornelissen and G. S. Katinas (1977). Glossary of chronobiology. Chronobiologia, 4, Suppl. 1, p. 7.

Haus, E., F. Halberg, L. E. Scheving, S. S. Cardoso, J. F. W. Kuhl, R. Sothern, R. N. Shiotsuka, D. S. Hwang and J. E. Pauly (1972). Increased tolerance of leukemic mice to arabinosyl cytosine with schedule adjusted to circadian system. Science, 177, 80-82.

Kanabrocki, E. L., L. E. Scheving, F. Halberg, R. L. Brewer and T. J. Bird (1973). Circadian variation in presumably healthy men under conditions of peace-time army reserve training. Space Life Sci., 4, 258-270.

Kanabrocki, E. L., L. E. Scheving, F. Halberg, R. L. Brewer and T. J. Bird (1974). Circadian Variation in Presumably Healthy Young Soldiers. Natl. Tech. Inf. Service, U.S. Dept. Commerce Doc. #PB228487, 56 pp.

Koehler, F., F. K. Okano, L. R. Elbeback, F. Halberg and J. J. Bittner (1956). Periodograms for study of physiological daily periodicity in mice and man. Exp. Med. Surg., 14, 5-30.

Kühl, J. F. W., E. Haus, F. Halberg, L. E. Scheving, J. E. Pauly, S. S. Cardoso and G. Rosene (1974). Experimental chronotherapy with ara-C; comparison of murine ara-C tolerance on differently timed treatment schedules. Chronobiologia, 1, 316-317.

Mayersbach, H. v. (1967). Seasonal influences on biological rhythms of standardized laboratory animals. In H. v. Mayersbach (Ed.), The Cellular Aspects of Biorhythms. Springer-Verlag, Berlin. pp. 87-99.

Moore Ede, M. C. (1973). Circadian rhythms of drug effectiveness and toxicity. Clin. Pharmacol. Thera., 14, 925-935.

National Center for Health Statistics, Division of Health Examinations Statistics (1964). Blood Pressure of Adults by Race and Area, United States, 1960-1962. U.S. Dept. Health, Education & Welfare, U.S. Govt. Printing Office, Washington, D.C.

Pauly, J. E., L. E. Scheving, E. R. Burns, J. Landon and J. E. Stone (1977). Studies of the circadian system in blind human beings. In XII International Conference Proceedings (Internat. Soc. Chronobiology). The Publishing House "Il Ponte", Milano, Italy. pp. 19-28.

Quay, W. B. (1963). Circadian rhythm in rat pineal serotonin and its modifications by estrous cycle and photoperiod. Gen. Comp. Endocrinology, 3, 473-479.

Reinberg, A., and F. Halberg (1971). Circadian pharmacology. Ann. Rev. Pharmacol., 2, 455-492.

Scheving, L. E. (1974). Chronobiology. In L. E. Scheving, F. Halberg and J. E. Pauly (Eds.), Chronobiology. Igaku Shoin Ltd., Tokyo. pp. 221-223.

Scheving, L. E. (1976). The dimension of time in biology and medicine - chronobiology. Endeavour, 35, 66-72.

Scheving, L. E. (1977). Temporal variation in man. In G. Lassman and F. Seitelberger (Eds.), Rhythmische Functionen in Biologischen Systemen. Facultas-Verlag, Vienna, pp. 49-74.

Scheving, L. E., and J. Dunn (1974). The cyclic nature of prolactin in mammals. In J. Aschoff, F. Ceresa and F. Halberg (Eds.), Chronobiologiaal Aspects of Endocrinology. Symposia Medica Hoechst, Vol. 9. Schattauer Verlag, Stuttgart. pp. 193-201.

Scheving, L. E., and J. E. Pauly (1974). Circadian rhythms: some examples and comments on clinical application. Chronobiologia, 1, 3-21.

Scheving, L. E., and J. E. Pauly (1976). Chronopharmacology - its implication for clinical medicine. In F. H. Clarke (Ed.), Annual Reports in Medicinal Chemistry, Vol. 11. Academic Press, New York. pp. 251-260.

Scheving, L. E., H. v. Mayersbach and J. E. Pauly (1974). An overview of chronopharmacology (a general review). J. Europeen Toxicol., 7, 203-227.

Scheving, L. E., D. F. Vedral and J. E. Pauly (1968a). A circadian susceptibility rhythm in rats to pentobarbital sodium. Anat. Rec., 160, 741-750.

Scheving, L. E., D. F. Vedral and J. E. Pauly (1968b). Daily circadian rhythm in rats to D-amphetamine sulfate: effect of blinding and continuous illumination on the rhythm. Nature, 219, 621-622.

Scheving, L. E., W. H. Harrison, P. Gordon and J. E. Pauly (1968). Daily fluctuation (circadian and ultradian) in the biogenic amines of the rat brain. Am. J. Physiol., 214, 166-173.

Scheving, L. E., S. S. Cardoso, J. E. Pauly, F. Halberg and E. Haus (1974a). Variation in susceptibility of mice to the carcinostatic agent arabinosyl cytosine. In L. E. Scheving, F. Halberg and J. E. Pauly (Eds.), Chronobiology. Igaku Shoin Ltd., Tokyo, pp. 213-217.

Scheving, L. E., C. Roig III, F. Halberg, J. E. Pauly and E. A. Hand (1974b). Circadian variations in residents of a "senior citizen's" home. In L. E. Scheving, F. Halberg and J. E. Pauly (Eds.), Chronobiology. Igaku Shoin Ltd., Tokyo. pp. 353-357.

Scheving, L. E., C. D. Enna, F. Halberg, R. R. Jacobson, A. Mather and J. E. Pauly (1975). Mean circadian cosinors of vital signs, performance, and of blood and urinary constituents in patients with leprosy. Internat. J. Leprosy, 43, 364-377.

Scheving, L. E., E. L. Kanaborcki, R. L. Brewer, T. J. Bird and J. E. Pauly (1976). Chronobiology and how it might apply to the problems of shift work. In P. G. Rentos and R. D. Shepard (Eds.), Shift Work and Health. HEW Publ. No. (NIOSH) 76-203. pp. 118-139.

Scheving, L. E., E. R. Burns, J. E. Pauly, F. Halberg and E. Haus (1977). Survival and cure of leukemic mice after optimization of treatment with cyclophosphamide and arabinosyl cytosine. Cancer Res., 37, 3648-3655.

Schuster, A. (1900). The periodogram of magnetic declination as obtained from the records of the Greenwich Observatory during the years 1871-1895. Trans. Cambridge Phil. Soc., 18, 107-135.

Sturtevant, F. M., R. P. Sturtevant, L. E. Scheving and J. E. Pauly (1976). Chronopharmacokinetics of ethanol. II. Circadian rhythm in rate of blood level decline in a single subject. Naunyn-Schmiedeberg's Arch. Pharmacol., 293, 203-208.

Tukey, J. W. (1949). The sampling theory of power spectrum estimates. In Proceedings of Symposium on Applications of Autocorrelation Analysis to Physical Problems, Woods Hole, MA. Office of Naval Research, Washington, D.C. pp. 46-67.

Wever, R. (1974). Different aspects of human circadian rhythms under the influence of weak electric fields. In L. E. Scheving, F. Halberg and J. E. Pauly (Eds.), Chronobiology. Igaku Shoin Ltd., Tokyo. pp. 694-699.

Acknowledgement: To Lederle Laboratories, American Cyanamid Company, Pearl River, NY, for travel support; and to Grant CA-14388 from National Cancer Institute.

Circadian Susceptibility Rhythm to Neuroleptics

HARUO NAGAYAMA, AKINORI TAKAGI, KENZABURO NISHIWAKI and RYO TAKAHASHI

Department of Neuropsychiatry, Nagasaki, University School of Medicine, Nagasaki, Japan

ABSTRACT

Experiments were carried out to study the differences in the effect of neuroleptics due to time of administration. Rats were administered chlorpromazine or haloperidol in a variety of combinations of dose and time and the sedation period was measured. Circadian fluctuation of sedative effect was observed in both the drugs. In order to elucidate the mechanism of these phenomena in two different experiments, one of the drugs, chlorpromazine or haloperidol was administered at two different times respectively, between which times there was a significant difference in the sedation period, and time-course changes of the drugs in plasma and brain concentration were followed. No difference was found between the two times of administration. In addition, it was found that there is circadian fluctuation in the anti-apomorphine effect of haloperidol. Those results are interpreted as indicating that the circadian fluctuation of sedative effect of haloperidol might be caused by the circadian fluctuation of sensitivity in the brain dopamine receptors.

Keywords : Circadian rhythm – Chronopharmacology – Chlorpromazine – Haloperidol – Sedation – Anti-apomorphine effect – Dopamine receptor

INTRODUCTION

It has been becoming clear that there exists circadian fluctuation in susceptibility to many kinds of drug (Reinberg, 1973).
The studies on such phenomenon as circadian fluctuation of effect of drugs are of great importance. First, they point out the importance of the time of administration in experiments and clinical treatments. Secondly, they may serve as a useful means for the clarification of the action mechanism of drug. Thirdly, if a biological "clock" does actually exist, they will be a useful means for studying its essential nature. In previous papers we reported that there is a circadian fluctuation in the effect of tetrabenazine, and that the circadian fluctuation of brain amine is involved with the onset mechanism of that phenomenon (Nagayama and others, 1974,1977).

In order to further the study, the circadian fluctuation of the effect of chlorpromazine and haloperidol was investigated.

MATERIALS AND METHODS

Male Sprague-Dawley rats weighing 300-400g were used. They were kept in a quiet dark room under controlled lighting conditions with a daily period of artificial light from 19:30 to 7:30 and darkness for the other 12 hours. The temperature of the animal house was maintained at 24-26°C. The animals were kept in the animal house for at least 5 weeks before experimentation began. Each rat was used only once in the experiment.

Circadian Fluctuation of Sedation Period

Each rat was placed in a sound-proof box and its behavior monitored with an Animex-DS apparatus. The temperature and lighting of the experimental box were the same as those of the animal house. Subjects were always placed in the experimental box at 16:30, and the next 27 to 48 hours was used to accustom the rat to the box. After this time chlorpromazine or haloperidol was administered i.p. Sedation appeared with 10-20 min after the administration of the drug. The sedation period was defined as the time from the onset of sedation to the time when a record of 90 counts/10 min was attained from the Animex-DS apparatus. The dosage of drugs was 1.2-40 mg/kg in chlorpromazine and 0.5-16 mg/kg in haloperidol. The times of administration were 7:30, 13:30, 19:30 and 1:30.

Changes of Level of Chlorpromazine and Haloperidol in the Plasma and Brain in the Course of Time

Either chlorpromazine or haloperidol was administered i.p. at different times to follow the time-course changes of the drug in their plasma and brain concentration. Administration was made at the two different times between which a significant difference in sedative effect was noted. The dosage of drugs was 10 mg/kg in chlorpromazine and 2 mg/kg in haloperidol.

Circadian Fluctuation of Anti-apomorphine Effect of Haloperidol

Haloperidol, 0.12-1.0 mg/kg, was administered i.p. at each of the times in a day, i.e. 7:30, 13:30, 19:30 and 1:30, and apomorphine, a dopamine agonist, was administered subcutaneously at the dose of 5 mg/kg 1 hour after the administration of haloperidol. After the administration of apomorphine, time duration of apomorphine-induced stereotyped behavior (AISB) were measured. The control group was given physiological saline instead of haloperidol.

RESULTS

Circadian Fluctuation of Sedation Period

The results are shown in Tables 1 and 2. It was found in both of the drugs that there is a circadian fluctuation in the sedative effect and that the pattern of the fluctuation differes depending on dosage. But the patterns of the circadian fluctuation curve were different in the two drugs. In chlorpromazine the crest of sedative effect moved gradually and smoothly, in accordance with an increase in dose of administration, from 1:30 (1.2 mg/kg), 19:30, and 13:30 to 7:30 (40 mg/kg). On the other hand, in haloperidol the crest in cases of small doses (0.5-1.0 mg/kg) and large doses (2-16 mg/kg) were at 19:30 and at 13:30, respectively.

TABLE 1 Sedation Period by Time and Dose of Chlorpromazine Administration

Time \ Dose	1.2	2.5	5	10	20	40 mg/kg
7:30		233±59*	260±36*	570±113*	1333±85	1713±114
13:30		223±29*	240±47*	1253±101	1090±25	
19:30	90±50	370±176	546±167	930±124	1050±35*	
1:30	166±86	700±151	713±144	773±17**		

Figures indicate mean ± S.E. (min)
Significant difference from the maximum value by dose (Student's t-test) * $P < 0.05$, ** $P < 0.01$
Each group consisted of 3 rats

TABLE 2 Sedation Period by Time and Dose of Haloperidol Administration

Time \ Dose	0.5	1	2	4	8	16 mg/kg
7:30	310±83	470±24*	487±54**	605±42**	865±32**	887±110
13:30	265±66	382±51*	890±42	982±31	1102±17	1117±70
19:30	465±79	665±62	840±58	912±19	960±67	
1:30	325±31	587±42	770±54	802±48*	795±50**	

Figures indicate mean ± S.E. (min)
Significant difference from the maximum value by dose (Student's t-test) * $P < 0.05$, ** $P < 0.001$
Each group consisted of 4 rats

Changes of Level of Chlorpromazine and Haloperidol in the Plasma and Brain in the Course of Time

There was no significant difference in the rise and fall of plasma level or brain concentration of either drug between any two time points of administration.

Circadian Fluctuation of Anti-apomorphine Effect of Haloperidol

The administration of haloperidol 1 hour before the administration of apomorphine was found to shorten the duration of AISB in a manner dependent on the dose of haloperidol. Inhibition percentage of AISB were obtained by taking the ratio of duration periods obtained at various times of administration and with various doses of haloperidol. The inhibition percentage was significantly different depending on the time of day of administration, regardless of the dose of the drug. The largest drug effect was observed after the administration at 19:30, followed by those at 1:30 and 7:30 in this order, then the smallest effect being observed with the administration at 13:30.

DISCUSSION

It was found that there is a circadian fluctuation in the sedative effect of chlorpromazine and haloperidol. What mechanism underlies the occurence of this phenomenon ? At the two different hours at which their sedative effects show significant differences, there is no difference in changes of the levels of drugs in the plasma and brain. Accordingly, the phenomenon can not be explained by the level of absorption, metabolism, excretion, and distribution of the drugs. It is reasonable to assume that the circadian fluctuation of the sedative effect may have been induced by the circadian fluctuation in the drug susceptibility of the acting site of the drugs. It is widely known that these drugs exert their action by blocking brain catecholamine receptors (Andén and others, 1970). Apomorphine, on the other hand, is supposed to stimulate the dopamine receptors directly (Andén and others, 1967; Ernst, 1967; Kehr and others, 1972; Lahti, McAllister, and Wozniak, 1972; Nybäck, Schubert, and Sedvall, 1970; Roos, 1969). The presence of the circadian fluctuation in the anti-apomorphine action of haloperidol was demonstrated in this study. This is considered to indicate the existence of the circadian fluctuation in the blocking activity of haloperidol to brain dopamine receptors. In addition, the pattern of the circadian fluctuation curve of anti-apomorphine action agreed with the pattern of the circadian fluctuation curve of sedative effect of haloperidol with small doses. In conclusion, the circadian fluctuation of the sedative effect of haloperidol in small doses might be caused by the circadian fluctuation in the blockage of brain dopamine receptors by this drug.

There might, however, be several questions about this conclusion.

Why is the pattern of circadian fluctuation of sedative effect with large doses of haloperidol different from that with small doses ? The following explanation seems to be valid in this connection. In the case of the administration of small doses, the circadian fluctuation is assumed to have been induced by the circadian fluctuation of affinity of brain dopamine receptors. On the other hand, in the case of the administration of large doses, the circadian fluctuation in the maximum response is assumed to have been induced by the circadian fluctuation in the number of binding sites of these receptors.

Is the same explanation applicable to chlorpromazine ? For this question it is required to study the circadian fluctuation of anti-apomorphine action of the drug and the possibility of a circadian fluctuation in the action of the drug on the brain norepinephrine receptors.

REFERENCES

Andén,N.-E., Rubenson,A., Fuxe,K., and Hökfelt,T.(1967). Evidence for dopamine receptor stimulation by apomorphine. J.Pharm.Pharmacol., 19, 627-629.

Andén,N.-E., Butcher,S.G., Corrodi,H., Fuxe,K., and Ungerstedt,V. (1970). Receptor activity and turnover of dopamine and noradrenaline after neuroleptics. Eur.J.Pharmacol., 11, 303-314.

Ernst,A.M.(1967). Mode of action of apomorphine and dexamphetamine on gnawing compulsion in rats. Psychopharmacologia, 10, 316-323.

Kehr,W., Carlsson,A., Lindqvist,M., Magnusson,J., and Atack,C.(1972). Evidence for a receptor-mediated feedback control of striatal tyrosine hydroxylase activity. J.Pharm.Pharmacol., 24, 744-747.

Lahti,R.A., McAllister,B., and Wozniak,J.(1972). Apomorphine antagonist of the elevation of homovanillic acid induced by antipsychotic drugs. Life Sci., 11, 605-613.

Nagayama,H., Takagi,A., Tateishi,T., and Takahashi,R.(1974). Studies on diurnal fluctuation of sedative effect of tetrabenazine. Jap.J.Pharmacol., 24, 112.

Nagayama,H., Takagi,A., Tateishi,T., and Takahashi,R.(1977). Circadian susceptibility rhythm to neuroleptics : tetrabenazine. Psychopharmacology, 55, 61-66.

Nybäck,H., Schubert,J., and Sedvall,G.(1970). Effect of apomorphine and pimozine on synthesis and turnover of labelled catecholamine in mouse brain. J.Pharm.Pharmacol., 22, 622-624.

Reinberg,A.(1973). Chronopharmacology. In J.N.Mills (Ed.), Biochemical aspects of circadian rhythms, Plenum Press, London. pp.121-152.

Roos,B.-E.(1969). Decrease in homovanillic acid as evidence for dopamine receptor stimulation by apomorphine in the neostriatum of the rat. J.Pharm.Pharmacol., 21, 263-264.

Behavioural Effects of Indoleamine and Catecholamine Precursors

Transmitter Precursor Loading - Uses and Limitations

G. CURZON

Department of Neurochemistry, Institute of Neurology, 33 John's Mews, London WC1N 2NS, England

ABSTRACT

Certain precursor amino acids can cause increased synthesis of their major indoleamine or catecholamine transmitter products at physiological sites of occurrence. When the hydroxylated precursors (5-hydroxytryptophan and dopa) are used synthesis can also occur at non-physiological sites and may lead to displacement of other transmitters from them. Furthermore, administration of non-hydroxylated precursors can raise levels of so-called trace amines, especially after MAOI treatment. Behavioural experiments suggest that these effects and also extracerebral metabolic changes must be considered when interpreting the behavioural consequences of precursor amino acid treatment.

KEYWORDS

Tryptophan, 5-hydroxytryptophan, tyrosine, dopa, 5-hydroxytryptamine, tryptamine, dopamine, noradrenaline, monoamineoxidase inhibitors, behaviour.

INTRODUCTION

Increasing transmitter synthesis by giving precursors has obvious attractions in that the kind of argument often used by protagonists of herbal and other natural remedies seems to be applicable i.e. that because life has survived ages of exposure to these substances we have guarantees of their safety that do not exist for synthetic drugs of recent origin. While such arguments are not without foundation, giving transmitter precursors may well lead to levels of precursors being raised to a quite non-physiological extent or to the presence of precursors or their products in compartments to which they normally do not gain access. Therefore it is as well to consider the effects of these substances critically when discussing their biochemical and behavioural effects. A number of questions pose themselves: e.g. Is transmitter synthesis increased in the brain? At other sites of normal occurrence? At non-physiological sites? Are there behavioural consequences? Do these depend on the previous state of neuronal systems normally containing the transmitter? Are there other biochemical effects which might influence behaviour?

EFFECT OF AMINO ACID PRECURSORS ON TRANSMITTER SYNTHESIS

Many workers have shown that in the rat, tryptophan hydroxylase, the rate-limiting enzyme for synthesis of 5-hydroxytryptamine (5HT) is normally not saturated with tryptophan so that giving the latter leads to increased brain concentrations of either 5HT itself or its metabolite 5-hydroxyindoleacetic acid (5HIAA) (Eccleston, Ashcroft and Crawford, 1965). Evidence in man is of necessity less direct e.g. the increase of 5HIAA in CSF after giving tryptophan (Eccleston and co-workers, 1970).

Professor Carlsson will present new evidence on the degree of saturation in the rat brain of tyrosine hydroxylase, the limiting enzyme for dopamine synthesis. However, in man while CSF studies point to increasing brain tryptophan altering 5HT turnover they fail to show that parallel tyrosine changes affect dopamine turnover. Thus, ventricular fluids from psychiatric patients without precursor loading showed a highly significant correlation between tryptophan and 5HIAA concentrations but not between tyrosine and HVA concentrations (Curzon and co-workers, 1976).

Limitation of transmitter synthesis at the hydroxylation stage no longer occurs when 5-hydroxytryptophan (5HTP) or dopa (the products of hydroxylation of tryptophan or tyrosine) are used as precursors. However,(as described below,) the location of transmitter synthesis varies according to whether the initial or hydroxylated amino acid precursors are used.

Tryptophan can be converted to brain 5HT only in 5HT containing neurones because brain tryptophan hydroxylase is present only at these sites. Similarily, tyrosine can be converted to catecholamines only in catecholamine containing neurones because brain tyrosine hydroxylase is present only at these sites. However, aromatic amino acid decarboxylase occurs in 5HT, dopamine (DA) and noradrenaline (NA) neurones (Christensen, Dairman and Udenfriend, 1972; Hokfelt, Fuxe and Goldstein, 1973) and also in brain capillaries (Bartholini, Tissot and Pletscher, 1971) and therefore the hydroxylated precursors can be decarboxylated to the corresponding amines at non-physiological as well as at physiological sites (Yunger and Harvey, 1976).

OTHER BIOCHEMICAL EFFECTS OF TRANSMITTER PRECURSORS OF POSSIBLE CNS IMPORTANCE

Not only the synthesis of major transmitter products may occur as a result of giving precursors but also other biochemical effects which may be relevant to behaviour. Firstly, possible interference by these amino acids with access to the brain of other amino acids of the same transport class should be mentioned and Professor Carlsson will be giving some new findings on this question - an important issue because both tryptophan and tyrosine are transported to the brain by a common mechanism. However, Smith and co-workers (1977) report that quite large doses of tryptophan did not affect rat brain DA or NA levels and that similar doses of tyrosine did not affect 5HT. (Tyrosine did not alter DA concentration significantly though small NA changes did occur.)

5HTP and dopa however interfere more seriously with transmitter metabolism probably largely because of their decarboxylation at various neuronal sites and the resultant displacement of transmitters from these sites. Thus, L-dopa + a peripheral decarboxylase inhibitor caused catecholamine to accumulate not only in DA but also in 5HT neurones and depleted 5HT from these neurones (Butcher, Engel and Fuxe, 1972). Similar treatment with DL-5HTP led to 5HT accumulating not only in 5HT neurones but also in DA and NA neurones and the depletion of these catecholamines. Work on rhesus monkeys suggests there may be considerable regional differences in the degree of depletion (Tsukada, Kishimoto and Nagai, 1975).

Another relevant effect of giving transmitter precursors is to increase synthesis of so-called trace amines normally present in the brain at very much lower concentrations than 5HT and the catecholamines. Unlike the major transmitter amines which normally can only be made within specific neuronal systems, the trace amines formed by decarboxylation can be made at any site containing aromatic amino acid decarboxylase though the subsequent side chain hydroxylation of phenylethylamines by dopamine β-hydroxylase is specific to NA neurones.

When tryptophan alone (up to 200 mg/kg i.p.) was given then brain 5HT rose considerably but the concentration of the trace amine tryptamine hardly altered, presumably because of its rapid turnover. [Higher tryptophan dosage (400 mg/kg) however does moderately increase brain tryptamine (Saavedra and Axelrod, 1973).] When tryptophan was given to rats pretreated with the MAOI pargyline then tryptamine rose to a proportionately much greater extent than 5HT though absolute concentrations were not as high (Marsden and Curzon, 1974). Qualitatively comparable results are reported by Tabakoff and co-workers (1977) although the mass spectral tryptamine method used gave much lower values than the radiochemical assay (Saavedra and Axelrod, 1973) used in our own work.

As might be predicted from the wide distribution of the aromatic amino acid decarboxylase required for synthesis of tryptamine from tryptophan this appears to take place not only in 5HT neurones but also in DA neurones. Synthesis of brain tryptamine in 5HT neurones is indicated by raphe lesions leading to parallel falls of both 5HT and tryptamine though results suggest that total destruction of the 5HT neuronal system does not completely deplete the brain of tryptamine. At least part of this tryptamine may be in DA neurones because when these were partly destroyed by intraventricular 6-hydroxydopamine then not only did DA fall but also tryptamine. Furthermore, extracerebral tryptamine (unlike 5HT or the catecholamines) appears to have relatively easy access to the brain as when peripheral decarboxylase was inhibited by RO4-4602 the rise of tryptamine in the brain after giving tryptophan to tranylcypromine treated rats was diminished (Marsden and Curzon, 1978).

The effects of tyrosine and phenylalanine on trace amine synthesis largely parallels that of tryptophan i.e. tyrosine increases brain octopamine (Harmar and Horn, 1976) and phenylalanine increases both octopamine (Harmar and Horn, 1976) and phenylethylamine (Saavedra, 1974) even without MAOI treatment though enormously higher levels are attained in the latter circumstances.

BEHAVIOURAL EFFECTS OF TRANSMITTER LOADING

Despite the above metabolic pathways, increased formation of major transmitter products at normal sites of synthesis in the brain is obviously the first mechanism to be considered for the behavioural effects of precursors. The occurrence of these effects either specifically or more strikingly in subjects with a pre-existing deficiency of the transmitter products is consistent with such mechanisms. Thus Dr Coppen's evidence that tryptophan is an anti-depressant may be linked with evidence for a pre-existing brain 5HT deficiency in depression while our own results on the behavioural effect of L-tryptophan in 5HT deficient rats (Marsden and Curzon, 1976) may be similarily explained. Also, despite much discussion and research activity the most generally accepted mechanism of action of L-dopa in Parkinson's disease still involves replacement of brain dopamine. Furthermore, the work Dr Engel will describe on the normalisation by L-dopa of the behaviour of catecholamine deficient animals implies consideration of mechanisms involving restoration of normal brain catecholamine levels. However, the different behavioural effects of 5HTP in endogenously depressed and normal subjects that Dr Puhringer will mention are less readily explained.

Some less obvious biochemical effects of precursor loading may also have behavioural consequences. Thus in the work of Butcher and co-workers (1972) the increased locomotor activity after giving L-dopa + the peripheral decarboxylase inhibitor RO4-4602 could well involve not only the increase of brain DA but also the decrease of 5HT which was noted. Furthermore, these workers found that the increased locomotor activity after giving 5HTP alone was probably related to extracerebral changes as it was prevented by RO4-4602.

Many observations suggest that tryptophan can affect behaviour through mechanisms other than those directly involving increased brain 5HT. For example, kynurenine which is formed from tryptophan in considerable amounts outside the brain and in smaller amounts inside it (Joseph, 1978) is reported to have behavioural effects (Lapin, 1971; 1972; Handley and Miskin, 1977) and it appears that the behavioural effects of tryptophan are altered if peripheral aromatic amino acid decarboxylase is inhibited. Thus Patkina and Lapin (1976) found that tryptophan or 5HTP given to cats inhibited self stimulation through hypothalamic electrodes and caused drowsiness and decreased motor activity but after pretreatment with RO4-4602 the drugs activated self-stimulation and did not cause drowsiness.

We have obtained similar results in rats using a procedure in which they are placed in an open field and ambulation measured after the initial motor responses to the new environment have subsided. Although the finding by Taylor (1976) that 20 mg/kg L-tryptophan considerably decreases ambulation was confirmed (Tricklebank and co-workers, 1978) this effect of tryptophan was completely blocked by RO4-4602 (Tricklebank and Curzon, unpublished). It probably however does involve 5HT receptors as it was also prevented by the blockers methysergide and cyproheptadine.

In other recent work we have investigated the behavioural effects of L-tryptophan + the MAOI tranylcypromine. These effects have been used extensively by Green and Grahame-Smith (1976) to study responses at 5HT post-synaptic receptors. Our results suggest that these receptors are involved but that the increase of brain tryptamine has major behavioural consequences.

Thus we found that the behavioural response to L-tryptophan of tranylcypromine treated rats was greatly decreased by giving RO4-4602 to inhibit peripheral tryptamine synthesis (Marsden and Curzon, 1978) (unlike 5HT, extracerebral tryptamine can enter the brain). Furthermore, subsequently (Marsden and Curzon, 1979) we found that a larger dose of the inhibitor sufficient to partly inhibit brain decarboxylase completely prevented the behavioural syndrome of reciprocal forepaw treading, lateral head weaving, straub tail and hindlimb abduction. This blockade of behavioural response occurred together with a large decrease of brain tryptamine accumulation but only slight or negligible decreases of accumulation of brain 5HT, striatal DA and hypothalamic NA. The full syndrome was restored by tryptamine. These results raise the question of whether tryptamine changes have a role in the anti-depressant effect of tryptophan-MAOI treatment.

ACKNOWLEDGEMENT

The Medical Research Council is thanked for financial support.

REFERENCES

Bartholini, G., R. Tissot and A. Pletscher (1971). Brain capillaries as a source of homovanillic acid in cerebrospinal fluid. Brain Res., 27, 163-168.

Butcher, L.L., J. Engel and K. Fuxe (1972). Behavioural biochemical and histochemical analyses of the central effects of monoamine precursors after peripheral decarboxylase inhibition. Brain Res., 41, 387-411.

Christensen, J.G., W. Dairman and S. Udenfriend (1972). On the identity of DOPA decarboxylase and 5-hydroxytryptophan decarboxylase. Proc. Nat. Acad. Sci. (USA), 69, 343-347.

Curzon, G., B.D. Kantamaneni, J.R. Bartlett and P.K. Bridges (1976). Transmitter precursors and metabolites in human ventricular cerebrospinal fluid. J. Neurochem., 26, 613-615.

Eccleston, D., G.W. Ashcroft and T.B.B. Crawford (1965). 5-Hydroxyindole metabolism in rat. A study of intermediate metabolism using the technique of tryptophan loading. J. Neurochem., 12, 493-503.

Eccleston, D., G.W. Ashcroft, T.B.B. Crawford, J.B. Stanton, D. Wood and P.H. McTurk (1970). Effect of tryptophan administration on 5HIAA in cerebrospinal fluid in man. J. Neurol. Neurosurg. Psychiat., 33, 269-272.

Green, A.R. and D.G. Grahame-Smith (1976). Effects of drugs on the processes regulating the functional activity of brain 5-hydroxytryptamine. Nature, 260, 487-491.

Handley, S.L. and R.C. Miskin (1977). The interaction of some kynurenine pathway metabolites with 5-hydroxytryptophan and 5-hydroxytryptamine. Psychopharmacology, 51, 305-309.

Harmar, A.J. and A.S. Horn (1976). Octopamine in mammalian brain: rapid post mortem increase and effects of drugs. J. Neurochem., 26, 987-993.

Hokfelt, T., K. Fuxe and M. Goldstein (1973). Immunohistochemical localisation of aromatic L-amino acid decarboxylase (DOPA decarboxylase) in central dopamine and 5-hydroxytryptamine nerve cell bodies of the rat. Brain Res., 53, 175-180.

Joseph, M.H. (1978). The determination of kynurenine, a simple GLC method applicable to urine, plasma, brain and CSF. J. Chromatog., 146, 33-41.

Lapin, I.P. (1971). Neurotropic activities of kynurenine and its metabolites. 1st Cong. Hungarian Pharmac. Soc., Hungarian Academy of Sciences, Budapest, 149-164.

Lapin, I.P. (1972). Interaction of kynurenine and its metabolites with tryptamine, serotonin and its precursors and oxotremorine. Psychopharmacology, 26, 237-247.

Marsden, C.A. and G. Curzon (1974). Effects of lesions and drugs on brain tryptamine. J. Neurochem., 23, 1171-1176.

Marsden, C.A. and G. Curzon (1976). Studies on the behavioural effects of tryptophan and p-chlorophenylalanine. Neuropharmacology, 15, 165-171.

Marsden, C.A. and G. Curzon (1978). The contribution of tryptamine to the behavioural effects of L-tryptophan in tranylcypromine-treated rats. Psychopharmacology, 57, 71-76.

Marsden, C.A. and G. Curzon (1979). The role of tryptamine in the behavioural effects of L-tryptophan + tranylcypromine. Neuropharmacology, submitted.

Patkina, N.A. and I.P. Lapin (1976). Effect of serotoninergic drugs on positive and negative reinforcing systems in cats. Pharmac. Biochem. Behav., 5, 241-245.

Saavedra, J.M. (1974). Enzymatic isotopic assay for and presence of β-phenylethylamine in brain. J. Neurochem., 22, 211-216.

Saavedra, J.M. and J. Axelrod (1973). Effect of drugs on the tryptamine content of rat tissue. J. Pharmac. Exp. Ther., 185, 523-529.

Smith, J.E., J.D. Lane, P.A. Shea and W.J. McBride (1977). Neurochemical changes following the administration of precursors of biogenic amines. Life Sci., 21, 301-306.

(REFERENCES - CONT.)

Tabakoff, B., S.R. Moses, S.R. Philips and A.A. Boulton (1977). Effects of tranylcypromine and pargyline on brain tryptamine. Experientia, 33, 380-381.
Taylor, M. (1976). Effects of L-tryptophan and L-methionine on activity in the rat. Br. J. Pharmac., 58, 117-119.
Tricklebank, M.D., J.L. Smart, D.L. Bloxam and G. Curzon (1978). Effect of chronic experimental liver dysfunction and L-tryptophan on behaviour in the rat. Pharmac. Biochem. Behav. In the press.
Tsukuda, Y., H. Kishimoto and K. Nagai (1975). Studies on amine metabolism in the monkey brain after the administration of amine precursors. In S. Kondo, M. Kawai and A. Ehara (Ed.), Contempory Primatology. Karger, Basle. 56-66.
Yunger, L.M. and J.A. Harvey (1976). Behavioural effects of L-5-hydroxytryptophan after destruction of ascending serotonergic pathways in the rat. The role of catecholamine neurones. J. Pharmac., 196, 307-315.

Behavioural Responses to L-Tryptophan and L-Dopa in Monoamine Oxidase Inhibitor Treated Rats

A. R. GREEN*, J. F. W. DEAKIN and D. W. COSTAIN***

*MRC Clinical Pharmacology Unit, Radcliffe Infirmary, Oxford OX2 6HE, England
**National Institute for Medical Research, Mill Hill, London NW7, England

ABSTRACT

Administration of L-tryptophan (L-Trp) to rats pretreated with a MAO inhibitor (MAOI) such as tranylcypromine (Tcp) results in the animals displaying characteristic behavioural changes including hyperactivity. A similar but different behavioural syndrome can be elicited by administration of L-dopa to Tcp pretreated rats. These syndromes are considered to result respectively from increased functional activity of 5-hydroxytryptamine (5-HT) and dopamine (DA) in the brain. Decreasing brain DA concentrations or blocking DA receptors inhibits the 5-HT syndrome, but decreasing brain 5-HT with p-chloramphetamine does not inhibit the dopamine mediated response. Increasing brain GABA concentrations by injection of amino-oxyacetic acid inhibits both syndromes. Many of the behavioural changes following Tcp/L-Trp appear to be hind-brain or spinally mediated. Propranolol totally inhibits the Tcp/L-Trp syndrome but not the Tcp/Dopa syndrome while methysergide and metergoline inhibit some of the behaviours in both syndromes. The possible neurotransmitter interactions suggested by these studies and action of the putative 5-HT and DA receptor blockers are discussed.

Keywords: Monoamine oxidase inhibitor, L-tryptophan, L-dopa, hyperactivity, behaviour, GABA, 5-hydroxytryptamine, dopamine, monoamine antagonists.

INTRODUCTION

In 1961 Hess and Doepfner reported that administration to rats of a monoamine oxidase (MAO) inhibitor and L-tryptophan resulted in a series of behavioural changes (the main features of which are listed in Table 1). Subsequently Everett (1966) noted similar but slightly different changes (for example the animals are much more reactive and appear somewhat aggressive) following MAO inhibition and L-dopa administration. It appears that the degree of behavioural hyperactivity is related to the rate of increase of synthesis and "spillover" into functional activity of brain 5-hydroxytryptamine (5-HT) and dopamine (DA) respectively as shown by Grahame-Smith (1971a) and Green and Kelly (1976).

Putative 5-HT agonists such as 5-methoxy N,N-dimethyltryptamine (Grahame-Smith, 1971b), quipazine (Green, Youdim and Grahame-Smith, 1976) and 5-methoxytryptamine (Green, Hughes and Tordoff, 1976) produce similar behavioural changes to those seen after MAO inhibition and L-tryptophan but with a different time course, while

TABLE 1 Behavioural Changes Seen in Rats Following Administration of Tranylcypromine Followed by L-tryptophan

Disperse	Shivering
"Explore"	Athetosis
Headweaving	Ataxia
Piloerection	Forepaw padding
Proptosis	Straubtail
Salivation	Weaving
Squeaking	Unresponsive to visual stimuli
Compulsive movements	- - - - - - - - - - - - - - - - Opisthotonus
Circling	Fits and death

The syndrome develops through the list, those behaviours below the dotted line only being seen after high doses of tryptophan.

somewhat different behavioural responses are produced by the dopamine releasing drug methamphetamine or the putative agonist apomorphine, although all these responses include a hyperactivity component.

Using these behavioural models, we have investigated the action of various drugs on monoamine synthesis and function and this is reviewed elsewhere (Green and Grahame-Smith, 1976a, 1978; also see Green and colleagues, this volume). In this communication we wish to report our recent findings on possible neurotransmitter interactions indicated by investigation of the action of putative 5-HT and DA antagonists on these behavioural syndromes.

RESULTS

It does not appear to matter which MAO inhibitor is used provided over 85% inhibition of both Type A and Type B MAO is produced. If only one form of the enzyme is inhibited the other form can apparently continue to metabolise the amine being formed. Without almost total MAO inhibition there is presumably still a large degree of intraneuronal metabolism by MAO and the amine does not "spill-over" from the nerve ending and produce a functional response; that is, the behavioural change (Green and Youdim, 1975; Green and colleagues, 1977). This is presumably also why no behavioural changes are seen following administration of L-tryptophan or L-dopa alone, in doses up to 100 mg/Kg (Grahame-Smith, 1971a).

Jacobs and Klemfuss (1975) have suggested that many of the behavioural components of the MAOI/L-tryptophan syndrome are hind-brain or spinally mediated and we would agree with this. Lesioning of the descending 5-HT pathways to the hind-brain and spinal cord with 5,7-dihydroxytryptamine results in degeneration of these tracts followed by post-synaptic receptor "supersensitivity" as first reported by Trulson and colleagues (1976). When these denervated animals are given the 5-HT agonist 5-MeODMT, many of the behavioural changes are enhanced (Table 2) indicating the responses are produced by the "supersensitive" spinal receptors.

The 5-HT-induced behavioural responses occur only when brain dopaminergic function is intact. This can be shown in several ways:

When brain dopamine concentrations are depleted by pretreatment of the animals with α-methyl p-tyrosine the tranylcypromine/L-tryptophan hyperactivity response is abolished for at least 60 min after the tryptophan administration (Deakin and

TABLE 2 Behavioural Effects of Tranylcypromine/5-MeODMT in Control and Spinal 5,7-Dihydroxytryptamine Lesioned Animals

	Control	Lesioned	p
No. of observations	10	5	
Head weaving	1.5 ± 1.0	2.8 ± 0.4	<0.02
Forepaw padding	1.8 ± 1.0	2.8 ± 0.4	N.S.
Hind limb abduction	1.7 ± 0.5	2.8 ± 0.4	<0.01
Straub tail	1.5 ± 0.7	2.8 ± 0.4	<0.01
Reactivity	1.4 ± 0.8	2.2 ± 0.4	N.S.
Locomotor counts/min	79.0 ± 19.0	123.0 ± 18.0	<0.01
Temperature ^{o}C	36.6 ± 0.4	38.0 ± 0.8	<0.02
Conc. of 5-HT in spinal cord	0.53 ± 0.10	0.14 ± 0.01	<0.01
Conc. of 5-HT in brain	1.01 ± 0.23	0.87 ± 0.12	N.S.

Behavioural score, 0 = absent, 3 = severe.
N.S.: not significantly different from control.

Green, 1978; Green and Grahame-Smith, 1974; Fig. 1). The gradual appearance of the behavioural changes after this time perhaps goes some way to explaining apparent discrepancies in the literature as to the effects of α-methyl p-tyrosine on the syndrome (Deakin and Green, 1978; Green and Grahame-Smith, 1974; Jacobs, 1974). The observation that disulfiram has no effect on the syndrome points to the importance of dopamine rather than noradrenaline in the syndrome. The dopaminergic system lies post-synaptic to the 5-HT neurones initiating the hyperactivity response since α-methyl p-tyrosine also inhibits the hyperactivity produced by the 5-HT agonist 5-methoxy N,N-dimethyltryptamine. Acute administration of neuroleptics will also inhibit the 5-HT-induced hyperactivity and, of course, the tranylcypromine/L-dopa responses (Heal and colleagues, 1976). Chronic administration of neuroleptics results in enhanced ("supersensitive") responses to tranylcypromine/L-dopa but not tranylcypromine/L-tryptophan, with the exception of chlorpromazine which when administered chronically enhanced both syndromes (Green, 1977; Heal and colleagues, 1976). This may indicate that this drug also blocks 5-HT receptors and there is some evidence for this (Bradley and colleagues, 1966; von Hungen, Roberts and Hill, 1975).

In contrast, we have not been able to show involvement of 5-HT in the DA-syndrome. Jacobs (1974) demonstrated that p-chlorophenylalanine (PCPA) pretreatment to decrease brain 5-HT concentrations markedly (Table 3) attenuated the MAOI/L-dopa syndrome and this was confirmed (Green and Kelly, 1975). However we showed that

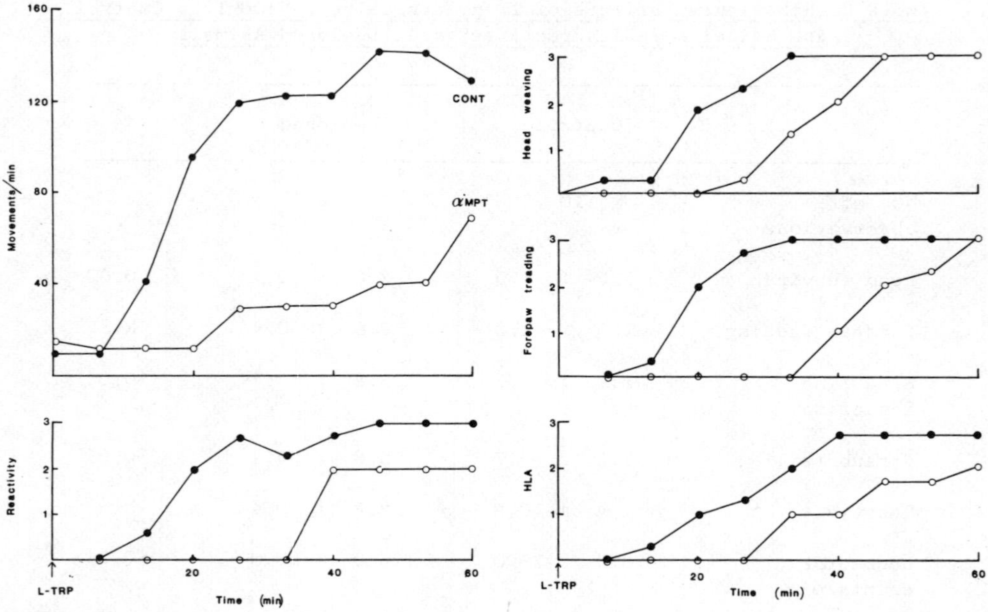

Fig. 1. Effect of α-methyl paratyrosine (αMPT) pretreatment on behaviour elicited by tranylcypromine and tryptophan. ●—● saline controls; O—O α-methyl paratyrosine 200 mg/kg 18 and 15 hr before tranylcypromine 20 mg/kg injection. Tryptophan 100 mg/kg 30 min after tranylcypromine. 3 animals per group. Differences between saline and αMPT pretreated animals significant on all measures for at least three time points ($p < 0.05$ Fishers exact probabilities test).

this drug also inhibited the uptake of L-dopa into the brain (Table 4) and when brain 5-HT concentrations were decreased by administration of p-chloroamphetamine (PCA; Table 3) no alteration of the tranylcypromine/L-dopa response was seen (Fig. 2, Table 4, Deakin and Green, 1978; Green and Kelly, 1976). This indicates that L-dopa, while perhaps being decarboxylated non-specifically in 5-HT neurones does not lead to a functional release of this amine. Thus we cannot say that the similarity of the two syndromes is because part of the behaviour seen in the tranylcypromine/L-dopa syndrome is the result of 5-HT release. Indeed the whole syndrome occurs when brain 5-HT concentrations are reduced by 75%.

The inhibitory transmitter γ-aminobutyric acid (GABA) also appears to play a modulatory role in both syndromes. Raising brain GABA concentrations inhibits both behavioural syndromes (Green, Hughes and Tordoff, 1976) and this inhibition occurs at some point post-synaptic to the monoamine neurones initiating the behavioural changes (Cott and Engel, 1977; Green, Hughes and Tordoff, 1976).

Finally we come to the question as to what drugs act as specific antagonists to the syndromes. As stated earlier, neuroleptics inhibit the MAOI/L-dopa syndrome. In contrast the putative 5-HT antagonists are remarkably ineffective in inhibiting the MAOI/L-tryptophan responses. While methysergide and metergoline inhibit the hind-brain or spinally mediated behavioural changes (forepaw padding, head weaving, Straub tail hind-limb abduction) the hyperactivity and hyper-reactivity are not

TABLE 3 Effect of p-chlorophenylalanine (PCPA) and p-chloroamphetamine (PCA) on Rat Brain 5-hydroxytryptamine (5-HT), Dopamine and Noradrenaline

Injected	Brain amine concentrations (μg amine/g brain (wet wt.)) 5-HT	Dopamine	Noradrenaline
Saline	0.51 ± 0.01 (4)	1.46 ± 0.08 (8)	0.24 ± 0.03 (6)
p-Chlorophenylalanine (200 mg/kg x 2)	0.14 ± 0.02 (4)*	1.14 ± 0.11 (4)	0.27 ± 0.02 (6)
p-Chloroamphetamine (10 mg/kg)	0.18 ± 0.02 (6)*	1.27 ± 0.04 (4)	0.28 ± 0.02 (4)

Rats were injected with PCPA 200 mg/kg on Day 1 and 2; 24 h later they were killed for brain amine determinations. PCA (10 mg/kg) was injected 24 h before rats were killed and brain amines determined. Results show mean ± s.e. mean with number of determinations in brackets. *Different from control ($P < 0.001$).

TABLE 4 Effect of p-chlorophenylalanine (PCPA) and p-chloroamphetamine (PCA) on Rat Brain L-Dopa, Dopamine and Noradrenaline Concentrations Following Subsequent Tranylcypromine (Tcp) and L-Dopa Administration

Injected	Brain Catechol Concentration (μg catechol/g brain (wet wt.)) L-Dopa	Dopamine	Noradrenaline
Saline	0.78±0.29(4)	1.46±0.08(8)	0.24±0.03(6)
Tranylcypromine(20 mg/kg)+L-dopa (100 mg/kg)	*55.1 ±7.4 (4)	11.74±1.29(7)	0.57±0.05(7)
PCPA(200 mg/kg x 2)+Tcp (20 mg/kg)+L-dopa (100 mg/kg)	11.5 ±4.0 (4)*	4.71±0.61(8)*	0.49±0.04(6)
PCA(10 mg/kg)+Tcp(20 mg/kg)+L-dopa (100 mg/kg)	N.D.	9.10±0.88(6)	0.53±0.03(6)

Rats were injected with PCPA or PCA as described in footnote to Table 2. Twenty-four hours after the PCA or second PCPA injection they were injected with tranylcypromine (20 mg/kg) and after a further 30 min with L-dopa (100 mg/kg). Rats were killed for brain noradrenaline and dopamine determinations 90 min after L-dopa and after 60 min for L-dopa determinations. Results show mean ± s.e. mean with number of determinations in brackets. N.D. - not determined. *Different from tranylcypromine/L-dopa values $P < 0.001$.

---

inhibited and indeed are enhanced with the animals showing bursts of locomotor activity (Fig. 3, Deakin and Green, 1978). (-)-Propranolol on the other hand is able to inhibit all the behavioural changes seen while (+)-Propranolol is ineffective in

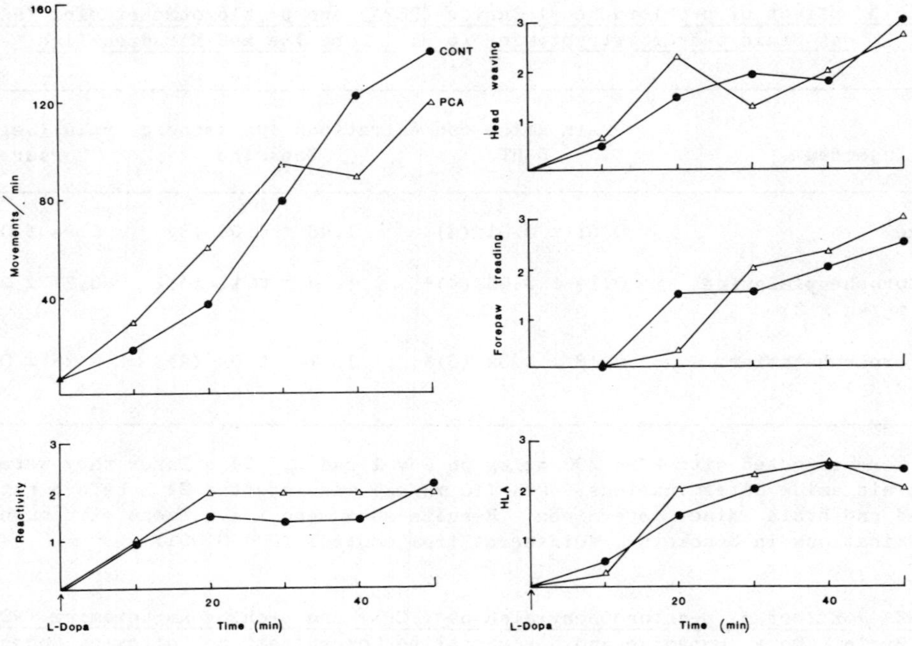

Fig. 2. Lack of effect of parachloroamphetamine pretreatment on behaviour elicited by tranylcypromine and L-dopa. ●—● saline controls; Δ—Δ parachloroamphetamine 10 mg/kg 24 hr before tranylcypromine 20 mg/kg injection. L-dopa 50 mg/kg injected 30 min after tranylcypromine. 3 animals per group.

inhibiting the syndrome (Costain and Green, 1978; Deakin and Green, 1978; Green and Grahame-Smith, 1976b).

(-)-Propranolol has no effect on the DA-mediated syndrome. Recent data have shown that all non-specific (i.e. $\beta_1+\beta_2$) β-adrenoceptor antagonists which penetrate the brain well are able to inhibit to some degree the 5-HT-syndrome whilst not affecting the DA-syndrome (Costain and Green, 1978). Our data on β-adrenoceptor antagonists is therefore consistent with the report of Middlemiss, Blakeborough and Leather (1977) that these drugs are potent inhibitors of the binding of 5-HT to synaptic membranes.

What complicated these observations considerably was the finding that methysergide and metergoline inhibit those components of the DA-syndrome which they block in the 5-HT-syndrome, namely, head weaving, hind limb abduction and forepaw treading (Deakin and Green, 1978). Since we cannot demonstrate the involvement of 5-HT in the DA-syndrome, we must perhaps speculate that these drugs have effects not only on some 5-HT systems but also on DA-receptors.

CONCLUSIONS

The behavioural changes induced by administration of L-tryptophan or L-dopa to MAO inhibitor treated rats are very similar. However while an involvement of DA could be shown in the 5-HT mediated response the involvement of 5-HT in the DA-mediated

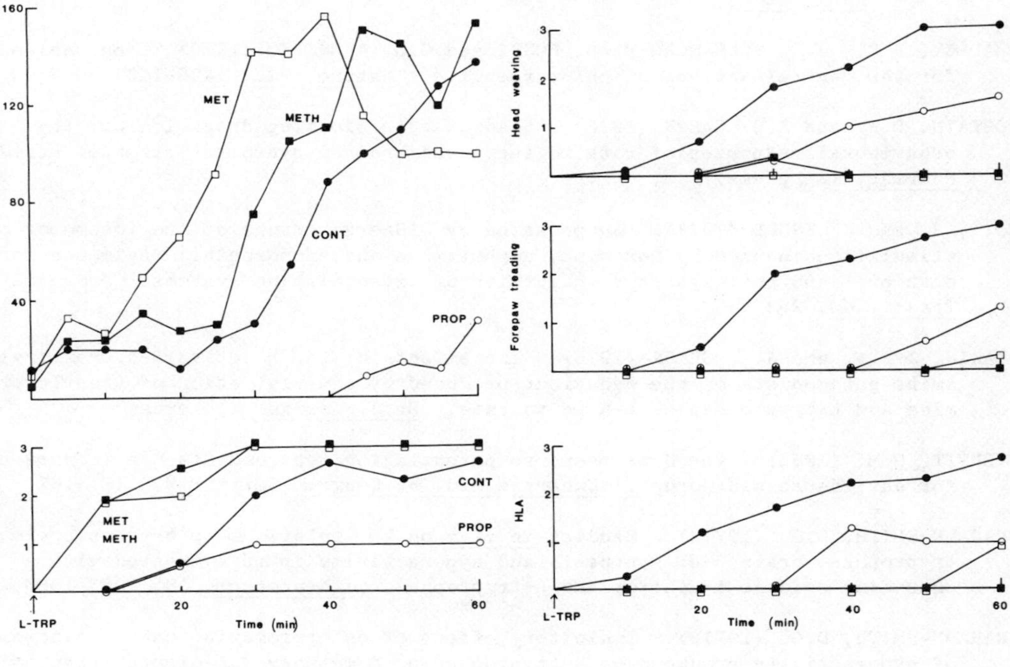

Fig. 3. Effects of methysergide, methergoline and propranolol on behaviour elicited by tranylcypromine and tryptophan. ●—● saline pretreated; O—O (-)-propranolol (20 mg/kg) 45 min before tranylcypromine (20 mg/kg); □—□ methysergide (MET) (10 mg/kg) with tranylcypromine (20 mg/kg); ■—■ methergoline (METH) (5 mg/kg) with tranylcypromine (20 mg/kg). Tryptophan (100 mg/kg) was injected 30 min after tranylcypromine in each group. Animals were grouped in threes for activity recording. Individual animals were rated at same time as activity recording. Behavioural ratings show means of six saline pretreated animals and three in each of the drug pretreated groups. Differences between saline and drug pretreated animals are significant ($p < 0.05$ Fishers exact probabilities test) for at least three time points on all measures except Straub tail.

changes was not found. The putative 5-HT antagonists methysergide and metergoline block only some of the 5-HT behavioural changes in agreement with their lack of central action shown by others (Haigler and Aghajanian, 1976). Propranolol and other β-adrenoceptor antagonists will inhibit the 5-HT response but not the DA-response. Neuroleptics inhibit both syndromes, the effect on the 5-HT behaviour presumably being an indirect effect since intact DA-function is necessary for the behavioural expression of the 5-HT-induced changes. Finally in agreement with the observations of Jacobs and Klemfuss (1975) it appears that, at least with the 5-HT syndrome, many of the behavioural changes are mediated by hind-brain or spinal neurones.

REFERENCES

BRADLEY, P.B., J.H. WOLSENCROFT, L. HÖSLI and G.L. AVANZINO (1966). Neuronal basis for the central actions of chlorpromazine. Nature, 212, 1425-1427.

COSTAIN, D.W. and A.R. GREEN (1978). β-Adrenergic blocking drugs inhibit the behavioural responses of rats to increased brain 5-hydroxytryptamine. Br.J. Pharmac. (in press).

COTT, J. and J. ENGEL (1977). Suppression by GABAergic drugs of the locomotor stimulation induced by morphine, amphetamine and apomorphine: evidence for both pre- and post-synaptic inhibition of catecholamine systems. J.Neural Trans., 40, 253-268.

DEAKIN, J.F.W. and A.R. GREEN (1978). The effects of the putative 5-hydroxytryptamine antagonists on the behaviour produced by administration of tranylcypromine and L-tryptophan or L-dopa to rats. Br.J.Pharmac. (in press).

EVERETT, G.M. (1966). The dopa response potentiation test and its use in screening for anti-depressant drugs. Excerpta Med.Int.Congr., Series 122, 164-167.

GRAHAME-SMITH, D.G. (1971a). Studies in vivo on the relationship between brain tryptophan, brain 5-HT synthesis and hyperactivity in rats treated with a monoamine oxidase inhibitor and L-tryptophan. J.Neurochem., 18, 1053-1066.

GRAHAME-SMITH, D.G. (1971b). Inhibitory effect of chlorpromazine on the syndrome of hyperactivity produced by L-tryptophan or 5-methoxy N,N-dimethyltryptamine and a monoamine oxidase inhibitor. Br.J.Pharmac., 43, 856-864.

GREEN, A.R. (1977). Repeated chlorpromazine administration increases the behavioural responses of rats to 5-hydroxytryptamine receptor stimulation. Br.J. Pharmac., 59, 367-371.

GREEN, A.R. and D.G. GRAHAME-SMITH (1974). The role of brain dopamine in the hyperactivity syndrome produced by increased 5-hydroxytryptamine synthesis in rats. Neuropharmacology, 13, 949-959.

GREEN, A.R. and D.G. GRAHAME-SMITH (1976a). The effects of drugs on the processes regulating the functional activity of brain 5-hydroxytryptamine. Nature, 260, 487-491.

GREEN, A.R. and D.G. GRAHAME-SMITH (1976b). (-)-Propranolol inhibits the behavioural responses of rats to increased 5-hydroxytryptamine in the central nervous system. Nature, 262, 594-596.

GREEN, A.R. and D.G. GRAHAME-SMITH (1978). Processes regulating the functional activity of brain 5-hydroxytryptamine: Results of animal experimentation and their relevance to the understanding and treatment of depression. Pharmacopsychiat., 11, 3-16.

GREEN, A.R., J.P. HUGHES and A.F.C. TORDOFF (1975). The concentration of 5-methoxytryptamine in rat brain and its effects on behaviour following its peripheral injection. Neuropharmacology, 14, 601-606.

GREEN, A.R. and P.H. KELLY (1976). Evidence concerning the involvement of 5-hydroxytryptamine in the locomotor activity produced by amphetamine or tranylcypromine plus L-dopa. Br.J.Pharmac., 57, 141-147.

GREEN, A.R., B.D. MITCHELL, A.F.C. TORDOFF and M.B.H. YOUDIM (1977). Evidence for dopamine deamination by Type A and Type B monoamine oxidase in rat brain _in vivo_ and for the degree of inhibition of the enzyme necessary for increased functional activity of dopamine and 5-hydroxytryptamine. _Br.J.Pharmac._, _60_, 343-349.

GREEN, A.R., A.F.C. TORDOFF and M.R. BLOOMFIELD (1976). Elevation of brain GABA concentrations with amino-oxyacetic acid; effect on the hyperactivity syndrome produced by increased 5-hydroxytryptamine synthesis in rats. _J.Neural Transmission_, _39_, 103-112.

GREEN, A.R. and M.B.H. YOUDIM (1975). Effects of clorgyline, deprenil and tranylcypromine on rat brain 5-HT concentrations, monoamine oxidase activity and hyperactivity following subsequent tryptophan administration. _Br.J.Pharmac._, _55_, 415-422.

GREEN, A.R., M.B.H. YOUDIM and D.G. GRAHAME-SMITH (1976). Quipazine: its effects on rat brain 5-hydroxytryptamine metabolism, monoamine oxidase activity and behaviour. _Neuropharmacology_, _15_, 173-179.

HAIGLER, H.T. and G.K. AGHAJANIAN (1977). Serotonin receptors in the brain. _Fedn. Proc._, _36_, 2159-2164.

HEAL, D.J., A.R. GREEN, D.J. BOULLIN and D.G. GRAHAME-SMITH (1976). Single and repeated administration of neuroleptic drugs to rats: effects on striatal dopamine sensitive adenylate cyclase and locomotor activity produced by tranylcypromine and L-tryptophan or L-dopa. _Psychopharmacology_, _49_, 287-300.

HESS, S.M. and W. DOEPFNER (1961). Behavioural effects and brain amine content in mice. _Arch.int.Pharmacodyn.Ther._, _134_, 89-99.

von HUNGEN, K., S. ROBERTS and D.F. HILL (1975). Serotonin sensitive adenylate cyclase in immature rat brain. _Brain Research_, _84_, 257-267.

JACOBS, B.L. (1974). Evidence for the functional interaction of two central neurotransmitters. _Psychopharmacologia_, _39_, 81-86.

JACOBS, B.L. and H. KLEMFUSS (1975). Brainstem and spinal cord mediation of serotonergic behavioural syndrome. _Brain Res._, _100_, 450-457.

MIDDLEMISS, D.N., L. BLAKEBOROUGH and S.R. LEATHER (1977). Direct evidence for an interaction of adrenergic blockers with the 5-HT receptor. _Nature_, _267_, 289-290.

TRULSON, M.E., E.E. EUBANKS and B.L. JACOBS (1976). Behavioural evidence for supersensitivity following destruction of central serotonergic nerve terminals by 5,7,dihydroxytryptamine. _J.Pharmac.exp.Ther._, _198_, 23-32.

Symposium on Behavioural Effects of Indoleamine and Catecholamine Precusors: Summary

G. CURZON

Department of Neurochemistry, Institute of Neurology, 33 John's Mews, London WC1N 2NS, England

This symposium dealt with behavioural and relevant biochemical effects of amino acid precursors of indoleamine and catecholamine transmitters- i.e. (1) the effects of tryptophan and 5-hydroxytryptophan on 5-hydroxytryptamine synthesis and action; (2) the effects of tyrosine and dopa on catecholamine synthesis and action. Drug treatments of this kind as well as providing useful experimental tools have intrinsic attractions from a therapeutic point of view. It is often assumed that because the biosphere has survived prolonged exposure to these substances we have guarantees of their safety that do not exist for synthetic drugs of recent origin. However, giving physiologically occurring transmitter precursors may lead to precursor levels being raised to a completely non-physiological extent or to the presence of precursors or their products in compartments to which they normally do not gain access. Furthermore - attempts to increase transmitter accumulation by giving precursors with a MAOI drug may also lead to striking accumulation of amines normally only present as traces. Indeed we have evidence that such a mechanism - the synthesis of tryptamine - mediates much of the behavioural response to tryptophan + the MAOI drug tranylcypromine in rats. This raises the question of the exact mechanism by which tryptophan + MAOI drugs produce the anti-depressant effects shown by Dr Coppen.

Nevertheless, many behavioural effects of the precursors under consideration do have an association with evidence of a pre-existing deficiency of the normal major transmitter product. This must incline us towards the belief that many behavioural effects of precursors result from increased synthesis of these major products. For example, evidence suggests that both 5-hydroxytryptamine deficiency and the therapeutic action of tryptophan in depressive illness can be considered in these terms. Drs Coppen and Wood gave substantial evidence that plasma free tryptophan was low in depression while our own work (presented elsewhere) indicates that plasma free tryptophan correlates with indices of brain 5-hydroxytryptamine metabolism in man.

While arguments about whether tryptophan is a treatment of choice for depression may well continue indefinitely there is now strong evidence that some depressed patients are helped by tryptophan. This increases the importance of studying how tryptophan causes behavioural effects. Even here, the simple replacement of brain 5-hydroxytryptamine is only one of a number of possibilities. Thus we find that the decreased motor activity of laboratory animals given tryptophan is prevented by a peripheral decarboxylase inhibitor.

Although relationships between the behavioural and biochemical effects of tryptophan may not be as simple as has often been assumed, it has long been accepted that giving it increases brain 5-hydroxytryptamine turnover. That tyrosine may increase catecholamine turnover has only been considered fairly recently. Professor Carlsson and Dr Lindqvist presented results showing that rat brain tryptophan hydroxylase and tyrosine hydroxylase (the rate limiting enzymes for 5-hydroxytryptamine and catecholamine synthesis respectively) are normally both unsaturated. This study was of particular interest as brain tryptophan and tyrosine were manipulated both upwards and downwards from their normal levels. It provides useful guide lines for future studies of behavioural effects of altered transmitter amine synthesis. In the specific work described however, brain amine levels were unaltered as metabolism beyond the hydroxylation step was prevented by decarboxylase inhibition.

In much of the work described by the other speakers, limitation of transmitter synthesis at the hydroxylation stage no longer occurred, as the hydroxylated amino acid products 5-hydroxytryptophan or dopa were used as precursors. This is an effective means of increasing transmitter synthesis although the widespread occurrence in the brain of the enzyme required - aromatic amino acid decarboxylase - leads to formation of transmitters at non-physiological as well as at physiological sites. A striking effect of infusing 5-hydroxytryptophan was reported by Drs Puhringer and Wirz-Justice - namely that mood was consistently elevated in normal but not in depressive subjects. This difference leads these authors to question any simple 5-hydroxytryptamine deficiency hypothesis of depressive illness. Such doubts are consistent with much other evidence on the nature of the biochemical disturbance in depression. Their resolution must await increased understanding of how different transmitter systems interact.

Dr Green's work provides a fruitful approach to such interactions. He has studied how behavioural responses to dopa or tryptophan in MAOI drug treated rats are affected by drugs which alter other neuronal systems. Results suggest that the response to tryptophan is decreased when dopaminergic function is impaired but the response to dopa still occurs when serotonergic function is impaired. Responses to both drugs are diminished when brain gamma-aminobutyric acid is increased. Such procedures provide us with clues about neuronal wiring diagrams but one must of course be cautious about making deductions about the normal behavioural roles of the transmitters from these experiments in which transmitters probably diffuse or flood out to receptors rather than being released to them by neuronal activity.

Differences of this kind were considered in the paper on behavioural effects of dopa given by Dr Engel. These were markedly different if the dopa replaced dopamine or noradrenaline neuronal stores depleted by tyrosine hydroxylase inhibition or if it was given in circumstances in which neuronal storage was either impaired by reserpine or exceeded by high dosage of dopa so that the catecholamine flooded out.

The symposium as a whole elucidated the experimental and therapeutic value of transmitter precursors. It provided a number of pointers towards future advances.

Addiction: Drugs of Abuse

Opiate Addiction - New Perspectives in Research

RÜDIGER SCHULZ and ALBERT HERZ

Department of Neuropharmacology, Max-Planck-Institut für Psychiatrie, Kraepelinstrasse 2, D-8000 München 40, Federal Republic of Germany

ABSTRACT

The demonstration of opiate receptors in nervous tissue and the subsequent identification of endogenous ligands, endorphins, for these receptors raised hopes for a better understanding of drug addiction. This article discusses some aspects of the concept of multiple opiate receptors and their supposed interaction with the known endorphins. Specific emphasis is given to the issue of how the nervous system adapts to the chronic inhibitory action of opiates and to how the endorphinergic system may be affected during the opiate tolerant/dependent state,as well as during withdrawal. From the data presently available, it may be concluded that an altered metabolism of endorphins could contribute to opiate addiction.

KEYWORDS

Multiple Opiate Receptors - Morphine - Endorphins - Naloxone - Tolerance/Dependence - Addiction - Withdrawal.

Two major findings have significantly influenced our understanding of how opiates interfere with the functioning of the central nervous system: First the demonstration of opiate receptors in 1973; and secondly, two years later, the discovery of the endogenous ligands for these receptors - the endorphins. These developments greatly affected modern biology, and particularly raised hopes for a better understanding of the biochemical mechanisms underlying opiate tolerance and dependence as well as of the general phenomenon of drug dependence. As of yet, the mechanism of opiate addiction is not well understood. However, some new developments are evident in the field of opiate research, which will be discussed here in the light of some aspects of our present understanding of addiction.

Multiple Opiate Receptors

In 1954 Beckett and Casy conceptualized an opiate receptor model based on the structure-activity relationship of morphine and its congeners. The receptor was thought to exhibit an anionic group, a flat surface and a cavity for accomodating the narcotic analgesic. However, the rigid Beckett and Casy model could not explain data obtained with other opiates, so that Porthogese (1965) subsequently postulated that different opiates might combine with more than one kind of opiate receptor. Such a concept of multiple receptors appears to be attractive, since one could then attribute specific receptor types to specific pharmacological actions of the opiates. During the following years the interest focussed mainly on the isolation and characterization of opiate receptors, which culminated in 1973 in the demonstration of opiate receptors in nervous tissue (Pert and Snyder; Simon and others). By means of the radio receptor assay technique, it was shown that, beside other criteria,

1. narcotic agonists as well as antagonists bind competitively to their receptors,
2. the binding is stereospecific, and
3. the receptors are unevenly distributed within the central nervous system.

Although these studies revealed different opiate binding sites (Lord and others, 1977; Lowney and others, 1974; Pasternak and Snyder, 1975), a heterogeneity of opiate receptors was not documented. This concept of multiple opiate receptors was advanced again in 1976 by Martin and associates on the basis of pharmacological data. Experiments with chronically spinalized dogs caused Martin to suggest at least three different types of opiate receptors:

1. μ-receptors (which mainly combine with morphine-like drugs),
2. κ-receptors (specific for ketocyclazocine, a drug with high antinociceptive potency, but which fails to suppress withdrawal symptoms in opiate-dependent monkeys (Hutchinson and others, 1975), and
3. σ-receptors (which mainly interact with N-allylnorcyclazocine).

Further strong support for the existence of multiple opiate receptors comes from studies with isolated preparations as well as with intact animals (Lord and others, 1976, 1977; Smith and others, 1976).

A major aspect of this concept is the hope of finding narcotic analgesics which combine with receptors mediating mainly the analgesic action, but which are less sensitive to the addictive capacity of opiates. So far, all investigations conducted along these lines have reaffirmed the close association between analgesic potency and addictive capacity of opiates. Moreover, there is little hope on theoretical grounds, for a separation of the two phenomena (Herz and Schulz, 1978).

Endorphins

The presence of highly specific opiate receptors caused an intense search for endogenous ligands for these receptors. Such ligands were eventually isolated (Hughes and others, 1975; Teschemacher, 1978),

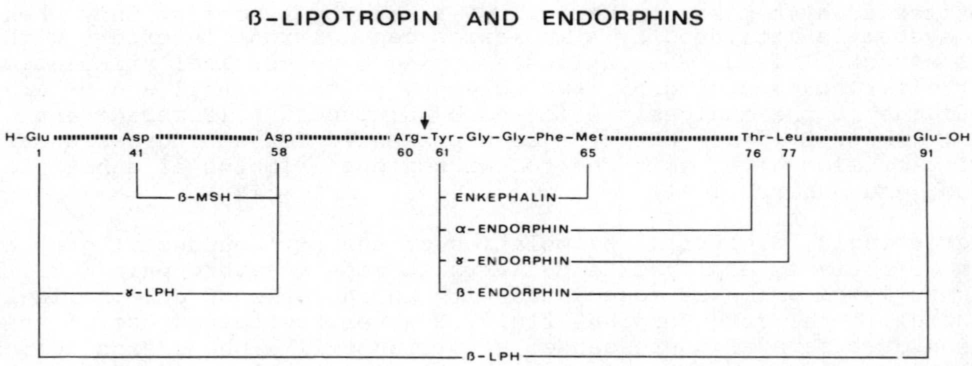

Fig. 1. The pituitary hormone ß-lipotropin (ß-LPH) comprises 91 amino acid residues. ß-LPH (sequence 1-91), as well as γ-LPH (1-58), possess lipolytic activity. The melanocyte-stimulating hormone (ß-MSH) is represented by the sequence 41-58. Cleavage of ß-LPH between arginine and tyrosin (arrow) generates ß-endorphin (61-91). Sequence 61-65 is identical with met-enkephalin.

and found to be peptides in nature. Figure 1 demonstrates that the identified endorphins (endogenous morphine), other than the pentapeptide leucine-enkephalin (H-Tyr-Gly-Gly-Phe-Leu-OH), are comprised in the polypeptide ß-lipotropin. This peptide is devoid of opiate-like activity, while cleavage between the amino acids 60 (arginine) and 61 (tyrosine) generates ß-endorphin (61-91), which has been suggested to be the precursor for smaller endorphins (Bradburry and others, 1976). Since the pituitary contains extremely high concentrations of ß-endorphin (Gramsch and others, 1978), it was thought that brain endorphins might be derived from the pituitary. However, hypophysectomy does not affect the concentration of endorphin in the brain (Cheung and Goldstein, 1976; Wesche and others, 1977). Recent research reveals that the brain by itself synthesizes endorphins in specific neurone whereby ß-endorphin on the one hand and the enkephalins on the other hand are located consistently in separate neurones.

Although the physiologic significance of the endorphins is largely unknown, a function as neurotransmitter (Kosterlitz and Hughes, 1975) appears likely. For example, electrical stimulation of specific regions of the brain causes release of enkephalins (Henderson and others, 1978; Iversen and others, 1978; Osborne and others, 1978), as does electrical stimulation of the periaqueductal grey (Akil and others, 1978) or the myenteric plexus (Schulz and others, 1977).

To elucidate the physiologic significance of endorphins it appeared helpful to block opiate receptors using the narcotic antagonist naloxone, so that the endorphins could not combine with those receptors. Unexpectedly, naloxone given to man or animals failed to bring about distinct pharmacologic actions, although the blood concentration of prolactin and growth hormone was reported to be reduced by the antagonist (Frederickson, 1977). This outcome suggests that the endorphinergic system may primarily have a standby function. Only when the system is activated by stimulation can naloxone interfere with this effect. Indeed, the analgesia caused by electrical stimulation of the periaqueductal grey is blocked by naloxone (Akil and others, 1976), as is the analgesia elicited by acupuncture (Pomeranz and Chiu, 1976). Evidence has also been presented for an increased sensitivity of mice given naloxone to the noxious stimulus of a hot plate (Jacob and others, 1974).

Interestingly, electrical stimulation of the periaqueductal grey has been effectively employed in patients to impair severe pain (Akil and others, 1978) which is associated with an increase of enkephalin-like material in the cerebrospinal fluid. However, sustained use of stimulation over several hours caused a tolerance-like phenomenon, which could be avoided by intermittent use of the stimulator. This development of tolerance is to be expected, since endorphins interact with opiate receptors, and the tolerance and dependence liability of these compounds is a well documented fact (Bläsig and Herz, 1976; Wei and Loh, 1976).

The Effect of Chronic Opiate Administration

Chronic opiate administration causes adaptive changes in the nervous system which compensate for the continuous inhibitory action of the drug (Herz and Schulz, 1978). Apparently, chronic exposure of animals to morphine does not change the number or affinity of opiate receptors (Höllt and others, 1975; Simon and Hiller, 1978).

The question arises, thus, if the opiate receptors fail to adapt, how does the neuronal system respond to the chronic inhibitory opiate action? From studies with the tolerant/dependent guinea pig ileum it is known that neurones adapt by changing their sensitivity. Apparently, the meyenteric plexus counteracts the chronic inhibitory action of morphine by increasing its sensitivity to excitatory compounds, for example to serotonin (Fig. 2). In a stable state of tolerance/dependence, however, an altered neuronal sensitivity cannot be detected,the myenteric plexus functions "normally". Only a disturbance of the newly established equilibrium by elimination of the inhibitory opiate input, such as by administration of the narcotic antagonist naloxone, reveals the altered sensitivity. Thus, the state of opiate withdrawal is associated with a change in neuronal sensitivity. Further studies demonstrated that supersensitivity also develops to prostaglandin E_1 and E_2 (Schulz and Herz, 1976), while subsensitivity was observed to the inhibitory action of catecholamines (Goldstein and Schulz, 1973). Analogous investigations conducted with tolerant/dependent rats yielded similar changes in the sensitivity of the central nervous system (Schulz and Herz, 1977).

The biochemical mechanism underlying the development of changes in neuronal sensitivity is unknown. Investigations of the adenylate cyclase system suggest, however, that cyclic adenosine monophosphate (cAMP) is probably involved. Studies with neuroblastoma x glioma hybrid cells demonstrated that morphine inhibits the adenylate cyclase activity which, in turn, decreases the cAMP level. During continuous exposure to morphine the adenylate cyclase activity increases, so that tolerant cells have cAMP levels close to normal in the presence of morphine. Withdrawal of the opiate increases the amount of cAMP

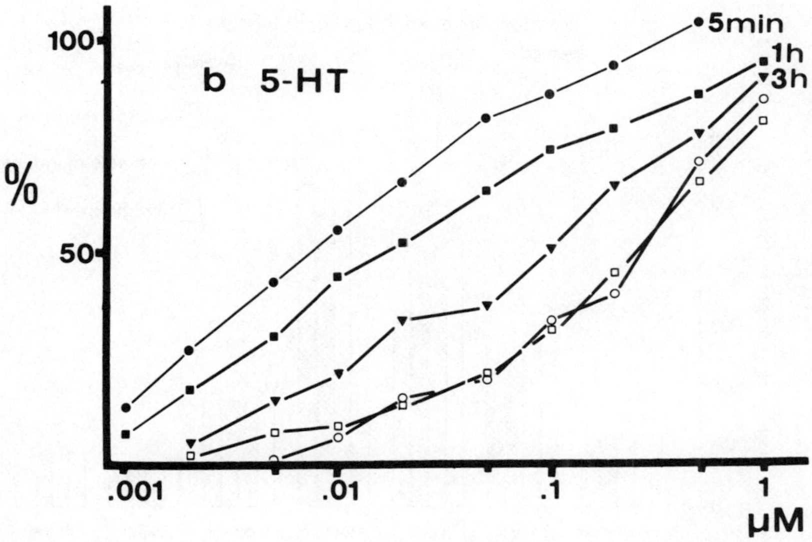

Fig. 2. Dose-response curves for serotonin (5-HT) on myenteric plexus-longitudinal muscle strips of naive or tolerant/dependent guinea pigs. Tolerant strips were exposed, after set up in Krebs-Ringer solution, to 200 nM normorphine to prevent withdrawal. Naive controls (○) were challenged with 5-HT. Tolerant strips were challenged in the presence of normorphine (□), 5 min after induction of withdrawal (50 nM naloxone) (●), and 1 (■) or 3 hrs (▼) after extensive washing in order to remove normorphine. The abscissa represents the drug concentration (μM) of 5-HT. The ordinate reflects tension in % of the preceding electrically induced twitches (Schulz and Herz, 1976).

to an abnormally high level (Sharma and others, 1975; Traber and others, 1975). Such high cAMP concentrations may affect the generation of excitatory action potentials (Gallagher and Shinnick-Gallagher, 1977). Efforts to demonstrate similar biochemical mechanisms in the central nervous system yielded less convincing results (Hamprecht, 1978).

These experiments disclose, however, that changes in neuronal sensitivity do become manifest during the state of opiate withdrawal. These facts have to be taken into consideration during the medical treatment of addicts undergoing withdrawal.

Endorphins and the State of Opiate Tolerance and Dependence

As a general rule, hormones and neurotransmitters are controlled by feed back mechanisms. Kosterlitz and Hughes (1975) proposed, therefore, that sustained administration of exogenous opiates would bring

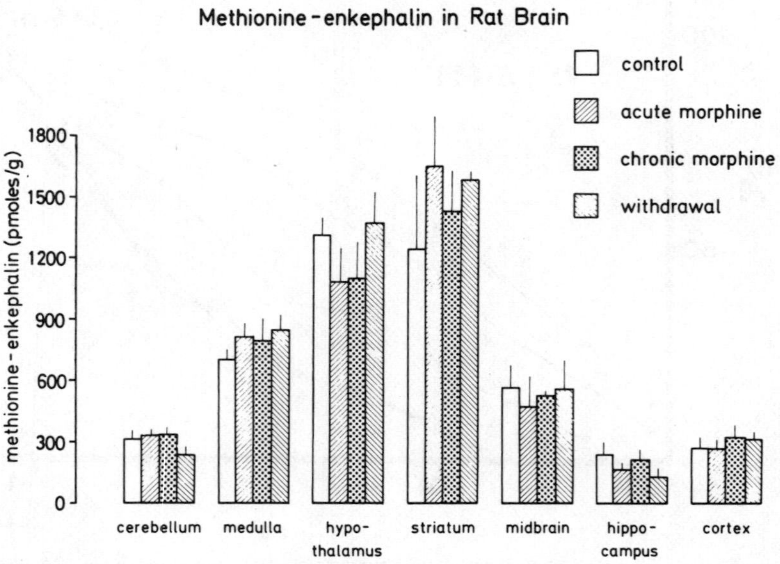

Fig. 3. Methionine-enkephalin in various regions of the rat brain. Each bar represents the mean value ± S.D. of 3-4 experiments. The radioimmunoassay was performed in triplicate (Wesche and others, 1977).

about reduced synthesis of endorphins. Examination of this hypothesis revealed that during the state of morphine tolerance and dependence the brain enkephalin concentration is unchanged (Childers and others, 1978; Wesche and others, 1977), as is also the case during withdrawal (Fig. 3). Nevertheless, since these experiments only investigated absolute levels, they provide no information about the turnover of enkephalins, which is essential to an evaluation of the functional state of the endorphinergic system.

Somewhat different results were obtained with respect to ß-endorphin. Although no changes were determined in the concentration of ß-endorphin immunoreactivity in plasma or pituitary of rats made tolerant/dependent within ten days, the induction of withdrawal in these animals significantly increased the concentration of ß-endorphin immunoreactivity in plasma and simultaneously decreased in the anterior lobe of the pituitary (Höllt and others, 1978). It appears likely that a release of ß-endorphin into the blood circulation occurs due to the stress of the rats undergoing withdrawal, as already reported in other stress situations (Rossier and others, 1977).

Further investigations focussed on the effect of long term opiate treatment on the content of ß-endorphin in the pituitary. Morphine given for four weeks considerably decreased ß-endorphin in the anterior as well as in the intermediate/posterior lobe of this organ (Fig. 4).

This finding is in line with postulated negative feed back loops caused by prolonged supply of an exogenous receptor agonist (that is, morphine). Thus, chronic opiate abuse may cause a deficiency of end-

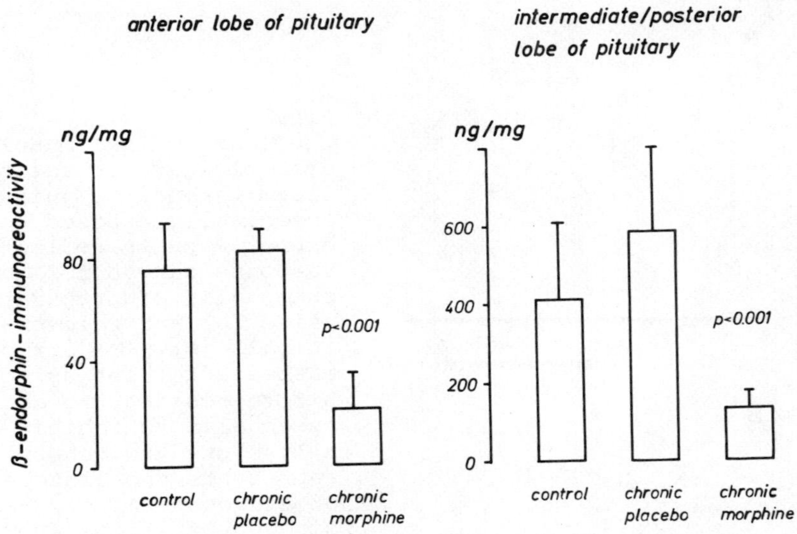

Fig. 4. Effect of long term administration of morphine to rats on the concentrations of ß-endorphin-like immunoreactivity in the anterior and intermediate/posterior lobes of pituitary. Bars indicate means ± S.D. (Höllt and others, 1978).

orphin (Goldstein, 1976), which might become manifest during acute and protracted abstinence. So far, the data support the concept that a "metabolic disease" may underly or at least contribute to the addictive state (Dole and Nyswander, 1967). One may speculate that the addict undergoing withdrawal requires a continuous supply or exogenous opiate in order to make up for the deficiency of ß-endorphin. One could imagine that such a deficiency may contribute to the high relapse rate of heroin addicts. However, if an insufficient endorphinergic system is already manifest in heroin addicts, then a blockage of opiate receptors by long term treatment with narcotic antagonists, suggested as a preventive measure against the resumption of heroin use (Martin, 1977), would be contraindicated. Recent investigations concerning long term treatment of animals with naloxone revealed significantly alterations in the endorphinergic system. Guinea pigs chronically exposed to naloxone exhibited an increased sensitivity of the myenteric plexus to opiates, which is due to an increase in the number of opiate receptors (Fig. 5). A similar phenomenon has been observed in rats which, after chronic exposure to naloxone, display an increased sensitivity to the antinociceptive effect of morphine (Tang and Collins, 1978). Thus, long term naloxone treatment could render heroin addicts even more susceptible to opiates, so that the need for endogenous (or exogenous) opiate would subsequently be increased. Parallel biochemical mechanisms upon chronic exposure to neuroleptics are obvious (Burt and others, 1977; Ezrin-Waters and Seeman, 1977).

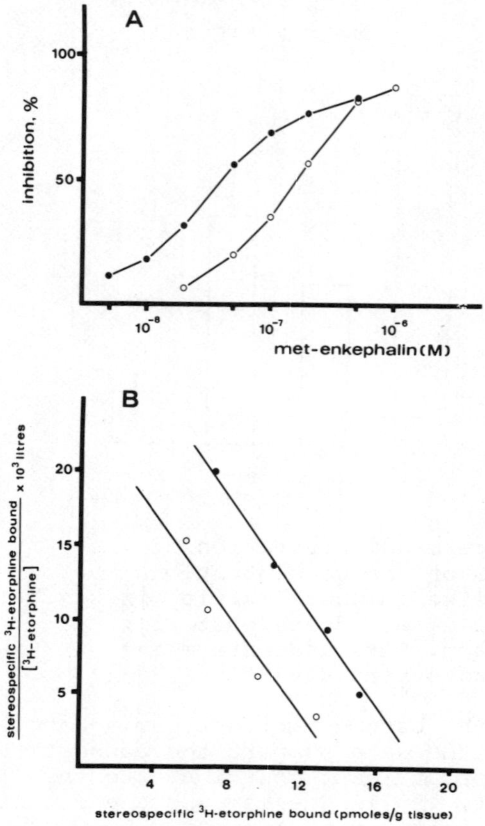

Fig. 5.
The longitudinal muscle/myenteric plexus preparation of the ileum taken from guinea pigs chronically exposed to naloxone. Panel A reflects dose-response curves for methionine-enkephalin of preparations from naive (o) and naloxone-treated animals (●). The strips were washed after set up for 3 hrs before testing the activity of enkephalin to inhibit electrically evoked twitches. Panel B represents the Scatchard plot of stereospecific ^{3}H-etorphine binding of strips from naive (o) and naloxone-treated animals undergoing the wash procedure described above (Schulz and others, submitted).

Conclusions

1. Pharmacological data have been provided indicating the existence of multiple opiate receptors. It is conceivable that specific opioids interact with specific opiate receptors. According to our present knowledge, however, the hope that synthetic derivatives of endorphins will combine with particular receptors which mediate analgesia but fail to induce tolerance and dependence appears unlikely.
2. Opiate tolerance and dependence are associated with a change in neuronal sensitivity. These changes become manifest only during the state of withdrawal. It is likely, therefore, that addicts undergoing withdrawal will exhibit unexpected responses to medical treatment affecting neuronal transmission.
3. Long term opiate treatment in rats causes a significant decrease of ß-endorphin immunoreactivity in the pituitary. By analogy, a similar deficiency of ß-endorphin may exist in heroin addicts, possibly contributing to the high relapse rate of such individuals. Prolonged treatment of patients with naloxone, originally proposed

as a preventative against resumption of heroin use, seems to be contraindicated, because chronic naloxone administration increases the sensitivity to opiates.

Acknowledgement

This work was supported by Deutsche Forschungsgemeinschaft.

REFERENCES

Akil, H., D. J. Mayer, and J. C. Liebeskind (1976). Antagonism of stimulation-produced analgesia by naloxone, a narcotic antagonist. Science, 191, 961-962.

Akil, H., D. E. Richardson, J. Hughes, and J. D. Barchas (1978). Enkephalin-like material elevated in ventricular cerebrospinal fluid of pain patients after analgetic focal stimulation. Science, 201, 463-465.

Beckett, A. H., and A. F. Casy (1954). Synthetic analgesics: Stereochemical considerations. J. Pharm. Pharmacol., 6, 986-1001.

Bläsig, J., and A. Herz (1976). Tolerance and dependence induced by morphine-like pituitary peptides in rats. Naunyn-Schmiedeberg's Arch. Pharmacol., 294, 297-300.

Bradbury, A. F., D. G. Smyth, C. R. Snell, N. J. M. Birdsall, and E. C. Hulme (1976). C fragment of lipotropin has a high affinity for brain opiate receptors. Nature, 260, 793-795.

Burt, D. R., J. Creese, and S. H. Snyder (1977). Antischizophrenic drugs: Chronic treatment elevates dopamine receptor binding in brain. Science, 196, 326-328.

Cheung, A. L., and A. Goldstein (1976). Failure of hypophysectomy to alter brain content of opioid peptides (Endorphins). Life Sci., 19, 1005-1008.

Childers, S. R., R. Schwarcz, J. T. Coyle, and S. H. Snyder (1978). Radioimmunoassay of enkephalins: Levels of methionine- and leucine-enkephalin in morphine-dependent and kainic acid-lesioned rat brains. In E. Costa, and M. Trabucchi (Eds.), Advances in Biochemical Psychopharmacology, Vol. 18, Raven Press, New York. pp. 161-173.

Dole, V. P., and M. Nyswander (1967). Heroin addiction - a metabolic disease. Arch. Intern. Med., 120, 19-24.

Ezrin-Waters, C., and P. Seeman (1977). Tolerance to haloperidol catalepsy. Europ. J. Pharmacol., 41, 321-327.

Frederickson, R. C. A. (1977). Enkephalin pentapeptides - a review of current evidence for a physiological role in vertebrate neurotransmission. Life Sci., 21, 23-42.

Gallagher, J. P., and P. Shinnick-Gallagher (1977). Cyclic nucleotides injected intracellularly into rat superior cervical ganglion cells. Science, 198, 851-852.

Goldstein, A., and R. Schulz (1973). Morphine-tolerant longitudinal muscle strip from guinea-pig ileum. Brit. J. Pharmacol., 48, 655-666.

Goldstein, A. (1976). Opioid peptides (Endorphins) in pituitary and brain. Science, 193, 1081-1086.

Gramsch, C., V. Höllt, P. Mehraein, A. Pasi, and A. Herz (1978). Endorphins in human brain. International Narcotic Research Conference, Noordwijkerhout, in press.

Hamprecht, B. (1978). Opiates and cyclic nucleotides. In A. Herz (Ed.), Developments in Opiate Research, Marcel Dekker, Inc., New York. pp. 357-406.

Henderson, G., J. Hughes, and H. W. Kosterlitz (1978). In vitro release of leu- and met-enkephalin from the corpus striatum. Nature, 271, 677-679.

Herz, A., and R. Schulz (1978). Changes in neuronal sensitivity during addictive processes. In J. Fishman (Ed.), The Bases of Addiction, Dahlem Konferenzen, Berlin. pp. 375-394.

Höllt, V., J. Dum, J. Bläsig, P. Schubert, and A. Herz (1975). Comparison of in vivo and in vitro parameters of opiate receptor binding in naive and tolerant/dependent rodents. Life Sci., 16, 1823-1828.

Höllt, V., R. Przewłocki, and A. Herz (1978). ß-Endorphin-like immunoreactivity in plasma, pituitaries and hypothalamus of rats following treatment with opiates. Life Sci., in press.

Hughes, J., T. W. Smith, H. W. Kosterlitz, L. A. Fothergill, B. A. Morgan, and H. R. Morris (1975). Identification of two related pentapeptides from the brain with potent opiate agonist activity. Nature, 258, 577-579.

Hutchinson, M., H. W. Kosterlitz, F. M. Leslie, A. A. Waterfield, and L. Terenius (1975). Assessment in the guinea-pig ileum and mouse vas deferens of benzomorphans which have strong antinociceptive activity but do not substitute for morphine in the dependent monkey. Brit. J. Pharmacol., 55, 541-546.

Iversen, L. L., S. D. Iversen, F. E. Bloom, T. Vargo, and R. Guillemin (1978). Release of enkephalin from rat globus pallidus in vitro. Nature, 271, 679-681.

Jacob, J. J., E. C. Tremblay, and M.-C. Colombel (1974). Facilitation de reactions nociceptives par la naloxone chez la souris et chez le rat. Psychopharmacologia (Berl.), 37, 217-223.

Kosterlitz, H. W., and J. Hughes (1975). Some thoughts on the significance of enkephalin, the endogenous ligand. Life Sci., 17, 91-96.

Lord, J. A. H., A. A. Waterfield, J. Hughes, and H. W. Kosterlitz (1976). Multiple receptors. In H. W. Kosterlitz (Ed.), Opiates and Endogenous Opioid Peptides, Elsevier/North-Holland Biomedical Press, Amsterdam. pp. 275-280.

Lord, J. A. H., A. A. Waterfield, J. Hughes, and H. W. Kosterlitz (1977). Endogenous opioid peptides: multiple agonists and receptors. Nature, 267, 495-499.

Lowney, L. J., K. Schulz, P. J. Lowery, and A. Goldstein (1974). Partial purification of an opiate receptor from mouse brain. Science, 183, 749-753.

Martin, W. R., C. G. Eades, J. A. Thompson, R. E. Huppler, and P. E. Gilbert (1976). The effect of morphine - nalorphine-like drugs in the nondependent and morphine-dependent chronic spinal dog. J. Pharmacol. exp. Ther., 197, 517-532.

Martin, W. R. (1977). In W. R. Martin (Ed.), Drug Addiction I, Springer Verlag, Berlin-Heidelberg-New York. pp. 298-312.

Osborne, H., V. Höllt, and A. Herz (1978). Potassium-induced release of enkephalins from rat striatal slices. Europ. J. Pharmacol., 48, 219-221.

Pasternak, G. W., and S. H. Snyder (1975). Identification of novel high affinity opiate receptor binding in rat brain. Nature, 253, 563-565.

Pert, C. B., and S. H. Snyder (1973). Opiate receptors: Demonstration in nervous tissue. Science, 179, 1011-1014.

Pomeranz, B., and D. Chiu (1976). Naloxone blockade of acupuncture analgesia: Endorphin implicated. Life Sci., 19, 1757-1762.

Porthogese, P. S. (1965). A new concept on the mode of interaction of narcotic analgesics with receptors. J. Med. Chem., 8, 609-616.

Rossier, J., E. D. French, C. Rivier, N. Ling, R. Guillemin, and F. Bloom (1977). Foot-shock induced stress increases ß-endorphin levels in blood but not brain. Nature, 270, 618-620.

Schulz, R., and A. Herz (1976). Aspects of opiate dependence in the myenteric plexus of the guinea-pig. Life Sci., 19, 1117-1128.

Schulz, R., and A. Herz (1977). Naloxone-precipitated withdrawal reveals sensitization to neurotransmitters in morphine tolerant/dependent rats. Naunyn-Schmiedeberg's Arch. Pharmacol., 299, 95-99.

Schulz, R., M. Wüster, R. Simantov, S. Snyder, and A. Herz (1977). Electrically stimulated release of opiate-like material from the myenteric plexus of the guinea pig ileum. Europ. J. Pharmacol., 41, 347-348.

Sharma, S. K., W. A. Klee, and M. Nirenberg (1975). Dual regulation of adenylate cyclase accounts for narcotic dependence and tolerance. Proc. Nat. Acad. Sci. USA, 72, 3092-3096.

Simon, E. J., J. M. Hiller, and J. Edelman (1973). Stereospecific binding of the potent narcotic analgesic ^{3}H-etorphine to rat brain homogenate. Proc. Nat. Acad. Sci. USA, 70, 1947-1949.

Simon, E. J., and J. M. Hiller (1978). In vitro studies on opiate receptors and their ligands. Fed. Proc., 37, 130-136.

Smith, A. A., R. Albin, and M. Crofford (1976). Heterogeneity of receptor for analgesia, respiration and lenticular effect. In H. W. Kosterlitz (Ed.), Opiates and Endogenous Opioid Peptides, Elsevier/North-Holland Biomedical Press, Amsterdam. pp. 289-294.

Tang, A. H., and R. J. Collins (1978). Enhanced analgesic effect of morphine after chronic administration of naloxone in the rat. Europ. J. Pharmacol., 47, 473-474.

Teschemacher, H. J. (1978). Endogenous ligands of opiate receptors (Endorphins). In A. Herz (Ed.), Developments in Opiate Research, Marcel Dekker, Inc., New York. pp. 67-151.

Traber, J., R. Gullis, and B. Hamprecht (1975). Influence of opiates on the levels of adenosine 3',5'-cyclic monophosphate in neuroblastoma x glioma hybrid cells. Life Sci., 16, 1863-1868.

Wei, E., and H. H. Loh (1976). Physical dependence on opiate-like peptides. Science, 193, 1262-1263.

Wesche, D., V. Höllt, and A. Herz (1977). Radioimmunoassay of enkephalins. Regional distribution in rat brain after morphine treatment and hypophysectomy. Naunyn-Schmiedeberg's Arch. Pharmacol., 301, 79-82.

Pharmacological Basis of Clinical Abuse of Sedative Drugs

H. COPER* and G. STILLE**

*Institut für Neuropsychopharmakologie der Freien Universität Berlin, Ulmenallee 30, 1000 Berlin 19, FRG
**Institut für Arzneimittel, Bundesgesundheitsamt, Berlin

ABSTRACT

In many industrialized countries 1 to 2 % of the population are misusing sedative drugs. Most addicts come to the abuse by prescription from their physician for a longer period. An intensive elucidation about the danger of chronical consumption can lead to a decreased use. Calculation of a "Relative Abuse Index" confirms the general experience that the dependence potential of opioids and stimulants is essentially higher compared to that of classical hypnotics and the latter is higher than that of benzodiazepines. Practically all substances which cause animals to perpetuate or increase self-injection are able to evoke psychic dependence in man and can be substituted by other similarly acting substances in order to avoid withdrawal symptoms. Under chronic use a mechanism must be set in motion which modifies not only vegetative reactions or motor-activity but feelings. These changes may be responsible for maintaining the consumption. Some arguments are collected on the hypothesis that one of the pharmacological bases of abuse of sedative drugs occurs by interference into the dopaminergic system.

INTRODUCTION

It is well-known that certain drugs evoke psychic effects which may cause an irresistable craving for these drugs.

Extensive research using pharmacological and psychological methods have been carried out in order to determine and to predict the dependence potential of therapeutically used drugs (for review see Isbell and Chrusciel, 1970; Kagan and others, 1975; Smith, 1977; Thompson and Unna, 1977). The main interest of these investigations still lies in the dependence on opioids.

As currently defined, abuse of sedative drugs does not raise distinctly social problems as abuse of opioids, stimulants or comparable drugs. Nevertheless, it is necessary to worry whether the present en masse-consumption, besides the consequences for the individuals, may create risks which have not yet been recognized. After all, in industrialized countries 1 to 2 % of the population is using sedative drugs and tranquilizers without medical indication (Allgulander, 1978;

Bayer, 1973; Falco, 1976; Maletzky and Klotter, 1976; Poser and others, 1974; Smith and Wesson, 1974; Stille, 1976; Thompson, 1977; Weise and Price, 1975). Nearly everywhere middle-class women about 45 years are most severely endangered (Bochnik, 1975; Chambers, 1972; Herud and others, 1975; Hofman and Kryspin-Exner, 1970; Laubenthal, 1964; Woodcock, 1970). Many dependents came to an abuse of sedative drugs by prescription from a physician for a longer period. Some studies therefore deal with the motivation in prescribing those substances. First of all, patients ask for a prescription and the physicians meet their demand. Additionally, very busy doctors want to shorten the consultation and/or avoid a confrontation with their patients' complaints and problems in prescribing those remedies (Kaufmann and others, 1972). In the meantime it could be demonstrated that after an intensive education about the dangers of chronic use, the number of prescriptions and, therefore, the use may diminish (Clift, 1972; Kaufmann and others, 1972; Maronde, 1969; Muller, 1972; v. Zerssen, 1968). On this occasion it was also demonstrated that many cases of dependence on sedative drugs are masked, even considering that the overlapping stage from use to abuse surely is flowing.

In man the evaluation of the dependence potential of abused drugs is based on experiences and on questionnaires. Even if considerable objections exist to the validity of an appropriate sequence for the different sedatives and also for other abused drugs, some observations give important references on that problem. Jones (1977) for example, has summarized in a list, collected by the "Drug Abuse Warning Networks", all reported cases of abuse and the total volume of prescriptions. From these data she formed a relative abuse-index. This index nearly corresponds to that established by Kielholz (1972), who has compared the number of all first-hospitalizations and first-consultations of drug-dependents from Swiss clinics in relation to the total volume of addictive drugs sold. Both studies came to nearly the same results; that means, diazepam is the drug most frequently abused, but it is also prescribed more often than other similarly acting substances. Jones (1977) reports a five-fold lower abuse-index for diazepam (0. 79) than for sekobarbital (4. 24), a substance which is more infrequently abused but also prescribed. The index for 4 benzodiazepines investigated does not differ significantly (diazepam 0. 79; flurazepam 0. 81, chlorazepate 0. 51 and chlordiazepoxid 0. 49) for methaqualon an index has been determined (2. 29) which is to be found between those of diazepam and sekobarbital.

These findings conform rather well with experimental self-application and substitution-studies in animals (Findley and others, 1972). It was also shown that the dependence potential of substances such as opiates and stimulants is much higher than that of the classical sedative drugs, and the potential of the latter is higher than that of benzodiazepines.

Despite development of new experimental models in animals and considerably extended detail-knowledge of symptomatology and epidemiology of dependence in man, the most important factors which initiate and maintain an abuse of drugs are unknown. Thus, the aim of all experimental research must be to find new conceptions and methods to elucidate causes and conditions of mastering the initiation of dependence.

Scientific progress does not only depend on more and more new data, but is also decided by examinating new hypotheses from already existing findings. Thus, in this review known results shall be summarized, arranged and critically evalua -

ted anew.

PHYSICAL DEPENDENCE

In a classical study of 1934, the abstinence symptoms of hypnotics in addicted man have been described by Pohlisch and Panse. It is noteworthy that in the American literature before 1950, only few similar descriptions are to be found. But in the fifties and sixties this problem gained more and more significance (Essig, 1964; Isbell, 1959; Smith and Wesson, 1974). In numerous investigations, different methods have been tested to quantify the particular symptoms in animals as well as to some extent in man, and to establish a standardized profile of abstinence syndromes with regard to intensity and duration, by varying dose and frequency of application (Bigelow and others, 1976).

It was found in these investigations that mode and intensity of abstinence syndromes are not so decisively determined by the pharmacodynamic of sedative drugs but more by their divergent elimination kinetics (Boisse and Okamoto, 1977; Stumpff and others, 1965; Wulff, 1960). For example, under same conditions, abstinence syndrome of pentobarbital is more distinctly marked than that of barbital. But, if the elimination of pentobarbital is retarded by respective substitution, the abstinence syndrome diminishes. Acceleration of the elimination of barbital by peritoneal dialysis, intensifies those abstinence syndromes (Okamoto, 1977). With regard to the kinetics, obviously all hypnotic drugs examined until now have the same physical dependence potential. Measured by the main indicators of abstinence (anorexia, irritability, loss of weight, and convulsions) Jones (1977) found the same dependence profile for pentobarbital and sekobarbital; that of methaqualon only deviates unsignificantly.

Although no comparative studies are available for the different benzodiazepines, it can be concluded from the frequency of withdrawal syndromes, the mode of the abstinence-symptomatology and the kinetics of these substances that the potential of physical dependence of minor tranquilizers does not differ significantly from that of barbiturates and non-barbiturate hypnotics (Essig, 1969). Surely, more additional specific information can be found, but new basic knowledge from the clinical point of view is scarcely to be expected in this field.

SUBSTITUTION

Also in applying substitution-tests not more than confirmation - perhaps certain modification - is to be achieved from the very often described finding that sedative drugs which cause physical dependence, may be substituted by other similarly acting substances in order to avoid withdrawal symptoms. Sedative drugs which do not show cross-tolerance or cross-dependence in substitution tests mostly possess a weak potential of dependence (Yanagita, 1977).

PSYCHIC DEPENDENCE

Even with knowledge about frequency and symptomatology of physical dependence of drugs and the ability to substitute them mutually, it cannot be determined which effect of the drug motivates man to take it compulsively and continously.
In animal experiments psychic dependence can only be imitated in analogue trials. Based on the hypothesis that the desire to take a drug non-medically is initiated

and maintained by pharmacodynamically induced psychic factors which also may be reproduced in animal experiments, it has been tested whether and under what conditions animals self-administer drugs, continue and even increase this self-application.

Practically all substances which cause animals to perpetuate or increase self-injection are able to evoke psychic dependence in man. Thus, through the application of such a test, the existence of abuse liability can be predicted, in principle. However, these procedures produce only a very limited range of quantitative data on the potential of psychic dependence, even if the abuse potential of sedative drugs and minor tranquilizers is distinctly less significant than that of opioids and stimulants.

Further considerations proceed from the thesis that all abused substances, even those which lead only to psychic dependence, have clearly defined dependence-producing pharmacodynamic actions. We think "liking", "craving" or "seeking" is the psychic expression of a pharmacologically induced disturbance in brain functions, which cannot yet be localized with certainty.

Although the quality of subjective feelings caused by sedative drugs, or by drugs, acting as depressants in certain doses (pentobarbital, chlorpromazin and alcohol -PCAG) differs from that of morphine and amphetamine (MBG) (Haertzen, 1966), it needs to be examined,whether they, after all, have some common pharmacological effects, which could explain their ability to cause dependence.

Positively coloured feelings after taking a drug are obviously not essential for their continuing use. Rather psychic dependence may develop on substances which produce reactions which are first considered as disagreable by non-addictive consumers. In this context, the investigations of Martin (1977) are very interesting. He found that people without drug-experience generally perceive the effects of amphetamine and pentobarbital as pleasing, but not those of morphine and heroine, whereas ex-users do not only perceive amphetamine and pentobarbital as pleasing but also morphine and heroine. Similar findings have been published by Lasagna and co-workers already in 1955.

Moreover, in self-application tests under certain conditions, monkeys continue or even increase aversive stimuli such as electro-shock (Kelleher and Morse, 1968). Also the postulate that alone the fear of abstinence-syndromes forces consumers to continue the use of drugs, seems to be doubtful, especially since at least "seeking" appears many hours before abstinence-symptoms begin.

In animals it is easy to demonstrate that the pattern of action of dependence-producing drugs changes after chronic treatment. In mice as well as in rats, tolerance to different depressant effects of morphine developed neither at the same rate nor to the same extent. Moreover, a much smaller shift of dose-response-curve to the right has been observed in case of several symptoms of stimulation as determined in the open field procedure (Fernandes and others, 1977 a; 1977 b). Similar observations have been reported by us using another experimental arrangement. When morphine is administered chronically to rats, the development of tolerance to catalepsy is accompanied with an increase of stereotypies and, in brain-lesioned animals, with appearance of intensive rotation. Also tolerance to two effects of diazepam and phenobarbital (anticonvulsant and incoordination in the rotarod test) develops to different degrees (Fuxe and others, 1975).

Already in 1950 Isbell and co-workers reported that subjects who chronically received increasing doses of barbiturates, became after an initial period of elation, disheveled, confused, irritable, quarrelsome, and belligerent. All these findings call to mind the fact that after chronic use in many cases sedative drugs are no longer sedating but stimulating.

In summary, under chronic use of addictive drugs a mechanism must be set in motion which modifies not only vegetative reactions or motor-activity but feelings. These changes may be responsible for maintaining the consumption, whereas in the individual case, it is not decisive, whether the effects are experienced as positive or not (review Mello, 1976).

Until now no review has been published in which the variations in the pattern of the particular qualities of drugs after chronic treatment are compared with the dependence potential of the respective substances.

In 1977 Dews again raised an old question which, however, has never been systematically examined: Why people do not abuse neuroleptics, antidepressants or even analeptics, although they have some effects which are also produced by hypnotics, tranquilizers, opioids, alcohol and stimulating drugs? A comparison of common and divergent qualities of action of those two groups results in the following: As far as has been investigated until now, abused sedative drugs (barbiturates, methaqualon, meprobamate, benzodiazepine) have four characteristics:

a) Administered acutely, they cause a dose-dependent anxiolysis, increased readiness to sleep and muscle relaxation (Stille and White, 1971).
b) Administered chronically they change the mode of action, namely the depressant components decrease.
c) The EEG shows a shift towards higher frequencies, especially in ß-rhythm; in man the frequencies of 15-20 Hz are affected (Fink, 1964; Itil, 1971; Saletu, 1976), in animals the higher frequencies (Giurgea and Moeyersoons, 1964; Joy and others, 1971; Schallek and others, 1965; Schallek and others, 1968). This accelerated activity starts in the forebrain area and then extends to the partietal and occipital region. This effect is interpreted by neurophysiologists as increased vigilance, and may explain the described stimulating effects of barbiturate, methaqualon and benzodiazepines.
d) They inhibit electric excitability of the limbic system, especially in the nucleus amygdala and hippocampus (inhibition of electric after-discharge and arousal after electric stimulation) (Arrigo and others, 1965; Olds and Olds, 1969; Schallek and Kuehn, 1965; Schallek and others, 1964; Tsuchiya and Kitagawa, 1976).

Thus, in a certain sense, barbiturates, methaqualon, meprobamate and benzodiazepines pronounce a dissoziation of different brain functions. Especially methaqualon users characterize the combination of relaxation and ecstatic feelings as seductively pleasant. In order to fully enjoy this effect, they try with all their energy to fight against sleep (Stille, 1976). It is remarkable in this context that a similar increase of ß-frequencies is also to be found in centrally anticholinergic substances (Fink, 1964; Klett and Johnson, 1957; Saletu, 1976) and antihistaminics (Goldstein and others, 1968; Saletu, 1976). After anticholinergics, the increased vigilance leads in extreme cases to restlessness accompanied with alterations in consciousness and delirant states (Vojtechovsky and others, 1966). Remarkably, Mandrax, a combination of methaqualon with diphenhydramine, is more frequently abused than methaqualon alone. Thus, an interesting question is to what extent central-anticholinergics intensify the stimulating effects of methaqualon and other sedative drugs on the ß-frequency in the EEG. Antipsychotics, especially neuroleptics, also possess, particularly in non-psychotic patients, depressant and anticholinergic properties. But, the inhibition of electric excitability of limbic systems and the increase of ß-frequencies in the EEG is missing (Saletu, 1976; Schallek and Kuehn, 1965). Rather a decrease of vigilance is observed. Instead, a raised excitability of the striatal system accompanied with akinesia, catalepsy, and rigor is predominent (Stille, 1971). General depression with such mode of motoric immobilization obviously does not lead to positively perceived relaxation and is even experienced as dysphoric.

Since the increased excitability of the striatal system after neuroleptics is based on blocking the dopaminergic inhibitory afferences it is to be considered whether this effect is connected with the missing abuse of these substances. Noteworthy, too, is the effect that dopaminergic substances like amphetamine or cocaine have a high potential of psychic dependence. Also morphine has, even if hidden, dopaminergic effects as well especially with repeated application (Kuschinsky, 1977), a finding that can be deduced from stereotypies and circling of unilaterally lesioned rats (Stille, 1978, unpublished). Carlsson and co-workers (1972) as well as Bustos and Roth (1976) described an enhanced impulse-flow in the nigrostriatal system with increased dopamine turnover with ethanol. Only benzodiazepines are incompatible with this system. They diminish in acute trial the dopamine turnover in corpus striatum (Taylor and Laverty, 1969). Probably in chronic treatment, the effect on the dopaminergic nigrostriatal system reverses.

In this context it is interesting that the strongly dopaminergic receptor blocking pimozide causes a dose-related (0.0625 to 0. 5 mg/kg) increase in the frequency of self-administration rate of cocaine; at higher doses self-administration did not occur. These effects of pimozide seem parallel to those of reward reduction and reward determination in general, and thus, suggest an important role of dopaminergic brain mechanisms in the mediation of cocaine reinforcement (DeWit and Wise, 1977).

However, with intervention in the dopaminergic systems alone no convincing concept of the whole mechanism of psychic dependence development can be deduced. But the discovery of a dopaminergic reward system in the medial forebrain bundle brought a further argument for a dopamine hypothesis of dependence (Stille, 1977; Ungerstedt, 1971).

Although not much noticed, the clinical observation seems important that the potential of psychic dependence on addictive drugs of patients with endogenous psychic diseases is significantly small compared to that of healthy persons or, for example, in patients with cancer.

During the pre-neuroleptic period, within which treatment of psychotic patients with relatively high doses of an extract of opium alkaloids or morphine occurred, only one single case of dependence came to be known (Burchard. 1967; Schmitz, 1926).

Gelma (1952) thought that he could interrupt the autism of longlasting heavy schizophrenics by inducing a morphine-craving in them. He presumed that they, like "normal" addicts, have to be forced by their dependence to provide morphine come what may. But disappointedly, Gelma had to realize that this presumption could not be substantiated. Moreover, he found that his patients in general showed only minor abstinence symptoms after withdrawal from the relatively high morphine doses.

This year these observations have been confirmed by Schrappe. Some of his patients reached doses of 300 mg morphine daily, a dose which in non-schizophrenics would provoke severe abstinence-symptomes after an immediate withdrawal. It remains to be considered that one characteristic of schizophrenic final states is a vegetative rigidity and torpidness; thus, counterregulations such as described in Himmelsbach's theory (1942; 1943) are hardly possible. However, Schrappe (1978) also has treated cyclic depressions (in former times the main indication for opiods) with methadone. In these patients the vegetative reactions are generally not changed, and the expected abstinence-symptoms appear. On the other hand, they never showed addictive behaviour like seeking and craving, i. e., a dissoziation of psychic and physical dependence occurs. It seems, therefore, that psychic diseases, and in particular parkinsonism, are connected to a resistence against development of psychic dependence on addictive drugs.

Another indication on the connexion between dopaminergic systems and addiction may be achieved from observations in treatment of alcoholics and addicts depending on other drugs with apomorphine (Amitai and others, 1972; Beil and others, 1977; Feldmann, 1952 a; 1952 b; Hedri, 1972; Schlatter and others, 1972). As Beil (1977) reported positive effects of apomorphine treatment are impressive: withdrawal symptoms which occur at the beginning are tolerated by the patient; the need for the drug (barbiturate, diazepam, tilidine) or alcohol vanishes after 4 days, anxieties are reduced and a general tranquility takes place. The personality of the patient tends to be reconstructed and all patients report an aversion against alcohol or the other drugs, respectively. In most cases normal sleep returned without sedatives in the course of the first two weeks. The apomorphine doses used are below the nausea threshold. Apomorphine stimulates dopamine-receptors. At least it seems to be possible that in psychic dependent patients apomorphine may provide a substitute for some dopaminergic effects of amphetamine, alcohol or tilidine. Probably, with such a "saturation" of the dopaminergic reward-system, the craving for the addictive drugs is attenuated.

Our persual of the pharmacological literature on the mechanism of the development of psychic dependence on sedative drugs led us to the dopaminergic system. Evidence for its participation remains to be found. Rather, it seems to be unlikely that the somatic causes of dependence are based on the influence of only one single transmitter system. The mediation and processing of impulses and, therefore, of information in the brain, involves various transmitters which are complexly interrelated with eachother. Thus, our hypothesis is to be understood as a stimulus to confirm, to modify or even to contradict such ideas.

REFERENCES

Allgulander, C. (1978). Dependence on Sedative and Hypnotic Drugs. A Comparative Clinical and Social Study. Acta Psychiat. Scand., Suppl. 270. Munksgaard, Copenhagen.

Amitai, M., H. Dickhaut, and P. Hasenknopf (1972). Behandlung des Entzugs-Syndromes bei "Fixern". Der Nervenarzt, 42, 157.

Arrigo, A., G. Jann, and P Tonali (1965). Some aspects of the action of valium and of librium on the electrical activity of the rabbit brain. Arch. int. Pharmacodyn., 154, 364.

Bayer, J. (1973). The abuse of psychotropic drugs. Bull. Narcotics, 25/3, 11-25.

Beil, H. and Trojan, A. (1977). The use of apomorphine in the treatment of alcoholism and other addictions:Results of a general practitioner. Brit. J. Add., 72, 129.

Bigelow, G., R. Griffiths, and I. Liebson(1976). Experimental Human Drug Self-Administration:Methodology and Application to the Study of Sedative Drugs. Pharmacol. Rev., 27/4, 523-531.

Bochnik, H. J. (1975). Zur Psychiatrie der Schlafstörungen. In H. Kaiser (ed.), Der gestörte Schlaf, Ärzteverlag, Köln. pp. 54-72.

Boisse, N. R. and M. Okamoto (1978). Physical Dependence to Barbital Compared to Pentobarbital. IV. Influence of Elimination Kinetics. J. Pharmacol. exp. Ther., 204/3, 526-539.

Burchard, J. M. (1967). Opiumtherapie und moderne Psychopharmaka. Arzneimittelforschung, 1-12, 557-561.

Bustos, G. and R. H. Roth (1976) Effect of acute ethanol treatment on transmitter synthesis and metabolism in central dopaminergic neurons. J. Pharm. Pharmac., 28, 580.

Carlsson, A., J. Engel, and Th. Svensson (1972). Inhibition of ethanol-induced excitation in mice and rats by α-methyl-p-tyrosine. Psychopharmacologia (Berl.), 26, 307.

Chambers, C. D. (1972). An assessment of drug use in general population. In J. Susman, Ed.), Drug Use and Social Policy:An AMS Anthology, AMS Press, New York. pp. 50-123.

Clift, A. D. (1972). Factors leading to dependence on hypnotic drugs. Brit. Med. J., III, 614-617.

Dews, P. (1977). Remarks. In T. Thompson and K. R. Unna (Eds.), Predicting Dependence Liability of Stimulants and Depressant Drugs. University Park Press, Baltimore, London, Tokyo. pp. 75-80.

Essig, C. F. (1964). Addiction to nonbarbiturate sedative and tranquilizing drugs. Clin. Pharmacol. Ther., 5/3, 334-343.

Essig, C. F. (1969). The potential risk of addiction to nonbarbiturate sedative and minor tranquilizing drugs. In F. Sjöqvist and M. Tottie (Eds.), Abuse of central stimulants, Almqvist and Wiksell, Stockholm. pp. 89-112.

Falco, M. (1976). Methaqualone misuse: Foreign experience and United States drug control policy. Int. J. Addictions, 11/4, 597-610.

Feldmann, H. (1952a). Le traitement de l'alcoolisme chronique par l'apomorphine -Etude de 500 cas. Praxis, 41, 571.

Feldmann, H. (1952b). L'equilibre humeral dans le traitement de l'alcoolisme chronique par l'apomorphine. Rev. Med. Suisse Romande, 72, 205.

Feldmann, H. (1959). The ambulatory treatment of alcoholic addicts-A study of 250 cases. Brit. J. Add., 55, 121.

Fernandes, M., S. Kluwe, and H. Coper (1977a). The development of tolerance to morphine in the rat. Psychopharmacology, 54, 197-201.

Fernandes, M., S. Kluwe, and H. Coper (1977b). Quantitative assessment of tolerance to and dependence on morphine in mice. Naunyn-Schmiedeberg's Arch. Pharmacol., 297, 53-60.

Findley, J. D., W. W. Robinson, and L. Peregrino (1972). Addiction to sekobarbital and chlordiazepoxide in the rhesus monkey by means of a self-infusion preference procedure. Psychopharmacologia (Berl.), 26, 93-114.

Fink, M. (1960). Effect of anticholinergic compounds on postconvulsive electroencephalogram and behavior of psychiatric patients. Electroenceph. clin. Neurophysiol., 12, 359.

Fink, M. (1964). A selected bibliography of electroencephalography in human psychopharmacology 1951-1962. Electroenceph. clin. Neurophysiol. suppl. 23.

Fuxe, K., L. F. Agnati, P. Bolme, T. Hokfelt, P. Lidbrink, A. Ljungdahl, M. Perez, and S. Ogren (1975). The possible involvement of GABA mechanisms in the action of benzodiazepines on central catecholaime neurons. Adv. Biochem. Psychopharmacol., 14, 45-61.

Gelma, E. (1952). Note sur la facon de réagir des schizophrènes à l'égard de la morphinisation. Cahiers psychiatr., 8, 15.

Giurgea, C. and F. Moeyersoons (1964). L'effet initial de certaines drogues psychotropes sur l'EEG:Phenomène d'amplification du rythme rapide. Int. J. Neuropharmacol., 3, 579.

Goldstein, L. (1968). Comparative study of EEG effects of antihistamines in normal volunteers. J. clin. Pharmacol., 8, 42.

Haertzen, C. A. (1966). Development of scales based on pattern of drug effects, using the addiction research center inventory (ARCI). Psychological Reports, 18, 163-194.

Hedri, A. (1972). Apomorphine bei der Opiat-Entziehungskur. Praxis, 61, 488.

Herud, W. F., W. Nickolai, and B. Schmidtbreick (1975). Erhebung über Gebrauch und Mißbrauch von Schlaf- und Beruhigungsmitteln. Suchtgefahren, 21, 56-61.

Himmelsbach, C. K. (1942). Clinical studies of drug addiction, physical dependence, withdrawal and recovery. Arch. int. Med., 69, 766-772.

Himmelsbach, C. K. (1943). With reference to physical dependence. Fed. Proc., 2, 201.

Hofman, G. and K. Kryspin-Exner (1970). Medikamentenabhängigkeit bzw. -sucht im Krankengut der Wiener Psychiatrisch-Neurologischen Universitätsklinik unter besonderer Berücksichtigung der Psychopharmaka. Arzneim. -Forsch., 7, 871-873.

Isbell, H. (1959). Addiction to hypnotic and sedative drugs. Association of Food and Drug Officials of the United States. Vol. XXIII, No. 1, 36-43.

Isbell, H., S. Altschul, C. H. Kornetzky, A. J. Eisenman, H. G. Flanary, and H. F. Fraser (1950). Chronic barbiturate intoxication. Arch. Neurol. Psychiat., July-vol., 1-27.

Isbell, H. and T. L. Chrusciel (1970). Dependence liability of "non-narcotic" drugs. Bull. Wld. Hlth. Org., Suppl. to Vol. 43, 1-111.

Itil, T., P. Gannon, R. Cora, S. Polvan, F. Akpinar, L. Veres, and E. Eskazan (1971). Sch-12. 041, a new anti-anxiety agent (Quantitative pharmaco-electroencephalography and clinical trials). Physicians' Drug Manual, 3, 26.

Jones, B. E. jr. (1977). Predicting abuse liability of depressant drugs. In T. Thompson and K. R. Unna (Eds.), Predicting Dependence Liability of Stimulants and Depressant Drugs. University Park Press, Baltimore, London, Tokyo. pp. 35-46.

Joy, R. M. (1971). A quantitative electroencephalagraphic comparison of some benzodiazepines in the primate. Neuropharmacology, 10, 483.

Kagan, F., T. Harwood, K. Rickels, R. Rudzik and H. Sorer (1975). Hypnotics, Methods of Development and Evaluation. Spectrum Publications, New York.

Kaufman, A., P. W. Brickner, R. Varner, and W. Mashburn (1972). Tranquilizer Control. J. Amer. Med. Ass., 221, 1504-1506.

Kelleher, R. T. and W. H. Morse (1968). Schedules using noxious stimuli. III. Responding maintained with response-produced electric shocks. J. Exp. Anal. Behav., 11, 819-838.

Kielholz, P. (1973). In Psychiatrie der Gegenwart, II. p. 504.

Klett, G. A. and M. W. Johnson (1957). Effect of atropine and scopolamine upon electroencephalographic changes induced by electro-convulsive therapy. Electroenceph. clin. Neurophysiol., 9, 217.

Kuschinsky, K. (1977). Opiate Dependence. G. Fischer Verlag, Stuttgart.

Lasagna, L., J. M. von Felsinger and H. K. Beecher (1955). Drug-induced mood changes in man. 1. Observations on healthy subjects, chronically ill patients, and "postaddicts". J. Amer. Med. Ass., 157, 1006-1020.

Laubenthal, F. (1964). Allgemeine Probleme um Mißbrauch, Süchtigkeit und Sucht. In F. Laubenthal (Ed.), Sucht und Mißbrauch, G. Thieme Verlag, Stuttgart.

Maletzky, B. M. and J. Klotter (1976). Addiction to diazepam. Int. J. Addictions, 11, 95-115.

Maronde, R. F., D. Burks II., P. V. Lee, P. Light, M. M. McCarron, M. McCary, and S. Seibert (1969). Physician Prescribing Practises. Amer. J. Hospital Pharmacy, 26, 566-572.

Martin, W. R. (1977). Assessment of depressant abuse potentiality. In T. Thompson and K. R. Unna (Eds.), Predicting Dependence Liability of Stimulant and Depressant Drugs, University Park Press, Baltimore, London, Tokyo. pp. 9-16.

Mello, N. K. (1977). Stimulus self-administration: Some implications for the prediction of drug abuse liability. In T. Thompson and K. R. Unna (Eds.), Predicting Dependence Liability of Stimulant and Depressant Drugs, University Park Press Baltimore, London, Tokyo. pp. 243-260.

Muller, C. (1972). The overmedicated society: Forces in the market-place for medical care. Science (Washington), 176/4034, 488-492.

Okamoto, M. (1977). Physical Dependency Characteristics of a Long-Acting Barbiturate, Barbital, Compared to the Short-Acting Pentobarbital. In T. Thompson and K. R. Unna (Eds.), Predicting Dependence Liability of Stimulants and Depressant Drugs, University Park Press, Baltimore, London, Tokyo. pp. 57-74.

Olds, M. E. and J. Olds (1969). Effects of anxiety-relieving drugs on unit discharges in hippocampus, reticular midbrain, and pre-optic area in the freely moving rat. Int. J. Neuropharmacol., 8, 87.

Pohlisch, K. and F. Panse (1934). Schlafmittelmißbrauch. Georg Thieme, Leipzig.

Poser, W., S. Poser, and M. Echternkamp (1974). Mißbrauch bromhaltiger Schlaf- und Beruhigungsmittel. Dtsch. med. Wschr., 99, 2489-2497.

Saletu, B. (1976). Psychopharmaka, Gehirntätigkeit und Schlaf. Bibliotheca Psychiatrica No. 155, G. Karger, Basel.

Smith, C. M. (1977). The pharmacology of sedative/hypnotics, alcohol and anesthetics: Sites and mechanisms of action. In W. R. Martin (Ed.), Drug Addiction I, Handbook of Experimental Pharmacology, Springer Verlag, Berlin, Heidelberg, New York. pp. 413-587.

Smith, D. E. and D. R. Wesson (1974). Drugs of Abuse 1973: Trends and Developments. Ann. Rev. Pharmacol., Vol. 14, 513-520.

Schallek, W., F. Zabransky, and A. Kuehn (1964). Effects of benzodiazepines on central nervous system of cat. Arch. int. Pharmacodyn., 149, 467.

Schallek, W. and A. Kuehn (1965). An action of mogadon on the amygdala of the cat. Med. Pharmacol. exp., 12, 204.

Schallek, W. and A. Kuehn (1965). Effects of benzodiazepines in spontaneous EEG and arousal responses of cats. In K. Akert (Ed.), Progress in Brain Research, Vol. 18, Sleep Mechanisms, Elsevier Publishing Company, Amsterdam.

Schallek, W., T. Levinson, and J. Thomas (1968). Power spectrum analysis as a tool for statistical evaluation of drug effects on electrical activity of brain. Int. J. Neuropharmacol., 7, 35.

Schlatter, E. K. E. and S. Lal (1972). Treatment of alcoholism with Dent's oral apomorphine method. Quarterly J. Study Alcohol, 33, 430.

Schmitz, H. (1926). Die Opiumbehandlung bei Geisteskrankheiten, insbesondere bei Melancholie, ihre Geschichte, ihr heutiger Stand und eigene Erfahrungen. Allg. Zschr. f. Psychiatr., 83, 92-113.

Schrappe, O. (1976). Abhängigkeit - Symptom oder Krankheit? In W. Keup (Ed.) Sucht als Symptom, 2. Wiss. Symp. der DHS, Bad Kissingen, Thieme, Stuttgart. pp. 29-37.

Stille, G. (1978), unpublished.

Stille, G. (1971). Zur Pharmakologie katatonigener Stoffe. Editio Cantor, Aulendorf.

Stille, G. (1976). Methaqualon-Mißbrauch, ein ernstes Problem. Dtsch. Ärzteblatt, 73, 959-962.

Stille, G. (1977). Früherfassung des Abhängigkeitspotentials bei neuen Arzneimitteln. In G. Fülgraff (Ed.), Bewertung von Risiken für die Gesundheit, Fischer Verlag.

Stille, G. and T. White (1971). Correlation between pharmacology and clinic. In O. Vinar, Z. Votava, and P. B. Bradley (Eds.), Advances in Neuro-Pharmacology, North-Holland Publishing Company, Amsterdam.

Stumpff, Ch. and J. Chiari (1965). Echte Gewöhnung an Hexobarbital. Naunyn-Schmiedeberg's Arch. exp. Path. Pharmak., 251, 275-287.

Taylor, K. M. and R. Laverty (1969). The chlordiazepoxide, diazepam and nitrazepam catecholamine metabolism in regions of brain. Europ. J. Pharmacol., 8,296

Thompson, T. (1977) Predicting abuse liability of sedatives and stimulants. In T. Thompson and K. R. Unna (Eds.), Predicting Dependence Liability of Stimulant and Depressant Drugs, University Park Press, Baltimore, London, Tokyo, pp. 1-8.

Thompson, T. and K. R. Unna (1977). Predicting Dependence Liability of Stimulant and Depressant Drugs, University Park Press, Baltimore, London, Tokyo.

Tsuchiya, T. and S. Kitagawa (1976) Effects of benzodiazepines and pentobarbital on the evoked potentials in the cat brain. Japan J. Pharmacol., 26, 411.

Ungerstedt, U. (1971). Stereotaxic mapping of the monoamine pathways in the rat brain. Acta Physiol. Scand., Suppl. 367.

Vojtechovsky, M., V. Vitek, and K. Rysanek (1966). Experimentelle Psychose nach Verabreichung von Benactyzin. Arzneim.-Forsch., 16, 240-242.

Weise, C. E. and S. F. Price (1975). The Benzodiazepines - Patterns of Use. In R. J. Hall (Ed.), Bibliographic Series No. 9, Addiction Res. Found., Toronto.

deWit, H. and R. A. Wise (1977). Blockade of cocaine reinforcement in rats with the dopamine receptor blocker pimozide, but not with the noradrenergic blockers phentolamine or phenoxybenzamine. Canad. J. Psychol./Rev. Canad. Psychol., 31/4, 195-203.

Woodcock, J. (1970). Long-term consumers of psychotropic drugs. In M. Balint, J. Hunt and others (Eds.), A Study of Repeat Prescriptions in General Practise, Tvistock Publications, J. B. Lippincott Co., Philadelphia, Appendix. pp. 147-176.

Wulff, M. H. (1960). The barbiturate withdrawal syndrome. A clinical and electroencephalographic study, In Electroencephalography and Clinical Neuropharmacology, Suppl. 14, Munksgaard, Copenhagen.

Yanagita, T. (1977). Methodological considerations in testing physical dependence potential of sedative-hypnotics in animals. In T. Thompson and K. R. Unna (Eds.) Predicting Dependence Liability of Stimulant and Depressant Drugs, University Park Press, Baltimore, London-Tokyo. pp. 47-55.

v. Zerssen, D., E. Stephan, and J. Kaiser (1968). Der Schlafmittelmißbrauch und seine Verhütung. Nervenarzt, 10, 459-464.

Reinforcement Mechanisms of Stimulant Drugs

L. P. GONZALEZ and E. H. ELLINWOOD, JR.

Behavioral Neuropharmacology Section, Department of Psychiatry,
Duke University Medical Center, Durham, N.C., U.S.A.

ABSTRACT

Studies of stimulant self-administration and electrical self-stimulation of central dopamine sites are reviewed as they relate to mechanisms of stimulant reinforcement. Pharmacological manipulations which alter dopaminergic function alter the reinforcement value of self-administered stimulants, suggesting that CNS stimulants reinforce behavior through their effects on central dopaminergic systems. A further implication of the involvement of dopamine pathways in the mediation of reinforcement is their ability to maintain responding for electrical stimulation. Although the methods of drug self-administration and electrical self-stimulation have been somewhat limited in their application to the study of stimulant reinforcement, these techniques do provide a useful means by which to study basic mechanisms of reinforcement as well as questions of substance abuse and drug-seeking behavior.

KEY WORDS reinforcement mechanisms, drug self-administration, electrical self-stimulation, CNS stimulants

INTRODUCTION

One of the most prominent characteristics of CNS stimulants is their ability to support self-administration behavior in animals and man. While the determinants of human drug abuse are complex interactions of psychological societal, and physiological factors, the specific characteristics of certain drug classes make these substances particularly amenable to abuse.

The mechanisms of action of the stimulant drugs have recently been reviewed by several authors, but few have examined the central mechanisms by which CNS stimulants act to reinforce behavior. This paper examines the role of central catecholamine systems in the mediation of the reinforcing properties of the stimulant drugs.

STIMULANT SELF-ADMINISTRATION

A variety of animal studies have demonstrated that injections of psychomotor stimulants which are contingent upon the occurrence of specific behavior patterns can serve to reinforce the acquisition and maintenance of those behaviors. This technique provides a useful means for indicating the abuse potential of new drugs and is uniquely suited for studies of the reinforcing properties of drugs.

While drug self-administration by oral (Zabik and Lal, 1970) and intragastric (Altshuler, Weaver, and Phillips, 1975) routes has been demonstrated, the majority of studies examining the psychomotor stimulants have used the intravenous route of administration. This procedure was first developed by Weeks (1962) to allow rats to self-infuse drugs through chronic indwelling vascular catheters. Thompson and Schuster (1964) then adapted the technique for use in the rhesus monkey. The self-administration of stimulants was reported soon thereafter (Deneau, Yanagita, and Seevers, 1964; Pickens and Thompson, 1968; Woods and Schuster, 1968).

The pattern of drug intake observed in animals self-administering intravenous cocaine or amphetamine (Deneau, Yanagita, and Seevers, 1969; Johanson, Balster, and Bonese, 1976) is similar to patterns of human drug use (Griffith, 1966; Kramer, Fischman, and Littlefield, 1967). Fenfluramine, a ring-substituted amphetamine analogue, is not self-administered by rats (Baxter, Gluckman, and Scerni, 1973; Gotestam and Anderson, 1975), monkeys (Woods and Tessel, 1974), or baboons (Griffiths and others, 1976), and its potential for human abuse seems low (Griffiths and others, 1976).

TABLE 1 Animal Self-administration of Stimulants and Sympathomimetic Amines

Administered	
d-Amphetamine	Methylenedioxyamphetamine
l-Amphetamine	Methylphenidate
Apomorphine	Nicotine
Caffeine	β-Phenylethylaminene
Clortermine	Phenmetrazine
Chlorphentermine	Phentermine
Cocaine	Pipradrol
Diethylpropion	Piribedil (EI-495)
Fencamfamin	SPA
Methamphetamine	Tranylcypromine
Not Administered	
Fenfluramine	
Pemoline	

This similarity between animal and human behavior has been presented as a verification of the use of animal self-administration as a model of human drug abuse (Balster and Schuster, 1977; Johanson and Schuster, 1977). In general, animals self-administer the same drugs (Table 1) that are abused by humans (Deneau, Yanagita, and Seevers, 1969; Schuster and Thompson, 1969; Schuster and Johanson, 1974; Woods and Tessel, 1974); however, animals will also initiate self-administration of drugs which are typically not abused by man. The dopamine-receptor stimulant apomorphine, for example, is self-administered by rats (Baxter and others, 1974; Roberts, Corcoran, and Fibiger, 1977; Yokel and Wise, 1978) and by squirrel monkeys (Gill, Holz, and Zirkle, 1975), but is not abused by man. Rats have also been shown to self-administer haloperidol (Glick and Cox, 1975) and chlorphentermine (Baxter, Gluckman, and Scerni, 1973), although neither drug is a major substance of abuse in man. Chlorphentermine, in fact, is reported to lack the euphoric effects that most CNS stimulants produce in man (Griffith, 1977).

The major uses of the self-administration technique have been in the establishment of procedures for determining the abuse potential of drugs (Brady, Griffiths, and Winger, 1975; Griffiths and others, 1975; Griffiths, Snell, and Brady, 1976; Johanson and Schuster, 1975; Thompson and Unna, 1977; Yanagita, 1973), and in studying the response characteristics of behavior reinforced by drug administration (Goldberg and Kelleher, 1977). In addition, some investigators have used the self-administration paradigm to compare the reinforcement characteristics of various drugs, or for studies of the mechanisms of action of psychoactive drugs.

The relative reinforcing potency of drugs has been examined in choice procedures in which animals can select between several drugs or drug doses (Balster and Schuster, 1977; Johanson and Schuster, 1975). Similar information has been provided by studies of response cost, or the breaking point of increasing work effort (that is, in the number of responses required for drug administration) beyond which an animal will no longer perform to obtain drug (Brady and Griffiths, 1977). These studies have confirmed the strength of amphetamine-like drugs as reinforcers, but they have not addressed questions of reinforcement mechanisms.

The results of self-administration studies which have examined the mechanisms of action of cocaine and amphetamine generally support the notion that the reinforcing properties of those drugs are mediated through central catecholaminergic systems. The effects of pharmacological manipulation of monoamine functioning are summarized in Tables 2 and 3.

TABLE 2 Effects of Monoamine Potentiation upon Stimulant Self-administration

	Effects on SA[1]	
Re-Uptake Blockade		
Imipramine	↓	Cocaine
MAO Inhibition		
Pargyline	↓	Cocaine
DBH Inibition		
Diethyldithiocarbamate (DDC)	↓	Amphetamine
1-phenyl-3-(2-thiazolyl)-2-thiourea (U-14,624)	↓	Amphetamine
Precursor Loading		
1-Dopa	N.E.	Amphetamine

1 ↑ indicates increase in self-administration
↓ indicates decrease in self-administration
N.E. indicates no effect on self-administration

The results of self-administration studies which have examined the mechanisms of action of cocaine and amphetamine generally support the notion that the reinforcing properties of those drugs are mediated through central catecholaminergic systems. The effects of pharmacological manipulation of monoamine functioning are summarized in Tables 2 and 3.

TABLE 3 Effects of Catecholamine Inhibition upon Stimulant Self-administration

	Effects on SA[1]
Tyrosine Hydroxylase Inhibition	
α-methyl-p-tryosine	↑ Amphetamine, Cocaine
Receptor Blockade	
Butaclamol	↑ Amphetamine
Haloperidol	↑ Cocaine
Pimozide	↑ Amphetamine, Cocaine, Apomorphine
	N.E. β-Phenylethylamine
Trifluoperzaine	↑ Cocaine,
Chlorpromazine	↑ Amphetamine, Cocaine Apomorphine, Methylphenidate, Pipradrol, β-Phenylethylamine, Phenmetrazine
Phenoxybenzamine	
Phentolamine	N.E. β-Phenylethylamine, Cocaine
Propranolol	
Degeneration of Catecholamine Terminals	
6-OHDA	
dorsal & ventral NA bundles	N.E. Cocaine
Nucleus Accumbens	N.E. Apomorphine
	↓ Cocaine

1 ↑ indicates increase in self-administration
↓ indicates decrease in self-administration
N.E. indicates no effect on self-administration

Pretreatment with the monoamine oxidase inhibitor pargyline, which reduces the metabolic degradation of norepinephrine, dopamine, and serotonin, is reported to significantly decrease the responding of rhesus monkeys for intravenous cocaine (Wilson and Schuster, 1974). Imipramine, which blocks catecholamine re-uptake, also decreases the self-administration of cocaine (Wilson and Schuster, 1973). Reduced responding presumably indicates a potentiation of the effects of cocaine, since animals tend to maintain stable drug intake by reducing self-administration responding with increases in the unit dose and by increasing responding with decreases in the unit dose (Goldberg and others, 1971; Pickens, 1968; Yokel and Pickens, 1974; Wilson, Hitomi, and Schuster, 1971). A similar interpretation can be applied to the results of Davis, Smith, and Khalsa (1975). These investigators have reported that inhibitors of dopamine-β-hydroxylase (diethyldithiocarbamate (DDC) and U-14,624), which raise whole-brain dopamine levels and reduce norepinephrine levels, decreases responding for d-amphetamine. Depletion of neuronal catecholamine stores by chronic reserpine treatment increases cocaine self-administration (Wilson and Schuster, 1974); responding returns to control levels, however, after several days. Acute treatment with alpha-methyl-para-tyrosine (AMPT), which inhibits the biosynthesis of dopamine and norepinephrine, has been shown to increase self-administration in rhesus monkeys responding for cocaine (Schuster and Wilson, 1972; Wilson and Schuster, 1974) or in rats responding for amphetamine (Pickens, Meisch and Dougherty, 1968). Davis and Smith (1972, 1973) have reported preventing the acquisition of amphetamine-reinforced responding in rats after eight hours of treatment with AMPT. Interestingly, amphetamine-induced euphoria is reportedly reduced or blocked in man by AMPT (Gunne, Anggard, and Jonsson, 1972; Jonsson, Gunne, and Anggard, 1969; Jonsson, Anggard, and Gunne, 1971). The euphoric effects of amphetamine-like drugs are regarded as the basis of their abuse by man (Eddy and others, 1965; Kramer, 1969). Treatment with AMPT does not alter self-administration of the dopamine receptor stimulant apomorphine (Baxter, Gluckman, and Scerni, 1976), suggesting that amphetamine and cocaine act indirectly rather than through a direct action on dopamine receptors.

Previous investigators have made a distinction between amphetamine-like and cocaine-like stimulants based upon the differential effects of AMPT in blocking some of the behavioral effects of these drugs in laboratory animals. AMPT inhibits the central stimulant behavioral effects of amphetamine, phenmetrazine, and ephedrine (Dominic and Moore, 1969a,b; Sayers and Handley, 1975; Scheel-Kruger, 1971; Scheel-Kruger and others, 1977; Thornburg and Moore, 1973), but not the stimulant effects of cocaine, methylphenidate, pipradol, or nomifensine (Dominic and Moore, 1969b; Kopinger, 1958; Scheel-Kruger, 1971, 1972; Thornburg and Moore, 1973; Wallach and Gershon, 1972). Since AMPT blocks self-administration of both amphetamine and cocaine, the two classes of stimulants may have a common mechanism of action with respect to their reinforcing properties. However, time course differences in the self-administration paradigm, i.e. chronic administration, may account for this effect.

Stimulant self-administration (amphetamine, phenmetrazine, methylphenidate, pipradol, and cocaine) is reported to increase--suggesting reduced drug potency--after treatment with the catecholamine receptor blockers chlorpromazine (Gill, Holz, and Zirkle, 1975; Risner and Jones, 1976; Wilson and Schuster, 1972), trifluoperazine (Wilson and Schuster, 1973), and particularly with the more specific dopamine receptor blockers pimozide (Baxter and others, 1974; Gill, Holz, and Zirkle, 1975; Risner and Jones 1976; Yokel and Wise, 1975; Yokel and Wise, 1976), haloperidol (Davis and Smith, 1974; Gill, Holz, and Zirkle, 1975; Smith and Davis, 1973), and butaclamol (Yokel and Wise, 1976). Pimozide is also reported to block amphetamine-induced euphoria in man (Gunne, Anggard, and Jonsson, 1972), and haloperidol blocks methylphenidate-induced euphoria in man (Belmaker, Wald, and Ebstein, 1978). -phenethylamine self-administration in dogs increases following chlorpromazine pretreatment but is unaltered by pimozide or phenoxybenzamine (Risner and Jones, 1977).

Reports that the noradrenergic blocking agents phentolamine,phenoxybenzamine, and propranolol do not alter stimulant self-administration suggest that noradrenergic systems are not important in the mechanisms by which stimulants reinforce behavior (Risner and Jones, 1976; Risner and Jones, 1977; Wilson and Schuster, 1974; Yokel and Wise, 1975; Yokel and Wise, 1976). Although there has been one report of phenoxybenzamine increasing the euphoria produced by amphetamine in human subjects (Gunne, Anggard, and Jonsson, 1972), the same investigators have reported no effect of similar treatment in another study (Jonsson, Anggard, and Gunne, 1971). In addition, propanolol does not alter amphetamine euphoria ratings in humans (Gunne, Anggard, and Jonsson, 1972). Amphetamine self-administration is also not affected by pre-treatment with the α-adrenergic agonist methoxamine, and methoxamine is not itself self-administered (Risner and Jones, 1976). Further, 6-hydroxydopamine (6-OHDA) lesions of ascending dorsal and ventral noradrenergic fiber tracts do not alter cocaine self-administration, although similar lesions of the presynaptic dopaminergic terminals of the nucleus accumbens significantly reduce responding for cocaine but not for apomorphine (Roberts, Corcoran, and Fibiger, 1977), a direct dopamine receptor stimulant.

While studies of self-administration have implicated catecholamine systems in the mediation of the reinforcing properties of stimulant drugs, some problems remain. Pretreatment with L-dopa, a dopamine and norepinephrine precursor, does not alter amphetamine administration (Pickens, Meisch, and Dougherty, 1968). The tricyclic antidepressants imipramine and amitriptyline are similar to cocaine in their ability to block the re-uptake of norepinephrine. Imipramine, however, is not self-administered by rhesus monkeys (Hoffmeister and Goldberg, 1973; Hoffmeister, 1977), and amitriptyline does not alter responding for cocaine (Gill, Holz, and Zirkle 1975). At present, no data is available on the self-administration of more potent dopamine re-uptake blockers (i.e., benztropine). Benztropine is not, however, widely abused by man.

No satisfactory hypothesis has yet been presented to account for these findings relative to those which suggest that the reinforcing properties of the psychomotor stimulants are mediated through dopamine or norepinephrine receptor stimulation. However, the evidence presented above, particularly findings that the dopamine receptor stimulant apomorphine is self-administered and that dopamine receptor blockers alter self-administration of CNS stimulants, strongly suggests the involvement of dopamine in stimulant reinforcement of behavior. More specific localization of stimulant reinforcement mechanisms has not been attempted with self-administration techniques.

ELECTRICAL SELF-STIMULATION

The hypothesis of dopamine involvement in the mediation of the reinforcing properties of stimulant drugs receives additional support from studies of electrical self-stimulation. Olds amd Milner (1954) first demonstrated that an animal would repeat a response that was followed by the delivery of electrical stimulation to the septal region of the brain. Since then, many studies have examined this phenomenom and the characteristics of brain stimulation which can serve to reinforce behavior.

Although the majority of studies have examined electrode placements within noradrenergic pathways, electrode sites within the nigrostriatal, mesolimbic, and mesocortical dopaminergic pathways are among those which support self-stimulation behavior. These sites include the substantia nigra pars compacta, caudate nucleus, nigro-striatal interconnecting pathway, ventral tegmental area (nucleus A10), nucleus accumbens, olfactory tubercle, the interconnecting pathway between nucleus A10 and the latter two sites, and the medial and sulcal prefrontal cortex.

Recent pharmacological evidence suggests an important role for dopamine, as well as norepinephrine, in the mechanisms by which electrical brain stimulation acts to maintain self-stimulation responding. The results of studies which have examined the effects of pharmacological manipulations upon self-stimulation of central dopamine sites are summmarized in Table 4.

Self-stimulation of dopaminergic sites is inhibited by the reduction of catecholamine synthesis with AMPT (Stinus and Thierry, 1973; Stinus, Thierry, and Cardo, 1976) or by depletion of transmitter stores by reserpine (Stinus, Thierry, and Cardo, 1976). Responding can also be reduced or eliminated by treatment with the receptor blocking agents chlorpromazine (Miliaressis, Bouchard, and Jacobowitz, 1975), spiroperidol (Rolls and others, 1974), and haloperidol (Liebman and Butcher, 1973; Phillips, Brooke, and Fibiger, 1975; Wauquier and Niemegieers, 1972) and pimozide (Liebman and Butcher, 1973; Liebman and Butcher, 1974; Phillips, Brooke, and Fibiger, 1975; Wauquier and Niemegieers, 1972).

TABLE 4 Effects of Catecholamine Agents upon Self-stimulation of Dopamine Sites

Treatment	Stimulation Site	Effects on S-S
Receptor Stimulation		
Apomorphine	Substantia Nigra	↑ or ↓
	Prefrontal Cortex	↓
	Far-Lateral Hypothalamus	↓
Clonidine	Substantia Nigra	↓
	Far-Lateral Hypothalamus	↓
Increased Release		
d-Amphetamine	Substantia Nigra	↑
	Nucleus Accumbens	↑
	Ventral Tegmentum	↑
	Caudate Nucleus	↑
l-Amphetamine	Substantia Nigra	↑
	Ventral Tegmentum	↑
	Nucleus Accumbens	↑
DBH Inhibition		
Diethyldithiocarbamate (DDC)	Substantia Nigra	↓
Fla-63	Ventral Tegmentum	no effect
U-14, 624	Ventral Tegmentum	no effect
Disulfiram	Ventral tegmentum	no effect
Tyrosine Hydroxylase Inhibition		
a-Methyl-p-tyrosine	Ventral Tegmentum	↓
Receptor Blockade		
Chlorpromazine	Ventral Tegmentum	↓
Haloperidol	Substantia Nigra	↓
	Nucleus Accumbens	↓
	Ventral Tegmentum	↓
Pimozide	Substantia Nigra	↓
	Nucleus Accumbens	↓
Spiroperidol	Nucleus Accumbens	↓
	Ventral Tegmentum	↓
Thymoxamine	Substantia Nigra	↓
	Far-Lateral Hypothalamus	↓
Degeneration of CA Terminals		
6-ohda:		
In Substantia Nigra	Caudate Nucleus	↓
In ventral tegmentum	Ventral Tegmentum	↓
In nigrostriatal pathway	Substantia Nigra	↓
In dorsal and ventral Noradrenergc bundles	Substantia Nigra	↑ or no long-term effect
Storage depletion		
Reserpine	Ventral Tegmentum	

6-OHDA lesions of dopamine pathways results in large reductions in responding for stimulation in the caudate nucleus (Phillips, Carter, and Fibiger, 1976a) and in the ventral tegmentum (Stinus, Thierry, and Cardo, 1975). Chemical lesions of the dorsal and ventral noradrenergic bundles either increase responding for nigral stimulation (Phillips, 1975) or produce a temporary biphasic response: decreased responding on the day of the lesion, and increased responding for several days thereafter, with a subsequent return to control levels of self-stimulation (Belluzi and others, 1975). 6-OHDA lesions of the nigrostriatal bundle in the lateral hypothalamus reduce nigral self-stimulation (Clavier and others, 1977).

α-adrenergic receptor blockade (Herberg, Stevens, and Franklin, 1976) results in decreased responding for nigral stimulation. Stimulation of α-adrenergic receptors with clonidine, however, also reduces responding for nigral stimulation and for stimulation of the far-lateral hypothalamus (Herberg, Stevens, and Franklin, 1976). Inhibition of dopamine-β-hydroxylase (DBH) with DDC reduced responding for nigral stimulation (Belluzi and others, 1975), suggesting the possible involvement of the nearby ascending noradrenergic pathway in maintaining responding in this region. The DBH inhibitors FLA-63, U-14,624, and disulfiram, however, had no effect on ventral tegmental self-stimulation (Stinus and Cardo, 1975), even when preceded by reserpine depletion of catecholamine stores (Stinus, Thierry, and Cardo, 1976).

Amphetamine causes dramatic increases in self-stimulation behavior with electrode placements in dopaminergic sites particularly when the stimulation current is near the threshold for maintaining responding (Herberg, Stephens, and Franklin, 1976; Liebman and Butcher, 1974; Liebman and Segal, 1976; Miliaressis, Bouchard, and Jacobowitz, 1975; Phillips and Fibiger, 1973; Phillips, Brooke, and Fibiger, 1975; Stein, 1964). Amphetamine-induced potentiation of nigral self-stimulation is not altered by reserpine depletion of catecholamine stores, nor is it affected by reserpine depletion plus inhibition of norepinephrine synthesis. However, reserpine plus AMPT inhibition of dopamine, as well as norepinephrine, synthesis completely suppresses the effect of amphetamine on self-stimulation (Breese, 1977). These findings are in accord with the presumption that amphetamine alters the characteristics of dopamine release. Direct receptor stimulation with apomorphine has produced variable results with some subjects showing increased responding for stimulation of dopamine sites and some reduced responding (Herberg, Stephens, and Franklin, 1976; Liebman and Butcher, 1974; Mora and others, 1976a; Phillips and others, 1976d; Broekamp and VanRossum, 1974). This variability seems to be independent of electrode site (Broekamp and VanRossum, 1974), and may be the result of apomorphine-induced stereotypy or the reinforcement of on-going behavior by apomorphine administration, or apomorphine-induced inhibition of transmitter synthesis.

Chemical lesions of the nigrostriatal pathway which reduce nigral self-stimulation, also eliminate the response potentiation induced by amphetamine (Clavier and others, 1977). This finding is a further confirmation of the role of dopaminergic systems in the mechanism of action of this drug, and highlights the importance of intact neurogenic processes in mediating the effects of amphetamine.

SUMMARY AND CONCLUSIONS

From the preceding, it is clear that dopaminergic systems are intimately involved in mediating the reinforcement derived from the administration of central stimulants. Electrical stimulation of dopamine sites can also serve to reinforce behavior; and pharmacological manipulations which alter stimulant self-administration also alter electrical self-stimulation of dopaminergic sites. The important potentiation of self-stimulation behavior observed following amphetamine administration is a further suggestion of a relationship between the mechanisms of stimulant reinforcement and those of electrical brain stimulation.

While studies of self-administration and self-stimulation have implicated the involvement of dopamine in reinforcement mechanisms, these techniques have not been extensively employed in investigations of mechanisms by which stimulants reinforce behavior. The CNS stimulants affect neurotransmitter function in several ways, including promoting release, blocking re-uptake, and inhibiting monoamine oxidase (MAO) activity. Which of these effects is of major importance in the mediation of stimulant reinforcement has yet to be determined. Neither benztropine (a potent dopamine re-uptake blocker), nor MAO inhibitors are major drugs of abuse. The mechanism with the highest gradient of activity would appear to be neurotransmitter release, with re-uptake blockade and MAO inhibition possibly acting to potentiate the effects of increased release.

The self-administration and electrical self-stimulation techniques are unique tools for the study of reinforcement mechanisms. Their continued application to questions of stimulant reinforcement may provide both basic information of reinforcement mechanisms and an understanding of the biobehavioral mechanisms, which maintain stimulant abuse.

REFERENCES

Altshuler, H., S. Weaver, and P. Phillips (1975). Intragastric self-administration of psycho-active drugs by the rhesus monkey. Life Sci., 17, 883-890.

Balster, R. L., and C. R. Schuster (1977). A preference procedure that compares efficacy of different intravenous drug reinforcers in the Rhesus monkey. In E. H. Ellinwood, Jr., and M. M. Kilbey (eds.), Cocaine and Other Stimulants. Plenum Press, New York. pp. 571-584.

Baxter, B. L., M. I. Gluckman, and R. A. Scerni (1973). Differential self-injection behavior produced by fenfluramine versus other appetite-inhibiting drugs. Fed. Proc., 32, 754.

Baxter, B. L., M. I. Gluckman, L. Stein, and R. A. Scerni (1974). Self-injection of apomorphine in the rat: Positive reinforcement by a dopamine receptor stimulant. Pharmacol. Biochem. Behav., 2, 387-391.

Baxter, B. L., M. I. Gluckman, and R. A. Scerni (1976). Apomorphine self-injection is not affected by alpha-methylparatyrosine treatment: Support for dopaminergic reward. Pharmacol. Biochem. Behav., 4, 611-612.

Belluzi, J. D., and others, (1975). Substantia nigra self-stimulation: Dependence on noradrenergic reward pathways. Behavioral Biology, 13, 103-111.

Belmaker, R. H., D. Wald, and R. Ebstein (1978). Haloperidol and lithium blocking of the mood response to intravenous methylphenidate. Collegium Internationale Neuro- psychopharmacolgicum Abs., 395.

Brady, J. V., R. R. Griffiths, and G. Winger (1975).Drug maintained performance procedures and the evaluation of sedative hypnotic dependency potential. In F. Kagan, T. Harwood, K. Rickels, A. Rudzik, and H. Sorer (eds.), Hypnotics: Methods of Development and Evaluation. Spectrum Publications, Inc., New York. pp. 221-235.

Brady, J. V., and r. R. Griffiths (1977). Drug-maintained performance and the analysis of stimulant reinforcing effect. In E. H. Ellinwood, Jr., and M. M. Kilbey (eds.), Cocaine and Other Stimulants. Plenum Press, New York. pp. 599-613.

Breese, G. R. (1977). Pharmacological evidence implicating dopamine in intracrania self-stimulation. Neurosci. Res. Prog. Bull., 15, 182-191.

Broekkamp, C. L. E., and J. M. Van Rossum (1974). Effects of apomorphine on self-stimulation behavior. Psychopharmacologia, 34, 71-80.

Clavier, R. M, H. C. Fibiger, and A. G. Phillips (1977). On the role of ascending catecholamine projections in intracranial self-stimulation of substantia nigra. Brain Res. 131, 271-286.

Davis, W. M., and S. G. Smith (1972). Alpha-methyltyrosine to prevent self-administration of morphine and amphetamine. Curr. Ther. Res., 14, 814-819.

Davis, W. M., and S. G. Smith (1973). Blocking effect of -methyltyrosine on amphetamine based reinforcement. J. Pharm. Pharmacol., 25, 174-177.

Davis, W. M., and S. G. Smith (1974). Positive reinforcing effects of apomorphine, d-amphetamine and morphine: Interaction with haloperidol. Pharmacologist, 16, 193.

Davis, W. M., S. G. Smith, and J. H. Khalsa (1975). Noradrenergic role in the self-administration of morphine or amphetamine. Pharmacol. Biochem. Behav., 3, 477-484.

Deneau, G. A., T. Yanagita, and M. H. Seevers (1964). Psychogenic dependence to a variety of drugs in the monkey. Pharmacologist, 6, 182.

Deneau, G., T. Yanagita, and M. H. Seevers (1969). Self-administration of psychoactive substances by the monkey. Psychopharmacologia(Berl.), 16, 30-48.

Dominic, J. A., and K. E. Moore (1969a). Acute effects of -methyltyrosine on brain catecholamine levels and on spontaneous and amphetamine-stimulant motor activity in mice. Arch. Int. Pharmacodyn. Ther., 178, 166-176.

Dominic, J. A., and K. E. Moore (1969b). Supersensitivity to the central stimulant actions of adrenergic drugs following discontinuation of a chronic diet of -methyltyrosine. Psychopharmacol., 15, 96-101.

Eddy, N. B.,H. Halbach, H. Isbell and M. H. Seevers (1965). Drug dependence: its significance and characteristics. Bull. Wld. Hlth. Org., 32, 721-733.

Gill, C. A., W. C. Holz, and C. Zirkle (1975). The role of dopamine in self-administration of psychomotor stimulants. Proceedings of the Committee on Problems of Drug Dependence, 37th anniversary meeting, 991-1006.

Glick, S. D., and R. S. Cox (1975). Self-administration of haloperidol in rats. Life Sci., 16, 1041-1046.

Goldberg, S. R., F. Hoffmeister, U. U. Schlicting, and W. Wuttke (1971). A comparison of pentobarbital and cocaine self-administration in rhesus monkeys: Effects of dose and fixed-ratio parameter. J. Pharmacol. Exp. Ther., 179(2), 277-283.

Goldberg, S. R., and R. T. Kelleher (1977). Reinforcement of behavior by cocaine injections. In E. H. Ellinwood, Jr., and M. M. Kilbey (eds.), Cocaine and Other Stimulants. Plenum Press, New York. pp. 523-544.

Gotestam, K. G., and B. E. Andersson (1975). Self-administration of amphetamine analogues in rats. Pharmacol. Biochem. Behav., 3, 229-234.

Griffith, J. D. (1966). A study of illicit amphetamine drug traffic in Oklahoma City. Am. J. Psychiat., 123, 560-569.

Griffith, J. D. (1977). Structure-activity relationships of several amphetamine drugs in man. In E. H. Ellinwood, Jr., and M. M. Kilbey (eds.), Cocaine and Other Stimulants. Plenum Press, New York. pp. 705-715.

Griffiths, R. R., J. D. Findley, J. V. Brady, K. Dolan-Gutcher, and W. W. Robinson (1975). Comparison of progressive-ratio performance maintained by cocaine, methylphenidate, and secobarbital. Psychopharmacologia, 43, 81-83.

Griffiths, R. R., G. Winger, J. V. Brady, and J. D. Snell (1976). Comparison of behavior maintained by infusions of eight phenylethylamines in baboons. Psychopharmacol., 50, 251-258.

Griffiths, R. R., J. D. Snell, and J. V. Brady (1976). Progressive-ratio performance in baboons and the assessment of the abuse liability of drugs:

Comparison of fenfluramine, chlorphentermine, diethylpropion, and cocaine. Proc. 38th Annual Meeting of the Comm. on Problems of Drug Dependence, Richmond, Va. pp. 546-551.

Gunne L. M., E. Anggard, and L. Jonsson (1972). Clinical trials with amphetamine-blocking drugs., Psychiat. Neurol. Neurochir., 75, 225-226.

Herberg, L. J., D. N. Stephens, and K. B. J. Franklin (1976). Catecholamines and self-stimulation: Evidence suggesting a reinforcing role for noradrenaline and a motivating role for dopamine. Pharmacol. Biochem. Behav., 4, 575-582.

Hoffmeister, F. (1977). Assessment of reinforcing properties of stimulant and depressant drugs in the rhesus monkey as a tool for the prediction of psychic dependence-producing capability in man. In T. Thompson and K. R. Unna (eds.), Predicting Dependence Liability of Stimulant and Depressant Drugs. University Park Press, Baltimore. pp. 185-201.

Hoffmeister, F., and S. R. Goldberg (1973). A comparison of chlorpromazine, imipramine, morphine, and d-amphetamine self-administration in cocaine-dependent Rhesus monkeys. J. Pharmacol. Exp. Ther., 187, 8-14.

Johanson, C. E., and C. R. Schuster (1975). A choice procedure for drug reinforcers: Cocaine and methylphenidate in the rhesus monkey. J. Pharmacol. Exp. Ther., 193, 676-688.

Johanson, C. E., R. L. Balster, and K. Bonese (1976). Self-administration of psychomotor stimulant drugs: The effects of unlimited access. Pharmacol. Biochem. Behav., 4, 45-51.

Johanson, C. E., and C. R. Schuster (1977). Procedures for the preclinical assessment of abuse potential of psychotropic drugs in animals. In T. Thompson and K. R. Unna (eds.), Predicting Dependence Liability of Stimulant and Depressant Drugs, University Park Press, Baltimore. pp. 203-229.

Jonsson, L. E., E. Anggard, and L. M. Gunne (1971). Blockade of intravenous amphetamine euphoria in man. Clin. Pharmacol. Ther., 12, 889-896.

Jonsson, L. E., L. M. Gunne, and E. Anggard (1969). Effect of -methyltyrosine in amphetamine-dependent subjects. Eur. J. Clin. Pharmacol., 2, 27-29.

Kopinger, W. (1958). Differentiation between the sedative actions of 5-hydroxytryptamine and reserpine in mice by means of two stimulating substances. Acta Pharmacol. Toxicol., 14, 138-147.

Kramer, J. C. (1969). Introduction to amphetamine abuse. J. Psychedelic Drugs, 2, 1-16.

Kramer, J. C., V. S. Fischman, and D. C. Littlefield (1967). Amphetamine abuse. J. Am. Med. Assoc., 201, 89-93.

Liebman, J. M., and L. L. Butcher (1973). Effects on self-stimulation behavior of drugs influencing dopaminergic neurotransmission mechanisms. Naunyn-Schiedeberg's Arch. Exp. Path. Pharmak., 277, 305-318.

Liebman, J. M., D. N. Stephens, and K. B. J. Franklin (1976). Comparative involvement of dopamine and noradrenaline in rate-free self-stimulation in substantia nigra, lateral hypothalamus, and mesencephalic central gray. Naunyn-Schiedeberg's Arch. Pharmacol., 284, 167-194.

Liebman, J. M., and D. S. Segal (1976). Lack of tolerance or sensitization to the effects of chronic d-amphetamine on substantia nigra self-stimulation. Behavioral Biology, 16, 211-220.

Miliaressis, E., A. Bouchard, and D. M. Jacobowitz (1975). Strong positive reward in median raphe: Specific inhibition by para-chlorphenylalamine. Brain Research, 98, 194-201.

Mora, F., A. G. Phillips, J. M. Koolhaas, and E. T. Rolls (1976). Prefrontal cortex and neostriatum. Self-stimulation in the rat: Differential effects produced by apomorphine. Brain Res. Bull., 1, 421-424.

Olds, J., and P. M. Milner (1954). Positive reinforcement produced by electrical stimulation of septal area and other regions of rat brain. J. Comp. Physiol. Psychol., 47, 419-427.

Phillips, A. G., and H. C. Fibiger (1973). Dopaminergic and noradrenergic substrates of positive reinforcement: Differential effects of D- and L-Amphetamine. Science, 179, 575-577.

Phillips, A. G.(1975). Dopaminergic substrates of reward: the role of the nigro-neostriatal system. Paper read at: 46th Annual Meeting of Eastern Psychological Association. New York.

Phillips, A. G., S. M. Brooke and H. C. Fibiger. Effects of amphetamine isomers and neuroleptics on self-stimulation from the nucleus accubens and dorsal noradrenergic bundle. Brain Res., 85, 13-22.

Phillips, A. G., D. A. Carter and H. C. Fibiger. (1976). Dopaminergic substrates of intracranial self-stimulation in the caudate-putamen. Brain Res., 104, 221-232.

Phillips, A. G., F. Mora, J. M. Koolhaas, and E. T. Rolls (1976d). Differential effects of apomorphine on self-stimulation of mesocortical and nigrostriatal systems in rat and rhesus monkey. Neurosci. Abstr., 2, 721.

Pickens, R., and T. Thompson (1968). Cocaine-reinforced behavior in rats: effects of reinforcement magnitude and fixed-ratio size. J. Pharmacol. Exp. Ther., 161, 122-129.

Pickens, R. (1968). Self-administration of stimulants by rats. Int. J. Addict., 3, 215-221.

Pickens, R., R. A. Meisch, and J. A. Dougherty (1968). Chemical interactions in methamphetamine reinforcement. Psych. Rep., 23, 1267-1270.

Risner, M. E., and B. E. Jones (1976). Role of noradrenergic and dopaminergic processes in amphetamine self-administration. Pharmacol. Biochem. Behav., 5, 477-482.

Risner, M. E., and B. E. Jones (1977). Characteristics of B-phenethylamine self-administration by dog. Pharmacol. Biochem. Behav., 6, 689-696.

Roberts, D. C. S., M. E. Corcoran, and H. C. Fibiger (1977). On the role of ascending catecholaminergic systems in intravenous self-administration of cocaine. Pharmacol. Biochem. Behav., 6, 615-620.

Rolls, E. T., B. J. Rolls, P. H. Kelly, S. G. Shaw, R. J. Wood, and R. Dale (1974). The relative attenuation of self-stimulation, eating and drinking produced by dopamine-receptor blockade. Psychopharmacologia, 38, 219-230.

Sayers, A. C., and S. L. Handley (1973). A study of the role of catecholamines in the response to various central stimulants. Eur. J. Pharmacol., 23, 47-55.

Scheel-Kruger, J. (1971). Comparative studies of various amphetamine analogues demonstrating different interactions with the metabolism of the catecholamines in the brain. Eur. J. Pharmacol., 14, 47-59.

Scheel-Kruger, J. (1972). Behavioral and biochemical comparisons of amphetamine derivatives, cocaine, benztropine and tricyclic antidepressant drugs. Eur. J. Pharmacol., 18, 63-73.

Scheel-Kruger, J., C. Braestrup, M. Nielson, K. Golembiowska, and E. Mogilnicka (1977). Cocaine: discussion on the role of dopamine in the biochemical mechanism of action. In E. H. Ellinwood, Jr. and M. M. Kilbey (Eds.), Cocaine and Other Stimulants. Plenum Press, New York. pp. 373-407.

Schuster, C. R., and C. E. Johanson (1974). The use of animal models for the study of drug abuse. In: R. J. Gibbins, Y. Israel, H. Kalant, R. E. Popham, W. Schmidt, and R. G. Smart (Eds.),Research Advances in Alcohol and Drug Problems, Vol. I. John Wiley and Sons, New York. pp. 1-31.

Schuster, C. R., and T. Thompson (1969). Self-administration of and behavioral dependence on drugs. Ann. Rev. Pharmacol., 9, 483-502.

Schuster, C. R., and M. C. Wilson (1972). The effects of various pharmacological agents on cocaine self-administration by rhesus monkeys. In E. Ellinwood, Jr., and S. Cohen (Eds.),

Schuster, C. R., and T. Thompson (1969). Self-administration of and behavioral dependence on drugs. Ann. Rev. Pharmacol., 9, 483-502.

Schuster, C. R., and M. C. Wilson (1972). The effects of various pharmacological agents on cocaine self-administration by rhesus monkeys. In E. H. Ellinwood, Jr., and S. Cohen (Eds.), Current Concepts on Amphetamine Abuse. National Institute of Mental Health, Rockville, Maryland. pp. 37-41.

Smith, S. G., nd W. M. Davis (1973). Haloperidol effects on morphine self-adminsitration testing for pharmacological modification of primary reinforcement mechanism. Psychol. Rec., 23, 215-221.

Stein, L. (1964). Self-stimulation of the brain and the central stimulant action of amphetamine. Federation Proceedings, 23, 836-850.

Stinus, L., and A. M. Thierry (1973). Self-stimulation and catecholamines ii. Blockade of self-stimulation by treatment with alpha-methylparatyrosine and the reinstatement by catecholamine precursor aadministration. Brain Research, 64, 189-198.

Stinus, L., A. M. Thierry, and B. Cardo (1975). Self-stimulation and local injections of 6-hydroxydopamine into the rat brain: enhanced behavioral depressive effects of alpha-methylparatyrosine. Pharmacology Biochemistry and Behavior, 3, 19-23.

Stinus, L., and B. Cardo (1975). Effect of various inhibitors of tyrosine hydroxylase and dopamine B-hydroxylase on self-stimulation behavior. Brain Res., 85, 196- .

Stinus, L., A. M. Thierry, and B. Cardo (1976). Effects of various inhibitors of tyrosine hydroxylase and dopamine beta-hydroxylase on rat self-stimulation after reserpine treatment. Psychopharmacologia, 45, 287-294.

Thompson, T., and C. E. Schuster (1964). Morphine self-administration, food reinforced and avoidance behaviors in rhesus monkeys. Psychopharmacologia, 5, 87-94.

Thompson, T., and K. R. Unna (1977). Predicting Dependence Liability of Stimulant and Depressant Drugs. University Park Press, Baltimore.

Thornburg, J. E., and K. E. Moore (1973). The relative importance of dopaminergic and noradrenergic neuronal systems for the stimulation of locomotor activity induced by amphetamine and other drugs. Neuropharmacol., 12, 853-866.

Wallach, M. B., and S. Gershon (1972). The induction and antagonism of central nervous system stimulant-induced stereotyped behavior in the cat. Eur. J. Pharmacol., 18, 22-26.

Wauquier, A., and C. J. E. Niemegieers (1972). Intracranial self-stimulation in rats as a function of various stimulus parameters. ii. Influence of haloperidol, pimozide and pipamperone on medical forebrain bundle stimulation with nomopolar electrodes. Psychopharmacologia(Berlin), 27, 284-294.

Weeks, J. R. (1962). Experimental morphine addiction: method for automatic intravenous injections in unrestrained rats. Science, 138, 143-144.

Wilson, M. C., M. Hitomi, and C. R. Schuster (1971). Psychomotor stimulant self-administration as a function of dosage per injection in the phesus monkey. Psychopharmacologia, 22, 271-281.

Wilson, M. C., and C. R. Schuster (1972). The effects of chlorpromazine on psychomotor stimulant self-administration in the rhesus monkey. Psychopharmacologia, 26, 115-126.

Wilson, M. C., and C. R. Schuster (1973). The effects of stimulants and depressants on cocaine self-administration behavior in the rhesus monkey. Psychopharmacologia, 31, 291-304.

Wilson, M. C., and C. R. Schuster (1974). Aminergic influences on intravenous cocaine self-administration by rhesus monekys.

Woods, J., and C. R. Schuster (1968). Reinforcement properties of morphine, cocaine, and SPA as a function of unit dose. Int. J. Addict., 3, 231-237.

Woods, and Tessel (1974). Fenfluramine: amphetamine congener that fails to maintain drug-taking behavior in the rhesus monkey. -2av Science, 185, 1068-1069.
Yanagita, T. (1973). An experimental framework for evaluation of dependence liability of various types of drugs in monkeys. Bull. Narcot., 25, 57.
Yokel, R. A., and R. Pickens (1974). Drug level of d- and l-amphetamine during intravenous self-administration. Psychopharmacologia, 34, 225-264.
Yokel, R. A., and R. A. Wise (1975). Increased lever pressing for amphetamine after pimozide in rats: implications for a dopamine theory of reward. Science, 187, 547-549.
Yokel, R. A., and R. A. Wise (1976). Attenuation of intravenous amphetamine reinforcement by central dopamine blockade in rats. Psychopharmacologia, 48, 311-318.
Yokel, R. A. and R. A. Wise (1978). Amphetamine -type reinforcement by dopaminergic agonists in the rat. Psychopharmacol., 58, 289-296. -5av
Zabik, J. E., and H. Lal (1972). Self-injection of dextroamphetamine under multiple-operant-contingencies in acute and chronically treated rats. In J. M. Singh, L. Miller, and H. Lal (Eds.), Drug Addiction: Experimental Pharmacology. Futura, Mt. Kisco, N. Y. pp. 269-291.

Present Use of Hallucinogens

LEO E. HOLLISTER

Professor of Medicine, Psychiatry and Pharmacology, Stanford University
School of Medicine and Veterans Administration Hospital, Palo Alto,
California 94304, U.S.A.

ABSTRACT

The use of hallucinogens in the United States has remained relatively constant at a modest level for the past several years. Patterns of use have shifted, with a decline in the use of lysergide (LSD) and other hallucinogens accompanied by a rise in the use of phencyclidine (PCP). The major source of PCP is from illicit manufacture, as the drug has no current human use and its veterinary use is limited. PCP differs from other hallucinogens in its spectrum of clinical manifestations, which are believed by some to resemble more closely those of schizophrenia. It is unique among hallucinogens in being self-administered by animals and in being directly lethal, from convulsions, hypertension, and respiratory depression. Overdoses may be treated by usual supportive measures as well as by continual gastric suction and acidification of the urine. It is impossible to tell how long PCP will remain the current fad hallucinogen.

INTRODUCTION

The great increase in interest about cannabis over the past decade has pushed the hallucinogens off the front pages of newspapers and has greatly reduced both public and scientific interest in these drugs. Both the number of scientific studies of cannabis and the availability of funds for research with this drug have been abundant, so that investigators who might normally study the hallucinogens now study cannabis. Virtually all current studies of hallucinogens, reduced as they are in number, involve animals or *in vitro* systems; human studies have virtually disappeared. Indeed, one wonders whether human studies with hallucinogens could ever again be done, so great are the current ethical constraints about studies in humans with drugs of abuse. We have the paradoxical situation in which all human studies of these drugs, meager as they are in providing useful data, occur in self-appointed, unsupervised volunteers.

A continuing aspect of hallucinogen abuse is that fad use of a particular drug is common. The rapid upsurge of use of hallucinogens during the 1960s had all the trappings of a fad. Lysergide (LSD) was promoted both by various gurus and by the press as a drug with remarkably beneficial properties. Within a few years, the young members of the drug cults came to believe that only natural materials were really good. LSD, being a product of the chemical laboratory, became a synthetic material to be avoided, but mescaline, nearly identical in its clinical effects, was an acceptable natural product. Alas, virtually all mescaline sold in the streets to drug users was mislabeled LSD; only those who actually bought peyote tops obtained the real drug. Now mescaline is out, and the synthetic drug, phencyclidine (PCP), is in. The more things change, the more they are the same.

TYPES OF HALLUCINOGENS

Basing a classification on chemical structures, one can separate seven groups of these drugs: (a) lysergic acid derivatives, of which LSD is the prototype; (b) phenylethylamine derivatives, of which 3,4,5-trihydroxyphenylethylamine (mescaline) is the prototype; (c) indolealkylamines, such as 4-phosporodimethyl-tryptamine (psilocybin); (d) other indolic derivatives, such as the harmine alkaloids or ibogaine; (e) piperidyl benzilate esters, such as N-ethyl-3-piperidyl cyclopentylphenyl gylcolate (JB-329 'Ditran'); (f) 1-phenylcyclohexyl compounds, such as phenylcyclidine ('Sernyl'); and (g) a miscellaneous group of varying chemical structures. Because the first three groups are virtually identical in their clinical effects, they are often lumped together as the LSD-mescaline-psilocybin group (Hollister, 1968).

The choice of drugs available to the user is limited. LSD is easily synthesized and has been far more available than either mescaline or psilocybin, although it is often labeled with the names of these other similar drugs. Piperidyl benzilate esters, being rather like scopolamine, are not especially attractive drugs, although a few non-critical users will take them. Phencyclidine (PCP) is very readily synthesized and its chemical precursors are so widely used that they are virtually impossible to control. Under the circumstances, therefore, it should not have been surprising that if LSD were to lose favor, PCP should gain it.

EPIDEMIOLOGIC ASPECTS

It is virtually impossible to determine the current frequency of use of hallucinogens. Epidemiologic studies of drug abuse are fraught with many difficulties. The data obtained are largely anecdotal, that is, what people say, and it is well known that what people say and what they do may be quite different. To compound the difficulty, even the most honest and cooperative respondent labors under the burden of not really knowing what drug was taken. Mislabeling of street drugs is more common than accurate labeling. Mislabeling of LSD as mescaline may not be of serious consequence for epidemiologic purposes, as the two drugs are quite similar and might well be classified together. On the other hand, mislabeling of THC as PCP is of serious consequence as the two categories of drugs are considered to be separate. The only bases that drug users have for correcting for mislabeling are their past experience with similar drugs, the opinions of fellow drug users or the reputation of their source of drugs. None of these factors are very likely to resolve ambiguity about what they really took. Thus, epidemiologic studies which lack any chemical verification of drugs (and these are virtually impossible to design) will only be crude indices of what drugs are really being used.

Despite these difficulties, the available data in the United States indicate that the rates of hallucinogen use, variable as they may be among separate epidemiologic surveys, have remained relatively constant over the past few years (Abelson and Atkinson, 1975). Within this general pattern of use, a substantial change has occurred in regard to the drugs chosen. LSD is less often used (at least so labeled) while PCP use probably has increased in recent years to what is now being called an epidemic. Differences in use by sex are also apparent; more women have tried these drugs than before, their rate of such use now approaching that of men. Perhaps this shift is due to the general move towards equality for women. Happily, the rates of frequent use of hallucinogens, always low in comparison to the number of experimenters with the drug, have not shifted.

Because the change of greatest importance has been the current popularity of a relatively new hallucinogen, PCP, with qualities distinctly different from those of conventional drugs, this paper will focus on various properties of this drug, rather than repeating the many reviews of hallucinogens of the more conventional types which have been well covered elsewhere (Freedman, 1969; Cohen, 1971; Brawley and Duffield, 1972; Radouco-Thomas and others, 1974; Sankar, 1975).

Phencyclidine

History. The history of PCP is of some interest, as the drug was first thought to be useful for medical practice. It was first studied in 1957 as a potential anesthetic agent ultimately to be marketed under the name 'Sernyl' (Greifenstein and others, 1958). Although it lacked muscle relaxation, it produced a state of analgesia without full loss of consciousness and without impairment of respiratory drive or impairment of pharyngeal and laryngeal reflexes. By 1959, however, it had become apparent that patients emerging from anesthesia with this drug experienced a mental state that in some ways resembled that of hallucinogenic drugs. As studies of its hallucinogenic effects grew, it became apparent that PCP had such properties, and that these were highly variable depending upon dose and route of administration (Luby and others, 1959). Further, they were distinctly different from those of LSD. In the opinion of many investigators, the PCP-induced mental state was a better model for schizophrenia than was the mental state produced by LSD. Verification of the hallucinogenic effects of the drug in man led to its withdrawal from the market as an anesthetic in 1965. Its hallucinogenic properties were of less consequence in animals, so that by 1967 it was re-introduced into the market as an anesthetic for veterinary use under the name 'Serylan.' This use of the drug has remained to the present, the drug being considered to be quite valuable for anesthesia of primates.

The first street use of the drug occurred in 1967, during the "summer of love", when the drug culture erupted on the streets of San Francisco. The drug's popularity was short-lived, as its unpredictable, unpleasant and often startling effects gave it a bad reputation. During the next several years PCP was hardly ever used knowingly by drug takers. By 1972 it had become a popular substance for being mislabeled as other drugs, or as an adulterant of other drugs (Hart and others, 1972). By 1974, however, the pendulum swung completely back; PCP now became an acceptable drug in its own right, despite its vagaries. From that point on, its use has grown to what is now called epidemic proportions. Because of the frequently dramatic consequences of its use, the actual rate of use may have been overestimated.

The drug is readily synthesized by illicit chemical laboratories and all the evidence suggests that virtually all PCP on the streets comes from such sources. Nonetheless, the panic that its rising use created has led to the proposal that the drug be re-scheduled into a more restricted category of controlled drug. Such re-scheduling would make the cost of assuring control of supplies so great that the manufacturer of PCP for veterinary anesthesia seems likely to abandon its sale, much to the concern and consternation of many investigators who rely heavily on it for their work involving primates. The desire to control drugs of abuse often leads to totally inappropriate actions just so long as some action is taken.

Pharmacology. As is the case with most centrally active drugs, the effects of PCP on various neurotransmitters has been most studied. PCP is believed to act by increasing the availability of dopamine, possibly both by increasing its release as well as by inhibiting its uptake (Smith and others, 1975). The increased locomotor activity produced by the drug in rodents is characteristic of that induced by other methods of increasing dopaminergic activity. It is enhanced by antimuscarinic drugs and antagonized by cholinergic agents. The effects on acetylcholine are ambiguous. In some situations it seems to be cholinergic and in others, anticholinergic. Many of the latter properties are evident from some of its clinical effects (Maayani and others, 1974). The drug blocks uptake of norepinephrine and this action is related to the sympathomimetic effects evident clinically (Hitzeman and others, 1973). Its effects on serotonin are uncertain.

Neurophysiologic studies indicate that the EEG effects in primates seem to show a possibly characteristic pattern of delta-theta mixed with low voltage fast activity. Sensory evoked potentials are also suppressed, leading to the postulation that the primary site of action is on the nonspecific thalamocortical projection (Miyasaki and Domino, 1968). The impairment of sensation, for pain, touch and proprioception, is consonant with its clinical use as an anesthetic. It may also be pertinent to the provocation of a schizophreniclike state, which many investigators have likened to that of sensory deprivation.

The drug is unique among hallucinogens in being self-administered (Balster and Johanson, 1973). This difference, as well as many clinical and pharmacologic differences from the LSD group of hallucinogens, has led some persons to suggest that PCP be considered as a separate class of drug, similar to the classification of cannabis. However, the definition of hallucinogen is broad enough to include drugs other than the LSD group. So far as the use of the drug on the streets is concerned, it is clearly being used by hallucinogen fanciers. Animals can discriminate the drug apart from morphine, chlorpromazine, tetrahydrocannabinol, ditran and pentobarbital, again indicating its rather unique set of enteroceptive cues. In man, the effects are said to be similar to those seen in schizophrenic patients, but the closeness of this model psychosis to the real thing has not been studied carefully for many years. It might again be appropriate for doing so, for were it to prove to be a viable model, it might be a valuable tool for research into the nature of schizophrenia.

PCP in man is generally considered to be a rather long-acting drug, yet its half-life in plasma is only about 11 hours even after large overdoses (Marshman and others, 1976). Due to a high degree of lipid solubility, it moves rapidly into the brain, so that concentrations in brain and in cerebrospinal fluid are more persistent. Thus, the toxicity of the drug may be greatest when the plasma levels are lowest. Some of the drug is secreted from the blood into the stomach, whose acid contents keep the weakly basic drug ionized. As it enters the more alkaline medium of the upper intestine, it again becomes unionized and is reabsorbed. Thus, a certain amount of gastroenteric recycling of the drug occurs. It is likely also that PCP produces active metabolites. Thus, three factors - active metabolites, sequestration in fat and recycling through the gastrointestinal tract - may account for its long duration of action, which is especially evident in cases of overdose.

Clinical effects. Distortion of body image, disorientation, detachment from surroundings and vivid dreaming are some of the most common mental effects of PCP. Those who take it seem to lose the ability to integrate sensory input, especially for touch and proprioception (Rosenbaum and others, 1959). This effect may, in turn, lead to the analgesia and paresthesias that are experienced, as well as produce a cataleptic state in some individuals. Such effects are generally produced by doses of the drug of 0.1 mg/kg up to 12 mg single doses, regardless of the route of administration. Some persons develop mania or hostility, but these are generally considered to be side effects, more related to the personality of the subject than to a direct effect of the drug. Although some similarities to the schizophrenic state are obvious, it is not clear that the mental state produced by PCP is an especially good model of that illness.

Physical symptoms include dizziness, dysarthria, ataxia and nystagmus, lid ptosis, tachycardia, sweating and increased deep tendon reflexes. Most subjects show some degree of hypertension, associated with increased minute and tidal volumes of respiration, increased formation of urine and increased muscle tone. The latter may lead to increased serum creatine phosphokinase concentrations. With very large doses, convulsions and respiratory arrest are the terminal events (Burns and others, 1975). The course of clinical symptoms and signs following various doses of PCP is shown in Table 1.

TABLE 1 Patterns of Clinical Effects from Increasing Oral Doses of PCP

Dose	Effects
5 - 10 mg	ataxia, nystagmus, mood changes, hallucinations, vomiting, analgesia, paresthesias Onset 1-2 hours; duration 4-8 hours
10 - 20 mg	stupor, eyes open, random movements, resting nystagmus, hyper-reflexia, hypertension Onset 1/2 - 1 hour; duration 8-24 hours
> 50 mg	deep coma, chills, nystagmus, eyes closed, hypertension, labored breathing, seizures Duration up to 4 days
> 100 mg	lethal - 3 to 10 days respiratory depression, hypertensive crisis, cerebral bleeding, loss of deep tendon reflexes, decreased renal function, decreased liver function

Most of the experiments with PCP, done in the early 1960s, gave the drug intravenously. On the street, however, the major method of administration is by inhalation (often smoked as a cigarette using parsley as the medium for smoking) or by oral route in a variety of formulations.

Overdoses. Overdoses of PCP have been directly fatal, which is somewhat different from the case of other hallucinogens, such as LSD. Hypertensive crises, convulsions and respiratory arrest are the major causes of death. Indirect fatalities, due to accidents caused by loss of critical judgment, are similar to those known to occur with LSD. For some reason or other, deaths by drowning are frequent with PCP.

No pharmacologic antidote exists for the effects of the drug. Chlorpromazine aggravates rather than ameliorates the behavioral effects. Diazepam adds to respiratory depression, but may be required for uncontrolled seizures. Experimentally, neither diphenhydramine, droperidol, tetrahydroaminacrine, physostigmine or scopolamine were useful in reversing the effects of PCP.

Acidification of the urine to pH 5.5, using either ammonium chloride or ascorbic acid, keeps the drug in the ionized form and hastens its excretion (Domino and Wilson, 1977). Gastric lavage is useful only when the drug has been taken orally and soon after intake. Continual gastric suction, however, may reduce the gastrointestinal recycling of the drug and is worth doing routinely. General supportive treatment and management of symptoms as they arise is most useful. Reduced sensory stimuli reduce the psychic effects of the drug, so patients should be treated in a quiet room with little extraneous sounds.

COMMENTS

Most attention has been given to PCP in this discussion simply because it is widely used at the moment. This popularity may be only transient, if one can judge by previous history about the use of hallucinogens. That such popularity ever developed at all is rather surprising, for on balance, the effects of PCP seem to be not nearly so pleasant as those of LSD. Yet, it has all the disadvantages of LSD, including the ability to precipitate rather long-lasting psychotic states in susceptible persons. In addition, it may directly cause death from overdose. Yet, it is the hallucinogen of the moment and therefore must be reckoned with.

REFERENCES

Abelson, H.I., and R.B. Atkinson (1975). Public Experience with Psychoactive Substances, Part I: Main Findings and Part III: Methods and Procedures. Report prepared for the National Institute of Drug Abuse, Division of Behavioral and Social Sciences, Rockville, Maryland.

Balster, R.L., and C.E. Johanson (1973). Phencyclidine self-administration in the rhesus monkey. Pharmacol. Biochem. Behav., 1, 167-172.

Brawley, P., and J.C. Duffield (1972). The pharmacology of hallucinogens. Pharmacol. Rev., 24, 31-66.

Burns, R.S., S.E. Lerner, R. Corrado, and others (1975). Phencyclidine - states of acute intoxication and fatalities. West. J. Med., 123, 345-349.

Cohen, S. (1971). The psychotomimetic agents. Prog. Drug Res., 15, 68-102.

Domino, E.F., and A.E. Wilson (1977). Effects of urine acidification in plasma and urine phencyclidine levels in overdose. Clin. Pharmacol. Ther., 22, 421-424.

Freedman, D.X. (1969). The psychopharmacology of hallucinogenic agents. Annu. Rev. Med., 20, 409-418.

Greifenstein, F.E., M. DeVault, J. Yoshitake, and others (1958). A study of a 1-aryl cyclo hexyl amine for anesthesia. Anesth. Analg., 37, 283-294.

Hart, J.B., J.D. McChesney, M. Greis, and others (1972). Composition of illicit drugs and the use of drug analysis in abuse abatement. J. Psychedelic Drugs, 5, 83-88.

Hitzeman, R.J., H.H. Loh, and E.F. Domino (1973). Effect of phencyclidine on the accumulation of ^{14}C-catecholamines formed from ^{14}C-tyrosine. Arch. Int. Pharmacodyn., 202, 252-258.

Hollister, L.E. (1968). Chemical Psychoses. LSD and Related Drugs. Charles C. Thomas, Springfield, Illinois.

Luby, E.D., B.D. Cohen, G. Rosenbaum, and others (1959). Study of a new schizophrenomimetic drug - Sernyl. Arch. Neurol. Psychiatry, 81, 363-369.

Maayani, S., H. Weinstein, N. Ben-Zvi, and others (1974). Psychotomimetics as anticholinergic agents - I. Biochem. Pharmacol., 23, 1263-1281.

Marshman, J.A., M.D. Ramsay, and E.M. Sellers (1976). Quantitation of phencyclidine in biological fluids and application to human overdose. Toxicol. Appl. Pharmacol., 35, 129-136.

Miyasaki, M., and E.F. Domino (1968). Neuronal mechanisms of ketamine-induced anesthesia. Int. J. Neuropharmacol., 7, 557-573.

Radouco-Thomas, S., T.H. Schwarz, and R. Michaud (1974). Psychotomimetics and cerebral cations. In S. Radouco-Thomas, A. Villeneuve and C. Radouco-Thomas (Eds.) Pharmacology, Toxicology and Abuse of Psychotomimetics (Hallucinogens). Les Presses De L'Universite Laval, Quebec. pp. 239-248.

Rosenbaum, G., B.D. Cohen, E.D. Luby, and others (1959). Comparison of Sernyl with other drugs. Arch. Gen. Psychiatry, 1, 113-118.

Sankar, D.V.Siva (1975). LSD - A Total Study. PJD Publications Ltd., Westbury, New York.

Smith, R.C., H. Meltzer, H. Dekirmenjian, and others (1975). Effects of phencyclidine on biogenic amines in rat brain. Neurosci. Abstr., 1, Number 468.

The Summaries of the Symposia: A Synthesis

MARTIN ROTH

The difficulty I have in attempting any kind of synthesis of the very large body of scientific observations presented during the symposia and summarised this afternoon reminds me of the story about Szent-Gyorgyi at about the time when he accidently discovered ascorbic acid. He knew that he was dealing with a water soluble and easily oxidisable carbohydrate-like substance but he had not appreciated that it had the properties of a vitamin. Accordingly he decided to christen his mysterious substance as 'ignose' and this is the name he used for it in the first paper he sent on the subject to an international journal. The editor returned to paper objecting that the name applied to the new substance was frivolous and unseemly in a scientific publication. Szent-Gyorgyi promptly renamed ascorbic acid as "Godnose" and returned the paper to the Editor.

Selection is unavoidable in a statement such as this and even the most learned and accomplished symposiast cannot be other than uncertain about his choices. Time may show him to have paid undue attention to ephemeral findings and to have overlooked the most significant contribution. Such hazards are inseparable from scientific activity; I shall therefore make my apologies for omissions here and not again.

I will turn then to the group of observations relating to electro convulsive therapy. It was appropriate that this subject should have been entered on the first day of the programme. For it was the first form of anti depressive treatment to be introduced and it remains the most effective and reliable therapy for the management of psychotic, acutely suicidal and seriously ill depressed patients. Within recent years it has been under heavy attack from many critics of psychiatry. It is alleged that this is a treatment without a known mode of action applied in a haphazard and even punitive manner without heed to the possibilities of brain damage. The findings at this meeting of the CINP have served to refute a number of these assertions. They have in this way vindicated what every experienced clinician knows to be a valuable and often life-saving remedy.

Findings have been adduced that in experimental animals this treatment enhances the response to drugs which act by stimulating the post synaptic receptors of 5-hydroxy-tryptamine and dopamine (Green et al). There is also evidence for increased synthesis and turnover of norepinephrine and enhanced sensitivity of post synaptic dopamine receptors (Modish). The treatment may thus serve to compensate for any decrease in synthesis of neuro transmitters or decreased sensitivity of receptors. Other changes described included increased blood flow and an enhancement of diffusion of small molecules from the blood into the brain during seizures. In psychiatric patients treatment is followed with a 10-20 minute interval by increased production of cortisol and prolactin.

Now it has been claimed recently that ECT works through its powerful suggestive effects. But some of the most striking biochemical changes such as the 5 HT mediated responses, fail to appear following sub convulsive shocks. The passage of an electric current is inessential for the inhalant flurothyl has exactly the same effects as shocks electrically induced. It would seem likely that the oldest anti depressive remedy works like the most recent ones by influencing the metabolism of the brain. We deal with a biochemical treatment (Fink et al) Nor is there any substance in the claim that brain damage is produced. Electron microscopy has failed to define any irreversible morphological alterations.

It is interesting to compare the character of these observations with those that were being adduced a little more than a quarter of a century ago in an attempt to account for the effects of ECT. Alterations in sleep rhythm, appetite, activity, menstrual cycle, sexual interest and striking changes in the EEG led to the hypothesis that effects stemmed from enhanced activity of regulating centres in the diencephalon. The contemporary language of biochemistry which can be used to described the effects is a much more precise one. Further comparison of the effects of anti depressive drugs and convulsive treatment might serve to bring to light phenomena common to them both and so pave the way for more fruitful hypotheses regarding the causation of depressive illness for which ECT seems so highly specific.

We have moved a long way from theories that gained currency in the 1950 International Congress of Psychiatry when much attention was given to "La joie de la renaissance" - or the joy of rebirth following the symbolic death induced by the convulsion which was held to be at the centre of the therapeutic effects.

Convulsive treatment has some measure of effectiveness in a very wide range of psychiatric disorders. It is not surprising that its actions on the brain proved to be complex. But in the field of genetics the investigator can reasonably hope to discover biochemical correlates of a much more specific and significant kind. If any of the psychoses for example were due to major gene differences we could live in hope of being able to describe their basic causes in parsimonious and elegant terms such as the lack or deficiency of a single specific enzyme. Major gene differences hav in fact been postulated as the underlying causes both in the case of the affective and the schizophrenic group of psychoses. If so their penetrance must be very low.

One difficulty about major gene theories in this area arises from the fact that with a few exceptions for which there is a clear explanation all diseases due to classical mendelian major genes have proved to be of very low prevalence. The reasons for this are obvious. In contrast in both the major groups of psychoses and even more so in neuroses we deal with some of the commonest maladies of man. For these among other reasons polygenes have been suggested as an alternative explanation for the hereditary basis of most major mental disorders. The problem about such hypotheses is that they are exceedingly difficult to test and refute being readily reconcilable with so many different kinds of data.

However, it is possible that the categories of psychiatric disorder with which we deal are heterogeneous and within them there will be sub groups due to major gene differences in which you can expect to discover biochemical correlates of a wholly distinctive kind. The recent finding that there are multiple forms of monoamine oxidase (Yondim) suggests that the search for biochemical sub groups is a useful strategy. Bellmaker and Ebstein have made the interesting point that conflicting reports regarding platelet MAO in schizophrenia may have stemmed from the existence of many genetic variants of platelet MAO. One of these would prove specific for schizophrenia, and if this could be established a major advance in heredity and biochemistry of this illness will have been registered.

Specificity in biochemical causation might also come to light through the demonstration that some sub groups of the mental disorder but not others respond to a given form of psychopharmacological treatment. In this connection the observations of Mendelewitz that lithium response in affective disorders is under genetic control represents a group of observations whose further development will be awaited with interest.

Similar claims have been made by Cazullo et al and Perris et al in respect of the relationship between antigens of the HLA system and the response to neuroleptic drugs and lithium respectively. It is too early to judge from these and other studies reported at this meeting the promise of enquiries into specificity of association with HLA antigens. As some of these are implicated in membrane function at specific receptor sites a discovery in this area would have wide implications.

Controversies about the inheritance of alcoholism and aggressive behaviour have a long and eventful history. The recent tendency to focus endeavour upon specific experimental models in which the effects of neuro transmitter systems can be examined (Mandel et al) and on specific drinking patterns (Garcin et al) appear to be promising strategies in relation to behaviour patterns that have a daunting complexity.

This leads naturally into the field of neuro transmitters and their role in the etiology of affective disorders. A number of competing hypotheses have been advanced at our symposia. Marie Asberg has reported the finding of bimodal distributions in the concentration of the serotonin metabolite 5 hydroxy indoleacetic acid (5-HIAA) in the cerebrospinal fluid in two independent series of endogenously depressed patients. The observations have predictive value in that those with low 5 HIAA are more prone to commit suicide and also differ in their response to treatment with tricyclic antidepressant drugs from other patients; substances which block uptake of norepinephrine are ineffective. She found CSF levels of the presumptive nor adrenalin metabolite MHPG to be similar between depressives and volunteers.

On the other hand Goodwin draws attention to the inconsistency of data on CSF levels and reports lower urinary levels of this compound in bipolar as compared with unipolar patients. Among the latter, lower MHPG levels may predict a favourable response to imipramine and non-response to amitryptiline. He concludes that an interaction between noradrenergic and dopaminergic systems might provide relatively clear lines of explanation for the differential effects of anti depressive drugs in disorders of affect.

Each of these last two groups of findings is in conflict at some point with those of Vestergaard et al who none-the-less decide in favour of involvement of catecholamines in affective disorders. We have to be grateful to these workers as also to Randrup et al and Agnoli for having so clearly and unequivocally committed themselves to theories in terms of serotoninergic nor adrenergic, dopaminergic or catecholamine hypotheses regarding the etiology of major depressive disorders or in relation to the mode of action of drugs efficacious in these disorders. It is plain that the problem is of great complexity. And only time can tell whether it will prove possible to make a clear choice between these hypotheses. Perhaps reconciliation of the conflicting findings will prove possible only after a new insight paves the way for some grand synthesis.

The need for a synthesis of existing knowledge becomes all the more pressing as the number of neuro transmitter systems defined in the brain continues to increase with the advance of knowledge. Observations on the recently identified peptide hormone have not for the present revealed the secret of their function in the brain. Nor is there clear indication for the present as to whether they are likely to prove of therapeutic value (Prange et al).

Inconsistencies between the findings of different observers also appeared in relation to the distribution of HLA antigen frequencies in affective disorders. Thus Rafaelsen et al reports significantly more frequent occurrence of HLAB-7 while Perris et al describes a decreased frequency of antigen.

Here as in relation to other biochemical investigations in patient populations differences in the classification of affective illness employed and the definition of specific disorders utilised probably serve to befog issues and perhps to obscure valuable results. Among investigators in the United States the bipolar-unipolar principle appears to have displaced all other concepts in the diagnosis and the taxonomy of depressive disorders. But Leonhard who originally suggested the unipolar-bipolar dichotomy had no intention of applying it beyond the realm of "endogenous" states. Once the concept of 'endogenous' depression (in a phenomenological-descriptive rather than an aetiological sense is judged as superfluous the unipolar group of depressive illnesses is in danger of becoming a receptacle for a heterogenous blend of many disorders. In some of these 'depression' will be merely one among many features of illness and not necessarily the clue to the central clinical syndrome present.

Biochemical investigations in human subjects with depressive disorders are indispensable if only because no wholly convincing animal model of a depressive state has been placed on record. But if consistent findings are to be registered a broad concensus will have to be reached regarding the classification of these disorders and the nomenclature to be used to designate them. To this end a new synthesis has been advanced which, integrates new diagnostic concepts that have proved fruitful in biological research with the older ones of proven value. It attempts to bring into a coherent relationship observations in relation to three issues usually studied in isolation; the neurotic-endogenous, the anxiety versus depressive and affective-schizophreniform diagnostic problems.

The extent to which the behaviour of monoamines in the blood platelets mirrors synaptic events in monoaminergic neurones in the brain remains uncertain. The fact that certain ligands relating to monoamine function bind to platelet receptors <u>in vitro</u> has led to investigations of various parameters of platelet response in the hope that drug receptor interactions might be illuminated in this way (Boullin). However, as in the case of the presynaptic alpha and beta adrenoceptors, the extent to which peripheral systems can be taken as a model for what is happening in the CNS is uncertain. The anxiolytic and sedative effects of these latter compounds endow investigations in this area (Langer) with importance from the point of view of psychiatry.

As Dr. Simeon pointed out the fact that a symposium has been devoted to the neuro psychopharmacology of childhood represented a new development. The striking contrasts between patterns of disordered behaviour in childhood and adult life provide ample scope for scientific explorations. Why are true schizophrenic and manic depressive psychoses so rare in childhood? How is it that manifestations of personality disorder so prominent in the second and third decades so often go into abeyance in the decades that follow. We know nothing about the neurological or biochemical correlates in such phenomena.

The development of a valid generally acceptable classification presents difficult problems which are being tackled with the aid of systems such as DSM3 (Campbell). The establishment with the aid of controlled trials of the superior therapeutic effects of psycho stimulant drugs as compared to neuroleptic substances and behaviour, therapy in hyperkinetic children (Gittleman-Kline) is an important development.

The refined methods of quantification introduced into EEG enquiries have made it possible to identify significant differences between psychotic and normal children in respect of the EEG and evoked potentials. Discriminant function analysis made it possible to achieve clear separation between the groups in respect of the electrophysiological phenomena. The electro-encephlogram may be mentioned here as the observations reported span topics that have been subject to discussion in a number of different symposia. In addition to its uses in child psychiatry modern EEG techniques have shed some light on problems of drug dependence, they have proved of value in the analysis of the effects of pharmacological preparations and they have brought about a revolution in the scientific investigation of sleep (Oswald). Yet although techniques such as power spectrum analysis and the use of computers have made these studies much more precise than could have been expected 25 years ago the EEG has had its failures as well as its successes. It looks doubtful at the present time whether it can by itself serve as the basis for the classification of drugs.

Some recent discoveries in the neuro-endrocrinology of childhood may prove to have far reaching implications for a wide range of problems in the field of adult mental health. The psycho-sexual development and behaviour of children who had been exposed to androgens or oestrogens prenatally proves to be measurably different from that of controls and it is possible that the effects are life long. The psycho-sexual dwarfism that stems from maternal deprivation may also be irreversible. On the other hand the arrest of growth induced by dl-amphetamine treatment of hyperkinetic children reverses on cessation of treatment.

New drugs for the relief of mental suffering appear to emerge at a more rapid rate than the ability of scientists to arrive at valid explanations for their mode of action. In the case of benzodiazepines there is an embarrassing richness of hypotheses. Their effects have been ascribed to an influence on serotonin transmission in the brains punishment system (Stein) to their action as post synaptic glycine agonists which is claimed to correspond closely to their clinical efficacy and to an influence on GABA-ergic inhibitory synapses perhaps by removal of an endogenous inhibitor of GABA binding. Other explanations include an affect on endorphins.

A plausible theory would have to subsume the anxiolytic, sedative anti convulsant, hypnotic and muscle relaxant effects of these substances. It would also be exprected to account for the relative specificity of their clinical actions. A synthesis capable of providing a parsimonious account of all such effects would constitute an important forward leap in knowledge.

The field of drug abuse which is also full of problems and paradoxes both bewildering and beguiling. As Dr. Hollister has pointed out approximately 1-2% of the population of advanced countries abuses drugs. If we focus attention on the most malignant forms of dependence the same individuals are found to take drugs with sedative effects at one time and stimulant ones at another or both of these together as in the combination of barbiturates with amphetamines. We do not clearly understand what these preparations have in common in the way of psychological and pharmacological effects.

In some preliminary studies of beta endorphin by intravenous injection some promising effects have been described in a number of psychiatric disorders (Kline). However, there is no indication for the present that changes in the function or metabolism of endogenous ligands or opiate receptors play a primary or significant role in the development of opiate addiction. A wide array of clinical and behavioural effects is observed in association with addiction to opiate and sedative drugs. They are seen in most striking form during acute withdrawal but each of the syndromes may be observed while drugs continue to be taken, acute delirium may develop or a state of severe anxiety with terrifying dreams. Alternatively an acute hallucinosis with visual or auditory hallucinations may be experienced, or a paranoid state with an affect of terror but without hallucinations. Epileptic fits which may evolve auto epilepticus are particularly liable to occur in barbiturate or alcohol withdrawal but are not unknown in the case of opiates. Some patients become depressed and the state of anguish engendered entails a serious suicidal risk. Finally the electro encephlogram may show indubitable epileptic features even though convulsions have not been noted. There must be neurological neurochemical and pharmacological systems that work in close integration. Only in this manner can their common derangement by a single drug be explained. It follows that satisfactory explanations of withdrawal phenomena would be likely to shed light not only on problems of drug dependence but also on the neurobiological basis of other psychiatric disorders.

Endorphins may provide the means of advance towards such understanding. But for the present both their functions and their physiological effects remain obscure (Hollister).

Biological monitoring of the treatment of patients receiving psychotropic drugs is in its early stages and with the exception of a few specific substances its value remains to be established. One reason for the difficulty of forming useful judgments from plasma levels is that variability in such levels is merely one factor that contributes to the total clinical effect. Pharmaco kinetic variation is of great importance. However six studies from three independent teams of workers have now adduced evidence that the optimal therapeutic effects of nortriptyline are exerted from plasma levels between 100-150 G/L and unsatisfactory results are obtained at levels above 150-200 G/L (gram). In impramine, here there is a similar threshold to be passed but no upper limit beyond which affects are adverse. It is in endogenous depressions that the relationship between plasma level and clinical effect appears to be most close.

In the case of lithium the value of monitoring is now firmly established. Without it treatment is neither safe nor optimal. The findings reported another section of this Congress that renal damage possibly irreversible in character may result in those taking lithium on a long term basis has cast a cloud over this valuable treatment. More observations are needed before the significance of the findings can be evaluated. In the final analysis a balance will have to be struck as between the risk of administering lithium and the suicidal and other hazards of not doing so.

A new form of prophylactic treatment has perhaps been adumbrated by Van Praag's preliminary finding that 5-HTP defective in averting attacks of both unipolar and bipolar depression. As the character of the CSF 5-HIAA response after probenecid loading appears to be a good prediction of the anti depressant effect of 5-HTP, the view that there may be a serotonin deficient form of depression receives confirmation from these studies (Van Praag) that this is a rational form of treatment is supported by the increasing evidence that amino acid precursors of dopamine nor-adrenaline and 5 hydroxy-tryptamine enter the brain from the blood. Dopa and to a lesser extent tyrosine increase the brain catecholamine concentration and tryptophan enhances the synthesis of brain 5HT (Curzon). The effects of the precursors are produced in an orderly manner and they are within limits predictable from pharmacokinetic and neurochemical data (Carlsson and Lindquist). However the therapeutic benefits described (Coppen and Wood) in relation to which more evidence is needed are not necessarily related to intracerebral changes since precursor loading causes a variety of metabolic effects in diverse systems within and outside the brain.

If it is accepted that some of the experimentally induced models of 'depression' in animals are relevant to the human form of disorder these observations will have created a foundation for investigating in a relatively stringent manner the hypothesis that depressive illnesses are due to the deficiency of one or more biogenic amines in the brain.

In contrast to the abundance of papers dealing with affective disorders there was a dearth of contributions in relation to schizophrenic illness in the course of the symposia. But the conference was noteworthy for the convergence of evidence from several centres pointing to the existence of a possible biochemical substrate for some forms of schizophrenic illness. Brief reference will be made to these studies to round off the picture. Dopamine and nor-epinephrine concentration has been described as significantly increased in the nucleus accumbens but normal in the caudate nucleus and putamen in one centre (Bird and Iversen). A distribution that was just the reverse of this was found in respect of dopanime in another controlled study (Owen, Longden and Crow). Perhaps of even greater interest is the finding that specific binding of both 3H-spiroperidol and 3H-haloperidol was higher by 70-75% of the caudate and 50-70% in the putamen of 20 schizophrenic brains studied post mortem (Seeman et al). Similar observations have been placed on record in another controlled study (Owen Longden and Crow) which found no clear relationship between increased binding and pharmacological treatment. As the binding of 3H-apomorphine did not differ in schizophrenics as compared with control brains the evidence suggested that there was an increase of post synaptic dopamine receptor sensitivity in schizophrenic subjects.

It has been a source of particular satisfaction to note the increasing tendency for collaborative work between neuropharmacologists, biochemists, psychiatrists, physiologists, psychologists in the attack upon specific problems. The complications and side effects of treatment with psychotropic drugs which may take some years to emerge have taught us to speak with caution when assessing the progress achieved in our field. One is also deterred from over optimistic pronouncements by Bertrand Russell's warning "Organic life, we are told, has developed gradually from the protozoon to the philosopher, and this development, we are assured, is indubitable an advance. Unfortunately it is the philosopher, not the protozoon who gives us this assurance."

Yet when all due qualifications have been made these symposia will I believe come to be judged as a record of significant progress and as notable contributions to the history of the CINP.

One omission mentioned by our President in his opening address is perhaps of sufficient importance to be mentioned here again. At a time when a proportion of aged people is increasing over a greater part of the world, and when psychiatric disorders among the aged represent major challenges for health and welfare services everywhere, it is anomolous that there should have been a symposium on child psychiatry but none devoted to the mental disorders of later life. The omission is all the more striking in that there has been a burgeoning of interest in the pharmacological treatment of geriatric mental disorders and some important growing points have emerged in the neurochemistry of the aging brain. But this gap will doubtless be filled in one of the forthcoming Congresses.

For the present all that remains is for me to thank all the contributors this afternoon for their succinct and valuable summaries and to express my appreciation of the Executive Committee for the honour they have done me in asking me to present this synthesis.

Index

The page numbers refer to the first page of the article in which the index term appears.

DATE DUE

GAYLORD PRINTED IN U.S.A.